Current Critical Problems
in Vascular Surgery

Current Critical Problems in Vascular Surgery

VOLUME 7

EDITOR

Frank J. Veith, M.D.

Professor and Director,
Vascular Surgical Services,
Montefiore Medical Center/
Albert Einstein College of Medicine,
New York, New York

with 309 illustrations

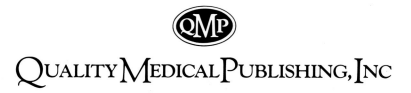

ST. LOUIS, MISSOURI
1996

Copyright © 1996 by Quality Medical Publishing, Inc.

All rights reserved. Reproduction of the material herein
in any form requires the written permission of the publisher.

Printed in the United States of America.

PUBLISHER Karen Berger
EDITOR Beth Campbell
PROJECT MANAGER Donna Rothenberg
PRODUCTION Judy Bamert
COVER DESIGN Diane M. Beasley

Quality Medical Publishing, Inc.
11970 Borman Drive, Suite 222
St. Louis, Missouri 63146

ISBN 0-942219-07-4
ISSN 1052-4436

GW/WW/WW
5   4   3   2   1

Contributors

William M. Abbott, M.D.
Chief of Vascular Surgery, Professor of Surgery, Division of Vascular Surgery, Massachusetts General Hospital/Harvard Medical School, Boston, Mass.

Ali F. AbuRahma, M.D.
Professor of Surgery, Chief, Vascular Section, Department of Surgery, Robert C. Byrd Health Sciences Center of West Virginia University, Charleston, W.V.

Samuel S. Ahn, M.D.
Associate Clinical Professor of Surgery, Division of General Surgery, Section of Vascular Surgery, UCLA Center for the Health Sciences; Chief of Vascular Surgery, Olive View Medical Center, Section of Vascular Surgery, Los Angeles, Calif.

Ale Algra, M.D., Ph.D.
Clinical Epidemiologist, Clinical Epidemiology Unit, University Hospital Utrecht, Utrecht, The Netherlands

Jose C. Alves, M.D.
Research Associate, Division of Vascular Surgery, Department of Surgery, University of Utah School of Medicine, Salt Lake City, Utah

J. Dennis Baker, M.D.
Professor of Surgery, Department of Surgery, UCLA School of Medicine, Los Angeles, Calif.

William H. Baker, M.D.
Professor of Surgery, Department of Surgery, Loyola University Medical Center, Stritch School of Medicine, Maywood, Ill.

Wiley F. Barker, M.D.
Professor Emeritus, Department of Surgery, UCLA School of Medicine, Los Angeles, Calif.

Robert W. Barnes, M.D.
Professor and Chairman, Department of Surgery, University of Arkansas for Medical Sciences, Little Rock, Ark.

H.J.M. Barnett, M.D.
Scientist, Department of Clinical Neurological Sciences, The John P. Robarts Research Institute, London, Ontario, Canada

Hugh G. Beebe, M.D.
Director, Jobst Vascular Center, The Toledo Hospital, Toledo, Ohio; Adjunct Professor of Surgery, University of Michigan Medical School, Ann Arbor, Mich.

Michael Belkin, M.D.
Assistant Professor of Surgery, Department of Surgery, Division of Vascular Surgery, Harvard Medical School/Brigham & Womens Hospital, Boston, Mass.

Ramon Berguer, M.D., Ph.D.
Professor of Surgery, Department of Vascular Surgery, Wayne State University, Detroit, Mich.

F. William Blaisdell, M.D.
Professor, Department of Surgery, University of California–Davis Medical Center, Sacramento, Calif.

Jan D. Blankensteijn, M.D., Ph.D.
Department of Surgery, University Hospital Utrecht, Utrecht, The Netherlands

John Blebea, M.D.
Assistant Professor of Surgery, Division of Vascular Surgery, University of Cincinnati Medical School, Cincinnati, Ohio

David C. Brewster, M.D.
Clinical Professor of Surgery, Harvard Medical School/Massachusetts General Hospital, Boston, Mass.

Keith D. Calligaro, M.D.
Chief, Section of Vascular Surgery, Pennsylvania Hospital, Philadelphia, Pa.

Allan D. Callow, M.D., Ph.D.
Research Professor, Department of Medicine and Surgery, Boston University Medical Center, Whitaker Cardiovascular Institute, Boston, Mass.

Robert A. Cambria, M.D.
Assistant Professor of Surgery, Department of Vascular Surgery, Medical School of Wisconsin, Milwaukee, Wis.

Sandra C. Carr, M.D.
Vascular Fellow, Division of Vascular Surgery, Northwestern University Medical School, Chicago, Ill.

Jean-Christophe Cavenaile, M.D.
Fellow, Department of Vascular Pathology, Erasme University Hospital, Brussels, Belgium

Elliot L. Chaikof, M.D., Ph.D.
Assistant Professor of Surgery, Department of Surgery, Emory University School of Medicine, Atlanta, Ga.

Benjamin B. Chang, M.D.
Assistant Professor of Surgery, Department of Surgery, Albany Medical College, Albany, N.Y.

Marie H.M. Chen, M.D.
Assistant Professor of Surgery, Department of Surgery, Albert Einstein College of Medicine/Long Island Jewish Medical Center, New Hyde Park, N.Y.

Timothy A.M. Chuter, M.D.
Assistant Professor, Department of Vascular Surgery, University of California, San Francisco, San Francisco, Calif.

G. Patrick Clagett, M.D.
Professor of Surgery, Chairman, Division of Vascular Surgery, Department of Surgery, University of Texas Southwestern Medical Center, Dallas, Tex.

Daniel G. Clair, M.D.
Assistant Professor of Surgery, Department of Surgery, USUHS/Malcolm Grow Medical Center, Andrews Air Force Base, Md.

Jon R. Cohen, M.D.
Professor of Surgery, Chairman, Department of Surgery, Albert Einstein College of Medicine/Long Island Jewish Medical Center, New Hyde Park, N.Y.

Anthony J. Comerota, M.D.
Professor of Surgery, Chief of Vascular Surgery, Department of Surgery, Temple University School of Medicine, Philadelphia, Pa.

Blessie Concepcion, B.S.
Research Associate, Division of General Surgery, Section of Vascular Surgery, UCLA Center for the Health Sciences, Los Angeles, Calif.

John E. Connolly, M.D.
Professor of Surgery, Chief of Vascular Surgery, Department of Surgery, University of California, Irvine, Irvine, Calif.

John D. Corson, M.B., Ch.B., F.R.C.S. (Engl.)
Professor of Surgery, Department of Surgery, The University of Iowa Hospitals and Clinics, Iowa City, Iowa

Kellie A. Coyle, M.D., J.D.
Resident in General Vascular Surgery, Department of Surgery, Emory University School of Medicine, Atlanta, Ga.

Frank J. Criado, M.D.
Chief, Division of Vascular Surgery, and Maryland Vascular Institute, The Union Memorial Hospital, Baltimore, Md.

Jack L. Cronenwett, M.D.
Professor of Surgery, Section of Vascular Surgery, Dartmouth-Hitchcock Medical Center, Lebanon, N.H.

Michael D. Dake, M.D.
Assistant Professor of Radiology and Medicine, Department of Radiology, Stanford University School of Medicine, Stanford, Calif.

Anthony J. D'Angelo, M.D.
Department of Surgery, Albert Einstein College of Medicine/Long Island Jewish Medical Center, New Hyde Park, N.Y.

R. Clement Darling III, M.D.
Associate Professor of Surgery, Department of Surgery, Albany Medical College, Albany, N.Y.

Dominic A. DeLaurentis, M.D.
Section of Vascular Surgery, Pennsylvania Hospital, Philadelphia, Pa.

Richard J. DeMasi, M.D.
Assistant Professor of Clinical Surgery, Department of General Surgery, Eastern Virginia Medicine School, Norfolk, Va.

Ralph G. DePalma, M.D.
Professor of Surgery and Associate Dean, Department of Surgery, University of Nevada School of Medicine, Reno, Nev.

Jean-Pierre Dereume, M.D.
Professor of Vascular Surgery, Department of Vascular Pathology, Free University of Brussels/Erasme University Hospital, Brussels, Belgium

James A. DeWeese, M.D.
Professor of Surgery, Chair Emeritus, Division of Cardiothoracic Surgery, Section of Vascular Surgery, Department of Surgery, University of Rochester, Rochester, N.Y.

Magruder C. Donaldson, M.D.
Associate Professor of Surgery, Department of Surgery, Division of Vascular Surgery, Harvard Medical School/Brigham and Women's Hospital, Boston, Mass.

Carlos Donayre, M.D.
Assistant Professor of Surgery, University of California, Los Angeles School of Medicine, Los Angeles; Harbor–UCLA Medical Center, Torrance, Calif.

Mehrez El Douaihy, M.D.
Fellow, Department of Vascular Pathology, Erasme University Hospital, Brussels, Belgium

Matthew J. Dougherty, M.D.
Section of Vascular Surgery, Pennsylvania Hospital, Philadelphia, Pa.

F. Felmont Eaves III, M.D.
Assistant Professor, Division of Plastic, Reconstructive, and Maxillofacial Surgery, Emory University School of Medicine, Atlanta, Ga.

Bert C. Eikelboom, M.D., Ph.D.
Vascular Surgeon, Department of Vascular Surgery, University Hospital Utrecht, Utrecht, The Netherlands

José Ferreira, M.D.
Fellow, Department of Vascular Pathology, Erasme University Hospital, Brussels, Belgium

Thomas J. Fogarty, M.D.
Professor, Department of Surgery, Stanford University, Stanford, Calif.

Richard J. Fowl, M.D.
Associate Professor of Surgery, Department of Surgery, Division of Vascular Surgery, University of Cincinnati Medical School, Cincinnati, Ohio

Robert G. Gayle, M.D.
Assistant Professor of Clinical Surgery, Department of General Surgery, Eastern Virginia Medicine School, Norfolk, Va.

Jonathan P. Gertler, M.D.
Associate Professor of Surgery, Division of Vascular Surgery, Harvard Medical School/Massachusetts General Hospital, Boston, Mass.

David L. Gillespie, M.D., MAJ, MC, USA
Assistant Professor, Department of Surgery, Uniformed Services University, Bethesda, Md.

Peter Gloviczki, M.D.
Professor of Surgery, Vice-Chairman, Division of Vascular Surgery, Mayo Medical School, Rochester, Minn.

Michael A. Golden, M.D.
Assistant Professor, Department of Surgery, University of Pennsylvania, Philadelphia, Pa.

Jamie Goldsmith, R.N.
Vascular Nurse, Division of Vascular Surgery, Montefiore Medical Center/Albert Einstein College of Medicine, New York, N.Y.

Jerry Goldstone, M.D.
Professor of Surgery, Department of Surgery, University of California, San Francisco, San Francisco, Calif.

Richard M. Green, M.D.
Professor of Surgery, Department of Surgery, University of Rochester School of Medicine and Dentistry, Rochester, N.Y.

Lazar J. Greenfield, M.D.
Frederick A. Coller Professor and Chairman, Department of Surgery, University of Michigan Medical Center, Ann Arbor, Mich.

Roger Malcolm Greenhalgh, M.A., M.D., M.Chir., F.R.C.S.
Professor, Department of Vascular Surgery, Charing Cross and Westminster Medical School, London, England

Roger T. Gregory, M.D.
Associate Professor of Surgery, Department of General Surgery, Eastern Virginia Medicine School, Norfolk, Va.

Sophie Guyot, M.D.
Fellow, Department of Vascular Pathology, Erasme University Hospital, Brussels, Belgium

Moshe Haimov, M.D.
Clinical Professor of Surgery, Department of Surgery, The Mount Sinai School of Medicine, New York, N.Y.

John W. Hallett, Jr., M.D.
Professor of Surgery, Director of Vascular Surgery Fellowship, Division of Vascular Surgery, Mayo Medical School, Rochester, Minn.

Elizabeth B. Harrington, M.D.
Associate Professor of Surgery, Department of Surgery, The Mount Sinai School of Medicine, New York, N.Y.

Martin Harrington, M.D.
Assistant Professor of Surgery, Department of Surgery, The Mount Sinai School of Medicine, New York, N.Y.

Robert C.J. Hicks, F.R.C.S.
Lecturer, Department of Surgery, Charing Cross and Westminster Medical School, London, England

Daniel J. Higman, F.R.C.S.
Senior Registrar, Department of Surgery, Charing Cross and Westminster Medical School, London, England

Jamal J. Hoballah, M.D.
Assistant Professor, Department of Surgery, The University of Iowa Hospitals and Clinics, Iowa City, Iowa

James W. Holcroft, M.D.
Professor, Department of Surgery, University of California, Davis Medical Center, Sacramento, Calif.

Thomas S. Huber, M.D., Ph.D.
Assistant Professor of Surgery, Department of Surgery, Section of Vascular Surgery, University of Florida College of Medicine, Gainesville, Fla.

Paul W. Humphrey, M.D.
Clinical Instructor of Surgery, Department of Surgery, University of Missouri Health Sciences Center, Columbia, Mo.

Mark R. Jackson, M.D., MAJ, MC, USA
Assistant Professor, Department of Surgery, Uniformed Services University of the Health Sciences, Bethesda, Md.

Tonya L. Jackson, B.A.
Jobst Vascular Center, The Toledo Hospital, Toledo, Ohio

Brian F. Johnson, M.D.
Consultant Vascular Surgeon, Royal Hull Hospitals, Hull Royal Infirmary, Hull, England

Kenneth Wayne Johnston, M.D., F.R.C.S.(C)
Professor of Surgery and Biomedical Engineering, Head, Division of Vascular Surgery, Department of Surgery, University of Toronto/The Toronto Hospital, Toronto, Ontario, Canada

William D. Jordan, Jr., M.D.
Assistant Professor, Department of Surgery, Section of Vascular Surgery, University of Alabama Hospital at Birmingham, Birmingham, Ala.

Dolores J. Katz, Ph.D.
Staff, Centers for Disease Control, Atlanta, Ga.

Richard F. Kempczinski, M.D.
Professor of Surgery, Division of Vascular Surgery, University of Cincinnati Medical School, Cincinnati, Ohio

Richard J. Knight, M.D.
Assistant Professor of Surgery, Department of Surgery, The Mount Sinai School of Medicine, New York, N.Y.

George E. Kopchok, B.S.
Biomedical Engineer, Harbor–UCLA Medical Center, Torrance, Calif.

Timothy F. Kresowik, M.D.
Associate Professor, Department of Surgery, The University of Iowa Hospitals and Clinics, Iowa City, Iowa

Patrick J. Lamparello, M.D.
Clinical Associate Professor of Surgery, Department of Surgery, Division of Vascular Surgery, New York University School of Medicine, New York, N.Y.

Peter F. Lawrence, M.D.
Professor of Surgery, Chief of Vascular Surgery, Department of Surgery, University of Utah School of Medicine, Salt Lake City, Utah

Robert P. Leather, M.D.
Professor of Surgery, Department of Surgery, Albany Medical College, Albany, N.Y.

Alan B. Lumsden, M.D.
Associate Professor, Department of Surgery, Emory University School of Medicine, Atlanta, Ga.

Ross T. Lyon, M.D.
Assistant Professor of Surgery, Department of Surgery, Montefiore Medical Center/Albert Einstein College of Medicine, New York, N.Y.

Shane T.R. MacSweeney, F.R.C.S.
Senior Registrar in Surgery, Department of Vascular Surgery, Charing Cross Hospital and Westminster Medical School, London, England

John A. Mannick, M.D.
Moseley Distinguished Professor of Surgery, Department of Surgery, Harvard Medical School/Brigham and Women's Hospital, Boston, Mass.

M. Ashraf Mansour, M.D.
Assistant Professor, Department of Surgery, Section of Peripheral Vascular Surgery, Loyola University of Chicago, Stritch School of Medicine, Maywood, Ill.

Michael L. Marin, M.D.
Assistant Professor of Surgery, Department of Surgery, Division of Vascular Surgery, Montefiore Medical Center/Albert Einstein College of Medicine, New York, N.Y.

Ben U. Marsan, M.D.
Fellow Vascular Surgery, Department of Surgery, Division of Vascular Surgery, State University of New York at Buffalo, Buffalo, N.Y.

Mark A. Mattos, M.D.
Assistant Professor, Department of Surgery, Section of Peripheral Vascular Surgery, Southern Illinois University School of Medicine, Springfield, Ill.

James May, M.S., F.R.A.C.S.
Bosch Professor of Surgery, Department of Surgery, University of Sydney, New South Wales, Australia

Heather E. Meldrum, B.A.
The John P. Robarts Research Institute, London, Ontario, Canada

Arnold Miller, M.B., Ch.B.
Assistant Clinical Professor of Surgery, Department of Vascular Surgery, Harvard Medical School, MetroWest Medical Center, Framingham, Mass.

D. Craig Miller, M.D.
Professor, Department of Cardiothoracic Surgery, Stanford University, Stanford, Calif.

R. Scott Mitchell, M.D.
Associate Professor, Department of Cardiothoracic Surgery, Stanford University, Stanford, Calif.

Wesley S. Moore, M.D.
Professor of Surgery and Chief, Section of Vascular Surgery, Department of Surgery, University of California, Los Angeles School of Medicine, Los Angeles, Calif.

Serge Motte, M.D.
Fellow, Department of Vascular Pathology, Erasme University Hospital, Brussels, Belgium

Eugene A. Murphy, M.D.
Department of Surgery, Albert Einstein College of Medicine/Long Island Jewish Medical Center, New Hyde Park, N.Y.

Roman Nowygrod, M.D.
Professor of Surgery, Department of Surgery, Columbia University School of Physicians and Surgeons, New York, N.Y.

Thomas F. O'Donnell, Jr., M.D.
Andrews Professor of Surgery and Chairman, Department of Surgery, Tufts University School of Medicine/New England Medical Center, Boston, Mass.

Kevin J. Ose, M.D.
Resident Physician, Department of Surgery, University of Cincinnati Medical School, Cincinnati, Ohio

Kenneth Ouriel, M.D.
Associate Professor of Surgery, Department of Surgery, University of Rochester, Rochester, N.Y.

John T. Owings, M.D.
Assistant Professor, Department of Surgery, University of California, Davis Medical Center, Sacramento, Calif.

Joseph E. Palascak, M.D.
Associate Professor of Medicine, Department of Medicine, University of Cincinnati Medical School, Cincinnati, Ohio

F. Noel Parent III, M.D.
Assistant Professor of Clinical Surgery, Department of General Surgery, Eastern Virginia Medicine School, Norfolk, Va.

Amit V. Patel, M.D.
Assistant Professor of Surgery, Department of Surgery, Division of Vascular Surgery, Montefiore Medical Center/Albert Einstein College of Medicine, New York, N.Y.

Peggy Patten, R.N.
Vascular Nurse Specialist, Maryland Vascular Institute, The Union Memorial Hospital, Baltimore, Md.

Donald E. Patterson, M.D.
Advanced Vascular Resident, Section of Vascular Surgery, Pennsylvania Hospital, Philadelphia, Pa.

Philip S.K. Paty, M.D.
Assistant Professor of Surgery, Department of Surgery, Albany Medical College, Albany, N.Y.

William H. Pearce, M.D.
Professor of Surgery, Division of Vascular Surgery, Northwestern University Medical School, Chicago, Ill.

Bruce A. Perler, M.D.
Associate Professor of Surgery, Department of Surgery, The Johns Hopkins University School of Medicine, Baltimore, Md.

Malcolm O. Perry, M.D.
Chairman, Department of Surgery, St. Paul Medical Center, Dallas, Tex.

William C. Pevec, M.D.
Assistant Professor of Surgery, Department of Surgery, University of California, Davis Medical Center, Sacramento, Calif.

John P. Pigott, M.D.
Associate Director, Endovascular Surgery, Jobst Vascular Center, The Toledo Hospital, Toledo, Ohio

Neil R. Poulter, M.R.C.P.
Senior Lecturer in Epidemiology, Charing Cross Hospital and Westminster Medical School, London, England

Janet T. Powell, M.D., Ph.D.
Professor, Department of Vascular Surgery, Charing Cross Hospital and Westminster Medical School, London, England

Mary C. Proctor, M.S.
Senior Research Associate, Department of Surgery, University of Michigan Medical Center, Ann Arbor, Mich.

Luis A. Queral, M.D.
Co-Director, Maryland Vascular Institute, Division of Vascular Surgery and Maryland Vascular Institute, The Union Memorial Hospital, Baltimore, Md.

Dieter Raithel, M.D., Ph.D.
Professor of Vascular Surgery, Head, Department of Vascular Surgery, Nuremberg Southern Hospital, Nuremberg, Germany

Seshadri Raju, M.D.
Professor Emeritus of Surgery, Department of Surgery, University of Mississippi Medical Center, Jackson, Miss.

Norman M. Rich, M.D.
Professor and Chairman, Department of Surgery, Uniformed Services University of the Health Sciences, Bethesda, Md.

John J. Ricotta, M.D.
Professor of Surgery, Chief, Division of Vascular Surgery, Department of Surgery, State University of New York at Buffalo, Buffalo, N.Y.

Thomas S. Riles, M.D.
Professor of Surgery, Department of Surgery, New York University School of Medicine, New York, N.Y.

Agustin A. Rodriguez, M.D.
Assistant Professor in Surgery, Department of Surgery, Tufts University School of Medicine/New England Medical Center, Boston, Mass.

David B. Roos, M.D.
Clinical Professor of Surgery, Department of Surgery, University of Colorado Health Sciences Center, Denver, Colo.

Robert B. Rutherford, M.D.
Professor of Surgery, Department of Surgery, Vascular Surgery Section, University of Colorado Health Sciences Center, Denver, Colo.

Juha P. Salenius, M.D., Ph.D.
Assistant Professor of Thoracic and Vascular Surgery, Department of Vascular Surgery, University Hospital, Tampere, Finland

Luis A. Sanchez, M.D.
Attending Surgeon, Department of Surgery, Division of Vascular Surgery, Montefiore Medical Center/Albert Einstein College of Medicine, New York, N.Y.

Steven M. Santilli, M.D., Ph.D.
Assistant Professor of Surgery, Department of Surgery, University of Minnesota, Minneapolis, Minn.

Harry Schanzer, M.D.
Clinical Professor, Department of Surgery, The Mount Sinai School of Medicine, New York, N.Y.

Lee G. Schulman, M.D.
Director, Vascular Diagnostic Laboratory, Great Neck; Little Neck Community Hospital, Little Neck, N.Y.

Martin L. Schulman, M.D.
Assistant Professor of Clinical Surgery, Department of Surgery, The State University of New York at Stony Brook, Stony Brook; Little Neck Community Hospital, Little Neck, N.Y.

Mark A. Schwartz, M.D.
Vascular Fellow, Department of Surgery, The Mount Sinai School of Medicine, New York, N.Y.

Michael L. Schwartz, M.D.
Fellow in Vascular Surgery, Division of Vascular Surgery, Montefiore Medical Center/Albert Einstein College of Medicine, New York, N.Y.

James M. Seeger, M.D.
Professor and Chief, Department of Surgery, Section of Vascular Surgery, University of Florida College of Medicine, Gainesville, Fla.

Charles Semba, M.D.
Assistant Professor, Department of Radiology, Stanford University, Stanford, Calif.

Joseph M. Serletti, M.D.
Associate Professor of Surgery, Department of Surgery, University of Rochester School of Medicine and Dentistry, Rochester, N.Y.

Dhiraj M. Shah, M.D.
Professor of Surgery, Department of Surgery, Albany Medical College, Albany, N.Y.

William J. Sharp, M.D.
Associate Professor, Department of Surgery, The University of Iowa Hospitals and Clinics, Iowa City, Iowa

Donald Silver, M.D.
W. Alton Jones Distinguished Professor and Chairman, Department of Surgery, University of Missouri Health Sciences Center, Columbia, Mo.

Milan Skladany, M.D.
Instructor, Department of Surgery, The Mount Sinai School of Medicine, New York, N.Y.

Milton Slocum, M.D.
Clinical Instructor of Surgery, Resident Physician in Vascular Surgery, Department of Surgery, University of Missouri Health Sciences Center, Columbia, Mo.

Robert B. Smith III, M.D.
Professor of Surgery and Head, General Vascular Surgery, Department of Surgery, Emory University School of Medicine, Atlanta, Ga.

Stanley O. Snyder, Jr., M.D.
Clinical Associate Professor of Surgery, Department of Surgery, Vanderbilt Medical School, Nashville, Tenn.

James C. Stanley, M.D.
Professor of Surgery, Head, Section of Vascular Surgery, Department of Surgery, University of Michigan Medical School, Ann Arbor, Mich.

W. Anthony Stanson, M.D.
Associate Professor of Radiology, Department of Radiology, Mayo Medical School, Rochester, Minn.

Jeffrey S. Stein, M.D.
Assistant Professor, Department of Surgery, The Mount Sinai School of Medicine, New York, N.Y.

D. Eugene Strandness, Jr., M.D.
Professor of Surgery, Department of Surgery, University of Washington School of Medicine, Seattle, Wash.

William D. Suggs, M.D.
Assistant Professor of Surgery, Department of Surgery, Division of Vascular Surgery, Montefiore Medical Center/Albert Einstein College of Medicine, New York, N.Y.

David S. Sumner, M.D.
Distinguished Professor of Surgery, Department of Surgery, Section of Peripheral Vascular Surgery, Southern Ilinois University School of Medicine, Springfield, Ill.

Marco J.D. Tangelder, M.D.
Research Fellow in Vascular Surgery, Department of Vascular Surgery, BOA Trial-Bureau, Utrecht University Hospital, Utrecht, The Netherlands

Jesse E. Thompson, M.D.
Clinical Professor of Surgery, University of Texas Southwestern Medical Center, Dallas, Tex.

Jonathan B. Towne, M.D.
Professor of Surgery, Chairman, Department of Vascular Surgery, Medical College of Wisconsin, Milwaukee, Wis.

Sandra J. Uhl, R.N.
Vascular Surgery Research Coordinator, Division of Vascular Surgery, University of Cincinnati Medical School, Cincinnati, Ohio

R. James Valentine, M.D.
Associate Professor of Surgery, Division of Vascular Surgery, University of Texas Southwestern Medical Center, Dallas, Tex.

Frank J. Veith, M.D.
Professor and Director, Vascular Surgical Services, Montefiore Medical Center/Albert Einstein College of Medicine, New York, N.Y.

Gisèle Vincent, M.D.
Assistant Clinical Professor, Department of Vascular Pathology, Erasme University Hospital, Brussels, Belgium

Jean-Claude Wautrecht, M.D.
Assistant Clinical Professor, Department of Vascular Pathology, Erasme University Hospital, Brussels, Belgium

Kurt R. Wengerter, M.D.
Chief of Vascular Surgery, Associate Professor of Surgery, Department of Surgery, Division of Vascular Surgery, Montefiore Medical Center/Albert Einstein College of Medicine, New York, N.Y.

Jock R. Wheeler, M.D.
Dean and Provost, Department of Vascular Surgery, Eastern Virginia Medicine School, Norfolk, Va.

Geoffrey H. White, M.D., F.R.A.C.S.
Associate Professor of Surgery, Department of Surgery, University of Sydney, New South Wales, Australia

John V. White, M.D.
Professor of Surgery, Department of Surgery, Temple University School of Medicine, Philadelphia, Pa.

Rodney A. White, M.D., F.R.A.C.S.
Professor of Surgery, Department of Vascular Surgery, University of California, Los Angeles School of Medicine, Los Angeles; Harbor–UCLA Medical Center, Torrance, Calif.

Anthony D. Whittemore, M.D.
Professor of Surgery, Department of Surgery, Division of Vascular Surgery, Harvard Medical School/Brigham and Women's Hospital, Boston, Mass.

G. Melville Williams, M.D.
Professor of Surgery, Department of Surgery, Johns Hopkins University School of Medicine, Baltimore, Md.

Joseph I. Zarge, M.D.
Vascular Research Fellow, Department of Surgery, Temple University School of Medicine, Philadelphia, Pa.

Christopher K. Zarins, M.D.
Professor, Department of Surgery, Stanford University, Stanford, Calif.

Gerald B. Zelenock, M.D.
Professor of Surgery, Section of Vascular Surgery, University of Michigan Medical School, Ann Arbor, Mich.

Robert M. Zwolak, M.D., Ph.D.
Associate Professor of Surgery, Section of Vascular Surgery, Dartmouth-Hitchcock Medical Center, Lebanon, N.H.

To the people who
make the annual symposium a reality

the leading vascular surgeons
who prepare and present papers
on important, thought-provoking topics

the attendees
who come to share their knowledge
and stimulate lively discussions

our hardworking staff
who plan, organize, and take part
in this event

without the enthusiasm and support of
each of these groups, neither the symposium
nor this book would be possible

F.J.V.

Preface

For most of the twentieth century and a good portion of the nineteenth, the small nation of Switzerland enjoyed the enviable and largely unchallenged position as the world's foremost manufacturer of watches. Swiss technology and craftsmanship, in fact, were so widely admired that if a piece of machinery—or even a process—functioned at optimal efficiency, it was said to run "as smoothly as a Swiss watch." As recently as 1967, the Swiss had translated technical superiority into an overwhelming 65% share of the international market and had garnered 80% of the profits derived from watch sales with their high-end timepieces. But then, in 1968, a dramatic shift began to take place; one that saw the United States and Japan supplant Switzerland as watchmaker to the world. The shift was both sudden and startling; the European nation's market share plummeted to less than 10% in the course of one short decade, and an industry that had employed 65,000 skilled Swiss workers was ultimately reduced in size by more than 75%.

Ironically enough, it was the Swiss invention of quartz movement that sparked the change. The new technology was first unveiled at the Neufchatel research laboratory in 1967 to major Swiss watch manufacturers, who thought so little of the idea that they did not even bother to apply for patent protection. Others were more appreciative. The use of quartz movement, you see, made it possible to build extraordinarily accurate, reliable watches at prices nearly everyone could afford—a fact that was not long lost on the Americans and the Japanese. The rest, as the saying goes, is history. Some three decades and (one supposes) billions of francs later, the Swiss watch industry is still trying to recoup a fraction of the market that was once theirs almost exclusively.

Today's vascular surgeon-specialist finds himself in a curiously similar situation to the watchmakers at Neufchatel. He and his colleagues have also developed a ground-breaking technology that others may more speedily bring to market. You will understand immediately that I refer to the widespread use of endovascular grafting techniques by other specialists. Although it is no great secret that the pioneering work of vascular surgeons such as Drs. Parodi, Marin and Veith, May and White, Chuter, and Moore created the current state of the art, their early work initially received a tepid and even sometimes hostile response from many established vascular surgeons. We discussed too much and researched too little, at least in the beginning. Meanwhile, those with far less specialized training and only a fragmentary knowledge of the basic science behind our discipline filled the large and ever-growing public demand for less invasive endovascular procedures.

If the issue were solely economic, further discussion would be unnecessary. Self-preservation is, after all, an entirely personal matter, and it is up to individuals to decide what is best for them and their practices. The more pressing and disturbing question is whether we, as medical professionals, are willing to let our patients receive inferior treatment simply because we are too stubborn or too timid to learn the new techniques. These are harsh but necessary words. Now, more than ever before, patients know that there may be attractive alternatives to open surgery for a host of vascular maladies. Hopefully these alternatives will also prove to be safe and effective, and such proof must be sought. However, as this proof becomes available, patients will analyze their options and in many instances choose the ones that minimize suffering, increase comfort, and give the best results after treatment. In the long run, many will probably choose the less invasive vascular approaches. And maybe they are right.

Current Critical Problems in Vascular Surgery has, for several years now, sought to introduce vascular surgeon-specialists to the latest developments in this rapidly advancing area of research and practice. It is my hope that readers will approach the first two sections of the present volume, which cover endovascular treatments and techniques, with a renewed sense of interest and involvement. For the uninitiated, the time to learn is now; for the experts, the call to push forward with new and innovative endovascular research and techniques could not be clearer. The remainder of the book deals with more traditional but no less relevant information such as management and surgery of aneurysms, grafting techniques, treatment of lower extremity ischemia, carotid surgery, venous repair, and advances in basic science.

As always, we have assembled a select group of the world's leading vascular authorities to bring you up-to-the-minute news on all fronts. I will not cite names and topics since you will discover them in the chapters and pages that follow. Their words, in any case, will testify much more eloquently than my own to the continuing vitality that not only enlivens our specialty, but more importantly also improves treatment outcomes for our patients.

Frank J. Veith

Contents

Introduction

The Way We Were, 3
WILEY F. BARKER, M.D.

SECTION I Endovascular Treatments and Techniques

1 Impact of Endovascular Technology on the Practice of Vascular Surgery, 11
FRANK J. VEITH, M.D., MICHAEL L. MARIN, M.D.

2 The Vascular Surgeon as an Endoluminal Interventionist: Why Is It Important and How Can It Be Achieved? 16
FRANK J. CRIADO, M.D., LUIS A. QUERAL, M.D., PEGGY PATTEN, R.N.

3 Relationships Between Vascular Surgery and Interventional Radiology: How Should Turf Wars Be Resolved? 27
JOHN D. CORSON, M.B., Ch.B., F.R.C.S. (Engl.), WILLIAM J. SHARP, M.D.,
JAMAL J. HOBALLAH, M.D., TIMOTHY F. KRESOWIK, M.D.

4 Intraoperative Iliac Balloon Angioplasty and Stenting in Combination With Infrainguinal Bypass: Indications, Techniques, and Results, 32
STANLEY O. SNYDER, Jr., M.D., RICHARD J. DeMASI, M.D., JOCK R. WHEELER, M.D.,
ROGER T. GREGORY, M.D., ROBERT G. GAYLE, M.D., F. NOEL PARENT III, M.D.

5 Clinical Experience With an Integrated Self-Expandable Stent Graft (Corvita) for the Treatment of Various Arterial Lesions, 37
JEAN-PIERRE DEREUME, M.D., JOSÉ FERREIRA, M.D., MEHREZ EL DOUAIHY, M.D.,
JEAN-CHRISTOPHE CAVENAILE, M.D., SOPHIE GUYOT, M.D., SERGE MOTTE, M.D.,
GISELE VINCENT, M.D., JEAN-CLAUDE WAUTRECHT, M.D.

6 Endoluminal Stented Grafts for Treatment of Limb-Threatening Arterial Occlusive Disease, 46
ROSS T. LYON, M.D., MICHAEL L. MARIN, M.D., FRANK J. VEITH, M.D.

7 Endovascular Stent-Grafts in the Management of Arterial Injuries, 56
MICHAEL L. SCHWARTZ, M.D., MICHAEL L. MARIN, M.D., FRANK J. VEITH, M.D.

8 Why Vascular Surgeons Should Be Involved in Endovascular Procedures, 63
JAMES A. DeWEESE, M.D.

9 Subcutaneous Video-Assisted Saphenous Vein Harvest: A Minimally Invasive Technique for Vein Procurement, 67
ALAN B. LUMSDEN, M.D., WILLIAM D. JORDAN, Jr., M.D., F. FELMONT EAVES III, M.D.

10 Current Status of Peripheral Atherectomy, 72
SAMUEL S. AHN, M.D., BLESSIE CONCEPCION, B.S.

11 Outcome of Femoropopliteal and Femorotibial Bypass After Failed Balloon Angioplasty: Is It a Reason to Avoid PTA in Some Patients? 85
DIETER RAITHEL, M.D., Ph.D.

12 Value and Limitations of Angioscopy and Intravascular Ultrasound, 91
RODNEY A. WHITE, M.D., F.R.A.C.S., GEORGE E. KOPCHOK, B.S., CARLOS DONAYRE, M.D.

13 Surgery vs. Thrombolysis for Lower Extremity Ischemia: Updates on STILE and TOPAS Randomized Studies, 102
KENNETH OURIEL, M.D.

SECTION II *Endovascular Treatment of Aneurysms*

14 Aortic Aneurysm Morphology for Planning Endovascular Aortic Grafts, 109
HUGH G. BEEBE, M.D., TONYA L. JACKSON, B.A., JOHN P. PIGOTT, M.D.

15 Endovascular Treatment of Arterial Aneurysms, 115
AMIT V. PATEL, M.D., MICHAEL L. MARIN, M.D., FRANK J. VEITH, M.D.

16 Problems Encountered With EVT Devices (Tube and Bifurcated) for Treatment of Abdominal Aortic Aneurysms, 124
WESLEY S. MOORE, M.D.

17 Endovascular Bifurcated Graft Insertion for Abdominal Aortic Aneurysm Repair, 127
TIMOTHY A.M. CHUTER, M.D., ROMAN NOWYGROD, M.D.

18 Laparoscopically Assisted Abdominal Aortic Aneurysm Repair: Technique and Early Clinical Experience, 133
JON R. COHEN, M.D., MARIE H.M. CHEN, M.D., EUGENE A. MURPHY, M.D., ANTHONY J. D'ANGELO, M.D.

19 Stanford Experience With Stent-Graft Repair of Thoracic Aortic Aneurysms, 135
MICHAEL D. DAKE, M.D., D. CRAIG MILLER, M.D., CHARLES SEMBA, M.D., R. SCOTT MITCHELL, M.D., CHRISTOPHER K. ZARINS, M.D., THOMAS J. FOGARTY, M.D.

20 Sydney Experience With Endovascular Stent-Graft Repair of Abdominal Aortic Aneurysms: New Findings and Limitations, 137
JAMES MAY, M.S., F.R.A.C.S., GEOFFREY H. WHITE, M.D., F.R.A.C.S.

SECTION III Surgery of Aneurysms, the Aorta, and Its Visceral Branches

21 Factors Associated With the Growth of Abdominal Aortic Aneurysm: The Importance of Smoking, 145
JANET T. POWELL, M.D., Ph.D., SHANE T.R. MacSWEENEY, F.R.C.S., NEIL R. POULTER, M.R.C.P., ROGER MALCOLM GREENHALGH, M.A., M.D., M.Chir., F.R.C.S.

22 Abdominal Aortic Aneurysm Surgery: Statewide Variations in Prevalence and Operative Mortality, 150
DOLORES J. KATZ, Ph.D., JAMES C. STANLEY, M.D., GERALD B. ZELENOCK, M.D.

23 Mortality After Elective Aortic Reconstruction, 160
JAMES M. SEEGER, M.D., THOMAS S. HUBER, M.D., Ph.D.

24 Prognosis for Thoracoabdominal Aortic Aneurysms Managed Nonoperatively, 165
ROBERT A. CAMBRIA, M.D., JOHN W. HALLETT, Jr., M.D., W. ANTHONY STANSON, M.D., PETER GLOVICZKI, M.D.

25 Use of Ligation Treatment for Abdominal Aortic Aneurysms, 172
WILLIAM C. PEVEC, M.D., JAMES W. HOLCROFT, M.D., F. WILLIAM BLAISDELL, M.D.

26 Late Complications of Standard Aortic Aneurysm Resection: What Is the Ultimate Fate of the Graft and of the Patient Based on a 35-Year Experience? 176
JAMES A. DeWEESE, M.D.

27 Ischemic Nephropathy and Concomitant Aortic Disease: When Should Renal Artery Repair Be Undertaken? 181
ELLIOT L. CHAIKOF, M.D., Ph.D., ROBERT B. SMITH III, M.D.

28 Transaortic Renal Endarterectomy: Techniques, Pitfalls, and Results, 187
DANIEL G. CLAIR, M.D., MICHAEL BELKIN, M.D., ANTHONY D. WHITTEMORE, M.D., MAGRUDER C. DONALDSON, M.D., JOHN A. MANNICK, M.D.

29 Management of Aortoenteric Fistula, 193
STEVEN M. SANTILLI, M.D., Ph.D., JERRY GOLDSTONE, M.D.

30 The Importance of Age, Sex, and Aortic Size on the Outcome of Aortofemoral Bypass, 197
R. JAMES VALENTINE, M.D., G. PATRICK CLAGETT, M.D.

31 Axillobifemoral Bypass: Current Indications, Techniques, and Results, 201
ROBERT B. RUTHERFORD, M.D.

32 Reconstruction of the Celiac, Superior Mesenteric, and Left and Right Renal Arteries Using an Extended Left Retroperitoneal Approach: Techniques and Results, 206
R. CLEMENT DARLING III, M.D., DHIRAJ M. SHAH, M.D., BENJAMIN B. CHANG, M.D., PHILIP S.K. PATY, M.D., ROBERT P. LEATHER, M.D.

SECTION IV *Advances in the Management of Lower Extremity Ischemia*

33 Randomized Prospective Comparison of Epidural and General Anesthesia for Infrainguinal Bypass Surgery, 217
BRUCE A. PERLER, M.D.

34 Optimal Treatment of Vein and Anastomotic Lesions Responsible for Failing Vein Grafts: When Is PTA Appropriate? 223
LUIS A. SANCHEZ, M.D., WILLIAM D. SUGGS, M.D., MICHAEL L. MARIN, M.D., KURT R. WENGERTER, M.D., FRANK J. VEITH, M.D.

35 The Superficial Femoral Vein as a Bypass Graft: Indications, Techniques, Results, Morbidity, and "Spinoffs," 228
MARTIN L. SCHULMAN, M.D., LEE G. SCHULMAN, M.D.

36 Free Flaps in Association With Distal Bypasses to Extend Limb Salvage, 237
RICHARD M. GREEN, M.D., JOSEPH M. SERLETTI, M.D.

37 Tibiotibial Bypass for Limb Salvage, 241
ROSS T. LYON, M.D., FRANK J. VEITH, M.D.

38 Is Routine Vein Graft Angioscopy Worthwhile in Infrainguinal Bypass Surgery? 245
DANIEL G. CLAIR, M.D., MICHAEL A. GOLDEN, M.D., JOHN A. MANNICK, M.D., ANTHONY D. WHITTEMORE, M.D., MAGRUDER C. DONALDSON, M.D.

39 Why Angioscopy Is Worthwhile in Infrainguinal Bypass Surgery: How to Make It Work, 250
ARNOLD MILLER, M.B., Ch.B., JUHA P. SALENIUS, M.D., Ph.D.

40 Diagnosis and Treatment of Paradoxical Arterial Emboli: An Unrecognized Entity, 260
ALI F. ABURAHMA, M.D.

41 Optimal Treatment of Intermittent Claudication: Role of Conservative Measures, Drugs, Angioplasty, Atherectomy, and Operation, 266
ANTHONY D. WHITTEMORE, M.D.

42 Avoiding Infrainguinal Bypass Wound Complications in Renal Failure Patients: Should Grafts Be Tunneled Subfascially or Subcutaneously? 271
JONATHAN P. GERTLER, M.D., JAN D. BLANKENSTEIJN, M.D., Ph.D., WILLIAM M. ABBOTT, M.D.

43 Value and Limitations of Percutaneous Transluminal Angioplasty, Stents, and Lytic Agents for Aortoiliac Disease, 275
KENNETH WAYNE JOHNSTON, M.D., F.R.C.S.(C)

SECTION V Noninvasive and Less Invasive Diagnostic and Therapeutic Modalities

44 Vascular Laboratory Funding and Reimbursement: Present Status and Future Directions, 285
J. DENNIS BAKER, M.D.

45 Controversies Regarding Low-Dose Heparin Regimens, 289
F. WILLIAM BLAISDELL, M.D., JOHN T. OWINGS, M.D.

46 Are Oral Anticoagulants Indicated in Vascular Surgical Patients? Do They Increase Graft Patency and Do They Lower the Death Rate? 295
MARCO J.D. TANGELDER, M.D., ALE ALGRA, M.D., Ph.D., BERT C. EIKELBOOM, M.D., Ph.D.

47 Vascular Applications of Pneumatic Tourniquet Occlusion Techniques, 301
STANLEY O. SNYDER, Jr., M.D.

SECTION VI Carotid and Vertebral Surgery

48 The Ongoing Progress of NASCET, 307
H.J.M. BARNETT, M.D., HEATHER E. MELDRUM, B.A.

49 Carotid Endarterectomy in Symptomatic and Asymptomatic Patients Over 80 Years of Age: Indications and Results, 312
BRUCE A. PERLER, M.D.

50 To Shunt or Not to Shunt? To Patch or Not to Patch? 318
JONATHAN B. TOWNE, M.D.

51 Adjunctive Techniques for the Management of Difficult Carotid Artery Endarterectomies, 322
PATRICK J. LAMPARELLO, M.D., THOMAS S. RILES, M.D.

52 Nd:YAG Laser Ablation of Carotid Endarterectomy Flaps, 327
MILTON SLOCUM, M.D., PAUL W. HUMPHREY, M.D., DONALD SILVER, M.D.

53 Indications and Optimal Techniques for Carotid Shortening During Carotid Endarterectomy, 331
KELLIE A. COYLE, M.D., J.D., ROBERT B. SMITH III, M.D.

54 Treatment of Perioperative Neurologic Deficits After Carotid Surgery, 337
WILLIAM H. BAKER, M.D.

55 Is Carotid-Subclavian Prosthetic Bypass a Durable and Effective Procedure for Subclavian Occlusive Disease? A 22-Year Experience, 343
ROBERT W. BARNES, M.D.

56 Revascularization Across the Neck Using the Retropharyngeal Route, 348
RAMON BERGUER, M.D., Ph.D.

SECTION VII *Scientific Findings With Clinical Applications*

57 Natural History of Moderate Internal Carotid Artery Stenosis in Asymptomatic and Symptomatic Patients, 359
DAVID S. SUMNER, M.D., M. ASHRAF MANSOUR, M.D., MARK A. MATTOS, M.D.

58 Natural History of Moderate Carotid Stenosis, 365
D. EUGENE STRANDNESS, Jr., M.D., BRIAN F. JOHNSON, M.D.

59 Progress in Understanding the Etiology of Paraplegia in Thoracoabdominal Aneurysm Repair: Possible Remedies, 369
G. MELVILLE WILLIAMS, M.D.

60 Update on Progress in the Reversal of Atherosclerotic Lesions, 373
ALLAN D. CALLOW, M.D., Ph.D.

61 Natural History of Iliac Artery Aneurysms: When Should They Be Treated? 379
PETER F. LAWRENCE, M.D., JOSE C. ALVES, M.D.

62 The Importance of Genetic and Biochemical Factors in the Practical Management of Aneurysms, 385
SANDRA C. CARR, M.D., WILLIAM H. PEARCE, M.D.

63 Is the Natural History of Intermittent Claudication Worse Than We Thought? 391
JACK L. CRONENWETT, M.D.

64 Effect of Gram-Positive and Gram-Negative Bacteria on Selective Preservation of Infected Prosthetic Arterial Grafts, 397
KEITH D. CALLIGARO, M.D., FRANK J. VEITH, M.D., MICHAEL L. SCHWARTZ, M.D., MATTHEW J. DOUGHERTY, M.D., DOMINIC A. DeLAURENTIS, M.D.

65 Adaptation of Vein Grafts to Arterialization in Infrainguinal Bypasses: Does This Play a Role in Development of Vein Graft Stenoses? 402
ROBERT M. ZWOLAK, M.D., Ph.D.

66 Bleeding Time as a Predictor of Early PTFE Graft Failure: Does It Work and Why? 409
RICHARD J. FOWL, M.D., KEVIN J. OSE, M.D., JOSEPH E. PALASCAK, M.D., SANDRA J. UHL, R.N., JOHN BLEBEA, M.D., RICHARD F. KEMPCZINSKI, M.D.

67 The Effect of Smoking and Fibrinogen on Vein Graft Failure, 416
DANIEL J. HIGMAN, F.R.C.S., ROBERT C.J. HICKS, F.R.C.S., JANET T. POWELL, M.D., Ph.D., ROGER MALCOLM GREENHALGH, M.A., M.D., M.Chir., F.R.C.S.

SECTION VIII *Trauma and Complex Problems in Vascular Surgery*

68 Update on Optimal Management of Trauma to Large- and Medium-Sized Veins, 423
NORMAN M. RICH, M.D., MARK R. JACKSON, M.D., MAJ, MC, USA,
DAVID L. GILLESPIE, M.D., MAJ, MC, USA

69 Current Principles for Managing Carotid and Vertebral Artery Trauma, 427
MALCOLM O. PERRY, M.D.

70 Surgical Treatment of Chronic Mesenteric Ischemia, 433
DONALD E. PATTERSON, M.D., KEITH D. CALLIGARO, M.D.,
MATTHEW J. DOUGHERTY, M.D., DOMINIC A. DeLAURENTIS, M.D.

71 Management of Aortic Graft Infection By Graft Excision and Extra-Anatomic Revascularization: Long-Term Results With the Standard Treatment, 437
DAVID C. BREWSTER, M.D.

72 Treatment of Infected Aortic Prostheses Using Deep and Superficial Lower Extremity Vein Grafts for In Situ Replacement, 443
G. PATRICK CLAGETT, M.D.

73 Long-Term Follow-Up of More Than 100 Infected Extracavitary Arterial Prosthetic Grafts, 453
KEITH D. CALLIGARO, M.D., FRANK J. VEITH, M.D., MICHAEL L. SCHWARTZ, M.D.,
JAMIE GOLDSMITH, R.N., MATTHEW J. DOUGHERTY, M.D.,
DOMINIC A. DeLAURENTIS, M.D.

74 Transaxillary First Rib Resection With Extrapleural T2 Ganglion Thoracic Sympathectomy, 459
DAVID B. ROOS, M.D.

75 Pathogenesis and Management of Upper Extremity Ischemia Following Angioaccess Surgery, 463
HARRY SCHANZER, M.D., MILAN SKLADANY, M.D., RICHARD J. KNIGHT, M.D.,
ELIZABETH B. HARRINGTON, M.D., MARTIN HARRINGTON, M.D.,
MOSHE HAIMOV, M.D.

76 Techniques and Results of Vascular Surgery for Impotence: Large and Small Vessel Options, 468
RALPH G. DePALMA, M.D.

77 Management of Venous Ulceration: The Relative Role of Radical Excision for Intractable Ulcers, 475
BEN U. MARSAN, M.D., JOHN J. RICOTTA, M.D.

78 Treatment of Lymphatic Complications: A Comparison of Conservative Therapy and Lymphazurin-Assisted Early Ligation Techniques, 484
HARRY SCHANZER, M.D., MARK A. SCHWARTZ, M.D., MILAN SKLADANY, M.D.,
MOSHE HAIMOV, M.D., JEFFREY S. STEIN, M.D.

79 Treatment Alternatives for Deep Venous Thrombosis in Pregnancy: Anticoagulation vs. Vena Caval Filtration Devices, 487
ALI F. ABURAHMA, M.D.

SECTION IX *Venous Disease Update*

80 Valve Repair Techniques for Chronic Venous Insufficiency: When, How, and By Whom Should They Be Performed? 495
THOMAS F. O'DONNELL, Jr., M.D., AGUSTIN A. RODRIGUEZ, M.D.

81 Optimal Technique for Venous Valve Repair: Which Patients Should Have the Procedure? 502
SESHADRI RAJU, M.D.

82 The Plantar Venous Plexus and Applications of A-V Impulse System Technology, 507
JOHN V. WHITE, M.D., JOSEPH I. ZARGE, M.D.

83 Aggressive Interventional Treatment for Acute Iliofemoral Venous Thrombosis: Are Surgical Thrombectomy and Regional Catheter-Directed Urokinase Beneficial? 517
ANTHONY J. COMEROTA, M.D.

84 Stents and Lytic Agents for Large Vein Occlusive Disease, 524
MICHAEL D. DAKE, M.D.

85 Update on Pulmonary Embolism, 531
LAZAR J. GREENFIELD, M.D., MARY C. PROCTOR, M.S.

SECTION X *Pioneers in Vascular Surgery*

86 Norman Freeman, 537
JOHN E. CONNOLLY, M.D.

87 Valentine Mott, 540
JESSE E. THOMPSON, M.D.

Index, 545

Current Critical Problems in Vascular Surgery

Introduction

The Way We Were
(Or, Why Did We Change, and Will Things Ever Be the Same?)

WILEY F. BARKER, M.D.

There's nothing so passionate as a vested interest disguised as an intellectual conviction.
Sean O'Casey

Had I been asked to write this 15 years ago, I would have felt compelled to present a dissertation on how things should be done on some strictly technical matter (or at least, the way I thought that they should!) replete with all manner of dubious data and obfuscating charts. I might have regaled you with my concept of why endarterectomy (as I performed it, of course) was such a good operation, and my belief that our operations held up so well because of the use of heparin—and as Dr. Alexander Clowes will tell you concerning heparin, we were possibly right, but for the wrong reason. However, I am going to refrain from discussing specific clinical matters and rather will discuss some of our foibles as surgeons. I hope you will see yourselves reflected in the light of some of the things I have to say.

One of the overused buzzwords of the present is "change." I had not meant to develop a political treatise when I started this paper, nor do I mean it to be that now—but change and how we react to change is my text for the day.

Although we as doctors pride ourselves generally on the progress we have made in medicine, it is paradoxical that physicians often seem to resent and resist a proposed change in the way they do specific things, and there are probably few groups initially so sensitive to change imposed on their activities as is a group of surgeons.

We are in the midst of earthshaking changes in our professional lives, and a lighthearted look at some examples of how we have reacted to impending changes in the past is in order.

The pattern is simple: when he hears of a dramatic new technical procedure the conservative doctor usually says, "Good Lord, what in the world makes anyone think that's a good idea?" and after a little (sometimes too little) evaluation, he finds himself subscribing to the new procedure or concept with enthusiasm. Perhaps it's only a manifestation of Newton's first law of motion applied to human nature. The second and third laws may be seen subsequently to apply as well. Let's see how it works in real life.

In the modern world there are several examples to which most of us have been very close. For example, how did the general surgeon *first* react to the suggestions that cholecystectomies might be performed through the laparoscopic approach? And then how long did it take him to buy a laparoscopic kit and learn to use it? Today, major teaching programs are plagued with the problem of finding enough cases *unsuited* for laparoscopic cholecystectomy to train residents in the classic procedure, which still must be used in many cases. To turn to a more pertinent parallel from the history of vascular surgery, let me remind you that the first truly successful vascular reconstruction in humans was the endarterectomy as introduced by João Cid dos Santos and popularized by Jack Wylie and by myself and Jack Cannon. How many residents leave their training today able to skillfully perform an aortoiliac endarterectomy: how many of you would still undertake this operation rather than "placing an old bloody rag in the wound," as William Sandusky used to say? I would submit that in properly chosen patients, and when properly performed, this operation is effective, safe, and at least as durable as any form of bypass or replacement grafting in the aorta and iliac system and even in the femoral artery. I will not force-feed you with argumentative documentation, but I keep seeing or hearing from patients from 20 or 30 years ago who may require another vascular operation (carotid or distal femoral, as a rule) but who still maintain a nearly perfect and fully satisfactory aortic-iliac reconstruction by this technique. And although it is hard to match cases and controls truly, I believe that even the results of the femoral reconstructions *above the knee* that we reported in 1966[1] compare favorably with the results of vein used in either the in situ or reversed mode. You will notice that I am exhibiting the very resistance to change I am describing in others!

I thought it might be more interesting, however, to look back at some other examples of this resistance to change in the more remote history of surgery.

In the sixteenth century, Ambroise Paré was the instrument for a proposed change. He, a mere surgeon, had had the temerity to challenge a physician, Étienne Gourmelen, the Dean of the Faculty of Medicine in Paris, after the latter had taken Paré to task for daring to try to control hemorrhage from battle injuries by the use of the ligature instead of cautery or hot oil.[2] In his Apologie and Treatise, Paré made it clear that Gourmelen, as a physician who was above such things, had probably never managed a wound in his life, nor had he even read the authorities of ancient times. Finally, after figuratively cutting him down to size, Paré dismissed him condescendingly as "my little master." And today it's Paré we remember, not Gourmelen. I doubt if many operating room suites today could provide you with boiling oil, although the cautery and the ligature remain.

For many years in this century, ablation of the sympathetic nerves was about the only tool the surgeon had for the treatment of occlusive arterial disease. It may not have been one that did much good, and it is said to have done occasional harm. The famous French surgical teacher, René Leriche, was one of the greatest proponents of this procedure with which he had become familiar because of its use in the treatment of pain syndromes not necessarily of vascular origin. To this he added arteriectomy, excision of the obstructed portion of the artery, in an effort to preclude noxious sympathetic discharge from the obstructed vessel. Parenthetically, I believe that Leriche's continued espousal of this operation—which can be considered as another example of resistance to change—was responsible for holding back for years direct vascular reconstruction as we know it today. Leriche knew about the use of vein grafts; the bypass graft had been described in 1907, and in 1924 there were presented at an international surgical congress two separate series of 50 patients each in whom there had been placed venous grafts for arterial occlusions of both traumatic and chronic origins, with excellent results.[3,4] To be sure, these had been mostly short grafts, usually no more than 6 cm, but sometimes as long as 10 cm (hence the title of one of Jean Kunlin's early papers, "The treatment of arterial obliteration by the long venous graft"[5]). Some of Leriche's residents in later years told me their professor commonly remarked that it would be wonderful to dare to use a graft, but it was too dangerous: "Better a partial success than a total failure." But sympathetic ablation and arteriectomy of the occluded vessel, performed to remove an irritating focus in the artery, became Leriche's stock in trade in vascular surgery, and he carried it so far as to resect the aortic bifurcation and perform a bilateral sympathectomy for the atherosclerotic lesion that carries his eponymic title.[6]

When João dos Santos of Lisbon realized his first thromboendarterectomies might indeed be opening a door to a momentous new world of reconstructive surgery, he went to René Leriche, his former mentor, and asked him how to present it. Leriche chose to read his (Leriche's) version of dos Santos' paper on thromboendarterectomy before the Académie de Chirurgie of France,[7] (dos Santos was not a member of that prestigious group). The report that Leriche presented, after he had edited it considerably, was quite different from dos Santos' simple observations; he was quite ambivalent. Clearly he took pride in the work of his former student, but Leriche was also clearly worried that if dos Santos' approach succeeded, it might supplant Leriche's own favorite procedures of sympathectomy and excision of the thrombosed artery. We do hate to give up an operation in which we have invested much effort, and one to which we have become accustomed. On a personal note, I can remember very well how foolish it seemed to me that this mad Portuguese surgeon should try to scratch the clot out of thrombosed arteries and expect blood to flow through the repaired area!

Leriche's reaction was very similar when Kunlin finally persuaded Leriche to let him try a long vein graft in one of the professor's patients after sympathectomy and arteriectomy had failed.[5] The patient had returned with spotty gangrene and a cold foot, despite Leriche's prior classic treatment. Leriche was strongly against Kunlin's proposal to place a long graft in the leg, but Kunlin argued until the professor finally said, "Oh, go ahead," and left the room. Many years later, Kunlin[8] described to me how Leriche's face turned white on rounds a day or two later when he examined the patient: there was now a strongly palpable pulse in the foot, which was warm and free of pain. The gangrenous patches were beginning to demarcate. Leriche finally admitted that this operation *might* be suitable for the femoral artery, but it surely could not ever replace arteriectomy and sympectomy for lesions of the aorta and iliac system.

Leriche[9] was once described by a close associate, however, as having a "very mystical attitude" toward statistics; that this description is fitting is suggested by a report he made of 898 unilateral (left) adrenalectomies and bilateral lumbar sympathectomies for Buerger's disease, in which he finally admitted that after 898 operations he believed the procedure had failed to benefit anyone. As Newton said, "A body in motion tends to remain in motion, etc." Sometimes we fail to appreciate the significance of statistical analysis.

One of the techniques that enabled us to begin to perform vascular surgery, arteriography, also received short shrift when first presented. The discussion of the first paper on arteriography of the extremities by Reynaldo dos Santos[10] gave it a bitter reception, even though the technique had already been applied to the vessels of the brain by Egas Moniz. Lècene, for instance, said "These are certainly very fine pictures, but I demand to know what use they can ever be for the surgeon. . . . What can be the possible clinical use of the injections into these arteries? . . . We did not meet here just to applaud without thinking . . . and I think it would be very wise if it were never done again."

I met a less vociferous but similar reaction when I first tried to get our radiology department to perform arteriography of the extremities in 1950. The chief of the service at Wadsworth Veterans Hospital informed me that that was not a procedure in which the radiologists ever wanted to be involved; he finally agreed to let us do it if we would pay the technician from the surgical budget (after regular working hours) and use the X-ray department machine as long as they didn't have to have anything to do with it! O tempora. . . .

After the radiologists learned about the potentials of arteriography, Dotter and Judkins[11] began the first arterial dilatations with the hard Teflon probe, which of course led to one of the great changes in vascular surgery today—the endoscopic approach to many of our vascular problems. I am, in fact, true to the nature of a conservative surgeon, surprised by the rapid acceptance of many of these procedures (I am again showing that I am a closet follower of Leriche, you see) by so many of our vascular colleagues. My reaction was typical of many vascular surgeons when they saw the first percutaneous endovascular arterial dilatations, even the balloon dilatations, and especially so after one saw what they did to an arterial wall: "It isn't possible; it will destroy the vessel; it can't remain patent (if you left that much debris in an endarterectomized artery in the open technique the operation would be doomed to prompt thrombosis), and so on." And yet, as we know, many of these percutaneous dilatations not only did work, but some of them are very durable—but some do fail, and fail early. Many newer techniques have not yet met our rigorous reporting and evaluation standards and cannot yet be recognized as worthwhile. Yet we have come to realize that there is a place for many of them, and we have learned how to use them in that appropriate setting.

Today there are a host of other endoscopic technical changes facing us; the endovascular placement of stented grafts for the treatment of abdominal aneurysms without laparotomy seems to me one of the most dramatic and possibly useful techniques, and one which may greatly change the face of vascular surgery. I was originally a very serious skeptic, but time is already answering most of my objections. Endoluminal placement of grafts is a procedure in its infancy, but it is going to find its proper niche.

When we adopt any new procedure, however, certain matters must be considered that pertain to your choices as the surgeon as well as to the choices made by a third party payor, be it the government or otherwise. These innovative procedures must truly offer a simpler and better way to do things in terms of outcome and benefit to the patient.

First, you must question the *applicability and suitability* of the procedure in question. If the results are truly equal, these "lesser" operations may be properly indicated for *all* patients. Very often, however, any new operation is apt to be applied to those who can't tolerate our classic operations easily, or possibly, for those who simply refuse to do so. But what do you risk by submitting a patient to a lesser procedure for these reasons, especially if you think the patient can't tolerate the classic operative approach, when you *must recognize that a failure of the lesser procedure* may force you to perform the major procedure under perhaps the worst of circumstances?

Second, cost: is the newer procedure truly less costly, case for case? Example: hernia repair, as presently done by laparoscopy in our area, in comparison to a well done repair under a local anesthetic, until very recently cost considerably more than the standard procedure. It took more operating room time, and since it required a general or spinal anesthetic, was much more upsetting to the patient. Today it seems that the laparoscopic repairs are not only equal but in many instances are superior to the open repair, despite the need for and cost of the anesthesia.

On occasion we must account for both direct and indirect costs rather than just the cost of the specific equipment necessary for these new procedures. One financial consideration that is often overlooked is the matter of backup support: must valuable operating space and/or the services of a different operator be held on a standby basis in case something goes wrong with the "lesser" procedure?

Third, one of the greatest problems of these "lesser" procedures is that they may be performed by *persons without adequate training in the classic mode of operation.* This is what many have seen when the radiologists and nephrologists attempt to do major endoscopic repairs without the background of classic vascular surgical training and without the technical abilities to carry out the classic procedure. The person who is not fully trained, qualified, and "privileged" to convert the lesser to the classic procedure is a hazard to the patient for several reasons:

1. He is very often apt not to fully understand the nature of the disease.
2. Perhaps more important is that he may be dangerously unwilling to stop when he is in trouble, partly because he doesn't even recognize what trouble he is in. He may also be influenced by thoughts of the damage a failed operation can do to one's ego and reputation, or perhaps even for pecuniary reasons.

I believe we have to ask ourselves honestly whether we are opposed to impending changes because we are resistant to change, or because we can prove the faults and deficiencies of the new approach.

I think that ultimately the right choices will be made, but that along the way many people will have to suffer: patients may be subjected to the wrong operation through direct or indirect governmental influences, and good operations may be discarded because of a difference in expense between one operation and a less satisfactory procedure as health care dollars continue to be stretched. I've often thought how government policies on medical economics may come to require us to give patients saline solution instead of digitalis for a failing heart because it is cheaper.

I wish I could offer comforting philosophic balm to ease the pain of excessive intrusion by government, insurance companies, and by other fuzzy-thinking do-gooders. As I see it, however, this is an evolving process: there will continue to be ill patients, and physicians will continue to take care of these patients, although things may not ever again be as they once were.

Sorting this all out and choosing the right course is somewhat reminiscent of chaos theory: there are so many minuscule details that can combine to trap the unwary, it is almost impossible to compare the new with the old. It's worse than trying to project next year's or even next month's weather. The gross problem matching patient discomfort, expense, time away from work, complications, liberation of operating room facilities, increased hazards, unwise and unskillful performance—all add up to the apt application of an admonition by L.J. Henderson, which I must explain before I quote it. As a college student I took a course in medical history from Professor Henderson. On any given day we would pursue the ramifications of some of the great theorems in the history of science, going in detail through the accumulation of evidence suggesting the formulation of a hypothesis, the development of methods to test the hypothesis, the accumulation of data, and the conclusions. Finally, the professor would say that by means of these appropriate "scientific methods" one should be able to say with some statistical surety that "All other things being equal, *A* is different from *B*. But don't forget, all other things are *never* equal."

So, having decided that all other things are never equal, we are left with uncertainties regarding impending changes; what course can we follow? First, I suppose, is that you should do your best. Have patience, and hope that the truth will appear and prevail in due time, and that in the meanwhile your best efforts have not done harm to too many patients, physically or financially. Recognize that there will always be conflicts about what you do and how you do it, and one can only argue for his own conscientious best course, deriving the best statistical justifications possible as soon as sufficient experience can provide this information. And accept that things will never be the way they once were.

On the other hand, even reliable statistics aren't everything: as the late Bert Dunphy said, "It doesn't take five statisticians and a randomized prospective trial to recognize a pretty girl when you see one."

REFERENCES

1. Barker WF. Peripheral Arterial Disease. Philadelphia: WB Saunders, 1966, pp 178-205.
2. Keynes G. The Apologie and Treatise of Ambroise Paré. London: Falcon Educational Books, 1951.
3. Weglowski R. Ueber die Gefässtransplantation. Zentralbl Chir 52:2241, 1925.
4. Lexer E. 20 Jahre Transplantations Forschung in der Chirurgie. Arch Klin Chir 138:251-302, 1925.
5. Kunlin J. Le traitement de l'artérite oblitérante par la greffe veineuse longue. Rev Chir 70:206-224, 1951.
6. Leriche R. De la résection du carrefour aortico-iliaque avec double sympathectomie lombaire pour thromboses artéritique de l'aorte: Le syndrome de l'obliteration termino-aortique par artérite. Presse Med 48:601-604, 1940.
7. dos Santos JC. Sur la désobstruction des thromboses artérielles anciennes. (Read by René Leriche.) Mem Acad Chir 73:409-411, 1947.
8. Kunlin J. Personal communication, 1988.
9. Leriche R. Des causes d'échec de la surrénalectomie et de la ganglionectomie dans la thromboangeite, d'après 898 operations. Presse Med 57:539-540, 1949.
10. dos Santos R, Lamas A, Caldas J. L'arteriographie des membres, de l'aorte et des ses branches abdominales. Bull Mem Soc Natl Chir 55:587-601, 1929.
11. Dotter CT, Judkins MP. Transluminal treatment of atherosclerotic obstruction: Description of a new technique and a preliminary report of its application. Circulation 30:654-670, 1964.

SECTION I

Endovascular Treatments and Techniques

This section deals with some of the implications of evolving endovascular technologies. These include interspecialty relationships and how vascular surgeons can broaden their skills in the area of endovascular intervention. It also details some of the specific vascular surgical procedures that can be facilitated by combining them with endovascular procedures. It discusses the use of endovascular grafts in the treatment of limb-threatening occlusive disease and in the management of arterial injuries. New techniques for video-assisted vein harvest, peripheral atherectomy, angioscopy, intravascular ultrasound, and intra-arterial thrombolysis are also presented.

1

Impact of Endovascular Technology on the Practice of Vascular Surgery

FRANK J. VEITH, M.D., and MICHAEL L. MARIN, M.D.

The treatment of arterial and venous disease has changed over the past 15 years and will change even more dramatically in the years to come. Catheter-guidewire–based techniques have already made significant contributions to the manipulative or surgical management of aortoiliac, superficial femoral, and renal artery stenoses as well as arterial thromboembolism, iliofemoral venous thrombosis, arteriovenous malformations, and some visceral artery aneurysms. Some of these lesions can now be treated effectively with percutaneous transluminal angioplasty (PTA), catheter-directed lytic drugs and aspiration, intracaval filters, or coil embolization. The common element in all these techniques is their use of endovascular pathways, accessed from remote sites, to treat the offending vascular lesion, usually under fluoroscopic guidance. Because these endovascular techniques have proved to be a simpler, safer means of treating some patients with vascular disease, they have been embraced by vascular surgeons and used increasingly by them. In some cases these catheter-based treatments have been used directly by the vascular surgeon; in other cases management has been by referral to a collaborating interventional radiologist or cardiologist.

Because these endovascular techniques are gaining increasing acceptance and their less invasive nature renders them attractive to referring physicians and patients alike, it is reasonable to ask how they have affected the practice of vascular surgery. The present article answers this question and speculates as to what impact these newer derivative endovascular techniques (e.g., stents and stented grafts) will have on the practice of vascular surgery in the future.

IMPACT OF ENDOVASCULAR TECHNOLOGY TO DATE

Widely available endovascular techniques currently include PTA, lytic agents, caval filters, and intravascular occluding devices such as coils. To date, these endovascular treatments can be applied to some but not most patients with a valid indication for an open vascular surgical procedure. Only short stenotic lesions causing minor symptoms have responded well to PTA, whereas longer occlusive lesions causing ischemic symptoms severe enough to warrant open surgery have generally yielded poor results from simple balloon angioplasty.[1] The addition of *laser techniques* or *atherectomy devices,* although theoretically promising, has not improved these poor results with long complex lesions. Thus, although PTA has replaced some open operations for aortoiliac and renal artery disease, it has largely proved to be a helpful adjunct to arterial reconstructive surgery rather than a competitive modality. PTA is generally used to treat lesions that produce symptoms insufficient to justify open surgery and to aid in or simplify the management of complicated or difficult patients.[2,3] For example, fewer than 20% of lower limb salvage surgical candidates are amenable to treatment by PTA alone.[4,5]

The same is true of other current widely used endovascular methods. Lytic agents, catheter aspiration thromboembolectomy, caval filters, and coil embolization are currently used in only a small fraction of vascular surgical candidates. Moreover, these endovascular techniques are frequently a helpful adjunct in rendering the surgical and overall treatment of vascular patients simpler and better. For these reasons, endovascular technology to date has not had an overwhelming impact on the practice of vascular surgery, although it facilitates the management of some complex problems, provides a simpler alternative treatment for some patients whose symptoms might not be severe enough to war-

---

Data from Veith FJ. Transluminally placed endovascular stented grafts and their impact on vascular surgery. J Vasc Surg 20:855-860, 1994; Veith FJ, Marin ML. Endovascular surgery and its effect on the relationship between vascular surgery and radiology [editorial]. J Endovasc Surg 2:1-7, 1995; and Veith FJ, Marin ML. Impact of vascular technology on the practice of vascular surgery. Am J Surg (in press).

rant open surgery, and replaces at most approximately 15% of all vascular operations.

FUTURE IMPACT OF ENDOVASCULAR TECHNOLOGY

The introduction of endovascular stents and, more importantly, stented grafts will significantly change this relatively comfortable state of affairs. The availability of balloon-expandable or self-expanding intraluminal endovascular stents has largely eliminated portosystemic shunt operations by making it possible to create intrahepatic portal-to-hepatic venous communications within the liver via a percutaneous internal jugular approach (TIPS procedure).[6] Stents have also increased the effectiveness of PTA for treating stenotic lesions in large arteries and veins. They have clearly improved the results of simple balloon angioplasty of iliac artery stenotic lesions and made it possible to treat short iliac occlusions by endovascular means.[7] Stents have also made it possible to treat without an open surgical procedure renal artery ostial stenoses, as well as symptomatic stenoses and short occlusions of the innominate, common carotid, and subclavian arteries. Efforts are underway to evaluate the effectiveness of these devices in the femoropopliteal system and even carotid bifurcation. Even if these efforts prove that stents are ineffective in these peripheral locations, it is likely that endoluminal stenting procedures will replace another 10% of open vascular operations in addition to the 15% already replaced by simple PTA and other current endovascular techniques.

Transluminally placed endovascular stented grafts (TPEGs) have the potential to replace an even higher percentage of current open vascular surgical procedures. TPEGs are a group of devices consisting of a new vascular conduit or graft and elements to fix this conduit in a suitable position within the vascular tree. These devices are inserted from an access site remote from the lesion to be treated, guided fluoroscopically over a wire within blood vessels, and fixed in position to repair the vascular anomaly in a less invasive fashion than would characterize a standard operative procedure.

The TPEG concept was first introduced in 1969 by Charles Dotter,[8] a pioneer in angioplasty and other catheter-directed techniques. Throughout the 1980s several investigators explored the use of TPEGs to treat experimental aneurysms in animals.[9-12] In 1985 Volodos et al.[13] first used a TPEG device to treat iliac occlusive disease. However, their work, published only in Russian, received scant attention until Parodi et al.[14] performed the first TPEG repair of an aortic aneurysm in a high-risk patient in 1990. To date, Parodi[15] has performed more than 50 TPEG repairs, mostly of abdominal aortic aneurysms, although he has treated several traumatic arterial lesions as well.

In addition, our group in New York, over the past 25 months, has inserted 96 TPEGs in 77 patients with a variety of aneurysmal, occlusive, and traumatic lesions at various sites within the arterial tree.[16-20] Most of these patients had some serious comorbid condition or a surgical problem (such as scarring or infection) that precluded standard surgical or interventional treatment. Many were not candidates for general or regional anesthesia. All but one patient had some open vascular surgical component to their procedure. Even though many of these patients had end-stage disease with multiple previous therapeutic failures, our results to date in most patients have been encouraging. However, this experience is still too limited to make any recommendations concerning widespread use of these endovascular methods or to suggest that our indications be broadened to include all but these patients who were otherwise very difficult or impossible to treat. Almost all of these TPEG procedures were complex and difficult to perform. Successful attainment of a satisfactory end-point sometimes required a major vascular surgical or catheter-guidewire "rescue" component to the procedure. All of these TPEG procedures were performed with an anesthesiologist in attendance and full invasive pressure monitoring. In several instances this venue and staffing were crucial to achieve a successful outcome since some of the procedures were long and complicated.

Despite these reservations, our preliminary observations plus those of others[15-25] suggest that TPEGs may prove to be effective. If they are, they will constitute a potentially better method for treating a major additional fraction of our vascular surgical cases. Because they offer the advantage of being less invasive, TPEGs will be inherantly attractive to patients and physicians. These devices also offer the potential advantages of lower mortality, fewer complications, shorter hospital stays, and consequent cost reductions. If these advantages, some of which have already been observed,[18,23] are further documented, TPEGs will certainly replace a substantial proportion of current standard vascular grafts. We estimate the extent of this proportion to range from 30% to 70% of the standard prosthetic grafts currently used to treat aneurysmal, traumatic, and occlusive arterial lesions. Since prosthetic grafts are used in approximately 60% of major arterial operations, TPEG procedures could replace 18% to 42% of all major vascular operations. If this figure is added to the 25% of major vascular operations that will be replaced by other endovascular techniques, it means that 43% to 67% of major vascular operations could be performed by an endovascular technique. In addition, many of the remaining operations, such as vein bypasses and graft and native artery thromboembolectomy, will be greatly facilitated by endovascular fluoroscopically guided adjuncts such as PTA of residual inflow and outflow lesions and guidewire-assisted passage of balloon thromboembolectomy catheters.

The potential impact of these possibilities on the practice of vascular surgery is substantial and has caused a great deal of concern among vascular surgeons. Clearly the effective use of all these endovascular techniques, although they sometimes require vascular surgical skills, always require catheter-guidewire imaging skills, which some vascular surgeons do not possess. How will these surgeons cope with endovascular techniques that may provide better treatment options than the standard open operations used in more than half of their patients? How can they avoid becoming obsolete and being replaced by other interventional specialists? Several possible courses of action exist for vascular surgeons.

One approach already taken by some is to adopt an attitude of skepticism and denial—that is, "no interventional endovascular technique has been any good and none will be." This "ostrich" approach is dangerous and erroneous. It will result in vascular surgeons being largely excluded from a leadership role in the use of endovascular devices that are likely to work increasingly well in the coming years as technology improves and experience is gained. This ostrich approach should be avoided by vascular surgeons. So too should the "wait and see" approach, which will allow other interventional specialists in the fields of radiology and cardiology to gain control of a technology that may be required to treat a majority of patients with vascular lesions that warrant intervention. These other interventional specialists sincerely believe that their catheter-guidewire imaging skills make them better qualified to use TPEGs and other endovascular techniques than do our vascular surgical skills and knowledge of vascular disease.

A third very acceptable approach, which provides vascular surgical and interventional skills, is to have patients with vascular disease cared for by a team comprised of collaborating vascular surgeons and interventional radiologists or cardiologists. Such teams, largely under the leadership of vascular surgeons, have been responsible for most of the successful TPEG developmental efforts to date. Indeed, since vascular surgeons usually supervise the care of most vascular disease patients at present, most current collaborative multispecialty groups dealing with these patients are led by vascular surgeons. However, we should be concerned about the stated goal of other interventional specialists, which is to change current practice and assume the major responsibility for all care of patients with vascular disease.[26-30] Of course interventional specialists with such significant patient care responsibilities should be mandated to have all the knowledge and judgment currently used by most vascular surgeons in the care of their patients. This is not presently the case since many nonsurgical vascular interventional specialists are largely trained in and oriented toward treating lesions and not patients.

A fourth and possibly the best approach for dealing with emerging endovascular technology such as TPEGs is for vascular surgeons to become sufficiently competent in catheter-guidewire-imaging-stent techniques so that they can perform these procedures independently. This creates a number of subsidiary problems for many vascular surgeons. Obtaining appropriate training in these basic endovascular techniques is a fundamental requirement. Fortunately the number of vascular surgeons who possess these skills is sufficient to make such training available with appropriate organization and an effective administrative structure. Alternatively, many of us have mutually beneficial relationships with colleagues in other specialties so that we could receive adequate training enabling us to perform endovascular procedures as part of a healthy collaboration. This does not imply that vascular surgeons should become interventional radiologists or attempt to replace them. It simply means that as vascular surgeons develop improved endovascular techniques for managing vascular lesions, they must also develop sufficient proficiency with catheter-guidewire-imaging-stent methods so that they will be able to safely and effectively use TPEGs and other endovascular methods that may replace standard arterial repairs and bypasses.

Another important area of concern is how two previously distinct specialties can be integrated into one entity when a new technique is introduced that overlaps both. Some of the newer endovascular techniques, and particularly TPEGs, are cases in point. Both vascular surgeons and interventional radiologists have justification for believing that they should control these new developments. As a result conflicts can arise. This has already occurred and many believe serious turf battles are inevitable. However, these will be costly and will result in casualties at both the physician level and, more important, at the patient level. These battles must be avoided. How to do so remains the challenge.

First, it must be appreciated that both vascular surgeons and interventional radiologists fear they will be displaced by the other group, and these fears are legitimate. If vascular surgeons develop catheter-guidewire skills, some interventional radiologists are afraid they will become expendable. On the other hand, if interventional radiologists can insert TPEGs independently and if these grafts work, a major portion of vascular surgery will be eliminated and some vascular surgeons fear they will be displaced. The crucial step in avoiding turf battles is for both groups to eliminate the fear factor and reassure one another by word and deed that mutual destruction is not a goal. Interventional radiologists must be reassured that vascular surgeons do not intend to take over diagnostic angiography, balloon angioplasty, and the many other interventional techniques within their domain. Vascular surgeons must be assured that they will be able to perform newer endovascular procedures including TPEG insertions as these begin to replace open vascular surgical procedures.

However, this will not be enough. The two specialties must become confederated at the highest levels and be willing to represent each other's interests. This will require creation of a combined executive committee of the Society for Vascular Surgery/International Society for Cardiovascular Surgery and the Society for Cardiovascular and Interventional Radiology. This new committee will have to deal with such difficult issues as defining acceptable practice guidelines across the specialties, training each other's members and trainees, and limiting the numbers of trainees so that excessive numbers of specialists are not produced in both fields.

The long-term goal of this collaborative leadership function would be to produce adequate numbers of optimally trained specialists so that our nation's needs for treating vascular disease could be appropriately met. This could work best if vascular surgeons and interventional radiologists of the future worked in combined services or departments of vascular disease treatment. This radical solution will not be implemented easily or quickly, and resistance will be encountered from a number of quarters. However, this solution is proper because it will not only provide optimal patient care and treatment but will reduce costs as well. It will do so by avoiding the splintering of care, financially motivated procedures, and choice of procedure based on an individual physician's training or skills or what resources he controls. Combined services will also facilitate more rapid evaluation of different treatments. And they will prevent painful, costly turf battles—the worst possible impact the introduction of improved endovascular technology such as TPEGs could have on the practice of vascular surgery.

REFERENCES

1. Johnston KW, Rae M, Hogg-Johnston SA, et al. Five-year results of a prospective study of percutaneous transluminal angioplasty. Ann Surg 206:403-413, 1987.
2. Veith FJ, Gupta SK, Samson RH, et al. Progress in limb salvage by reconstructive arterial surgery combined with new or improved adjunctive procedures. Ann Surg 194:386, 1981.
3. Brewster DC, Cambria RP, Darling RC, et al. Long-term results of combined iliac balloon angioplasty and distal surgical revascularization. Ann Surg 210:324-333, 1989.
4. Veith FJ, Gupta SK, Wengerter KR, et al. Changing arteriosclerotic disease patterns and management strategies in lower-limb-threatening ischemia. Ann Surg 212:402-414, 1990.
5. Veith FJ, Gupta SK, Wengerter KR, Rivers SP, Bakal CW. Impact of nonoperative therapy on the clinical management of peripheral arterial disease. Circulation 83(Suppl 1):1-137–1-142, 1991.
6. La Berge JM, Ring EJ, Gordon RL, et al. Creation of transjugular intrahepatic portosystemic shunts with the Wallstent intravascular prosthesis: Results of 100 patients. Radiology 187:413-420, 1993.
7. Palmaz JC, Laborde JC, Rivera FJ, Encarnacion LE, Lutz JD, Moss JG. Stenting of the iliac arteries with the

Palmaz stent: Experience from a multicenter trial. Cardiovasc Intervent Radiol 15:291-297, 1992.
8. Dotter CT. Transluminally-placed coilspring endarterial tube grafts. Long-term patency in canine popliteal artery. Invest Radiol 4:329-332, 1969.
9. Balko A, Piaseck GS, Shah DM, Carney WI, Hopkins RW, Jackson BT. Transfemoral placement of intraluminal polyurethane prosthesis for abdominal aortic aneurysm. J Surg Res 40:305-309, 1986.
10. Mirich D, Wright KC, Wallace S, et al. Percutaneously placed endovascular grafts for aortic aneurysms: Feasibility study. Radiology 170:1033-1037, 1989.
11. Laborde JC, Parodi JC, Clem MF, et al. Intraluminal bypass of abdominal aortic aneurysm: Feasibility study. Radiology 184:185-190, 1992.
12. Chuter TAM, Green RM, Ouriel K, Fiore W, DeWeese JA. Transfemoral endovascular aortic graft placement. J Vasc Surg 18:185-197, 1993.
13. Volodos NL, Shekhanin VE, Karpovich IP, Troyan VI, Guriev YA. Self-fixing synthetic prosthesis for endoprosthetics of the vessels. Vestn Khir 137:123-125, 1986.
14. Parodi JC, Palmaz JC, Barone HD. Transfemoral intraluminal graft implantation for abdominal aortic aneurysms. Ann Vasc Surg 5:491-499, 1991.
15. Parodi JC. Endovascular repair of abdominal aortic aneurysms. Adv Vasc Surg 1:85-106, 1993.
16. Marin ML, Veith FJ, Panetta TF, et al. Transfemoral endoluminal stented graft repair of popliteal artery aneurysm. J Vasc Surg 19:754-757, 1994.
17. Marin ML, Veith FJ, Panetta TF, et al. Transfemoral stented graft treatment of occlusive arterial disease for limb salvage: A preliminary report [abst]. Circulation 88(Suppl):1-11, 1993.
18. Marin ML, Veith FJ, Panetta TF, et al. Transluminally placed endovascular stented graft repair for arterial trauma. J Vasc Surg 168:156-161, 1994.
19. Marin ML, Veith FJ, Cynamon J, et al. Transfemoral endovascular stented graft treatment of aortoiliac and femoropopliteal occlusive disease for limb salvage. Am J Surg 20:466-473, 1994.
20. Marin ML, Veith FJ. Endoluminal stented graft aortobifemoral reconstruction. In Greenhalgh RM, ed. Vascular and Endovascular Surgical Techniques, An Atlas, 3rd ed. Philadelphia: WB Saunders, 1994, pp 100-104.
21. Cragg AH, Dake MD. Percutaneous femoropopliteal graft placement. Radiology 187:643-648, 1993.
22. May J, White GH, Waugh R, Yu W, Harris JP. Transluminal placement of a prosthetic graft-stent device for treatment of subclavian aneurysm. J Vasc Surg 18:1056-1059, 1993.
23. Moore WS, Vescara CL. Repair of abdominal aortic aneurysm by transfemoral endovascular graft placement. Ann Surg 220:331-341, 1994.
24. May J, White G, Waugh R, Yu W, Harris J. Treatment of complex abdominal aortic aneurysms by a combination of endoluminal and extraluminal aortofemoral grafts. J Vasc Surg 19:924-933, 1994.
25. Dake MD, Miller DC, Semba CP, Mitchell RS, Walker PJ, Liddell RP. Transluminal placement of endovascular stent-grafts for the treatment of descending thoracic aortic aneurysms. N Engl J Med 331:1729-1734, 1994.
26. Kinnison ML, White RI, Auster M, et al. Inpatient admissions for interventional radiology: Philosophy of patient management. Radiology 154:349-351, 1985.
27. DeMaria AN. Peripheral vascular disease and the cardiovascular specialist. J Am Coll Cardiol 12:869-870, 1988.
28. Katzen BT, van Breda A. Developing an interventional radiology practice. Semin Intervent Radiol 5:99-102, 1988.
29. Kerlan RK, Marone T, Ring EJ. The clinical role of the interventional radiologist. Semin Intervent Radiol 5:103-104, 1988.
30. Cook JP, Dzau VJ. The time has come for vascular medicine. Ann Intern Med 112:138-139, 1990.

2

The Vascular Surgeon as an Endoluminal Interventionist: Why Is It Important and How Can It Be Achieved?

FRANK J. CRIADO, M.D., LUIS A. QUERAL, M.D., and PEGGY PATTEN, R.N.

Despite opinions (nonsurgical) to the contrary, surgeons have played a significant role in the development of the catheters used in vascular technology. dos Santos et al.[1] and Fogarty et al.[2] among others have contributed much to the conception and evolution of transluminal vascular diagnostic and therapeutic methodology. That notwithstanding, it was the contributions of Dotter and Judkins[3] and Gruentzig and Hopff[4] that did the most to usher in the era of endovascular therapy. Percutaneous angioplasty gradually emerged as an important treatment modality, with the potential to compete with established conventional vascular approaches. However, surgeons relinquished control of this evolving subspecialty because of two catastrophic miscalculations: (1) the abandonment of angiography as a diagnostic technique and (2) the almost universal rejection of balloon angioplasty as a valid therapeutic modality for occlusive vascular disease. As a result, we are now desperately trying to "catch up" with nonsurgical vascular specialists—radiologists in particular—who are the "natural leaders" in this exciting new field of endovascular therapy. The situation is not hopeless, however, as vascular surgeons remain the only physicians with the basic training and clinical skills necessary to qualify as "complete vascular specialists"; these basic requirements include evaluation, treatment, management of complications, and follow-up care of all peripheral vascular disorders. In addition—and appropriately so—vascular patients are referred to the surgeon who is responsible for overall clinical management.

Some of us may wistfully reflect upon a time, not that long ago, when things were much simpler—that is, the radiologist performed and interpreted diagnostic studies and the surgeon then treated the patient. However, this is no longer the case. Radiologists, and to a lesser extent cardiologists, perform most diagnostic angiographic studies; they uncover vascular lesions, which they may then be able to treat almost immediately. They rationalize that since the wire may already be across the lesion, it is simple enough to insert a balloon catheter, dilate the atheroma, and be done with it! And in fact, this may at times constitute the optimal course of action, especially when dealing with a tight focal iliac stenosis. In general, however, it is our opinion that such a modus operandi presents two serious dilemmas: (1) why shouldn't the surgeon be the one to perform the therapeutic procedure when it was he or she who referred the patient to the radiologist in the first place, and (2) is the best time to treat such a lesion really after the patient has been sedated and is not in a position to discuss the various options? Such a scenario, however, is unlikely in our present practice because the initial patient evaluation, which includes duplex surveillance of the lower extremity arteries, identifies in most instances the presence of significant focal lesions, especially in the iliac arteries.[5] Diagnostic angiography is prescribed in such a way that the most diseased side, if possible, is avoided during the catheterization, and the therapeutic decision is preferably made after appropriate discussion with the patient following angiography. Recognizing that at times it may be more cost-effective to undertake the therapeutic intervention during diagnostic angiography, we would surmise that diagnosis and therapy should optimally constitute two separate procedures.

THE SURGEON AS AN ENDOVASCULAR INTERVENTIONIST: WHY IS IT IMPORTANT?

In the United States approximately 200,000 peripheral angioplasties were performed in 1993. Furthermore, and despite opinions to the contrary,[6] the field of minimally invasive endovascular therapy will continue to grow and

evolve. It is inevitable that many vascular conditions and procedures, traditionally within the realm of conventional vascular surgery, will in the future become the focus of catheter-based methodology. A partial list of these would likely include the following:
  Arterial occlusion
  Venous obstruction
  Aneurysms
  Aortic dissections
  Arteriovenous fistulas
  Traumatic lesions
  Clot management
  Portosystemic shunts
  Inferior vena cava interruption
  Superior vena cava syndrome

Some of those who are unalterably opposed to this technology claim that it is ineffective, gimmicky, industry driven, and/or financially motivated. This opposition, however, will be overcome by the inexorable tide of reality. A few of us "endovascular surgeons" have accepted and practiced this subspecialty of catheter intervention for several years now and recognize the advantages of incorporating these skills into the various protocols used in the treatment of vascular disease. However, most present-day vascular surgeons find themselves in the intermediate position of becoming more receptive, perhaps performing an occasional angioplasty, but not knowing how to proceed further.

HOW DOES ONE BECOME AN ENDOVASCULAR SURGEON?

A satisfactory response to this complex question requires brief consideration of three important areas: endovascular training/credentialing, basic catheterization/interventional skills, and the catheterization laboratory setup.

The issues surrounding the incorporation of endovascular skills into vascular surgical training are foremost in the minds of all of us today. The "ultimate" solution will only be attainable through the inclusion of catheterization techniques into vascular fellowship programs, as is already beginning to occur.[7,8] Realistically, however, such evolution is still many years—perhaps even one or two generations—away. The more pressing question today relates to the trained/practicing vascular surgeon: How does he or she acquire the catheterization skills necessary to initiate an endovascular practice, and what minimum requirements should be met for credentialing purposes before hospital clinical privi-

Table 1 Endovascular credentialing recommendations

Society	Angioplasties	Angiograms
SVS/ISCVS	10-15	50
SCVIR	25	200
ACC	50	100
AHA	50	100
SCAI	50	100

SVS/ISCVS = Society for Vascular Surgery/International Society for Cardiovascular Surgery; SCVIR = Society of Cardiovascular and Interventional Radiology; ACC = American College of Cardiology; AHA = American Heart Association; SCAI = Society for Cardiac Angiography and Interventions.

leges are granted for the practice of endovascular surgery? Most of the major cardiovascular societies in the United States have published position papers and recommendations regarding minimum requirements for credentialing in percutaneous endovascular therapy[9-15] (Table 1). Not unexpectedly these standards vary widely. How do these serve the experienced, specialty-trained vascular surgeon? The authors' perspective, which stems from 7 years' experience performing well over 1000 endoluminal procedures as part of a busy private vascular surgery practice, differs from the published guidelines in the following ways: (1) it is unnecessary for experienced vascular surgeons to embark on a full 1-year endovascular fellowship; (2) the requirement of 50 to 200 diagnostic angiograms is completely unrealistic and, more important, of no practical value to the surgeon who wishes to perform endoluminal therapeutic procedures[15]; and (3) the minimum number of peripheral angioplasties recommended varies from 10 (SVS/ISCVS) to 50 (cardiology societies), and a number somewhere in between is more likely to be closer to the true requirement. Whether the surgeon is a "participant" or the "primary operator" is not critical as long as the experience is certified by a bonafide endovascular specialist who serves as the trainee's preceptor. Knowledge of thrombolysis alone is sufficient for initial credentialing and these qualifying experiences, when achieved, should entitle the applying vascular surgeon to be granted provisional endovascular privileges for 1 year during which time his endovascular cases will be reviewed with respect to indications, technical proficiency, and outcome. We would also recommend direct supervision/proctoring of the applicant's first 5 to 10 endoluminal cases, especially those performed percutaneously; such supervision should be carried out by a recognized endovascular expert, preferably with the same specialty background (i.e., vascular surgeon).

One "minor" aspect remains—that is, where can the surgeon attain such exposure and hands-on training? Indeed, very few opportunities exist. Our own experience with a tutorial hands-on training program in the recent past demonstrated the considerable interest and need that exist among surgeons in the United States and abroad. It is clear then that the establishment of surgical endovascular training centers should be among the highest priorities in this regard. Later on, as discussed previously, endovascular skills will surely be gradually incorporated into fellowship programs as major university centers and the directors of these programs will come to view current developments in endovascular techniques as critical to the practice of vascular surgery and to the future of our specialty.

Basic Catheter/Interventional Skills[16]

These skills can best be described by individually considering the various technical steps that must be followed in sequence when performing a given endovascular intervention. These steps include access, navigation, treatment, and imaging.

Access. Access to the vascular lumen can be achieved both percutaneously and by a surgical cutdown approach. The basic techniques are illustrated in Figs. 1 to 4. The surgeon aspiring to become a fully qualified endovascular interventionist should understand that proficiency with percutaneous access techniques is absolutely paramount. The decision as to whether a given procedure should be performed percutaneously or via an open approach should be based on the patient's needs and the type of lesion at hand, but not on the training and experience of the interventionist. It is not acceptable to simply state that "a small femoral cutdown adds very

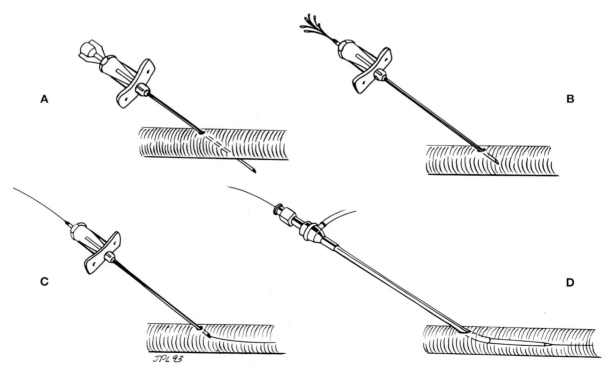

Fig. 1 Arterial needle puncture using the Potts-Cournand needle. Transfixing a needle puncture (**A**) is preferred in most instances, the exception being in cases where thrombolysis is anticipated or when performing open needle puncture of the artery. As the needle is withdrawn (**B**), the lumen is entered and a steerable, soft-tipped guidewire (**C**) is introduced into the arterial lumen and advanced antegrade or retrograde under direct fluoroscopic visualization. The introducer sheath (**D**) is then inserted, tracking over the guidewire and into the arterial lumen.

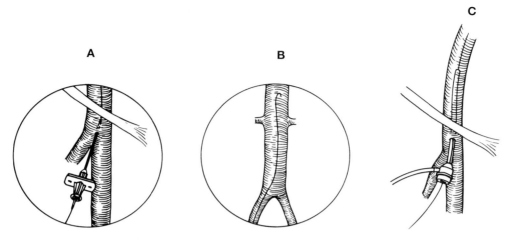

Fig. 2 Retrograde percutaneous puncture of the common femoral artery (**A**) with insertion of a guidewire into the abdominal aorta (**B**) and insertion of an introducer sheath (**C**). Note the infrainguinal course of the needle.

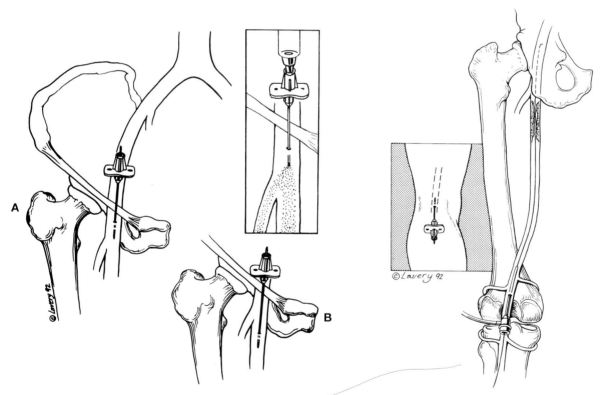

Fig. 3 Antegrade femoral puncture is performed preferentially in the common femoral artery (**A**), but occasionally it is necessary to directly puncture the upper superficial femoral artery (**B**). Inset: Test injection of dye is recommended to delineate the anatomy of the femoral bifurcation before proceeding with insertion of the guidewire.

Fig. 4 Percutaneous retrograde puncture of the popliteal artery. First, a small anterior common femoral sheath is inserted in retrograde fashion. Then the patient is turned over into the prone position. As dye is injected proximally, the popliteal artery is punctured under direct fluoroscopic visualization (inset), and this is followed by insertion of the introducer sheath in the usual fashion. It is customary to remove the popliteal sheath immediately on completion of the procedure and avoid systemic heparinization when this access technique is used.

little if any morbidity" to justify one's lack of percutaneous skills. In our experience more than 90% of transluminal interventions are performed percutaneously. Nevertheless, it should also be made clear that an open surgical approach is a suitable alternative in a number of relatively uncommon situations. The surgical cutdown, when done solely for the purpose of direct needle puncture of the vessel, is limited to minimal exposure of the anterior surface of the artery (Fig. 5). At other times the indication for a surgical approach rests with the need to introduce a large device requiring formal arteriotomy or perform a combined endoluminal/reconstructive procedure (Fig. 6). In either case a longer incision and wider exposure are necessary.

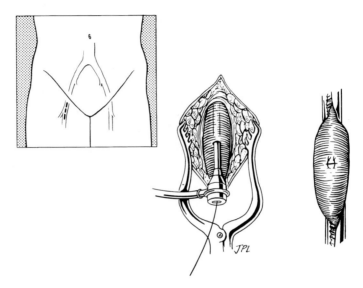

Fig. 5 Limited femoral cutdown and exposure for direct needle puncture of the common femoral artery.

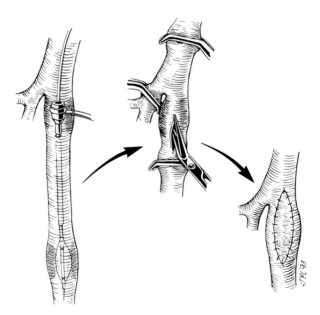

Fig. 6 When a combined endovascular and reconstructive procedure is contemplated, more extensive circumferential exposure of the femoral vessels is necessary.

Wire Introduction, Transluminal Navigation, and Lesion Crossing. Next to percutaneous puncture, wire manipulation and transluminal navigation are among the most difficult skills to learn and master. A certain finesse and "feel" are necessary and can only be achieved through proper initial training and sufficient ongoing endovascular experience. Good-quality fluoroscopy and angiography and a competent radiologic technologist with good understanding of the basics of the procedure will go a long way toward maximizing the surgeon's skills. A few important principles are described and illustrated in Figs. 7 to 9.

Treatment of the Target Lesion. This of course constitutes the very reason for the inter-

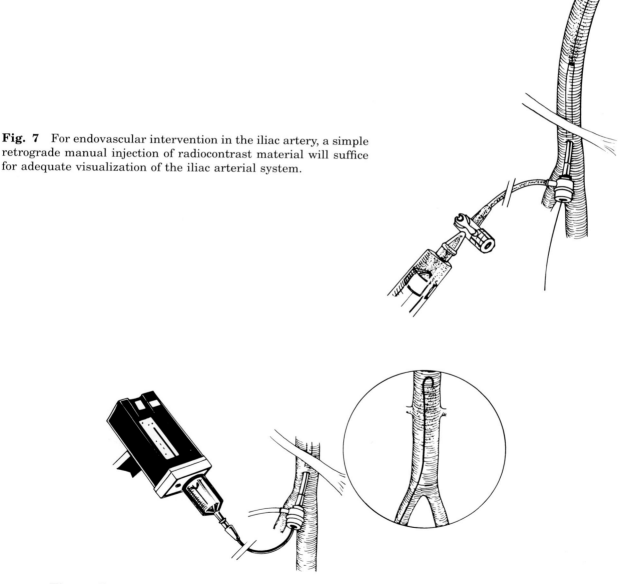

Fig. 7 For endovascular intervention in the iliac artery, a simple retrograde manual injection of radiocontrast material will suffice for adequate visualization of the iliac arterial system.

Fig. 8 For more complete angiographic delineation, or during procedures involving the abdominal aorta and its bifurcation, a technique consisting of introduction of a pigtail angiographic catheter with antegrade intra-aortic injections using a power injector is preferred.

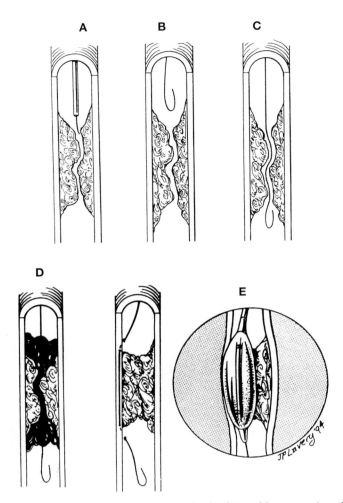

Fig. 9 Crossing the lesion with a guidewire can be facilitated by centering the wire with the aid of a small angiographic catheter (**A**). The "J maneuver" is often very helpful in wire crossing of difficult stenotic lesions (**B** and **C**). Short total occlusions can often be crossed in much the same way (**D**). One technical option is the creation of a subintimal plane of dissection to reach the more normal lumen beyond the lesion (**E**). Subintimal recanalization and angioplasty (inset) are generally but not universally viewed as undesirable by most interventionists.

vention. The possibilities are numerous. In most recanalization procedures, balloon angioplasty and stenting represent the best endoluminal procedures in the various vascular segments. Recent advances in catheter technology have been instrumental in improving the versatility of these devices while simultaneously lowering the incidence of complications that are predominantly access related. The following are examples of these improvements: (1) very low-profile catheters, which allow most angioplasties to be performed through an introducer sheath 6 Fr, or smaller; (2) hydrophilic coatings, which almost guarantee the passage of the catheter "anywhere" a wire has been placed; (3) the Terumo Glidewire (Terumo Medical Corp., Somerset, N.J.), which permits crossing of most lesions, even those that are totally occluded, with tremendous ease; (4) improved flexibility; and (5) better balloon materials, which offer a range of options in terms of trackability, inflation pressures, and resistance to puncture by atheromas and metallic stents. A few examples serve to illustrate important points in endoluminal therapy (Figs. 10 to 14). The following guiding principles can be elucidated: (1) transluminal

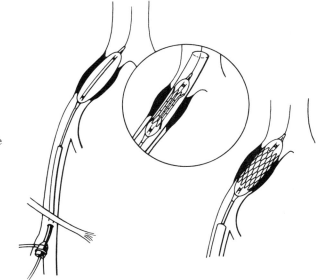

Fig. 10 Sequence of Palmaz stent deployment in the common iliac artery.

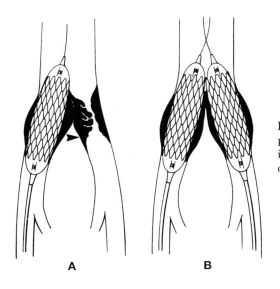

Fig. 11 A, Angioplasty and stenting on one side only may precipitate obstruction on the contralateral side. **B,** The "Kissing" technique can be helpful in cases of bilateral common iliac ostial lesions.

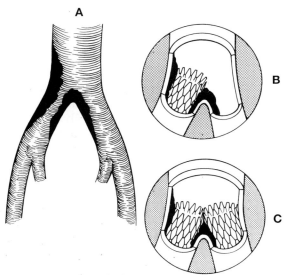

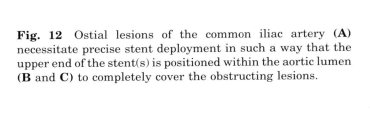

Fig. 12 Ostial lesions of the common iliac artery (**A**) necessitate precise stent deployment in such a way that the upper end of the stent(s) is positioned within the aortic lumen (**B** and **C**) to completely cover the obstructing lesions.

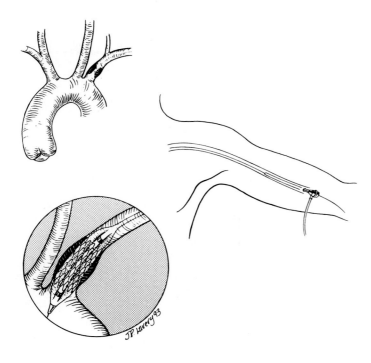

Fig. 13 Angioplasty and stenting of proximal subclavian artery lesions is performed via a retrograde transluminal approach.

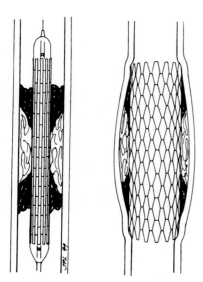

Fig. 14 Primary stenting is becoming the method of choice for recanalization of short total occlusions in iliac and femoropopliteal segments.

maneuvers and therapy should be limited to the minimum necessary to achieve the pre-established treatment goals; (2) one should resist the temptation to correct every defect/lesion visualized on angiography; (3) the guidewire placed across the lesion should not be removed until the end of the intervention; (4) transle-sional pressure measurements constitute the best guide as to the success and completeness of the procedure; and (5) balloon/stent lengths should be chosen so as to completely encompass the lesion. The latter is especially critical when treating ostial lesions, which are often extensions of disease in the main artery (see Fig. 12).

Imaging: Fluoroscopy and Angiography.[17] Performing endovascular interventions without adequate imaging is like performing conventional surgery with blurred vision—that is, it just does not work! "Fluoroscopic image-hand coordination" is one of the most difficult and important aspects of the endovascular learning experience. Exposure to practices in the angiography suite and/or catheterization laboratory can be very helpful to the surgeon in this regard. Ultimately, however, it is the surgeon's responsibility to ascertain that he or she will have the necessary imaging facilities in the operating room or wherever the endovascular therapeutic procedure is to take place. These considerations bring us to the final chapter of our scenario regarding the making of the endovascular surgeon.

The Catheterization Laboratory

From the hospital/institutional perspective, catheterization is perhaps the most frequently encountered limitation to the establishment of an endovascular surgery service. Although it is true that excellent vascular imaging capabilities currently exist in most hospitals in the United States, vascular surgeons are likely to find significant impediments to using the angiography suite as a workshop for endoluminal therapy for the following reasons: (1) the facility is controlled by the department of radiology; (2) sterility standards leave much to be desired; (3) it is extremely difficult to work with personnel who are completely unfamiliar with the surgeon's routines and idiosyncrasies; and (4) it is difficult and even risky to perform combined endoluminal/surgical procedures because of unsuitability of the table and the environment. Finally, endovascular grafting procedures, a definite future reality in the field of vascular surgery,[18] will require the type of sterility and readiness to operate that only the operating room can provide. We anticipated these difficulties early on (in 1988) and decided to convert one of our operating rooms into a catheterization laboratory of sorts. Utilization, improved procedural capabilities, optimization of conventional vascular operations, and future perspectives are all factors that have more than amply justified the initial expenditure of approximately $600,000. It is our firm belief that vascular surgery groups and institutions with a sufficient caseload should strive for this setup—the best of all solutions to the imaging dilemma—the creation of an endovascular surgical suite (Fig. 15), where surgeons can perform all of the following conventional and endoluminal techniques with a maximum of precision and efficacy:

- Endovascular surgery
- Prereconstruction angiography
- Completion angiography
    - Distal bypass
    - Carotid endarterectomy
    - Visceral/renal reconstruction
- Inferior vena caval filter placement
- Vascular catheterization
    - Dialysis access
    - Venous access
    - Intra-aortic balloon pump

Of course, in addition to high-quality fluoroscopy/angioscopy, other guidance and endodiagnostic technologies such as angioscopy and intravascular ultrasound may have to be incorporated. Intravascular ultrasound in particular promises to assume a critical role in future advances in endovascular interventions.[19]

In conclusion, there should be no questioning

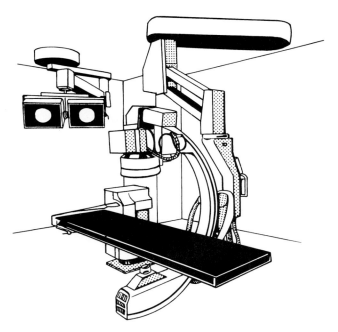

Fig. 15 Example of an endovascular suite, which is considered the ideal setup for all conventional reconstructive and endovascular procedures.

the fact that endoluminal techniques are critically important to the vascular surgeon who can indeed learn the necessary catheterization skills. Of no less importance, however, is the undeniable reality that becoming an endovascular surgeon at present may involve a somewhat unclear and tortuous pathway. Hence it is incumbent upon all practicing vascular surgeons and academic leaders to bring these issues to the forefront and rapidly set the stage to ensure the surgeon's leadership in this exciting field of endoluminal therapy.

REFERENCES
1. dos Santos R, Lamas A, Pereira CJ. L'arteriographie des membres de l'aorte et ses branches abdominales. Bull Soc Natl Chir 55:587-601, 1929.
2. Fogarty TJ, Cranley JJ, Krause RJ, et al. A method for extraction of arterial emboli and thrombi. Surg Gynecol Obstet 116:241-245, 1963.
3. Dotter CT, Judkins MP. Transluminal treatment of arteriosclerotic obstruction: Description of a new technique and a preliminary report of its application. Circulation 30:654, 1964.
4. Gruentzig A, Hopff H. Perkutane Rekanalixation Chronischer Arterieller: Verschlusse Miteinem Nellen Dilatation-Katheter Modification de Dotterchinik. Dtsch Med Wochenscher 9:2502, 1974.
5. Kohler TR, Nance DR, Cramer MM, et al. Duplex scanning for diagnosis of aorto-iliac and femoropopliteal

disease: A prospective study. Circulation 76:1074-1080, 1987.
6. Dalman RL, Taylor LM, Porter JM. Current status of extracoronary endovascular procedures. Perspect Vasc Surg 3:1-24, 1990.
7. Hodgson KJ, Mattos MA, Sumner DS. Canine or chameleon: The vascular surgeon's role in percutaneous endovascular therapy. Vasc Forum 1:237-247, 1993.
8. Fogarty TF. Personal communication, 1994.
9. Society of Cardiovascular and Interventional Radiology. Credentials criteria for peripheral, renal, and visceral percutaneous transluminal angioplasty. Radiology 167:452, 1988.
10. Ad Hoc Committee on Endovascular Surgery Credentialing and Training for Vascular Surgeons, Society for Vascular Surgery/International Society for Cardiovascular Surgery, North American Chapter. Endovascular surgeon credentialing and training for vascular surgeons. J Vasc Surg 17:1095-1102, 1993.
11. Van Breda A, Becker GJ. Endovascular credentialing. JVIR 5:90-92, 1994.
12. Special Writing Group of AMA Scientific Councils of Cardiovascular Radiology, Cardiothoracic and Vascular Surgery, and Clinical Cardiology. Training standards for physicians performing peripheral angioplasty and other percutaneous peripheral vascular interventions. Circulation 86:1348-1350, 1992.
13. Interventional Cardiology Committee, Subcommittee on Peripheral Interventions. Guidelines for performance of peripheral percutaneous transluminal angioplasty. Cathet Cardiovasc Diagn 2:128-129, 1990.
14. American College of Cardiology Peripheral Vascular Disease Committee. Recommendations for peripheral transluminal angioplasty: Training and facilities. J Am Coll Cardiol 21:546-548, 1993.
15. Diethrich EB. Endovascular surgery credentials [letter]. J Vasc Surg 18:1073-1074, 1993.
16. Criado FJ, Queral LA, Patten P. Transluminal recanalization, angioplasty and stenting in endovascular surgery: Techniques and applications. In Greenhalgh RM, ed. Vascular and Endovascular Surgical Techniques. Philadelphia: WB Saunders, 1994, pp 49-70.
17. Criado FJ, Queral LA, Patten P. Fluoroscopy and angiography of the aortoiliac segment in the operating room. In Greenhalgh RM, ed. Vascular Imaging For Surgeons. Philadelphia: WB Saunders, 1995, pp 213-225.
18. Parodi JC, Palmaz JC, Barone HD. Transfemoral intraluminal graft implantation for abdominal aortic aneurysms. Ann Vasc Surg 5:491-499, 1991.
19. Cavaye DM, White RA. Intravascular Ultrasound Imaging. New York: Raven Press, 1993.

3

Relationships Between Vascular Surgery and Interventional Radiology: How Should Turf Wars Be Resolved?

JOHN D. CORSON, M.B., Ch.B., F.R.C.S. (Engl.), WILLIAM J. SHARP, M.D., JAMAL J. HOBALLAH, M.D., and TIMOTHY F. KRESOWIK, M.D.

Our radiologist colleagues and other cardiovascular interventional specialists are presently challenging the previously uncontested position of vascular surgeons as experts in the pre- and postoperative care, diagnosis, and treatment of patients with peripheral vascular disease.[1-9] Radiologists are expressing concern that surgeons now wish to perform many endovascular procedures which, interestingly, they seem to perceive as their sole prerogative. In comparison to surgeons, interventional radiologists are relative novices in the treatment of patients with vascular disease. Interventional radiology, an evolving subspecialty of radiology, flourished with the development of percutaneous techniques that changed and expanded the potential role of the radiologist from one of pure diagnostician to that of therapist. Many of these new percutaneous techniques were applicable to general surgical, urologic, transplant, and vascular patients. The willingness of many surgeons to refer their patients to radiologists when percutaneous therapy was an option opened the door for the expansion of interventional radiology. Some radiologists would now have everyone believe that only they are capable of applying peripheral vascular percutaneous catheter-based technology![10] This is a widely held misconception and nothing could be further from the truth. These techniques are not specific to interventional radiologists but are appropriate for use by other specialists as well.

The establishment of the *Journal of Endovascular Surgery* as the official journal of the International Society of Endovascular Surgery in 1994 has helped to legitimize the concept of endovascular surgery. In addition, the importance of the subject to surgeons was further underlined by the fact that the *European Journal of Vascular Surgery*, the official journal of the European Society for Vascular Surgery, was recently renamed the *European Journal of Vascular and Endovascular Surgery*. Several recent articles have addressed the potential conflicts occasioned by the expansion of interventional radiology and the increasing interest of vascular surgeons in endovascular techniques.[1-4,10,11] In this chapter we seek solutions to these conflicts and analyze the basis for the current concern of vascular surgeons over retaining control of their specialty.

HISTORY

What began as surgical treatment of hemostasis and limb amputation centuries ago has now matured into a well-organized and important surgical specialty.[12] In the modern surgical era, techniques for vascular repair have been refined. The treatment of choice for vascular injuries of the extremities evolved from immediate amputation as practiced during World War I to pioneering revascularization procedures for limb salvage during the Korean conflict.[13] These improved and refined vascular surgical techniques have since been successfully applied to the civilian population not only for management of blunt and penetrating trauma but also for treatment of acute and chronic ischemia of the extremities and aneurysmal and cerebrovascular disease. The field of vascular surgery continues to undergo further expansion and change. The development of transluminally placed endovascular stented grafts is one example of this rapid change.[11] Many lessons have been learned, new technologies utilized, and still more innovative treatment methods continue to evolve. The time frame from research concept to state-of-the-art procedure is alarmingly short.

Vascular surgery is a specialty replete with well-trained clinical and academic surgeons entrusted with the responsibility for quality and progress in patient care, education, and research in the field of vascular disease.

ENDOVASCULAR PROCEDURES

It should be apparent to any observer that catheter-based technology is a cornerstone of many modern advances in medicine. In reality, catheter technology is not new. The use and development of catheter technology has not been limited to the field of radiology. Many other specialties utilize catheter-based technology and have done so for years. One example is cardiology where coronary angiography and balloon angioplasty are routine procedures. Interestingly, these procedures were initially developed in departments of radiology. New devices such as stents, atherectomy catheters, and lasers are also being used by cardiologists. Urologic surgeons perform both percutaneous and open, catheter-based, diagnostic, and therapeutic procedures. Gastrointestinal surgeons and gastroenterologists also use lasers and perform balloon dilatation in the management of their patients. Cardiovascular surgeons place intra-aortic balloon pumps percutaneously and frequently use guidewire technology for placement of pacemakers and monitoring devices in their patients. Similarly, vascular surgeons have the opportunity to perform many endovascular surgical procedures either percutaneously or with an open technique as an adjunct to conventional vascular surgical procedures. The use of percutaneous catheter technology is nothing new to vascular surgeons or other clinicians involved in the care of critically ill patients with significant multiorgan system disease. For years surgeons have placed percutaneous peripheral arterial catheters in small arteries such as the radial or larger arteries such as the femoral. In addition, they frequently place percutaneous transvenous catheters for hemodynamic monitoring, parenteral nutrition, and other applications. Surgeons are experienced in percutaneous approaches to the internal jugular, subclavian, and femoral veins for intravenous access for fluid resuscitation, monitoring, temporary dialysis access, and vena caval filter placement. The appropriate use of guidewires and dilators is second nature to those involved in these procedures. Surgeons have one unmistakable advantage when performing endovascular surgical procedures. They have seen and directly handled these vessels and have intimate knowledge of the associated anatomy and pathology. They have made those subtle connections and correlations between what is "seen" on an arteriogram or venogram and what actually exists inside the vessel. Additionally surgeons are very familiar with fluoroscopy, which is used in association with these guidewire techniques. The use of these skills is merely an extension of their experience with fluoroscopy for intraoperative cholangiography and angiography and other similar procedures acquired during their surgical training. One must also remember that there is still a cohort of senior surgeons in practice who were used to performing all of their own diagnostic angiographic studies prior to the development of a special procedures section in the department of radiology. Although most surgeons have relinquished control of diagnostic angiographic studies, there remain a number of surgeons who still perform their own diagnostic angiographic studies.

As experienced vascular surgeons, we have a responsibility to ensure proper use of new vascular technology. We are excited about the rapid rate of development of new vascular techniques but as a group we mostly remain cautious about their application and are concerned about their widespread and often indiscriminate use, especially by those individuals who have no other alternative therapy to offer.[14-19] Unfortunately, quality control is not always determined by those most qualified to see that it is enforced. Through the news media and advertising, along with the push of industry, medical "cutting edge" technology is frequently overmarketed. Some of this influence may well be reflected in the rising cost of health care. Vascular surgeons should be closely involved in all issues relating to cost containment in their specialty because they are the ones with a true appreciation of the real cost of new technology.

As vascular surgeons we continue to seek safe, cost-effective, efficient, and durable treatment for our patients. We have many therapeutic options. These must be individualized to any given patient. Whether it is a problem best suited for a percutaneous or open endovascular procedure or a traditional revascularization procedure should be of no consequence to the modern "state-of-the-art" vascular surgeon. The best option must be chosen for each patient. For interventional radiologists, when the only option is a percutaneous approach, this option may be inappropriately utilized.

CREDENTIALING

Subspecialization within medicine has caused self-interest groups to attempt to restrict and limit the practice of others. This is clearly reflected by the current situation that exists between radiologists and surgeons. Who should perform endovascular procedures?[15-17] Should only radiologists use percutaneous techniques? Criteria for the performance of many new and evolving vascular endovascular procedures have not been universally established. Vascular surgeons, radiologists, and cardiologists all favor their own criteria.[20-25] In addition, individual institutions, practitioners, and various ruling bodies or committees have suggested separate criteria. Credentialing criteria are usually specialty or institutionally dependent and tend under most circumstances to be rather self-serving. Clearly, standards need to be set for all interested parties that should not be designed to be restrictive or prohibitive to those persons who treat vascular disease who are specifically interested in using these new techniques. It seems that the optimal approach should be to allow trained physicians to do what they are capable of doing, provided the results achieved are consistent with those of other colleagues performing these procedures. Credentialing criteria may vary depending on individual experience and training. Hence the requirements for surgeons and radiologists may differ. The Association of Vascular Program Directors has determined that endovascular procedures should be a component of vascular fellowship training. The implementation of this concept at those institutions with vascular surgery training programs should allow vascular fellowship–trained individuals to be appropriately credentialed in the future for the independent performance of endovascular procedures. It remains to be determined how much time a trainee needs to devote to this endeavor. The paranoia of some interventional radiologists may limit appropriate exposure of the vascular surgical trainees to endovascular training. Interventional radiologists are concerned that the graduating endovascular trained vascular fellow will put them out of business. The reality, however, is that surgeons will obtain endovascular training either with or without the assistance of interventional radiology. Surely it is better for radiologists to take the high road in this matter and provide optimal training to maintain the type of relationship with surgeons that will maintain and expand their specialty?

ADMITTING PRIVILEGES

Another area of prime contention has been the granting of admitting privileges to interventional radiologists.[6-9,11,26] It has always been the conviction of most surgeons that this idea is not in the best interests of the patient. The concept of primary access radiologists has been proposed as a reasonable alternative to the current clinical referral system.[27] To justify the granting of admitting privileges for radiologists, they surely would first need to receive adequate clinical training in patient care. An interventional radiologist with admitting privileges could theoretically perform angioplasty, thrombolysis, atherectomy, or other procedures with no vascular surgical consultation or backup. This is a dangerous concept. It puts the patient at risk if complications occur and it favors the decline of painstakingly acquired clinical judgment. This clinical judgment is not achieved through declaration!

Vascular patients frequently have significant multiorgan system disease, particularly with regard to the cardiovascular system. Because of this complexity, patients with vascular disease often require significant clinical care and prolonged hospitalization regardless of the treatment modality employed. The quality of care would surely be compromised by allowing the patient to be managed primarily by a person who has been trained "in a field that exists only as a hodgepodge of catheter-related techniques."[28] The responsibility for patient care should be in the hands of those physicians who have established *clinical* expertise. Many interventional radiologists feel that what they need is equality in the management of patients. One must remember that the current training modes for surgery and radiology residents are completely different. In the training of a peripheral vascular surgeon the emphasis is on patient management and surgical technique. Surgeons are responsible for managing all aspects of severely ill patients including the subtleties of intensive care. Radiology residents by and large are not exposed to similar, often stressful clinical situations. Hence we believe they would not be the appropriate physicians to manage first hand complex and emergency clinical problems.

THE FUTURE

It is possible but unlikely that future modifications in training may place interventional radiology trainees on a par with residents in medicine or surgery programs. If this happens, interventional radiologists could equip themselves with clinical skills similar to those possessed by present-day vascular surgeons, thus allowing them to have more say in patient management.[27,29] This clinical exposure would certainly require several additional years of training. We believe it would be premature to claim that we are at that stage of development for current interventional radiology training programs.

Vascular surgeons should all be skilled and knowledgeable in endovascular surgical techniques and remain clinically active in this new field. Directors of vascular surgical residency programs should bear the responsibility for providing endovascular training for vascular residents in their programs. Vascular surgeons do not wish to abolish interventional radiology as a subspecialty. It is also not our intention to perform routine diagnostic angiographic studies except under exceptional circumstances. Diagnostic studies may best be performed by radiologists who are dedicated to the performance of these tests and have the time to carry out these studies. There will be many complex therapeutic and diagnostic procedures that will require consultation with an interventional radiologist before treatment of vascular, urology, transplantation and gastrointestinal patients is initiated. This work will maintain the viability of the field of interventional radiology. As surgeons we will always provide surgical support to patients for the management of interventional radiologic complications but in return we will always need prior involvement in any therapeutic decision. This arrangement should avoid problems with future patient management when complications arise. Interventional radiologists must work in a supportive fashion with established clinical services. Interventional radiologists should ideally function as cooperative consultants working on an endovascular team rather than as independent, competitive practitioners. This approach will provide an improved level of care for our patients and guarantee the survival and growth of interventional radiology as a specialty! A pitched battle between the two specialties can only be harmful to the institution, to the individual departments, and ultimately to the patient. Radiology would have much to lose.

No one group has exclusive rights to evolving medical technology and new innovations. Attempts to prevent a group of skilled physicians such as vascular surgeons from utilizing percutaneous or open endovascular techniques is clearly inappropriate. Nonetheless, they continue to arise, most frequently as credentialing or imaging equipment access issues.

We suggest developing an institutional "vascular center" within the framework of current clinical programs. At The University of Iowa we have had a very positive experience with a "digestive disease center." This is run jointly by members of the gastrointestinal surgical and medical sections. All patients with vascular problems could be followed in one central clinic and appropriate specialty consultations made as needed. Clinicians in other disciplines who wish to follow their patients with vascular disease would also be able to do so through this clinic. This unified multidisciplinary approach would limit the numerous frustrating clinic visits that are traditionally required of many vascular patients. Therapeutic areas for endovascular therapy should be jointly available to a team of surgeons and radiologists. More complex procedures would require the use of sophisticated imaging equipment in an operating room environment. A "one-stop shopping" approach has a marked appeal for the patient. This approach may also be the most efficient with regard to utilization of time and resources and may allow institutions to more successfully compete for health care contracts for these types of patients. This concept is adaptable to both university centers and private practice situations.

Endovascular surgery is an important growing area of vascular surgery and will evolve further in the future. The continued involvement of vascular surgeons in the endovascular field is critical and leadership positions must be maintained. Training programs should continue to incorporate more catheter-based training and ensure that this area is not neglected. The best option for limiting conflict and turf wars between surgery and radiology departments is to more closely integrate interventional radiologists into surgical services and to apply a team approach to patient care. This plan should provide a win-win solution for surgeons and radiologists as well as for vascular patients.

REFERENCES

1. Wexler L, Ginsburg R, Mitchell RS, Mehigan JT. The vascular war of 1988. JAMA 261:418-419, 1988.
2. Hollier LH. Presidential address: Influence of nonsurgical intervention on vascular surgical practice. J Vasc Surg 9:627-629, 1989.
3. Rutherford RB. Endovascular surgery: The new challenge. J Vasc Surg 10:208-210, 1989.
4. Zarins C. The vascular war of 1988: The enemy is met. JAMA 261:416-417, 1989.
5. Demaria AZ. Peripheral vascular disease and the cardiovascular specialist. J Am Coll Cardiol 12:869-870, 1988.
6. Kinnison ML, White RI, Auster M, et al. Inpatient admission for interventional radiology: Philosophy of patient management. Radiology 154:349-351, 1985.
7. Katzen BT, Van Breda A. Developing an interventional radiology practice. Semin Intervent Radiol 5:99-102, 1988.
8. Kerlan RK, Marone T, Ring EJ. The clinical role of the interventional radiologist. Semin Intervent Radiol 5:103-104, 1988.
9. Katzen BT, Kaplan JO, Dake MD. Developing an interventional radiology practice in a community hospital: The interventional radiologist as an equal partner in patient care. Radiology 170:955-958, 1989.
10. Smith TP, Cragg AH, Berbaum KS. Political trends in vascular and interventional radiology: A randomized survey. Radiology 170:941-944, 1989.
11. Veith F. Presidential address: Transluminally placed endovascular stented grafts and their impact on vascular surgery. J Vasc Surg 20:855-860, 1994.
12. Friedman DG, ed. A History of Vascular Surgery. New York: Futura Publishing, 1989.
13. Rich NM. Military surgery: "Bullets and blood vessels." Surg Clin North Am 58:995-1003, 1978.
14. Moosdorf R. Endovascular surgery—the state of the art. Cardiovasc Surg 2:319-323, 1994.
15. Capdevilla JM. Endovascular surgery: Who should perform it? Cardiovasc Surg 2:327-328, 1994.
16. D'Addato M. The future of vascular surgery. Cardiovasc Surg 2:329-330, 1994.
17. Bell PRF. Endovascular versus conventional surgery: Competitive or complementary methods? Cardiovasc Surg 2:324-326, 1994.
18. Bernstein EF, Dilley RB, Thomas WS, et al. Changing practice patterns in peripheral arterial disease. Ann Vasc Surg 8:186-194, 1994.
19. Hodgson KJ, Mattos MA, Sumner DS. Canine or chameleon? The vascular surgeon's role in percutaneous endovascular surgery. Vasc Forum 1:237-247, 1993.
20. Waltman AL, Katzen BT, Ring EJ, et al. Society of Cardiovascular and Interventional Radiology: Credential criteria for peripheral, renal and visceral percutaneous transluminal angioplasty. Radiology 167:452, 1988.
21. String ST, Brener BJ, Ehrenfeld WK, et al. Interventional procedures for the treatment of vascular disease: Recommendations regarding quality assurance, development, credentialing criteria, and education. J Vasc Surg 9:736-739, 1989.
22. Society for Cardiac Angiography and Interventions: Credentials for percutaneous transluminal peripheral angioplasty. Cathet Cardiovasc Diagn 21:128-129, 1990.
23. American Society of Cardiovascular Interventions: Credentials for percutaneous transluminal peripheral interventions. J Intervent Cardiol 3:181-182, 1990.
24. Levin DC, Becker GJ, Dorros G, et al. Training standards for physicians performing peripheral angioplasty and other percutaneous peripheral vascular interventions. Circulation 86:1348-1350, 1992.
25. White RA, Fogarty TJ, Baker WH, et al. Endovascular surgery credentialing and training for vascular surgeons. J Vasc Surg 17:1095-1102, 1993.
26. White RI, Denny DF, Osterman FA, et al. Logistics of a university interventional practice. Radiology 170:951-954, 1989.
27. Meaney TF. The decline of diagnostic radiology: Call to action. Radiology 172:889-892, 1989.
28. Cragg AH. The future of interventional radiology [letter]. AJR 148:1273-1274, 1987.
29. Levin DC. Role of the department chairman in the future of interventional radiology. Radiology 170:947-949, 1989.

4

Intraoperative Iliac Balloon Angioplasty and Stenting in Combination With Infrainguinal Bypass: Indications, Techniques, and Results

STANLEY O. SNYDER, Jr., M.D., RICHARD J. DeMASI, M.D., JOCK R. WHEELER, M.D.,
ROGER T. GREGORY, M.D., ROBERT G. GAYLE, M.D., and F. NOEL PARENT III, M.D.

Patients with symptoms of lower extremity ischemia often have multilevel hemodynamically significant arterial occlusive lesions requiring both suprainguinal inflow and infrainguinal outflow procedures. Correction of both lesions may be required to achieve limb salvage or maintain infrainguinal bypass graft patency, but a combined direct operative abdominal and lower extremity approach may have unacceptably high resultant morbidity and mortality. Transluminal angioplasty (TA) has been established as an effective alternative to conventional bypass procedures in patients with limited iliac disease.[1] Numerous reports in the vascular literature have confirmed the utility and durability of this approach combined with infrainguinal procedures.[2-6]

Vascular stents have become an important adjunct to TA for improving suboptimal angiographic or hemodynamic results.[7] Limitations of balloon angioplasty that can be alleviated by intraluminal stent placement include prevention of both elastic recoil and arterial wall dissection. Asymmetric cracked plaques can be pressed against the arterial wall to provide a larger more cylindrical lumen that will decrease subsequent thrombus formation (Fig. 1).[8] Standard indications for stent placement include the following:

- Residual stenosis >30%
- Residual trans-stenotic pressure gradient (>5 mm after TA)
- Dissection visualized after TA
- TA performed for restenosis
- Initial TA of completely occluded lesions

The excellent clinical results achieved with the use of stents, by Palmaz et al.[7] and others,[9,10] raised the issue of the possible superiority of routine stent placement following iliac TA procedures. Initial 5-year results of a randomized

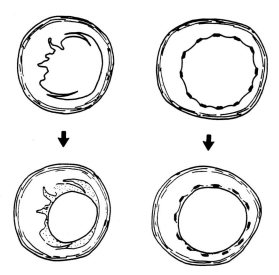

Fig. 1 Schematic representation of post–balloon angioplasty surface irregularities leading to early thrombus deposition and late myointimal replacement (left). Stent placement provides a smooth cylindrical lumen by compressing irregularities eccentrically. This favors nonturbulent flow, less thrombus deposition, and ultimately, a larger lumen (right). (From Palmaz JC. Intervascular stenting: From basic research to clinical application. Cardiovasc Intervent Radiol 15:279-284, 1992.)

multicenter trial of iliac artery stenting vs. percutaneous transluminal angioplasty (PTA) alone indicated both higher initial technical success rates and obliteration of lesion gradients as well as improved long-term angiographic patency and clinical success (Table 1).[11] The mean restenosis rate in the first 185 patients was lower in the stent group, and at 36 months only 2% of the stent group required therapeutic

Table 1 Prospective randomized trial of PTA alone vs. PTA combined with stent placement

	PTA alone	PTA + stent
Technical success	113/124 (91%)	121/123 (98%)
Gradient	29.5 → 6.7	29.4 → 1.4
5 yr patency	64.6%	93.6%
Clinical success	69.7%	92.7%

Data from Richter et al. Abstract presented at the 1992 European meeting of the Society of Cardiovascular Interventional Radiologists.

Table 2 Patient demographics and atherosclerotic risk factors

Male : Female → 10 : 4
Age (range) 65.5 ± 10.7 years (47 to 79 years)
Tobacco use 81%
Cardiac disease 45%
Hypertension 45%
Diabetes 36%
Carotid disease 27%
Renal disease 9%
Pulmonary disease 9%
Hyperlipidemia 9%

reintervention compared to 28% of the PTA-only group.

Follow-up data from various radiologic reports provide a second list of "potential" stent indications that includes the following:

- External iliac lesions (which have a high incidence of elastic recoil and subsequent restenosis)
- Ostial lesions at aortic bifurcations (which are difficult to dilate and often require bilateral stent techniques)
- Eccentric stenoses (recoil problems)
- Emboli-producing lesions (irregular plaque and subsequent blue toe syndrome)

Based on reports in the literature[7,11,12] and a 12-year personal experience with percutaneous and intraoperative TA, we thought that TA results could be enhanced with stent utilization, thus providing an improved and perhaps more durable inflow for distal bypass procedures. The purpose of this report is to review our preliminary experience with synchronous intraoperative TA and stent placement combined with distal revascularization procedures.

NORFOLK EXPERIENCE
Patients and Methods

During the interval from April 1992 through May 1994, 29 patients underwent 32 stent procedures. Of these, 14 patients underwent 16 procedures combining iliac balloon angioplasty and stent placement with a simultaneous distal revascularization. The patient population included 10 men and four women (average age 65½ years) with the standard atherosclerotic risk factors (Table 2).

The indications for surgery included limb salvage in 12 patients, disabling claudication in three patients, and an absent femoral pulse in one patient prior to an elective orthopedic surgical procedure. Eighteen lesions were treated with intraoperative balloon angioplasty and stent placement. A stent was required in the common iliac artery in seven cases and in the external iliac artery in 11, with two patients having tandem lesions requiring stent placement at both sites. All lesions were hemodynamically significant stenoses, but in no case was treatment of complete occlusion attempted. Early in this series, stents were placed only after inadequate results of common iliac angioplasty or in the case of focal external iliac lesions. However, as iliac stent placement became more universally accepted, we expanded the scope of iliac lesions suitable for dilatation, as demonstrated by the two patients with tandem lesions and dilatation of two lesions of sufficient length to require two adjacent stents to traverse the entire lesion. Fig. 2, *A* demonstrates tandem hemodynamically significant lesions in the common and external iliac arteries with both sites shown to be widely patent on a 10-month follow-up angiogram (Fig. 2, *B*).

The synchronous 16 distal revascularization procedures included eight femoropopliteal and six femorotibial bypasses. There was one common femoral endarterectomy proximal to a patent femoropopliteal graft and one stent was placed in conjunction with a thrombectomy of a femoropopliteal bypass.

Technique

Patients were preoperatively positioned on the operating table to enable fluoroscopic visualization from the distal aorta throughout the arterial tree of the lower extremities. Spinal anesthesia was employed and an arterial line was placed for continuous upper extremity pressure monitoring. The femoral vessels were exposed through groin incisions and controlled

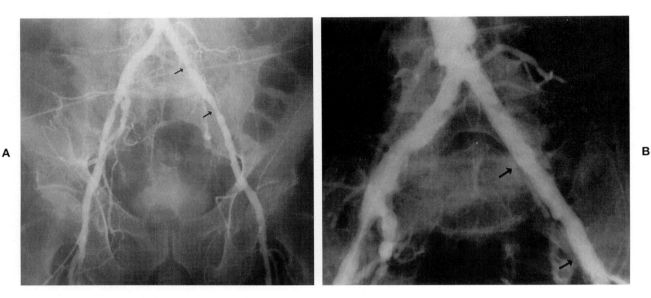

Fig. 2 A, Tandem common and external iliac artery stenosis. Arrows indicate stenotic sites before **(A)** and after **(B)** transluminal angioplasty and stent placement. **B,** Patent stented angioplasty sites at 10 months' follow-up.

with vessel loops and appropriate exposure of the distal anastomotic site; in addition, saphenous vein conduit was prepared as necessary. A 16-gauge angiocatheter was used for direct puncture of the common femoral artery at the site where the proximal anastomosis for the distal bypass procedure would be performed. A 0.35-gauge Glidewire (Medi-Tech/Boston Scientific Corp., Watertown, Mass.) was then passed under fluoroscopic control into the vessel and through the stenotic lesion, if possible. A 7 Fr introducer was inserted over the Glidewire, and the intra-arterial pressure below the lesion was measured and compared with the arm pressure (in some instances the aortic pressure above the lesion was used for comparison). If less than a 10 mm gradient was noted, the patient was given 60 mg of papaverine intra-arterially through the side port of the introducer to simulate the vasodilatory effect of exercise and the pressure gradient was again measured. Half-strength radiographic contrast material was then injected into the iliac artery with road-mapping techniques used to capture the image and facilitate subsequent passage of the guidewire if required. Intravenous heparin, 100 mg/kg, was administered once guidewire passage across the lesion was achieved. (Clamping the distal common femoral artery during contrast injection allows better visualization of the distal aorta and iliac system with smaller volumes of contrast material.)

Vessels were measured preoperatively to ascertain arterial diameters, and balloon dilatation was usually performed immediately before stent placement. Palmaz stents (Johnson & Johnson Interventional Systems Co., Warren, N.J.), 30 mm in length, preloaded onto either 6 or 8 mm ultrathin Meditech balloons with a 5 Fr catheter base were used in most cases. Road mapping enabled precise balloon and stent placement, and operative angiograms and intra-arterial poststent iliac pressure measurements were obtained. The introducer sheath was then removed and the femoral vessels were cross clamped for placement of the distal bypass graft using standard lower extremity reconstruction techniques. Postoperative anticoagulation consisted only of 5 grains of aspirin daily unless poor runoff distal to the lower extremity reconstruction procedure warranted intravenous heparin therapy.

Results

Initial stent placement was technically successful in all patients. The ankle/brachial index was raised from a preoperative mean of 0.43 to 0.91 postoperatively. The trans-stenotic systolic pressure gradient was diminished from 28.2 preoperatively to 3.0 postoperatively. Complications included one death resulting from a postoperative myocardial infarction that occurred on postoperative day 10. There have been two femoropopliteal graft occlusions, one related to a midvein graft stenosis that was repaired at thrombectomy and remained patent at 20 months. The second graft occlusion was in a patient with claudication and did not require further revascularization as the stent angioplasty site in the iliac artery remained patent and alleviated the claudication symptoms. A third patient demonstrated noninvasive evidence of a hemodynamically failing femoroperoneal graft at 5 months and underwent revision of the still-patent, less than 2 mm diameter graft, by replacing a 5-inch segment with contralateral saphenous vein. One groin lymphocele required reexploration for persistent drainage and one minor wound infection occurred but was managed successfully with antibiotic therapy.

During follow-up intervals ranging from 4 to 24 months, with a mean of 14.4 months, all stents remained patent as shown by physical examination and femoral Doppler waveform analysis. All patients with threatened limbs have had sustained clinical benefits with no limb loss. All three patients with claudication remained asymptomatic on follow-up despite femoropopliteal occlusion in one who, as mentioned previously, has maintained a patent stented iliac angioplasty site.

DISCUSSION

There are advantages and disadvantages to either the staged-procedure technique (i.e., PTA and stent placement as a separate preliminary procedure in the angioplasty suite) vs. synchronous intraoperative TA/stent placement combined with distal bypass. Advantages of the staged procedure include optimal imaging equipment available in the angioplasty suite and a time interval to allow evaluation of the adequacy of the PTA stent inflow procedure prior to the distal bypass. Disadvantages include either two visits to the angioplasty suite vs. the potential for too great a contrast load with a combined diagnostic and therapeutic angiographic procedure and the need for the presence of a vascular surgeon to evaluate the films and make appropriate clinical recommendations.[13] In addition, there is a definite complication rate associated with the percutaneous approach for stent placement. In a 1988 report on PTA, Brewster et al.[2] advocated a staged approach in 79 patients but encountered five major complications requiring an emergency operation, and three additional groin hematomas could also have been averted with intraoperative stent placement. The Canadian study of Johnston et al.[1] reported a 9.5% complication rate with percutaneous balloon angioplasty, and Palmaz et al.[7] demonstrated excellent clinical success in 587 procedures with a 9.9% complication rate. Many of these complications were procedure related and could have been averted with a femoral cutdown stent placement approach.

Advantages of intraoperative stent placement include the fact that the procedure-related complications associated with percutaneous stent placement can be avoided or dealt with immediately. Complete revascularization can be accomplished in a single procedure, thus avoiding delays and possibly shortening the hospital stay, thereby conserving hospital resources. In addition, it increases the treatment options and improves the decision-making processes available to the vascular surgeon at the time of definitive reconstruction.[13]

Intraoperative stent placement may play an increasingly significant role in vascular reconstruction in the future. Endoluminal procedures for aortic aneurysm repair, bypass of aortoiliac or femoropopliteal occlusive disease, and repair of traumatic lesions are already undergoing clinical trials and applications. Stents are routinely used for many renal, aortic, venous, and various other sites throughout the vascular tree.

The issue of training and credentialing of vascular surgeons for the various intraoperative endovascular techniques has been previously addressed by the vascular societies,[14] and it is important that vascular surgeons continue to play a leadership role in evaluating and developing new technology. Various subspecialty organizations have suggested criteria for interventional credentialing,[15] and it is imperative that appropriate training for endovascular procedures be incorporated into vascular surgery training programs. Not everyone agrees with this policy and in a recent debate in the British literature, Beard and Gaines[16] stated that "not surprisingly these recommendations have caused considerable disquiet."

CONCLUSION

Intraoperative stent placement is effective in abolishing hemodynamically significant lesions of the iliac artery and should be considered in lesions treated to provide inflow for distal reconstruction. In addition, stent placement can be safely and effectively combined with synchronous distal revascularization procedures in the operating room.

REFERENCES

1. Johnston KW, Rae M, Hogg-Johnston SA, et al. Five-year results of a prospective study of percutaneous transluminal angioplasty. Ann Surg 206:403-413, 1987.
2. Brewster DC, Cambria RP, Darling RC, et al. Long-term results of combined iliac balloon angioplasty and distal surgical revascularization. Ann Surg 210:324-331, 1989.
3. Alpert JR, Ring EJ, Freiman DB, et al. Balloon dilation of iliac stenosis with distal arterial surgery. Arch Surg 118:1289-1292, 1983.
4. Lowman BG, Queral LA, Holbrook WA, et al. Transluminal angioplasty during vascular reconstructive procedures. Arch Surg 116:829-832, 1981.
5. Corey CJ, Bush HL, Widrich WC, Nabseth DC. Combined operative angiodilation and arterial reconstruction for limb salvage. Arch Surg 118:1289-1292, 1983.
6. Peterkin GA, Belkin M, Cantelmo NL, et al. Combined transluminal angioplasty and infrainguinal reconstruction in multilevel atherosclerotic disease. Am J Surg 160:277-279, 1990.
7. Palmaz JC, Laborde JC, Rivera FJ, et al. Stenting of the iliac arteries with the Palmaz stent: Experience from a multicenter trial. Cardiovasc Intervent Radiol 15:291-297, 1992.
8. Palmaz JC. Intravascular stenting: From basic research to clinical application. Cardiovasc Intervent Radiol 15:279-284, 1992.
9. Strecker EPK, Hagen B, Liermann D, et al. Iliac and femoropopliteal vascular occlusive disease treated with flexible tantalum stents. Cardiovasc Intervent Radiol 16:158-164, 1993.
10. Wolf YG, Schatz RA, Knowles HJ, et al. Initial experience with the Palmaz stent for aortoiliac stenoses. Ann Vasc Surg 7:254-261, 1993.
11. Richter GM, Roeren T, Noeledge G, et al. Prospective randomized trial: Iliac stenting versus PTA [abst]. Angiology 43:268, 1992.
12. Firn D. Fifteenth Congress of the European Society of Cardiology. Clinica 569:16-17, 1993.
13. DeMasi RJ, Snyder SO, Wheeler JR, et al. Intraoperative iliac artery stents: Combination with infra-inguinal revascularization procedures. Am Surg 60:854-859, 1994.
14. String ST, Brener BJ, Ehrenfeld WK, et al. Interventional procedures for the treatment of vascular disease: Recommendations regarding quality assurance, development, credentialing criteria, and education. J Vasc Surg 9:736-739, 1989.
15. White RA, Fogarty TJ, Baker WH, et al. Endovascular surgery credentialing and training for vascular surgeons. J Vasc Surg 17:1095-1102, 1993.
16. Beard JD, Gaines PA. The future of vascular surgery. Br J Surg 80:185-186, 1993.

5

Clinical Experience With an Integrated Self-Expandable Stent Graft (Corvita) for the Treatment of Various Arterial Lesions

JEAN-PIERRE DEREUME, M.D., JOSÉ FERREIRA, M.D., MEHREZ EL DOUAIHY, M.D.,
JEAN-CHRISTOPHE CAVENAILE, M.D., SOPHIE GUYOT, M.D., SERGE MOTTE, M.D.,
GISÈLE VINCENT, M.D., and JEAN-CLAUDE WAUTRECHT, M.D.

Surgical treatment of various arterial diseases is now a well-established regimen since the introduction of synthetic arterial substitutes in the 1950s.[1] Clinically they are used worldwide with fairly good results. Nevertheless, it is generally recognized that the ideal prosthetic material has not yet been perfected, despite many recent improvements, and thrombogenicity, compliance, porosity, and healing properties remain a challenge for further developmental efforts.

Despite modern vascular surgical techniques and progress in anesthesiology and intensive care, mortality and morbidity are mostly related to associated cardiac and pulmonary diseases and remain a problem even in the most specialized centers.[2]

In addition, weakness of dissected arterial tissue and progression of disease often endanger the function of vital organs and preclude the success of a conventional surgical approach. Furthermore, even in fairly simple cases of arterial disease, a standard surgical approach can become hazardous as a result of multiple previous operations in the same anatomic area, concomitant neoplastic disease, or spontaneous or acquired fistulas in other organs.

To resolve these problems several groups began work on the development of minimally invasive techniques for the treatment of vascular disease whereby intraluminally introduced devices could function as vascular prostheses. In 1983 Krause et al.[3] described a sutureless aortic graft technique that consisted of a modified Dacron prosthesis with polypropylene rings at both ends. The prosthesis can be inserted manually through a longitudinal incision in the diseased vessel and the proximal ring can be attached to proximal healthy tissue with nylon tape. The technique does not require the use of surgical sutures, which is especially advantageous in the case of severely diseased and weakened tissue. Another type of intraoperatively introduced self-healing prosthesis was developed several years ago by Volodos et al.[4] at the Kharkov Research Institute.

All of these techniques had the disadvantage of requiring direct surgical exposure of the vessel near the diseased arterial segment. A more recent technique in which endovascular prostheses were used for treatment of arterial disease was described by Parodi et al.[5] These investigators used a composite endoprosthesis made from one or two balloon-dilatable metallic Palmaz-type stents that were attached to a Dacron prosthesis with surgical sutures. Marin et al.[6] also described the use of a composite endoprosthesis consisting of balloon-dilatable metallic stents with synthetic grafts attached to them. Chuter et al.[7] described an endoprosthesis consisting of barbed, self-expanding stents attached to a woven polyester fabric. A similar type of composite endoprosthesis has been developed (EVT; Endovascular Technologies, Inc., Menlo Park, Calif.), which is presently being implanted clinically in a phase I evaluation study in the United States and Europe. A composite endoluminal graft based on a different type of metallic stent has been developed by Cragg et al.[8] It is comprised of a metallic zigzag-type structure that is self-expandable because of the thermal memory of the alloy (nitinol) and an external Dacron sheath fixed to the metallic structure with surgical sutures (Mintec, Freeport, Grand Bahamas). May et al.,[9] Marin et al.,[10] Cragg and Dake,[11] and others have worked with a composite endoprosthesis made from balloon-expandable (e.g., Palmaz type) stents attached to a polytetrafluoroethylene (PTFE) graft.

Results of studies using an integrated endoprosthesis were recently presented by Piquet et al.[12] This endoprosthesis (Boston Scientific Corp., Watertown, Mass.) consists of a co-knit between a metallic component (tantalum wire) and a textile component (Dacron fibers). Studies in animals have yielded promising results and trials in a series of clinical implants are presently underway in Marseille, France. The integrated endoprosthesis needs to be in place for a few days before clotting in its large pores occurs; its efficacy in reducing the risks associated with aneurysmal enlargements remains to be demonstrated.

Recently developed endoluminal techniques for the treatment of arterial diseases including percutaneous transluminal angioplasty (PTA), atherectomy, laser therapy, and reinforcement of a diseased arterial wall with metallic stents are being widely used. Our experience combined with these techniques and the experience we have gained with the clinical use of a new, compliant, and highly porous peripheral vascular graft (Corvita Corp., Miami, Fla.)[13] led us to the concept of treating various arterial lesions with an integrated, self-expandable endoprosthesis that can be compressed into a small enough profile to permit vascular access from a remote vessel. The design of this endoprosthesis was patented in December 1992.

MATERIALS AND METHODS
The Stent and the Coating Components

In 1992 we first attempted to manufacture an integrated endoprosthesis with a coating made from elastic spun polycarbonate urethane fibers (Corethane, Corvita Corp.) and an iliac balloon-expandable Palmaz stent (Johnson & Johnson Interventional Systems Co., Warren, N.J.). The coating consisted of 300 layers of Corethane fibers spun on a mandrel at a low pitch angle. The endoprosthesis could be balloon expanded to four times the initial diameter with no signs of fiber rupture. This experimental endovascular graft was first tested in an animal model (eight dogs with a surgically created aortocaval fistula). The endovascular grafts were introduced via the transfemoral route and advanced to the aorta where they were successfully balloon dilated to close the fistulas. Complete healing of the endovascular graft with invasion of living tissue and neoendothelialization could be proved after 1 month in all eight dogs.

The limitations of both the length and diameter of the Palmaz stent led us to explore other metallic supports for our endovascular graft: the self-expandable metallic Wallstent (Schneider Europe AG, Bülach, Switzerland) and the thermal memory nitinol stent (Angiomed AG, Karlsruhe, Germany) were both tested for their coating qualities using Corethane fibers. The two devices were coated with 100 layers of Corethane fibers with a spinning (pitch) angle that was adjusted individually to the metallic structure of each stent in its relaxed state. Animal experiments with coated Wallstents demonstrated perfect healing and reendothelialization of the luminal surface of the endovascular grafts.

In these experiments, however, the metallic stents also demonstrated their technical limitations:

1. The Wallstent had an elongation ratio of 2 to 3 between its length in the compressed and the expanded (relaxed) state. The limited radiopacity made accurate endovascular graft placement difficult. Compressed endovascular grafts made from Wallstents sometimes encountered a great deal of friction between the delivery sheath and the Corethane coating (especially when the coating was applied to the outside of the stent). This friction rendered the release of the endovascular graft difficult, being greater with longer endovascular grafts.
2. When a nitinol stent was used as a component of the endovascular graft, the Corethane fibers could be applied evenly and effectively; however, we encountered practical difficulties in bringing the endovascular graft to a low-profile compressed state at the low temperature required. A further limitation of the nitinol stent was the length limitation and the inability to cut it to the desired length in the operating room.

Because of the aforementioned limitations, we decided to manufacture our own metallic support. We chose a stent design that was first described by Didcott[14] for esophageal applications. This stent is made from Elgiloy (Fort Wayne Metals, Fort Wayne, Ind.) or Phynox (Sprint Métal, Paris, France) wires with diameters ranging from 0.10 to 0.23 mm. Twenty-four to 76 wires are braided simultaneously with specially adjusted braiding machines to a double-helix spring structure. The double-helix structure is fixed by crimping the wires (bending the wires at their crossing points with each other) under high pressure, thus preventing the wires from slipping against each other between a compression and relaxation cycle and becoming dislodged (Fig. 1). This geometric fixation of the stent structure is critical for the stent performance; it ensures that the stent returns to its full expanded diameter completely and immediately after being released from its compressed state in the delivery sheath. The spring properties of the metal wire are further enhanced by using a heat treatment process. Afterward, a special surface treatment is applied to ensure a surgical implant grade surface quality with low surface contamination.

To achieve secure placement in the artery without migration and to ensure a blood-tight seal against the native artery, the metallic stent must exert a radial pressure against the vessel wall. This radial pressure is dependent on several of the following physical parameters:

1. The chosen ratio for oversizing the endovascular graft above the vessel diameter (i.e., how much larger the selected endovascular graft is than the diameter of the native host vessel) (usually an oversize ratio of 20% was chosen)
2. The diameter of the wires
3. The number of wires
4. The chosen braiding angle for the stent
5. The type of braiding: 1/1 or 2/2
6. The crimping and heat treatment process

The Corvita Endovascular Graft (CEVG) needs to be securely fixed (anchored) at the predetermined release site. Besides the friction fit created by the radial pressure, an additional mechanism ensures site fixation—that is, the wires at the ends of the CEVG are slightly flared (see Fig. 1). The flare functions as an anchor and can be controlled in the stent manufacturing process by adjusting the wire tension applied during braiding, by the method of crimping, or by artificially creating a mechanical defect.

The coating is made from several hundred layers of polycarbonate urethane fibers (Corethane), each fiber having a diameter of approximately 15 µm. These fiber layers are bonded to the metallic stent structure by means of an adhesive layer consisting of fibers made from a slightly modified polycarbonate urethane polymer. The coating can be fixed to the inner and/or outer wall of the metallic stent, whatever is optimal for the medical application; it can also be

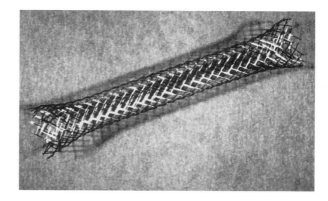

Fig. 1 Didcott stent with outside-flaring wire ends.

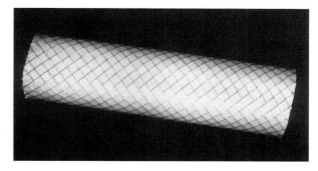

Fig. 2 Corvita Endovascular Graft with an internal coating.

fixed between two metal stents. The number of fiber layers and the location of the coating (inner or outer) can be adapted to the clinical needs (Fig. 2). For example, an "aneurysmal disease CEVG" with 800 fiber layers and an inside coating can withstand high pressures over a long period of time. An endovascular graft with 200 layers and an outside coating is optimal for closing an arteriovenous fistula or an arterial wound.

The fiber spinning angle must be precisely adjusted to the angle of the wire braids to permit a wrinkle-free compression of the CEVG and thus permit the use of a small-profile delivery system. We now use CEVGs with diameters ranging from 5 to 40 mm to correspond to the geometric requirements of various clinical situations. They can be easily cut to the desired length with scissors in the operating room just before they are mounted in the delivery system. The exact required length can be determined either by "on-table" angiography or more precisely with an invasive endoluminal sizing device. The type of coating (inside and/or outside) is available to meet the clinical needs. Special stent configurations have been developed to ensure, for example, a locally extra-high radial expansion force exerted by the endoprosthesis at the level of a short neck of an aneurysm. The design consists of a modified braiding angle, which induces an outright flare of the proximal portion of the CEVG. Flared CEVGs have been implanted successfully in aneurysms with very short necks.

A bifurcation endoprosthesis will soon be available. It consists of an integrated short CEVG with a high-recoil metallic stent on the outside. The inside of the CEVG is coated with a short bifurcated Corvita endoprosthesis with two short legs (3 cm in length). In each of the two legs, a longer externally coated iliac CEVG can be easily inserted transluminally. Once released inside the short bifurcation graft legs, the intimate contact between the two Corethane coatings creates a blood-tight seal along their entire length.

The Delivery System

Ideally the highest ratio between the expanded and compressed diameters of the CEVG is the best. It permits the smallest profile for the delivery system and thus placement of the CEVG via the most remote peripheral access vessels and often percutaneously. In practice, physical restrictions limit the compression ratio. These include the number and diameter of the metal wires used, the coating thickness, and the thickness of the delivery system itself.

Our first experiments were conducted with a simple delivery system comprising an external sheath with a diameter ranging from 7 to 18.5 Fr (depending on the size of the CEVG) with an inside "holding catheter." The task of the holding catheter is to stabilize the distal portion of the CEVG while the external sheath is pulled back during release of the CEVG. The stent is cut to the desired length in the operating room by the physician himself and is manually compressed and introduced over a guidewire into the external sheath. Once the CEVG is fully mounted within the delivery sheath, the distal portion of the sheath is closed with a soft cone-shaped tip (Fig. 3). This separate tip can be retrieved at the end of the procedure by placing a surgical knot near the distal extremity of the guidewire.

This delivery system has recently been modified to permit easier CEVG loading and an easier, better-controlled catheter advancement and CEVG release. It is made of three coaxial catheters; the soft tip is integrated into the distal portion of the internal thin catheter that fits in and precisely closes the external sheath. The intermediate catheter acts as a "holder" and blocks the distal part of the CEVG during release. The distance between the tip and the distal part of the "holder" can be adjusted manually to the length of that individual CEVG. The third catheter is the external sheath that holds the CEVG compressed during the release procedure. The use of an invasive sizing device ("sizer") helps to accurately define the anatomically required length for the CEVG. Furthermore, a retrieval catheter is presently being developed that will permit early retrieval of the CEVG in case of misplacement.

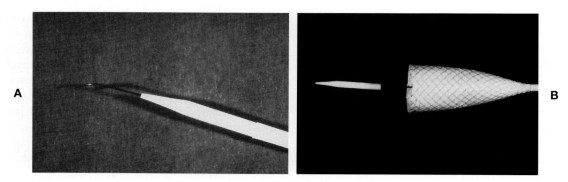

Fig. 3 **A,** The endovascular graft is fully mounted (over a guidewire) within the delivery sheath, which is closed with a soft tip. **B,** The endovascular graft in a partially opened position during the deployment procedure.

Method of Placement

Placement of the CEVG takes place under the following external conditions:

1. The procedure is performed in an operating room in the presence of a team of anesthesiologists who can adapt the type of anesthesia to any difficulties encountered in individual clinical cases.
2. A good-quality C-arm fluoroscope with vascular imaging capabilities (road mapping) must be available.
3. The team consists of a vascular surgeon(s) and an interventional radiologist(s). This team approach was found to be especially useful when difficulties with catheters or interventional techniques arose.
4. Whenever possible, an injection pump should be available to obtain accurate angiograms when controls are needed.

Preoperative requirements include careful evaluation of vital signs (cardiac, pulmonary, renal, and cerebrovascular function) and the precise anatomic location of the diseased vascular segment into which the endoprosthesis will be placed, as determined by angiography, spiral CT scan, reconstruction, and MRI and duplex scans.

The placement method should be as simple as possible. The vascular access site is chosen according to the location where the endoprosthesis is to be placed (i.e., brachial, axillary, carotid, subclavian, or femoral artery). The CEVG can be inserted via a percutaneous access route but the size of the delivery sheath is limited to 12 Fr; with larger sizes the risk of local complications becomes too high. For larger diameters an arteriotomy is preferred. Insertion and advancement of a hydrophylic guidewire into the diseased vessel segment was often easy, but we noticed that frequently this type of guidewire was not stiff enough to permit advancement of the delivery system. In the case of very tortuous vessels we found switching to a different type of guidewire to be helpful, especially a stiff Amplatz guidewire. When technical difficulties were encountered, especially those pertaining to tortuous iliac vessels, gaining access to the more proximal portion of the iliac artery by a retroperitoneal route was helpful. This technique permitted us, with the use of a Dacron side arm, to insert larger diameter delivery catheters with no difficulty.

The accurate placement of the endoprosthesis was controlled with "on-table" angiography. The effectiveness of CEVG treatment was evaluated in the days following the intervention; the effective exclusion of residual leaks in aneurysmal sacs or iatrogenic trauma was determined by repeat angiography. CT scans or MRI provided proof of total exclusion of an aneurysmal sac and gave the precise maximum transverse diameter of the aneurysm. CT scans were repeated every 3 months to ensure that the diameter of the aneurysm was not increasing.

RESULTS

Between February 1993 and September 1994, 23 patients were selected to undergo placement of our integrated CEVG according to the following inclusion criteria:

1. *Compassionate use: Fifteen cases.* In these patients, associated cardiac and/or pulmonary diseases precluded traditional surgical treatment because of a prohibitively high operative risk.
2. *Deliberate choice: Eight cases.* In this group technical difficulties (hostile abdomen, high-flow arteriovenous fistulas, "redo" operations) rendered traditional surgical treatment significantly more risky than the placement of a CEVG.

Technical success (successful deployment of the CEVG at the intended release site) was achieved in 17 patients. Unsuccessful placement (no deployment of CEVG at the intended release site) or failure of the delivery system to gain access to the intended release site was observed in six patients. In four cases we were unable to advance the delivery system because of tortuous iliac vessels. In two cases misplacement during the release procedure was observed. Five patients in that group subsequently underwent successful surgical procedures and one patient is still awaiting placement of a new CEVG.

Seventeen patients (14 men and three women) whose mean age was 60 years were successfully treated with a CEVG: 11 patients for compassionate-use inclusion and six patients for deliberate-choice inclusion. The arterial lesions included four high-flow fistulas, four false aneurysms, five true aneurysms, three ulcerated embolizing stenoses, and one aortourethral fistula (Fig. 4).

Deployment sites for the CEVG included the thoracic aorta in two patients, the abdominal aorta in five, the iliac artery in seven, and the

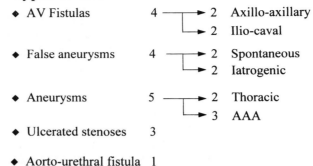

Fig. 4 Types of arterial lesions and technical success achieved in each.

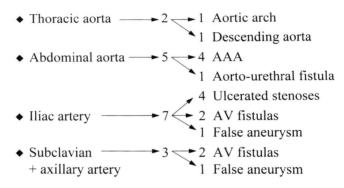

Fig. 5 Sites of endovascular graft placement.

subclavian and axillary arteries in three. The treatment sites are summarized in Fig. 5. Seven insertion procedures were easily performed under local anesthesia and 10 required general anesthesia.

Adequate CEVG placement required additional perioperative balloon angioplasty of the CEVG in four patients. An associated surgical vascular procedure was necessary in three patients: saphenous vein femoropopliteal bypass in one, femorofemoral crossover prosthetic bypass in one, and a temporary iliac Dacron side branch sutured to the external iliac artery for easier insertion of the CEVG in one. One patient died 40 days postoperatively of acute myocardial infarction; autopsy and histologic examination of the explant demonstrated invasion of the CEVG by living tissue and firm attachment of the CEVG to the healthy aortic wall. One patient sustained a thrombosis of the brachial artery at the entry site and remained asymptomatic. In one patient with two iliac CEVGs, acute thrombosis occurred postoperatively in one of the two iliac arteries and required a PTFE femorofemoral crossover graft.

Follow-up ranged from 1 to 20 months with a mean of 8 months. The effectiveness of the CEVG treatment has been evaluated by serial angiography and CT and MRI scans (Figs. 6 and 7). In 13 patients CEVG treatment has proved to be effective.

One abdominal aortic aneurysm that had been treated with a CEVG showed a distal residual leak at follow-up, which will be treated at a later date with balloon angioplasty or placement of a new device. One patient developed leg ischemia as a result of distal embolization from the CEVG and required, 14 months later, an aortofemoral Dacron bypass. In one patient delamination of the external coating was suspected after angiog-

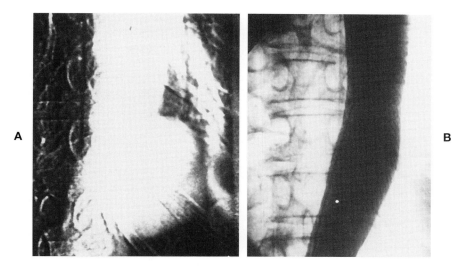

Fig. 6 Thoracic aortic aneurysm "fistulized" into the bronchial tree. Angiography before (**A**) and after (**B**) placement of an endovascular graft.

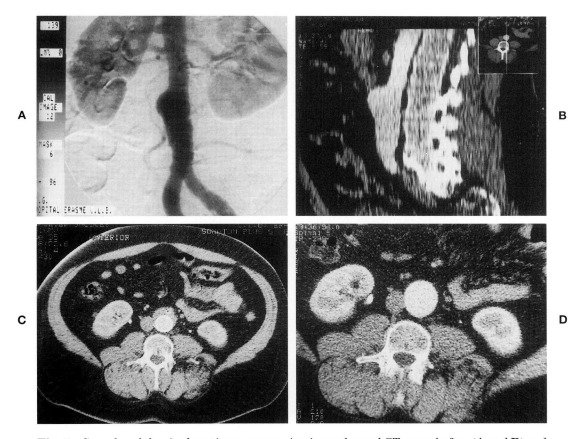

Fig. 7 Saccular abdominal aortic aneurysm. Angiography and CT scans before (**A** and **B**) and CT scans after (**C** and **D**) placement of an endovascular graft.

raphy showed an additional dye-filled hourglass-shaped image outside of the CEVG.

DISCUSSION

Despite the limited number of implants in this series and the relatively short follow-up period, this integrated endovascular graft has already proved its effectiveness in treating life-threatening arterial disease with a minimally invasive method at a comparatively low cost in relation to conventional surgical treatment. The main advantages of the integrated endoprosthesis described herein are:

1. The high compression ratio permits a small-profile delivery system and allows for the treatment of lesions up to the thoracic aorta from a remote entry vessel.
2. The CEVG can be cut to the desired length by the surgeon in the operating room according to measurements made from preoperative or perioperative images or after determining the required anatomic length with an invasive sizing device.
3. CEVGs are available with diameters ranging from 5 to 40 mm and with a coating on the inner and/or outer surface of the metallic support; this permits individual adaptation to each clinical case.
4. The coating is completely invaded by living tissue with good neointima formation and evidence of endothelial cells. This has been proved by the results of a multicenter study with the peripheral vascular graft. The CEVG healing properties have already been confirmed on one autopsy specimen after an implant time of 40 days.
5. With the development of a bifurcation endoprosthesis, the technique can be extended to clinical cases in which the abdominal aneurysm reaches into the iliac vessels. The design consists of a short aortic portion with two short legs that can be fitted with two iliac CEVGs of the desired lengths.
6. The "tubular" type of CEVG has the capability to accommodate large variations in vessel diameter (e.g., aortoiliac location) in one endovascular graft.
7. The fixation of the CEVG in the host arteries has been adequate with no signs of migration during short- and midterm follow-up.
8. An early retrieval technique for fully expanded and released CEVGs from a remote vascular access site is technically feasible and is currently being developed.

Some drawbacks have also been noted during this clinical implant series:

1. The anchoring of the proximal portion of the CEVG remains a challenge, especially when the neck of the aneurysm is less than 3 cm in length. A partial solution to this problem has already been found with reinforcement of the recoil at the proximal end of the CEVG by modifying the braiding angle or using a tapered CEVG. In the future some anchoring hooks or further improvement of the flaring characteristics could solve the problem.
2. The long-term biostability of the CEVG and its long-term clinical functionalism remain to be proved. Our 4-year follow-up of the Corvita peripheral graft has confirmed long-term biostability despite some signs of late biodegradation of the polymer. The long-term structural integrity of the peripheral graft is enhanced by the Dacron mesh. The metallic component of the CEVG should play the same role but this must be proved by future follow-up assessments.

REFERENCES

1. Voorhees AB, Jaretzke AL, Blakemore AH. The use of tubes constructed from Vinyon-N cloth in bridging arterial defects. Ann Surg 136:459, 1952.
2. Gardner RJ, Gardner NL, Tarnay TJ, Warden HE, James ED, Watne AL. The surgical experience and a one to sixteen year follow-up of 277 abdominal aortic aneurysms. Am J Surg 135:226, 1978.
3. Krause AH, Chapman RD, Bigelow JC, Salomon NW, Okles JE, Page US. Early experience with the intraluminal graft prosthesis. Am J Surg 145:619, 1983.
4. Volodos NL, Karpovich IP, Troyan VI, Kalashnikova YV, Shekanin VE, Ternyuk NE, Neoneta AS, Ustinov NI, Yakovenko LF. Clinical experience of the use of self-fixing synthetic prostheses for remote endoprosthetics of the thoracic and the abdominal aorta and iliac arteries through the femoral artery and as an intraoperative endoprosthesis for aortic reconstruction. Vasa Suppl 33P:93, 1991.
5. Parodi JC, Palmaz JC, Barone HD. Transfemoral intraluminal graft implantation for abdominal aortic aneurysms. Ann Vasc Surg 5:491, 1991.
6. Marin ML, Veith FJ, Panetta TF, Cynamon J, Bakal CW, Wengertner KR, Suggs WD, Parodi JC, Barone HD, Schonholtz C. Transfemoral stented graft treatment of occlusive arterial disease for limb salvage. A preliminary report. Circulation 88:I-11, 1993.
7. Chuter TM, Green RM, Ouriel K, Fiore WM, DeWeese JA. Transfemoral endovascular aortic graft placement. J Vasc Surg 18:185, 1993.

8. Cragg AH, Lund G, Rysavy JA, Salomonowitz A, Castaneda-Zuniga WR, Amplatz K. Percutaneous arterial grafting. Radiology 150:45, 1984.
9. May J, White G, Waugh R, Yu W, Harris J. Transluminal placement of a prosthetic graft-stent device for treatment of subclavian artery aneurysm. J Vasc Surg 18:1056, 1993.
10. Marin ML, Veith FJ, Panetta TF, Cynamon J, Barone H, Schonholz C, Parodi JC. Percutaneous transfemoral insertion of a stented graft to repair a traumatic femoral arteriovenous fistula. J Vasc Surg 18:299, 1993.
11. Cragg AH, Dake MD. Percutaneous femoropopliteal graft placement. J Vasc Intervent Radiol 4:455, 1993.
12. Piquet P, Bartoli JM, Rolland PH, Tranier P, Mercier C. Experience in using co-knit stent grafts for aortic and iliac aneurysms. Presented at the Sixth Annual Miami Vascular Institute at Baptist Hospital of Miami International Symposium on Vascular Diagnosis and Intervention. Miami, Fla.: Jan. 12, 1993.
13. Dereume JP, Van Romphey A, Vincent G, Engelmann E. Femoropopliteal bypass with a compliant, composite polyurethane/Dacron graft: Short-term results of a multicenter trial. Cardiovasc Surg 1:499, 1993.
14. Didcott CC. Oesophageal strictures: Treatment by slow continuous dilatation. Ann R Coll Surg 53:112, 1973.

6

Endoluminal Stented Grafts for Treatment of Limb-Threatening Arterial Occlusive Disease

ROSS T. LYON, M.D., MICHAEL L. MARIN, M.D., and FRANK J. VEITH, M.D.

Treatment of advanced lower extremity occlusive disease remains the most common challenging problem faced by vascular surgeons.[1] Lengthy revascularization procedures, performed primarily in elderly patients with multiple comorbid conditions, carry substantial risks.[2,3] In addition, the presence of multilevel occlusive disease, previous arterial revascularization procedures, anastomotic pseudoaneurysms, infection, and poorly accessible surgical sites make traditional operative approaches technically difficult and unappealing to the patient and surgeon alike. Unfortunately, some of the newer less invasive techniques such as percutaneous atherectomy and laser ablation have failed to provide a satisfactory solution and balloon angioplasty alone is only applicable in a small proportion of limb salvage situations.[4,5] Recently the development of endoluminal stent-graft procedures for arterial disease has allowed less invasive techniques to be used for revascularization of long-segment arterial occlusions and appears to simplify the approach and solutions in selected cases of limb-threatening ischemia[6-8] (Figs. 1 and 2).

Recanalization of occluded arteries is an old concept that is the basis of endarterectomy and balloon angioplasty, which are effective treatments for short-segment stenoses or occlusions in large or medium-sized arteries.[9-11] Supplementary use of intravascular stents has improved the results compared to balloon angioplasty alone in patients with iliac artery lesions.[12-14] These procedures, however, are less effective for longer segment stenoses or occlusions, especially of the infrainguinal arteries.[15] Endoluminal stent grafting is an extension of the recanalization concept and uses a combination of intraluminal techniques and therapies including real-time cinefluoroangiography, guidewire directioning, balloon dilatation, intravascular stenting, and arterial bypass grafting. When applied together for the purpose of stent-graft placement, these techniques have enabled treatment of longer occlusions that had previously required more extensive arterial bypass procedures to reestablish vascular continuity.[7,16] They have also been used to salvage previously failed standard arterial bypasses.[17] Coupling stent-graft procedures with conventional arterial bypass has also facilitated the treatment of patients needing simultaneous inflow and outflow revascularization.[18]

CLINICAL APPLICATIONS

Stent-graft procedures have recently been used in a variety of clinical situations including arterial trauma, and for aneurysms of the aorta, iliac, popliteal, and subclavian arteries and for treatment of lower extremity arterial occlusive disease.[6-8,19-23] Stented grafts used for occlusive lesions are of greatest benefit for relieving long aortoiliac artery occlusions. The large size of these vessels, the paucity of critical side branches, and the availability of a direct local access site (via the groin) make these vessels highly suitable for this procedure. The stent-graft technique has also been used for femoropopliteal occlusions, but the advantages at this location are less dramatic because of greater technical difficulties and problems with restenosis and because of the existing facility of standard noncavitary lower extremity bypass procedures. Therefore we primarily use endoluminal stented grafts for aortoiliac lesions and combine aortofemoral or iliac-femoral stented grafts with standard infrainguinal arterial bypass procedures for the treatment of multilevel lower extremity occlusive disease.[7,18]

Symptomatic upper extremity arterial occlusive disease is rarely the result of long-segment large-vessel occlusion; therefore stent-graft placement at these locations has mostly been limited to acute traumatic arterial injuries

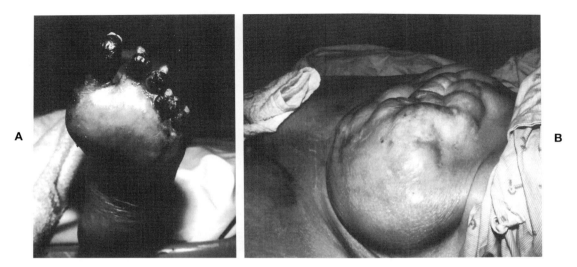

Fig. 1 Ischemic gangrene of the toes **(A)** and a "hostile abdomen" **(B)** in a patient with multilevel lower extremity arterial occlusive disease prior to revascularization using endoluminal surgical techniques instead of a transabdominal approach.

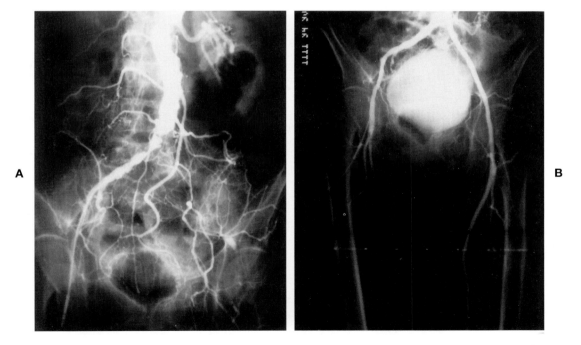

Fig. 2 A, Pre- and **B,** postprocedure angiograms from same patient as in Fig. 1, who underwent right iliac artery balloon angioplasty and stenting and a left iliac-to-profunda femoris artery stent-graft procedure and simultaneous femoral popliteal bypass.

and aneurysmal disease of the extremity inflow vessels.

Because of the risk of embolization and the short focal nature of cerebral vascular occlusive disease, coupled with the ease and reliability of current operative techniques in this region, stented grafts have not been aggressively applied for occlusive lesions of the carotid arteries. Other cerebral arterial lesions such as acute carotid cutaneous fistulas or aneurysms may be treated with a stented graft if a traditional repair is problematic.

TURF ISSUES

At the present time these procedures should be performed in an operating room setting because of the need for surgical cutdown, large arteriotomy, sterility, anesthesia, monitoring, blood replacement, and temperature control in addition to the need for adjunctive open surgical procedures.

Although most surgeons are skilled at simple catheterization, guidewire insertion, and angiographic procedures, stent-graft procedures require additional expertise with multiple guidewires, specialized catheters, fluoroscopy, angiography, balloon angioplasty, and intravascular stent devices (Figs. 3 and 4). These skills are brought to the operating suite by involving the interventional radiologist. Together, the vascular surgeon and the interventional radiologist form a complementary team that is optimally suited to maximizing the use of diagnostic and therapeutic techniques. The relationship between the vascular surgeon and the interventional radiologist is not necessarily problematic since the relative roles and hierarchy for decision making in this setting have already been established through the previous interaction between these specialists in treating patients requiring angiography and balloon angioplasty.

TECHNIQUES FOR STENT-GRAFT PLACEMENT

Stent grafting for occlusive disease is different in several respects from those techniques used for endoluminal repair of aneurysms or vascular trauma. Each application has distinct problems

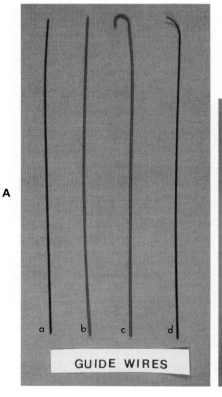

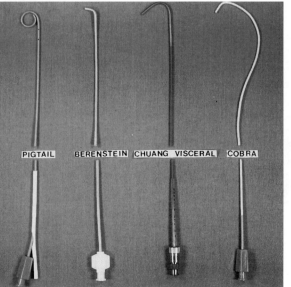

Fig. 3 A, Specialized angiographic wires. a = straight guidewire; b = straight Benston wire; c = J-tipped Benston wire; and d = curved Glidewire (Medi-Tech/Boston Scientific Corp., Watertown, Mass.). **B,** Specialized angiographic catheters.

and issues that must be anticipated, recognized, and dealt with to allow successful treatment. For example, predeployment arterial balloon dilatation is essential only for stent-graft treatment of occlusive lesions. Intramural dissection planes are important in occlusive disease to reestablish an arterial lumen but should be avoided with aneurysm repair and in the treatment of traumatic vascular injuries. On the other hand, fixation of and leakage around proximal and distal ends of stented grafts is not a problem in occlusive situations but is a major concern with aneurysms.

The technical aspects of endoluminal stent grafting for occlusive disease involves the following stages: access and pathfinding, path dilatation, stent-graft positioning, deployment, and assessment.

Access and Pathfinding

Arterial access must be obtained as the initial step for both imaging and diagnostic purposes and for introducing and deploying the stent-graft device. This can be accomplished by means of a single arterial cutdown site or with the addition of a separate percutaneous puncture that is used only for diagnostic and pathfinding purposes (Fig. 5). We prefer the two-site option because of its versatility in allowing simultaneous angiography and device manipulation. In addition, a second remote access site (diagnostic access site) allows for prograde arterial recanalization for the development of a new vessel lumen, which is needed to accomodate a patent graft. The deployment access site does not have to be via a patent artery. This allows the surgical team the freedom to choose a location for this site that is away from troublesome areas, severe scarring, infection, or open wounds.

Pathfinding is the process of initiating and defining the path where the stented graft will reside after deployment. Typically the arterial lumen is obliterated over a long segment prior to this step. Although the path can be created in a retrograde fashion by advancing a wire from the same arterial cutdown site used for introducing the graft, this does not allow precise control of the point of reentry into the native arterial lumen proximally. Therefore prograde recanalization is preferred during the pathfinding step (Fig. 6).

The new path negotiated by the guidewire is frequently located in the subadventitial plane, which is the most common path of least resistance. This is the same anatomic plane along which balloon angioplasty fracture lines occur and is similar to the plane that is normally created when a standard surgical endarterectomy is performed (Fig. 7).[24,25] However, over a

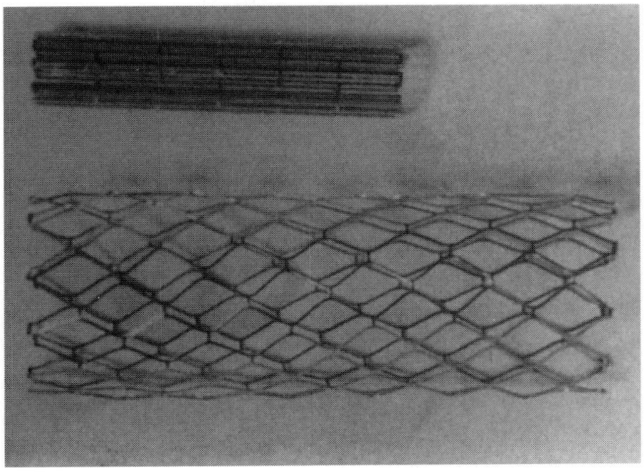

Fig. 4 Collapsed (**A**) and expanded (**B**) Palmaz endovascular stents.

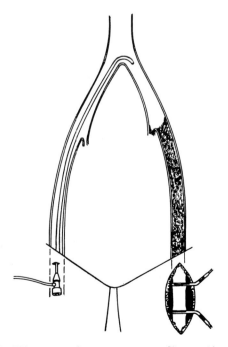

Fig. 5 Diagram of percutaneous diagnostic access site and arterial cutdown for deployment access site.

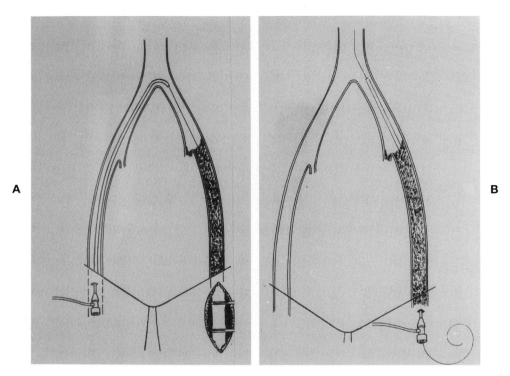

Fig. 6 Diagram of prograde (**A**) vs. retrograde (**B**) pathfinding techniques.

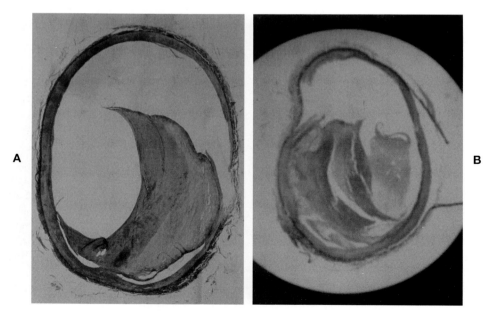

Fig. 7 Photomicrographs of stenotic (**A**) and occluded (**B**) arterial segments following balloon angioplasty.

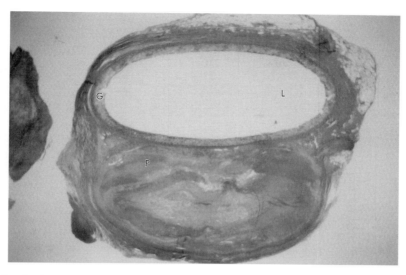

Fig. 8 Histologic cross section of endoluminal graft *(G)* and bypass lumen *(L)* in a previously occluded artery with excluded atherosclerotic plaque *(P)*.

long segment of diseased artery, the dissection plane may pass among the different layers of the arterial wall.[26] The resulting irregularity of the recreated arterial lumen is probably the principal factor that has limited the successfulness of balloon angioplasty when applied to long-segment occlusions. Although variable in depth and radial orientation along the artery, when lined by a stented graft, this lumen becomes continuous and uniform (Fig. 8).

Path Dilatation

Once established, the newly created path needs to be enlarged to accommodate the stent-graft delivery device and ultimately the patent stent graft. Dilatation is accomplished throughout the length of the path using standard 8 mm diameter balloon angioplasty catheters.

Device Placement and Positioning

Using a Seldinger technique, the stent graft (6 mm diameter polytetrafluoroethylene [PTFE] graft and attached Palmaz stent), deployment balloon catheters, and surrounding introducer sheath are inserted through a longitudinal arteriotomy (usually via a femoral vessel) and advanced under fluoroscopic guidance into the previously occluded vessel (Fig. 9).

Deployment

When the device is appropriately positioned, the introducer sheath and lead balloon are carefully withdrawn, the device position is rechecked, and the lead stent is deployed by balloon dilatation. The graft itself is then dilated along its length to seat it against the arterial wall. The remaining portion of the device sheath and distal portion of the stent graft are then brought out through the existing arteriotomy. The distal portion of the graft is then transected and sewn to the outflow vessel or to a standard more distal bypass in one of several configurations (Fig. 10).

Assessment

The last step in the process is to evaluate the final artery-stent-graft-lumen configuration. This is usually accomplished intraoperatively by means of fluoroscopic angiography, which allows qualitative assessment of flow and lumen configuration. We have also used intravascular ultrasound to define the resulting luminal configuration and have found that this allows a more precise three-dimensional evaluation of the new lumen (Fig. 11). Identified sites of significant residual stenosis can be treated by balloon dilatation and/or stent placement.

Montefiore Experience

Seventeen patients with limb-threatening multilevel aortoiliofemoral arterial occlusive disease have undergone endoluminal stent-graft repair in combination with a standard infrainguinal bypass at Montefiore Medical Center.

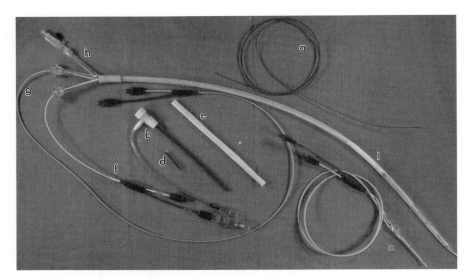

Fig. 9 Endovascular devices used for placement of intra-arterial stented grafts. a = Glidewire; b = introducer sheath; c = balloon angioplasty catheter; d = endovascular stent; e = PTFE graft; f = lead balloon catheter; g = deployment catheter; h = hemostatic valves; and i = stented graft loaded within an introducer sheath with lead and deployment balloons.

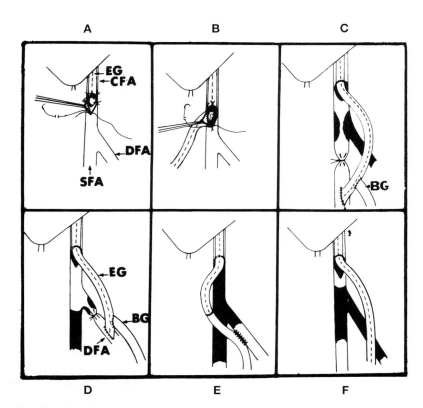

Fig. 10 The distal end of an endoluminal graft *(EG)* originating in the aorta or iliac arteries is anastomosed to a patent distal artery or graft in the groin in one of several ways. **A,** Endoluminal hand-sewn anastomosis to the inside of the common femoral artery *(CFA)* with runoff via the superficial femoral *(SFA)* and deep femoral *(DFA)* arteries. **B,** Endoluminal anastomosis with overlying patch angioplasty via the hood of a more distal bypass. **C,** Continuation of the bypass as an extraluminal bypass graft *(BG)*, which is then terminated in a standard end-to-side anastomosis to the SFA or **(D)** the DFA. **E,** End-to-end anastomosis to a more distal bypass. **F,** Direct continuation of bypass as an extraluminal conduit to a more distal artery. (From Marin ML, Veith FJ, Sanchez LA, et al. Endovascular aortoiliac grafts in combination with standard infrainguinal arterial bypasses in the management of limb-threatening ischemia: Preliminary report. J Vasc Surg 22:316-325, 1995.)

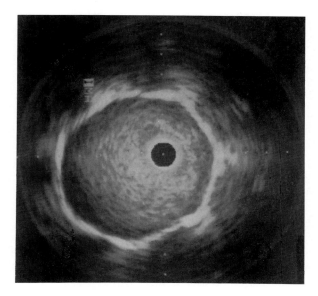

Fig. 11 Intravascular ultrasound image of deployed stented graft and surrounding artery.

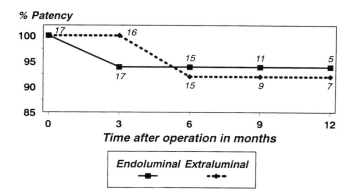

Fig. 12 Life-table graph of primary patency for endoluminal stented grafts and associated standard extraluminal bypass procedures. (From Marin ML, Veith FJ, Sanchez LA, et al. Endovascular aortoiliac grafts in combination with standard infrainguinal arterial bypasses in the management of limb-threatening ischemia: Preliminary report. J Vasc Surg 22:316-325, 1995.)

Fifteen of them had ischemic gangrene and two had severe ischemic rest pain. All had either severe symptomatic coronary artery disease and/or congestive heart failure (n = 14) or prior failed standard aortofemoral reconstructions (n = 8). Anesthesia was either epidural (n = 11), general (n = 5), or local (n = 1). Endoluminal stented grafts were used for inflow revascularization and originated from the aortoiliac junction (n = 7) or the common iliac artery (n = 10) and terminated at the common femoral (n = 9), superficial femoral (n = 4), or deep femoral (n = 4) artery. Simultaneous outflow procedures were performed using a standard open technique. Distal bypass conduits were PTFE (n = 15) or saphenous vein (n = 2) and extended to the popliteal (n = 12), tibial (n = 2), or contralateral femoral (n = 3) arteries. The primary and secondary patency rates for endoluminal stent-graft procedures were 94% ± 10% and 100%, respectively, at 1 year. Patency of the standard bypasses was 92% ± 10% and 100%, respectively (Fig. 12). There were no deaths associated with this series of patients. Minor complications occurred postoperatively in four cases (23%) and consisted of myocardial infarction in one, lymphocele in one, and groin hematomas in two. One patient required amputation at 16 months as a result of a necrotizing foot infection.

PERSPECTIVES

Endoluminal stent-graft procedures are in an evolutionary phase at present. Technical and device-related limitations including size, steerability, device slippage, balloon rupture, and pathfinding currently complicate deployment. The associated short-term successes and complications are only beginning to be appreciated and are likely to change and improve as experience is gained. Although there is considerable enthusiasm for these procedures, their application should be carefully selected and balanced against the currently known favorable results of standard open arterial revascularization procedures.

CONCLUSION

Although relatively recent in development and use, stent grafting for difficult arterial occlusive conditions has supplemented the existing limb salvage options and has allowed otherwise complicated arterial bypasses to be done through limited surgical incisions and with minimal morbidity. This operation should be considered as an alternative to or in conjunction with more traditional revascularization procedures.

REFERENCES

1. Veith FJ, Gupta SK, Wengerter KR, et al. Changing arteriosclerotic disease patterns and management strategies in lower-limb-threatening ischemia. Ann Surg 212:402-414, 1990.
2. Yaeger RA. Basic data related to cardiac testing and cardiac risk associated with vascular surgery. Ann Vasc Surg 4:193-197, 1990.
3. McCann RL, Clements FM. Silent myocardial ischemia in patients undergoing peripheral vascular surgery: Incidence and association with perioperative cardiac morbidity and mortality. J Vasc Surg 9:583-587, 1989.
4. Ahn SS, Eton D, Yeatman LR, Deutsch LS, Moore WS. Intraoperative peripheral rotary atherectomy: Early and late clinical results. Ann Vasc Surg 6:272-280, 1992.
5. McLean GK. Percutaneous peripheral atherectomy. J Vasc Interv Radiol 4:465-480, 1993.
6. Marin ML, Veith FJ, Panetta TF, et al. Transfemoral stented graft treatment of occlusive arterial disease for limb salvage: A preliminary report. Circulation 88:1-11, 1993.
7. Marin ML, Veith FJ, Cynamon J, et al. Transfemoral endovascular stented graft treatment of aorto-iliac and femoropopliteal occlusive disease for limb salvage. Am J Surg 168:156-162, 1994.
8. Cragg AH, Dake MD. Percutaneous femoropopliteal grafting: Report of a new technique. J Vasc Interv Radiol 4:64-65, 1993.
9. Cannon JA, Barker WF. Successful management of obstructive femoral artery arteriosclerosis by endarterectomy. Surgery 38:48-60, 1955.
10. Doller CT, Judkins MP. Transluminal treatment of arteriosclerotic obstruction. Description of a new technique and a preliminary report of its applications. Circulation 30:654-670, 1964.
11. Kadir S, White RI Jr, Kaufman SL, et al. Long-term results of aortoiliac angioplasty. Surgery 94:10-14, 1983.
12. Gunther RW, Vorwerk D, Bohndorf K, et al. Iliac and femoral artery stenoses and occlusions: Treatment with intravascular stents. Radiology 172:725-730, 1989.
13. Palmaz JC, Laborde JC, Rivera FJ, Encarnacio CE, Lutz JD, Moss JG. Stenting of the iliac arteries with the Palmaz stent: Experience from a multicenter trial. Cardiovasc Intervent Radiol 15:291-297, 1992.
14. Gunther RW, Vorwerk D, Antonucci F, et al. Iliac artery stenosis or obstruction after unsuccessful balloon angioplasty: Treatment with a self-expandable stent. AJR 156:389-393, 1991.
15. Johnston KW. Femoral and popliteal arteries: Reanalysis of results of balloon angioplasty. Radiology 183:767-771, 1992.
16. Dalman RL, Taylor LM Jr, Moneta GL, Yaeger RA, Porter JM. Simultaneous operative repair of multilevel lower extremity occlusive disease. J Vasc Surg 13:211-221, 1991.
17. Marin ML, Veith FJ. The role of stented grafts in the management of failed arterial reconstructions. Semin Vasc Surg 7:188-194, 1994.
18. Marin ML, Veith FJ, Sanchez LA, et al. Endovascular aortoiliac grafts in combination with standard infrainguinal arterial bypasses in the management of limb-threatening ischemia: Preliminary report. J Vasc Surg 22:316-325, 1995.
19. Volodos NL, Karpovich IP, Troyan VI, et al. Clinical experience of the use of self-fixing synthetic prostheses for remote endoprosthetics of the thoracic and the abdominal aorta and iliac arteries through the femoral artery and as intraoperative endoprosthesis for aorta reconstruction. Vasa Suppl 33:93-95, 1991.
20. Parodi JC, Palmaz JC, Barone HD. Transfemoral intraluminal graft implantation for abdominal aortic aneurysms. Ann Vasc Surg 5:491-499, 1991.
21. Palmaz JC, Laborde JC, Rivera FJ, Encarnacio CE, Lutz JD, Moss JG. Stenting of the iliac arteries with the Palmaz stent: Experience from a multicenter trial. Cardiovasc Intervent Radiol 15:291-297, 1992.
22. Marin ML, Veith FJ, Panetta TF, et al. Transfemoral endoluminal stented graft repair of a popliteal artery aneurysm. J Vasc Surg 19:754-757, 1994.
23. Marin ML, Veith FJ, Panetta TF, et al. Transluminally placed endovascular stented graft repair for arterial trauma. J Vasc Surg 20:466-473, 1994.

24. Lyon RT, Runyon-Haas A, Davis HR, Glagov S, Zarins CK. Protection from arteriosclerotic lesion formation by inhibition arterial wall motion. J Vasc Surg 5:59-67, 1987.

25. Lyon RT, Lu CT, Glagov S, Zarins CK. Arterial wall disruption by balloon dilatation: Quantitative comparison of normal, stenotic and occluded vessels. Surg Forum 32:386-388, 1981.

26. Marin ML, Veith FJ, Cynamon J, et al. Human transluminally placed endovascular stented grafts: Preliminary histopathologic analysis of healing grafts in aortoiliac and femoral artery occlusive disease. J Vasc Surg (in press).

7

Endovascular Stent-Grafts in the Management of Arterial Injuries

MICHAEL L. SCHWARTZ, M.D., MICHAEL L. MARIN, M.D., and FRANK J. VEITH, M.D.

The frequency with which penetrating arterial injuries occur from knives and handguns has paralleled the increase in civilian trauma. These vascular injuries may initially present as acute arterial occlusions, expanding pseudoaneurysms, or arteriovenous fistulas. Without prompt, appropriate therapy, these lesions may result in limb loss, exsanguinating hemorrhage, or congestive heart failure. Experiences with high-velocity missiles during World War II, the Korean War, and the Vietnam War have established the optimal treatment necessary to repair arterial injuries.[1-7] These principles form the basis by which we currently treat civilian arterial wounds. Unfortunately, the following factors make the direct surgical repair of these injuries a formidable challenge: (1) large, local hematomas make surgical proximal control more difficult, especially for central or truncal vessels; (2) associated vein, nerve, bone, and muscle injuries complicate dissection of the vessels; and (3) false aneurysms and arteriovenous fistulas can lead to venous hypertension, which distorts local anatomy, resulting in an operative intervention associated with significant blood loss.

A new therapeutic option employs recently developed endovascular stent-graft devices for the treatment of penetrating vascular injuries.[8-11] The use of this exciting new technology permits repair of the injured vessel via a remote access site, eliminating the need for operative proximal control and difficult arterial dissections.

This chapter will describe the technique used and Montefiore Medical Center's early clinical experience with endovascular stented grafts in the treatment of arterial pseudoaneurysms and arteriovenous fistulas secondary to iatrogenic and traumatic penetrating injuries.

HISTORY

The evolution of stent-graft technology is based on the initial work of Dotter, the developer of balloon angioplasty.[12,13] This early work resulted in the development of a number of different intravascular stents.[14-19] These stents were readily applied to occlusive lesions, but because of their porous quality they were not applicable in the management of other types of arterial pathologic conditions. Aneurysms, pseudoaneurysms, and arteriovenous fistulas typically require vascular grafts or direct surgical repair. The stent-graft, a combination of intravascular stents and vascular grafts, combined the fixation properties of a stent with the hemostatic properties of a graft (Fig. 1). The stent-graft can be used to treat occlusive, aneurysmal, and traumatic arterial lesions.[20-24] One of the first clinical cases using the stent-graft concept was reported by Volodos et al.[25,26] who used a Dacron graft covered self-expanding stent. These early experiences were refined in experimental canine models and clinical research.[8,27] In 1993, Parodi

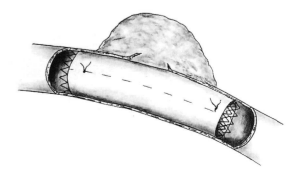

Fig. 1 Conceptualization of the use of the stent-graft for the treatment of a traumatic pseudoaneurysm.

Supported by grants from the U.S. Public Health Service (HL 02990-02), the James Hilton Manning and Emma Austin Manning Foundation, The Anna S. Brown Trust, and the New York Institute for Vascular Studies.

et al.[8] reported the use of stent-grafts to repair two traumatic arteriovenous fistulas.

TECHNIQUES AND DEVICES

At Montefiore Medical Center we currently use a balloon-expandable stent covered with polytetrafluoroethylene (PTFE) (W.L. Gore & Associates, Inc., Flagstaff, Ariz.). Although we have used PTFE in all cases, experimental and early clinical evidence demonstrates that the external covering of the stent does not appear to be critical for the appropriate function of the device. Although we use stainless steel Palmaz stents (Fig. 2) that vary between 20 and 30 mm in length, the size of the stent is tailored to the type of lesion being treated. An appropriate length of thin-walled 6 mm PTFE is suture-fixated to the outside of the stent with fine polypropylene sutures (Fig. 3). The stent-graft is then placed on a balloon angioplasty catheter (8 to 10 mm) and loaded into a 12 Fr introducer sheath. A "nose cone" dilator tip tapers the catheter to the sheath (Fig. 4). After the access artery is dissected and controlled, the patient is given systemic anticoagulation therapy and the artery is cannulated with a wire. The device is then coaxially threaded over the wire and, under fluoroscopic guidance, placed across the lesion (Fig. 5). After arteriographic confirmation, the sheath is retracted and the stent-graft is deployed by balloon inflation. Completion

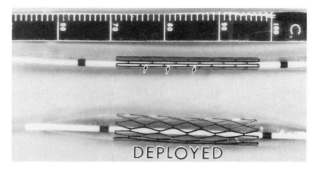

Fig. 2 The Palmaz stent before and after deployment by a balloon angioplasty catheter. The stent provides the fixation seal for the stent-graft.

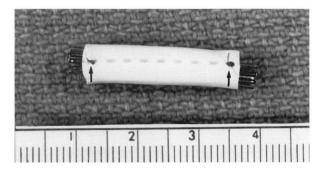

Fig. 3 Actual stent-graft before coaxial loading on a balloon angioplasty catheter. (Note the two "U" stitches that fix the 2.5 cm PTFE graft to the Palmaz stent.)

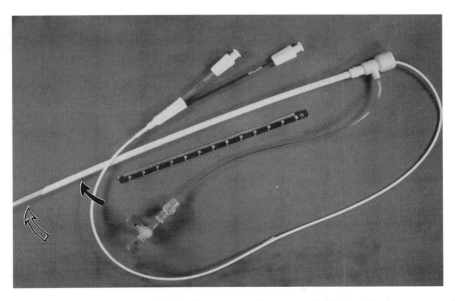

Fig. 4 Stent-graft deployment device features a "nose cone" dilator tip *(open arrow)* that tapers the angioplasty catheter to the 12 Fr introducer sheath *(black arrow)*.

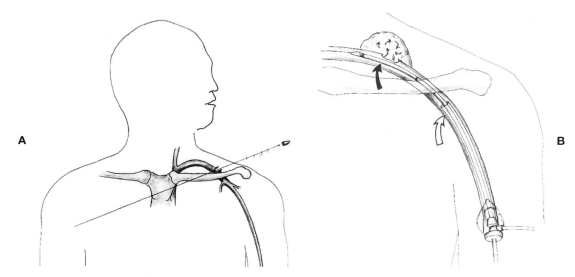

Fig. 5 A, Gunshot wound to the left axillosubclavian arterial segment. **B,** The stent-graft device is placed via a remote access site (brachial artery). The sheath is retracted *(white arrow)*, exposing the stent-graft surface *(black arrow)* to the pseudoaneurysm. The balloon is subsequently inflated, deploying the stent-graft, and the pseudoaneurysm is excluded from the circulation.

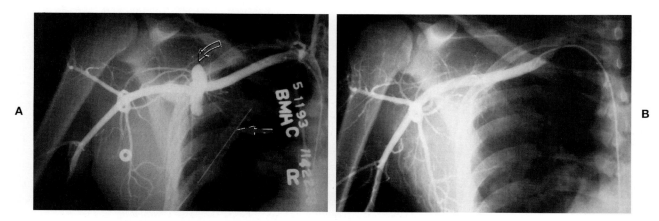

Fig. 6 A, Preoperative angiogram demonstrating a pseudoaneurysm *(curved arrow)* from a stab wound to the right chest. Note the chest tube placed for hemothorax *(straight arrow)*. **B,** Completion arteriogram of the same patient after treatment with a stent-graft device.

arteriograms are performed to document adequate therapy (Fig. 6). Duplex ultrasonography at regular follow-up intervals is used to confirm patency (Fig. 7).

RESULTS

Between December 1992 and February 1995, nine patients with traumatic or iatrogenic arterial injuries were treated with nine stent-grafts. Eight of these patients were male, ranging in age from 18 to 78 years (mean, 38 years). The mechanisms of injury included six bullet wounds, two vascular catheterization injuries, and one knife wound (Table 1). Two patients presented with arteriovenous fistulas (Fig. 8) and the remaining seven with associated large pseudoaneurysms (Fig. 9). Most of the patients had other injuries in addition to the arterial damage. The time interval between injury and repair varied from 3 hours to 4 months (Table 2).

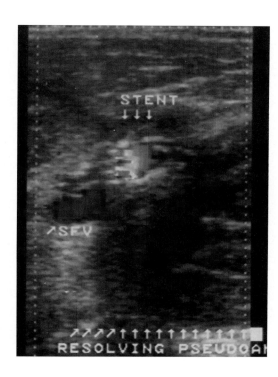

Fig. 7 Postoperative duplex examinations are performed at regular intervals to confirm patency of the repair. This duplex scan demonstrates closure of an arteriovenous fistula from the superficial femoral artery to the superficial femoral vein *(SFV)*.

Table 1 Injury characteristics

Sex/age	Mechanism of injury	Vessel involved*	Pseudoaneurysm	Arteriovenous fistula	Associated injuries
Male/20	Bullet	L SFA, SFV	Yes	Yes	Soft tissue
Male/28	Bullet	R SFA	Yes	No	Open femur fracture
Male/22	Bullet	L SFA	Yes	No	Soft tissue, DVT
Male/24	Knife	L ASA	Yes	No	Hemothorax
Male/35	Bullet	R ASA	Yes	No	Brachial plexus
Female/78	Catheter	R SA	Yes	No	Hemothorax
Male/78	Catheter	L CIA	Yes	No	None
Male/18	Bullet	R SA	Yes	Yes	Hemothorax
Male/21	Bullet	R ASA	Yes	No	Humerus

*R, right; L, left; SFA, superficial femoral artery; SFV, superficial femoral vein; ASA, axillary subclavian artery; SA, subclavian artery; CIA, common iliac artery.

Table 2 Repair, outcome, and follow-up

Sex/age	Interval until repair	Access vessel*	Stent-graft size (cm)	Balloon diameter (mm)	Hospital stay	Patency (months)
Male/20	36 hr	L SFA†	3	8	5 days	27
Male/28	12 hr	R SFA	3	7	9 days	24
Male/22	12 hr	L SFA	3	8	6 days	2‖
Male/24	4 hr	L brachial	3	8	7 days	21
Male/35	3 wk	R brachial	3	7	4 days	18
Female/78	24 hr	R brachial	3	8	2 mo‡	15
Male/78	4 mo	L CFA	2	10	2 days	15
Male/18	48 hr	R brachial	3	6	4 days	15
Male/21	24 hr	R brachial	3	8	2 mo§	2

*L, left; R, right; SFA, superficial femoral artery; CFA, common femoral artery.
†Percutaneous approach.
‡Hospitalized for multiple medical problems.
§Currently receiving in-hospital rehabilitation.
‖Died 2 months after the procedure (homicide).

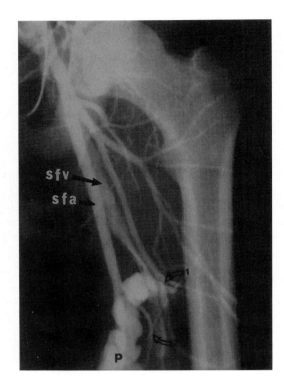

Fig. 8 Arteriovenous fistula resulting from a gunshot wound to the superficial femoral artery *(sfa)* in the thigh. Early filling of the superficial femoral vein *(sfv)* via the pseudoaneurysm *(p)* is noted.

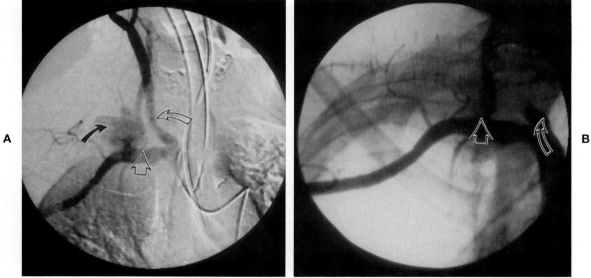

Fig. 9 A, Large iatrogenic subclavian artery pseudoaneurysm *(curved black arrow)* sustained from an attempted Swan-Ganz catheterization. Proximity of the vertebral *(open arrow)* and right common carotid *(curved open arrow)* arteries must be noted for correct deployment. **B,** Completion arteriogram shows exclusion of the pseudoaneurysm and preservation of the vertebral *(straight arrow)* and common carotid *(curved arrow)* arteries.

Access was by a percutaneous method in one case and by arterial cutdown in the remaining eight. We currently favor a small cutdown because it maximizes control of the vessel and eliminates puncture site complications that might occur with use of the large 12 Fr device.

The mean hospital length of stay for seven of the eight patients who underwent stent-graft procedures for arterial trauma was 5.5 days. One patient required intensive care unit management while being treated for multiple comorbid illnesses. Another patient remained hospitalized with a concomitant neurologic injury undergoing in-house rehabilitation. Follow-up in eight of the nine patients ranged from 2 to 29 months (mean, 17 months) with 100% patency and no early or late stent-graft occlusions. One patient died by homicide 2 months after the procedure. There were no perioperative mortalities. Except for one patient who required a vein patch angioplasty to assist in closure of the access site arteriotomy, there were no complications.

DISCUSSION

Enthusiasm for endovascular therapy of aneurysmal and occlusive arterial disease has increased over the past few years, as has interest in the potential application of this new modality to the treatment of arterial injury. Previously, arterial trauma required direct surgical repair to prevent immediate and delayed complications.[28-31] Unfortunately, in many cases the arterial injury is associated with large local hematomas or other associated injuries. This results in a surgical repair fraught with challenging arterial dissections and significant blood loss. This difficulty is magnified if the injury involves central or truncal vessels. Endovascular therapy has rapidly gained popularity, since it avoids the pitfalls associated with direct operative intervention.[32] The advantage of using stent-grafts for trauma is that they can be deployed at an area remote from the injury. The use of stented grafts also offers a less invasive intervention associated with reduced anesthesia and transfusion requirements. In appropriate instances, the device can be inserted under local or regional anesthesia. These procedures can be done safely with minimal in-hospital length of stay provided there are no comorbid illnesses.

There is concern about the use of prosthetic material in an area of potential contamination.[33] Classically, vein has been the conduit of choice for repair of traumatic arterial injuries in the extremities. However, to minimize potential infectious complications, there is enthusiasm for the use of prosthetic grafts as well.[34] We continue to use PTFE-covered stents in our protocol. Although we have not experienced infectious complications in our series, treatment of a greater number of patients and a longer follow-up period are necessary to fully evaluate this risk. Alternatively, the stents could be covered with vein segments.

Another theoretical disadvantage to the use of PTFE-covered stent-grafts is the lower patency achieved with prosthetic conduits. This is borne out by the fact that long prosthetic bypasses do not function as well as autogenous material for the treatment of atherosclerotic occlusive disease. Although it is likely that short segments of PTFE (3 cm) placed in high-flow vessels will result in satisfactory function, further follow-up is required. At its worst, late stent-graft failure can convert an emergency procedure into an elective procedure performed with autogenous tissue. At the time of the secondary procedure, patency of the ipsilateral vein should have been confirmed, associated injuries appropriately dealt with, and swelling diminished.

Further questions need to be answered. Can the stent-graft be used in a critically injured patient who is in shock? What is the stent-graft's role in a minimally injured artery (i.e., small pseudoaneurysms and noncritical intimal flaps)? Who should ultimately be performing these procedures? Although the answers to these questions are vague at this time, clarification will come with further experience, longer follow-up, and well-developed, controlled trials.

REFERENCES

1. Drapanas T, Hewitt RL, Weichert RF, et al. Civilian vascular injuries: A critical appraisal of three decades of management. Ann Surg 172:351-360, 1970.
2. Burnett HF, Parnell CL, Williams GD, et al. Peripheral arterial injuries: A reassessment. Ann Surg 183:701-709, 1976.
3. Feliciano DV, Bitondo CG, Mattox KL, et al. Civilian trauma in the 1980s: A 1-year experience with 456 vascular and cardiac injuries. Ann Surg 199:717-724, 1984.
4. Perry MO, Thal ER, Shires GT. Management of arterial injuries. Ann Surg 173:403-408, 1971.
5. Jahnke EJ Jr, Seeley SF. Acute vascular injuries in the Korean war: An analysis of 77 consecutive cases. Ann Surg 138:158-177, 1953.
6. Rich NM, Spencer FC. Vascular Trauma. Philadelphia: WB Saunders, 1978.

7. Winegarner FG, Baker AG Jr, Bascom JF, et al. Delayed vascular complications in Vietnam casualties. J Trauma 10:867-873, 1970.
8. Parodi JC, Barone HD, Schonholz C. Transfemoral endovascular treatment of aortoiliac aneurysms and arteriovenous fistulas with stented Dacron grafts. In Veith FJ, ed. Current critical problems in vascular surgery, vol 5. St. Louis: Quality Medical Publishing, 1993, p 264.
9. Marin ML, Veith FJ, Panetta TF, et al. Transluminally placed endovascular stented graft repair for arterial trauma. J Vasc Surg 20:466-473, 1994.
10. Marin ML, Veith FJ, Panetta TF, et al. Percutaneous transfemoral insertion of a stented graft to repair a traumatic femoral arteriovenous fistula. J Vasc Surg 18:299-302, 1993.
11. May J, White G, Waugh R, et al. Transluminal placement of a prosthetic graft-stent device for treatment of subclavian artery aneurysm. J Vasc Surg 18:1056-1059, 1993.
12. Dotter CT. Transluminally-placed coilspring endarterial tube grafts. Long-term patency in canine popliteal artery. Invest Radiol 4:329-332, 1969.
13. Dotter CT, Judkins MP. Transluminal treatment of arteriosclerotic obstruction. Description of a new technic and a preliminary report of its application. Circulation 30:654-670, 1964.
14. Hausegger KA, Cragg AH, Lammer J, et al. Iliac artery stent placement: Clinical experience with a nitinol stent. Radiology 190:199-202, 1994.
15. Henry M, Beron R, Chastel R, et al. Endoprothèsis vasculaires de Palmaz: Rèsultats prèliminaires. Presse Med 19:1401-1402, 1990.
16. Henry M, Beyar R. Initial clinical experience with the instent nitinol permanent and temporary stents. Circulation 88:I-586, 1993.
17. Joffre F, Puel J, Imbert C, et al. Use of a new type of self-expanding vascular stent prosthesis: Early clinical results. Proceedings of the 72nd Scientific Assembly of the Radiology Society of North America, Chicago, November 30, 1986.
18. Liermann D, Strecker EP, Peters J. The Strecker stent: Indications and results in iliac and femoropopliteal arteries. Cardiovasc Intervent Radiol 15:298-305, 1992.
19. Palmaz JC, Garcia OJ, Schatz RA, et al. Placement of balloon-expandable intraluminal stents in iliac arteries: First 171 procedures. Radiology 174:969-975, 1990.
20. Chuter TAM, Green RM, Ouriel K, et al. Transfemoral endovascular aortic graft placement. J Vasc Surg 18:185-197, 1993.
21. Marin ML, Veith FJ, Panetta TF, et al. Transfemoral stented graft treatment of occlusive arterial disease for limb salvage: A preliminary report. Circulation 88:I-11, 1993.
22. Marin ML, Veith FJ. The role of stented grafts in the management of failed arterial reconstructions. Semin Vasc Surg 7:188-194, 1994.
23. Marin ML, Veith FJ, Panetta TF, et al. Transfemoral endoluminal stented graft repair of a popliteal artery aneurysm. J Vasc Surg 19:754-757, 1994.
24. Parodi JC, Palmaz JC, Barone HD. Transfemoral intraluminal graft implantation for abdominal aortic aneurysms. Ann Vasc Surg 5:491-499, 1991.
25. Volodos NL, Shekhanin VE, Karpovich IP, et al. Self-fixing synthetic prosthesis for endoprosthetics of the vessels. Vestn Khir (Russia) 137:123-125, 1986.
26. Volodos NL, Karpovich IP, Troyan VI, et al. Clinical experience of the use of self-fixing synthetic prostheses for remote endoprosthetics of the thoracic and the abdominal aorta and iliac arteries through the femoral artery and as intraoperative endoprosthesis for aorta reconstruction. Vasa Suppl 33:93-95, 1991.
27. Boudghene F, Anidjar S, Allaire E, et al. Endovascular grafting in elastase-induced experimental aortic aneurysms in dogs: Feasibility and preliminary results. J Vasc Intervent Radiol 4:497-504, 1993.
28. Feliciano DV, Cruse PA, Burch JM, et al. Delayed diagnosis of arterial injuries. Am J Surg 154:579-584, 1987.
29. Richardson JD, Vitale GC, Flint LM Jr. Penetrating arterial trauma: Analysis of missed vascular injuries. Arch Surg 122:678-683, 1987.
30. Ben-Menachem Y. Vascular injuries of the extremities: Hazards of unnecessary delays in diagnosis. Orthopedics 9:333-338, 1986.
31. Escobar GA, Escobar SC, Marquez L, et al. Vascular trauma: Late sequelae and treatment. J Cardiovasc Surg 21:35-40, 1980.
32. Panetta TF, Sclafani SJA, Goldstein AS, et al. Percutaneous transcatheter embolization for arterial trauma. J Vasc Surg 2:54-64, 1985.
33. Keen RR, Meyer JP, Durham JR, et al. Autogenous vein graft repair of injured extremity arteries: Early and late results with 134 consecutive patients. J Vasc Surg 13:664-668, 1991.
34. Feliciano DV, Mattox KL, Graham JM, Bitondo CG. Five-year experience with PTFE grafts in vascular wounds. J Trauma 25:71-82, 1985.

8

Why Vascular Surgeons Should Be Involved in Endovascular Procedures

JAMES A. DeWEESE, M.D.

Dotter and Judkins[1] in 1964 reported an endovascular procedure that is best described as a percutaneous transluminal angioplasty (PTA). Through retrograde percutaneous catheterization of the contralateral femoral artery they introduced 0.1- and 0.2-inch outside diameter Teflon catheters over guidewires that were positioned through stenotic lesions of femoral arteries to enlarge the lumen. Six of 11 extremities "improved markedly" during short-term follow-up of less than 10 months. Outside Dotter's institution, few such procedures were performed in the United States during that period, although large numbers were performed in Europe.

In 1979 Grüntzig and Kumpe[2] introduced a noncompliant balloon catheter with a maximum diameter of 4 to 6 mm for the superficial femoral artery and 6 to 10 mm for the iliac artery, which improved the capabilities of the procedures. Grüntzig and Kumpe observed 2-year patency rates of 86% for balloon angioplasty of femoropopliteal lesions as compared with a 64% patency rate for those treated by the Dotter technique.

With the development of the balloon by Grüntzig, PTA has become a commonly used procedure for treatment of localized arterial stenoses, particularly those of the iliac artery. The procedures were usually performed by interventional radiologists and cardiologists, with varying degrees of involvement by vascular surgeons. In 1980 Ring et al.,[3] with the "close cooperation of vascular surgeons," reported early success in 57 of 62 balloon angioplasty dilatations of 54 iliac and femoral arteries and eight vein grafts. Veith et al.,[4] working closely with Sprayregen in 1981, reported the adjunctive use of PTA in 115 of 1196 patients requiring reconstructive arterial procedures for limb salvage. Johnston et al.[5] in 1987 reported the 5-year results of 984 PTAs performed or supervised by experienced vascular radiologists. Significantly better results were observed when (1) the common iliac artery was treated, rather than the external iliac or femoropopliteal arteries, (2) the operations were performed for claudication rather than limb salvage, (3) the lesion was treated for stenosis and not occlusion, (4) the runoff was good, (5) the patient was not diabetic, (6) the operation was not complicated, and (7) only a single site was dilated. Brewster et al.[6] in 1989 reported the use of 79 PTAs performed by radiologists before distal arterial reconstructions were performed.

In other reports, surgeons were performing the balloon angioplasties themselves. These procedures were usually performed in the operating room with or without fluoroscopic control. They were usually performed after surgical exposure of the femoral artery and in conjunction with other vascular reconstructions. Lowman et al.[7] in 1981 reported 16 intraoperative transluminal angioplasties of the iliac and femoropopliteal arteries with Grüntzig balloons during vascular reconstructive procedures. The femoral artery was exposed in the groin and the procedure performed without fluoroscopic control. Fogarty et al.[8] in 1981 reported 18 iliac angioplasties through the exposed femoral artery in the groin in the operating room at the time of distal arterial reconstructions. A newly developed dilating balloon was used that was introduced to the site of the stenosis and then the balloon extruded through the stenosis and dilated to a predetermined volume. Fluoroscopy was not found to be necessary. Pfieffer and String[9] in 1986 performed 80 proximal or distal balloon angioplasties in conjunction with vascular reconstructions. The procedures were performed in the operating room with the aid of fluoroscopy.

The results of PTA, particularly for stenotic arterial lesions and for short occlusions, were quite good for iliac lesions and satisfactory for femoral and distal lesions. Longer occlusions prevented the performance of angioplasty in most patients. It was postulated that the thermal energy of the laser might be used to penetrate these longer occlusions. Initial attempts with the technique resulted in a high rate of vessel perforations.[10] Sanborn et al.[11] developed an optical fiber with a cone-shaped metal cap on the end that reduced the rate of thermal injuries from misdirection. Initial clinical trials supported the experimental studies and in 1987 the Food and Drug Administration approved the use of lasers to enhance the efficiency of balloon angioplasty. Within a year, laser thermal angioplasty programs were established in more than 200 centers and more than 7000 cases were performed.[12] An increased number of cases were performed over the next 1 to 2 years. The procedures consisted of laser recanalization without angioplasty and laser-assisted balloon angioplasties. It was possible to recanalize some vessels with the laser tip without applying thermal energy and then perform balloon angioplasty alone. The 12- to 15-month actuarial reported patency rate for all lower extremity laser reconstructions varied from 7% to 77%, but was less than 15% in three of five reports.[12-16] Complication rates as high as 32% and 39% were also reported.[13,14] Although it had been hoped that the laser could recanalize long occlusions, it was not satisfactory if the occlusions were more than a few centimeters long. The procedure is now rarely used. The procedure did, however, increase surgeons' interest in endovascular techniques. Many of the procedures were used as adjuncts to other vascular reconstructions and were performed in the operating room with suitable tables and imaging equipment. Many surgeons sought additional training and performed the laser-assisted balloon angioplasties in suites in or out of the operating room. Some of the reported series were from these surgeons.[12,14-19]

There has been some interest in the use of atherectomy devices to treat arteriosclerotic occlusions. A number of such devices have been evaluated, and initial success rates of 61% to 92% have been reported. Rotablator atherectomies were recently evaluated by teams of cardiologists, radiologists, and surgeons.[20] The procedures were performed on arteries of the lower extremity, either through percutaneous or direct arterial insertions. The results were evaluated clinically by duplex scanning, noninvasive hemodynamic studies, and angiography. Complications occurred after approximately 50% of the procedures. Cumulative patency rates at 12 months were 31% and at 24 months were only 18.6%. The authors concluded that other devices must be similarly evaluated before atherectomy is routinely offered to patients as an alternative to vascular reconstruction or balloon angioplasty.

The next advance in endovascular techniques for treatment of arterial occlusive disease was the development of intraluminal stents. Palmaz et al.[21] in 1990 reported the results of a multicenter clinical trial in which 171 stenting procedures were performed. The procedures were performed on patients who had had an inadequate response to balloon angioplasty. The stent was a stainless steel, slotted tube that could be mounted on a balloon angioplasty catheter and introduced into the stenotic area and expanded by the balloon. After a short-term follow-up period, the patency rate was 100%. With longer follow-up, thrombosis and complication rates were acceptably low.

The newest advance in endovascular technology is the combination of a stent and graft as a transluminally placed endovascular graft (TPEG). Intraluminal stents within grafts have been successfully used to treat aortoiliac and femoral occlusive lesions.[22] In addition, however, they can be used to treat true aneurysms as well as false aneurysms and arterial injuries. A number of devices have been evaluated in the laboratory for transluminal repair. The first were performed in 1990.[23] Tube grafts anchored in place by Palmaz balloons and expandable stents were used to treat abdominal aortic aneurysms. Parodi[23] in 1995 reported results of 50 such procedures. Five patients developed proximal leaks; one died in the hospital, one died 2 months postoperatively of a ruptured aneurysm, and one died 7 months after operation of congestive heart failure. Another patient's leak responded successfully to a standard operation, and the last leak healed spontaneously. Two distal leaks did not affect the outcome. There were three patients who had embolization and died as a result of multiorgan failure. (Three other patients were later shown to have proximal or distal leaks.)

The use of stents such as the barbed Gianturco stent by Chuter and the modified Lazarus self-expanding device with fixation pins used by Endovascular Technologies may decrease the complication of migration and proximal and distal leaks.[24,25] TPEGs are being successfully used to treat peripheral aneurysms, false aneurysms, and arteriovenous fistulas.[22,23]

It is obvious that endovascular arterial reconstructions are here to stay. How much they will affect the volume of surgical arterial reconstructions is still unknown, but some information is available. In the period 1980 through 1989, Veith's group saw 2221 patients with threatened limbs.[26] PTAs alone were performed on 426 (19%) of the patients. A PTA and operation was performed on 331 (15%) of the patients. On the basis of a careful evaluation of abdominal aneurysms with three-dimensional CT scans, Chuter's group found 9% who had proximal and distal cuffs suitable for a tube TPEG.[27] There were 59% suitable for bifurcation TPEGs. Veith and Marin[28] have stated that they believe that TPEG procedures will replace 30% to 70% of current standard graft operations for aneurysmal, traumatic, and occlusive arterial lesions. This means that they would replace 20% to 40% of the major vascular operations now being performed. In addition, other endovascular techniques may replace another 25% of current vascular procedures. In other words, 45% to 65% of major vascular operations might be performed by endovascular techniques. Classic surgical expertise, however, will still be required for the primary treatment of many patients as well as for management of the complications of the endovascular procedures.

It is my opinion that vascular surgeons should be involved in endovascular procedures. They should either be an integral part of a multidisciplinary team or, with suitable training, become competent to meet all the requirements of such a team. The requirements of a multidisciplinary team are these:

1. Clinical experience with all vascular lesions, the knowledge of their natural history, and acquaintance with the role of all possible means of managing them
2. A high level of skill in catheter-guidewire-imaging techniques for performing endovascular procedures
3. Vascular surgical skills
4. Competency in evaluation of the outcomes of procedures that are performed.

Clinical experience with all vascular lesions has been part of the training of almost all physicians practicing vascular surgery and vascular medicine, compared with the limited exposure received by most cardiologists and radiologists.

Catheter-guidewire-imaging procedures are currently part of the experience of most general surgical and vascular surgical residents. The Residency Review Committee for Surgery recognizes the importance of the experience by recommending training in vascular access procedures and by requiring general surgical residents to list the number of procedures performed. Radiologists and cardiologists may get similar experiences during rotation on interventional services. Vascular surgical residents are currently performing endovascular procedures in some centers or attaining additional experiences in courses that include experience with insertion of devices in large animals or mock circulatory models.[29] Recommendations for the requirements for credentialing of vascular surgeons who want to perform endovascular procedures suggest that 50 diagnostic *or* therapeutic angiograms and 10 to 15 angioplasties be performed.[30]

A multidisciplinary team requires a surgeon with vascular surgical skills for the management of most unsuccessful endovascular procedures or complications of the procedures.

Another important role for a member of the team is the ability and desire to carefully follow and objectively evaluate the outcome of the procedure. Most vascular surgeons, cardiologists, and vascular internists are trained for and accept this responsibility.

A vascular surgeon who has received additional training and experience with endovascular techniques can assume any or all roles of a multidisciplinary team. In circumstances in which no such team is available and the equipment and assistance are present, the vascular surgeon can and should perform endovascular operations.

Many vascular surgeons have been and are currently involved in endovascular procedures. Some have invented new devices and procedures. Others have developed or revised existing equipment and techniques. Others have critically evaluated outcomes of the procedures and others have established guidelines for the indications for and performance of the procedures. Vascular surgeons should continue to be involved in endovascular procedures.

REFERENCES

1. Dotter CT, Judkins MP. Transluminal treatment of arteriosclerotic obstruction. Circulation 30:654-670, 1964.
2. Grüntzig A, Kumpe DA. Technique of percutaneous transluminal angioplasty with the Grüntzig balloon catheter. AJR 132:547-555, 1979.

3. Ring EJ, Alpert JR, Freiman DB, et al. Early experience with percutaneous transluminal angioplasty using a vinyl balloon catheter. Ann Surg 191:438-444, 1980.
4. Veith FJ, Gupta SK, Samson RH, et al. Progress in limb salvage by reconstructive arterial surgery combined with new or improved adjunctive procedures. Ann Surg 194:386-401, 1981.
5. Johnston KW, Rae M, Hogg-Johnston SA, et al. 5-year results of a prospective study of percutaneous transluminal angioplasty. Ann Surg 206:403-413, 1987.
6. Brewster DC, Cambria RP, Darling RC, et al. Long term results of combined iliac balloon angioplasty and distal surgical revascularization. Ann Surg 210:324-330, 1989.
7. Lowman BG, Queral LA, Holbrook WA, et al. Transluminal angioplasty during vascular reconstructive procedures. Arch Surg 116:829-832, 1981.
8. Fogarty TJ, Chin A, Shoor PM, et al. Adjunctive intraoperative arterial dilation. Arch Surg 116:1391-1398, 1981.
9. Pfeiffer RB Jr, String ST. Adjunctive use of the balloon dilatation catheter during vascular reconstructive procedures. J Vasc Surg 3:841-845, 1986.
10. White RA, White GH. Laser thermal probe recanalization of occluded arteries. J Vasc Surg 9:594-604, 1989.
11. Sanborn TA, Faxon DP, Haudenschild C, et al. Experimental angioplasty-circumferential distribution of laser thermal energy with a laser probe. J Am Coll Cardiol 5:934-938, 1985.
12. White RA, White GH, Mehringer MC, et al. A clinical trial of laser thermal angioplasty in patients with advanced peripheral vascular disease. Ann Surg 212:257-265, 1990.
13. Perler BA, Osterman FA, White RI Jr, et al. Percutaneous laser probe femoropopliteal angioplasty: A preliminary experience. J Vasc Surg 10:351-357, 1989.
14. Blebea J, Ouriel K, Green RM, et al. Laser angioplasty in peripheral vascular disease: Symptomatic versus hemodynamic results. J Vasc Surg 13:222-230, 1991.
15. Rosenthal D, Pesa FA, Gottsegen WL, et al. Thermal laser-assisted balloon angioplasty of the superficial femoral artery: A multicenter review of 602 cases. J Vasc Surg 14:152-159, 1991.
16. Feinberg RL, Gregory RT, Parent FN, et al. Rotational atherectomy and laser angioplasty: Do they have a role in the treatment of infrainguinal atherosclerosis? In Veith FJ, ed. Current Critical Problems in Vascular Surgery, vol 4. St. Louis: Quality Medical Publishing, 1992, pp 163-171.
17. Matsumoto T, Okamura T, Rajyaguru V. Laser arterial disobstructive procedures in 148 lower extremities. J Vasc Surg 10:169-177, 1989.
18. Criado FJ, Queral LA, Patten P, et al. Laser angioplasty in the lower extremities: An early surgical experience. J Vasc Surg 11:532-535, 1990.
19. Dietrich EB, Timbadia E, Bahadir I. Applications and limitations of laser-assisted angioplasty. Eur J Vasc Surg 3:61-70, 1989.
20. The Collaborative Rotablator Atherectomy Group (CRAG). Peripheral atherectomy with the rotablator: A multicenter report. J Vasc Surg 19:509-515, 1994.
21. Palmaz JC, Garcia OJ, Schatz RA, et al. Placement of balloon-expandable intraluminal stents in iliac arteries: First 171 procedures. Radiology 174:969-975, 1990.
22. Veith FJ. Presidential address: Transluminally placed endovascular stented grafts and their impact on vascular surgery. J Vasc Surg 20:855-860, 1994.
23. Parodi JC. Endovascular repair of abdominal aortic aneurysms and other arterial lesions. J Vasc Surg 21:549-557, 1995.
24. Chuter TAM, Green RM, Ouriel K, et al. Transfemoral endovascular aortic graft placement. J Vasc Surg 18:185-197, 1993.
25. Moore WS, Vescera CL. Repair of abdominal aortic aneurysm by transfemoral endovascular graft placement. Ann Surg 220:331-341, 1994.
26. Veith FJ, Gupta SK, Wengerter KR, et al. Changing arteriosclerotic disease patterns and management strategies in lower-limb-threatening ischemia. Ann Surg 212:402-414, 1990.
27. Chuter TAM, Green RM, Ouriel K, et al. Infrarenal aortic aneurysm structure: Implications for transfemoral repair. J Vasc Surg 20:44-50, 1994.
28. Veith FJ, Marin ML. Endovascular surgery and its effect on the relationship between vascular surgery and radiology. J Endovasc Surg 2:1-7, 1995.
29. Veith FJ, Abbott WM, Yao JST, et al. Guidelines for development and use of transluminally placed endovascular prosthetic grafts in the arterial system. J Vasc Surg 21:670-685, 1995.
30. White RA, Fogarty TJ, Baker WH, et al. Endovascular surgery credentialing and training for vascular surgeons. J Vasc Surg 17:1095-1102, 1993.

9

Subcutaneous Video-Assisted Saphenous Vein Harvest: A Minimally Invasive Technique for Vein Procurement

ALAN B. LUMSDEN, M.D., WILLIAM D. JORDAN, Jr., M.D., and F. FELMONT EAVES III, M.D.

Approximately 330,000 coronary artery bypass grafts were performed in the United States in 1987, an increase from 190,000 in 1983. The saphenous vein was used as the conduit in 98% of cases. An additional 100,000 saphenectomies are carried out annually for lower extremity revascularization. Indeed, saphenous vein harvest is one of the most commonly performed procedures. Removal of the vein is, however, only an adjunct to the principal procedure (i.e., performing the bypass). This perhaps is the reason why there have been essentially no significant developments in vein procurement.

There are scant data on complications of saphenous vein harvest in either the cardiac or peripheral vascular literature. Major wound complications following vein harvest are relatively rare (1% to 2%), but minor complications are very common yet rarely discussed. Complications associated with saphenous vein harvest are listed below:

Immediate
    Hematoma
    Saphenous nerve injury
    Leg pain
Intermediate
    Skin necrosis
    Fat necrosis
    Wound drainage
    Wound infection
    Wound separation
    Lymph leakage
Late
    Recurrent cellulitis
    Recurrent lymphangitis
    Limb swelling

The impact of harvest site complications is variable. Common complications including delayed healing, limb swelling, and incision pain affect poorly documented parameters such as length of hospital stay, ability to ambulate, and return to employment. Less common complications such as wound necrosis, gangrene, and amputation are more conspicuous and better documented. Impaired wound healing, defined as inflammation, wound separation, necrosis, or drainage, has been reported to range from 1.1% to 24.3% of patients and has been closely associated with female sex, obesity, diabetes, peripheral arterial disease, and elevated left ventricular end-diastolic pressure. The 24.3% incidence of healing impairment at the harvest site comes from the only prospective study to examine complications in the harvest of greater saphenous vein (GSV). In this series, wounds were inspected daily until the patient was discharged from the hospital and then weekly until complete healing was documented. Based on the same criteria for impaired wound healing of the saphenous harvest site compared to sternotomy, only 0.8% of sternal wounds were affected.

Laparoscopic procedures, particularly cholecystectomy, have demonstrated to the surgical community the impact of eliminating a large skin and muscle incision on postoperative pain, immobility, and length of hospitalization. Initial laparoscopic operations were limited to those locations where a natural optical cavity (e.g., pleural space, peritoneal space, bladder, or joints) provided ease of instrument insertion, visualization, and device manipulation. However, it has become increasingly apparent that an adequate optical cavity can be created by exploiting tissue interfaces (e.g., subcutaneous tissue-deep fascia or deep fascia-muscle) and surgically creating a space in which procedures can be performed. Furthermore, it has recently become feasible to create an optical cavity where no such natural tissue plane exists or is at best poorly defined. Such techniques have been made possible by the development of appropriate mechanical retractor systems that obviate the need for insufflation.

During the past 2 years, there has been increasing interest in the development of subcutaneous endoscopic surgery. Such techniques have been employed particularly in the field of plastic surgery, at locations in the body where remote incisions and reduced incision size have minimized scarring and improved cosmetic results. These operations have been conducted using gasless techniques, with a mechanical retractor system providing appropriate exposure. Such pioneering procedures have demonstrated the feasibility of subcutaneous dissection techniques and have the potential for widespread application throughout the surgical subspecialties. We have developed a subcutaneous video-assisted technique for harvest of saphenous vein using a technique described herein.

OPERATIVE TECHNIQUE

The patient is placed supine on the operating table and the entire leg is prepared. The saphenofemoral junction is surface marked 5 cm below and 2 cm lateral to the pubic tubercle. If a femoropopliteal graft is to be performed, the skin incision begins over the common femoral artery and angles inferomedially toward the saphenofemoral junction. When vein harvest is being performed for a remote bypass or for the opposite leg, the incision begins more medially and inferiorly, directly over the saphenofemoral junction.

If the surgeon is right-handed, then dissection distally from the groin wound is most comfortably performed with the surgeon standing on the left side of the patient. The retractor is held in the surgeon's left hand and the scissors are held in the right hand. For a right-handed surgeon, dissection in a cranial direction from the popliteal incision is best performed with the surgeon on the patient's right side, viewing a monitor positioned on the patient's left.

Through the groin incision the saphenous vein is identified, and the saphenofemoral junction is dissected using traditional open techniques with self-retaining retractors to provide exposure. Once the saphenofemoral junction has been carefully defined and the branches ligated, the dissection is begun in a caudal direction along the GSV. The vein is exposed using small Richardson retractors. After a tunnel has been developed anterior to the GSV distally for approximately 4 cm, the Emory endoplastic retractor (Snowden-Pencer, Tucker, Ga.) (Fig. 1) is introduced into the tunnel anterior to the GSV. Video imaging is achieved through a 30-degree angled

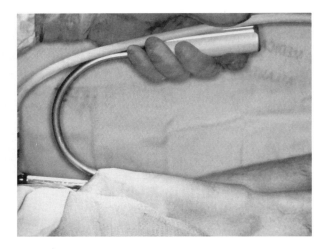

Fig. 1 Snowden-Pencer retractor with Hopkins rod scope.

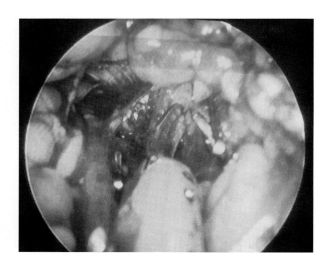

Fig. 2 View of the vein down the tunnel.

Hopkins rod scope inserted into the retractor (Fig. 2). The image is displayed with an Olympus three-chip camera (Olympus America, Inc., Lake Success, N.Y.) on a 19-inch monitor. The optimal operating arrangement calls for dual monitors to be placed at eye level on opposite sides of the patient for ease of viewing by both the surgeon and his or her assistant. Dual monitors are particularly timesaving when the direction of dissection changes from caudal to cranial during the switch from the inguinal to the popliteal incision.

Dissection is then continued along the vein in

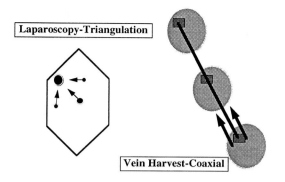

Fig. 3 Comparison of vein harvest with laparoscopy.

a coaxial fashion (Fig. 3), initially using standard open surgical instruments, while viewing the monitors, to the limit of comfortable dissection. At this point laparoscopic instruments are introduced. It is most expeditious to begin the dissection anterior to the GSV. The vein is roofed over by transverse fascial bands. There are very few anterior branches; consequently dissection in this plane progresses rapidly. Upward retraction on the tunnel permits the vein to fall posteriorly, which is readily viewed from above with the 30-degree scope. Once the anterior aspect has been freed for a distance of approximately 6 inches, the lateral and posterior margins are dissected.

Vein harvest is largely a one-person procedure. For a right-handed surgeon, the Emory endoplastic retractor is held in the left hand, elevating the roof of the tunnel, while dissection proceeds with the scissors held in the right hand. An assistant may place gentle traction on the vein or hook the vein to one side of the tunnel to facilitate exposure. Metzenbaum and 5 mm endoscissors (Ethicon Endo-Surgery, Cincinnati, Ohio) are the primary dissection instruments used. The latter are particularly useful because they may be bent to an appropriate shape for ease of use in the thigh.

Side branches greater than 3 mm in diameter are clipped with 5 mm Allclips (Ethicon Endo-Surgery) and divided with scissors. Smaller branches are cauterized with microbipolar cautery forceps and then divided. Division of fat adjacent to the vein is frequently necessary to maintain the width of the tunnel, which should be approximately 3 cm wide. Occasionally, in the distal thigh, the vein appears tethered to the roof of the tunnel. In this case further dissection superficial to the vein demonstrates a small anterior branch; division of this branch permits the vessel to drop back to the floor of the tunnel.

As additional lengths of vein are dissected, the retractor and its contained scope are advanced into the developing wound. Caudal dissection continues until the limits of the retractor are reached. At that point a separate counterincision is made over the vein above the knee. Accurate positioning of this incision in an obese leg may be facilitated by preoperative vein mapping using color-flow duplex ultrasound. This incision is initially deepened using traditional methods until the vein is identified. Cranial and caudal dissection is then begun until the tunnels are developed to permit introduction of the retractor system. Dissection then continues cranially until the proximal and distal tunnels connect. At that point the vein lies free in the posterior aspect of the tunnel. Caudal dissection across the knee and down into the calf then begins using an identical technique. Depending on the length of vein needed, a separate counterincision in the midcalf may be required. When the vein is dissected below the knee, care must be taken to avoid injuring the saphenous nerve. This is a sensory nerve that joins the vein at a variable location in the upper third of the leg, piercing the deep fascia between the tendons of the sartorius and gracilis muscles. It runs inferiorly on the medial side of the saphenous vein and is readily identified through the videoscope.

Once an adequate length of vein has been dissected, clips may be applied across the GSV and then divided. Frequently a few posterior fascial attachments tether the vein and must be divided prior to removal. The vein is then retracted up through the proximal incisions, divided at the saphenofemoral junction, and removed. Following removal, the distal end of the vein is cannulated, and heparinized saline solution is injected into the vein to check for leaks. Clips are removed from the side branches and ligated with 4-0 silk. Nonligated side branches are also tied and any leaks close to the vein wall are repaired with 6-0 Prolene.

Harvest site wounds are left open until the bypass procedure has been completed. The Emory endoplastic retractor is then reinserted into the wound and the entire tunnel is inspected for adequacy of hemostasis. Any bleeding points are grasped and cauterized using the bipolar forceps. Larger vessels may be grasped and endoclips applied. The tunnel is then irrigated and rolled with a gauze pad from its midpoint in a cranial and caudal direction to evacuate any hematoma. Seven-millimeter Jackson-Pratt drains are placed in the tunnel prior to closure through separate stab incisions. Recently we have opted to reverse the anticoagulation with protamine, recheck the tunnel with the endoscope following the reversal, and omit placement of a drain.

Wounds are then closed with one to two layers of continuous 3-0 subcutaneous Vicryl sutures, with 4-0 subcuticular Vicryl and Steri-Strips for skin closure. The harvest site is loosely wrapped with a 6-inch elastic bandage for 24 hours.

Harvest of the vein below the knee to the level of the ankle is more difficult (Fig. 4) with presently available instrumentation because of the lack of subcutaneous space. It does, however, avoid a skin incision below the distal third of the leg and obviates the need for parallel ankle incisions when a distal bypass is performed (Fig. 5).

PROBLEMS WITH THE CURRENT APPROACH AND FUTURE DEVELOPMENTS

Although we have demonstrated the feasibility of subcutaneous saphenous vein harvest, the preceding method represents an initial attempt to carry out the procedure. The principal problems with the technique include passing instruments down a long tunnel, holding open the optical cavity, manipulating the vein in a long narrow tunnel, and navigating the tight confines of the subcutaneous space below the knee.

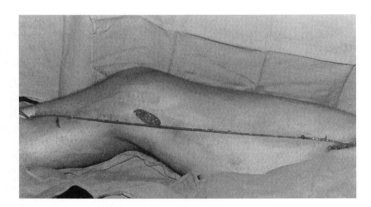

Fig. 4 Leg following removal of the vein to midcalf level.

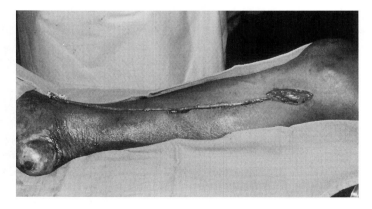

Fig. 5 Harvest of the vein below the knee.

All of these factors contribute to what we consider to be excessive harvest times—45 minutes for the thigh and 1½ hours for extension to the midcalf. This we believe limits widespread acceptance of the procedure, particularly for coronary artery bypass grafting. Our target harvest time for the entire leg is 45 minutes. Achieving this goal will be a function of improved instrumentation and expanded surgical experience. A second generation of instruments is currently under development.

BIBLIOGRAPHY

Adar R, Meyer E, Zweig A. Saphenous neuralgia: A complication of vascular reconstructions below the knee. Ann Surg 190:609-613, 1979.

American Heart Association. Heart and Stroke Facts. Dallas, Texas, 1990.

Baddour LM, Bisno AL. Recurrent cellulitis after saphenous venectomy for coronary bypass surgery. Ann Intern Med 97:493-496, 1982.

Baddour LM, Bisno AL. Recurrent cellulitis after coronary bypass surgery. JAMA 251:1049-1052, 1984.

Bailey RW, Zucker KA, Flowers JL, et al. Laparoscopic cholecystectomy: Experience with 375 consecutive patients. Ann Surg 214:531-541, 1991.

Carr RD, Rau RC. Dermatitis at vein graft site in coronary artery bypass patients. Arch Dermatol 117:814-815, 1981.

Chauhan BM, Kim DJ, Wainapel SF. Saphenous neuropathy following coronary artery bypass surgery. NY State J Med 81:222-224, 1981.

Dan M, Shapira I, Yakirewitch, et al. Erysipelas after venectomy for coronary bypass surgery. Isr J Med Sci 19:1100-1101, 1983.

DeLaria GA, Hunter JA, Goldin MD, Serry C, Javid H, Najafi H. Leg wound complications associated with coronary revascularization. J Thorac Cardiovasc Surg 81:403-407, 1981.

Dowden RV, Anain S. Endoscopic implant evaluation and capsulotomy. Plast Reconstr Surg 91:283-287, 1993.

File TM, Tan JS, Maseelal EA, Snyder RO. Recurrent cellulitus after bypass surgery associated with psoriasis. JAMA 252:1681, 1984.

Greenburg J, DeSanctis RW, Mills RM. Vein-donor-leg cellulitis after coronary artery bypass surgery. Ann Intern Med 97:565-566, 1982.

Harrington EB, Harrington ME, Schanzer H, et al. End-stage renal disease—Is infrainguinal limb revascularization justified? J Vasc Surg 12:691-696, 1990.

Hill SL. Relationship between ankle/arm blood pressure indices and healing of the harvest vein incision in coronary artery bypass patients. J Vasc Tech 11:232-235, 1987.

Hinder RA, Filipi CJ, Wetscher G, et al. Laparoscopic Nissen fundoplication is an effective treatment for gastroesophageal reflux disease. Ann Surg 220:472-483, 1994.

Ho LCY. Endoscopic assisted transaxillary augmentation mammoplasty. Br J Plast Surg 46:332-336, 1993.

Hurwitz RM, Tisserand ME. Streptococcal cellulitis proved by skin biopsy in a coronary artery bypass graft patient. Arch Dermatol 121:908-909, 1985.

Jugenheimer M, Junginger TH. Endoscopic subfascial sectioning of incompetent perforating veins in treatment of primary varicosis. World J Surg 16:971-975, 1992.

Lavee J, Schneiderman J, Yorav S, Shewach-Millet M, Adar R. Complications of saphenous vein harvesting following coronary artery bypass surgery. J Cardiovasc Surg 30:989-991, 1989.

Laws HL, McKernan BM. Endoscopic management of peptic ulcer disease. Ann Surg 217:548-556, 1993.

Lee KS, Reinstein L. Lower limb amputation of the donor site extremity after coronary artery bypass graft surgery. Arch Phys Med Rehabil 67:564-565, 1986.

Liehr P, Todd B, Rossi M, Culligan M. Cardiac surgical care: Effect of venous support on edema and leg pain in patients after coronary artery bypass graft surgery. Heart Lung 21:6-11, 1992.

Lumsden AB, Besman A, Jaffe MB, MacDonald MJ, Allen RC. Infrainguinal revascularization in end-stage renal disease. Ann Vasc Surg 8:107-112, 1994.

Lumsden AB, Eaves FF. Subcutaneous, video-assisted saphenous vein harvest. Perspect Vasc Surg 7:43-55, 1994.

Lumsden AB, Eaves FF. Vein harvest. In Bostwick J, Eaves FF, Nahai F, eds. Endoscopic Plastic Surgery. St. Louis: Quality Medical Publishing, 1995, pp 535-543.

Meldrum-Hanna W, Ross D, Johnson D, Deal C. Long saphenous vein harvesting. Aust N Z J Surg 56:923-924, 1986.

Narayanan K, Liang MD, Chandra M, Grundfest WS. Experimental endoscopic subcutaneous surgery. J Laparoendosc Surg 2:179-183, 1992.

Saltz R, Stowers R, Smith M, Gadacz TR. Laparoscopically harvested omental free flap to cover a large soft tissue defect. Ann Surg 5:542-547, 1993.

Scher LA, Samson RH, Ketosugbo A, Gupta SK, Ascer E, Veith F. Prevention and management of ischemic complications of vein harvest incisions in cardiac surgery—Case reports. Angiology 37:119-123, 1986.

Schnall B, Luis ES. Saphenous neuropathy following coronary bypass. Orthop Rev 8:121-122, 1979.

Southern Surgeons Club. A prospective analysis of 1518 laparoscopic cholecystectomies. N Engl J Med 324:1073-1078, 1991.

Teimourian B, Kroll SS. Subcutaneous endoscopy in suction lipectomy. Plast Reconstr Surg 74:708-711, 1984.

U.S. Department of Health and Human Services. Detailed diagnoses and surgical procedures for patients discharged from short stay hospitals. Public Health Service, National Center for Health Statistics: Vital and Health Statistics Series 13. DHHS publication No. (PHS) 85-1743, Rockville, Md.: National Center for Health Statistics, 1983.

Utley JR, Thomason ME, Wallace DJ, Mutch DW, Staton L, Brown V, Wilde CM, Bell MS. Preoperative correlates of impaired wound healing after saphenous vein excision. J Thorac Cardiovasc Surg 98:147-149, 1989.

Weewood JM, Cox SJ, Martin A, et al. Sensory changes following stripping of the long saphenous vein. J Cardiovasc Surg 16:123-124, 1975.

Weisman EB. Veins for coronary bypass surgery and cellulitis. Ann Intern Med 98:113, 1983.

Whittemore AD, Donaldson MC, Mannick JA. Infrainguinal reconstruction for patients with chronic renal insufficiency. J Vasc Surg 17:32-41, 1993.

10

Current Status of Peripheral Atherectomy

SAMUEL S. AHN, M.D., and BLESSIE CONCEPCION, B.S.

Recent advances in endovascular technology have generated a variety of alternative procedures and instruments for treating peripheral arterial occlusive disease. Mechanical atherectomy has been developed as an alternative to conventional percutaneous transluminal angioplasty (PTA) because of its limitations, which include dissection of the vessel wall and acute occlusion in 3% to 5% of cases,[1-3] difficulty in treating long, complex stenotic or occluded lesions,[4] and high restenosis rates of 30% to 40% within 6 months.[5-10] Atherectomy devices can selectively remove an atheroma by cutting or pulverizing it in atherosclerotic diseased arteries percutaneously with angiographic guidance or openly through a small arteriotomy distant from the diseased site under fluoroscopic or angioscopic control. Theoretically, atherectomy offers the following advantages over PTA: (1) greater immediate success with lower rates of intimal dissection and acute occlusion as a result of controlled removal of atheroma from the lumen; (2) wider application to complex lesions not readily amenable to PTA; and (3) reduction in restenosis rates as a result of the debulking of atheromatous mass.

There are currently two types of atherectomy procedures: extirpative and ablative. Extirpative atherectomy is characterized by shaving, cutting, or directly removing the atheroma and collecting the excised material from the vessel lumen and wall. Ablative atherectomy, on the other hand, uses a high-speed rotational device to pulverize the atheroma into fragments small enough to be aspirated or removed through the reticuloendothelial system. Among the numerous atherectomy devices currently available, only four have undergone extensive clinical trials: extirpative catheters including the Simpson Atherocath and the transluminal extraction catheter, and ablative devices including the Trac-Wright catheter and the Auth Rotablator. This chapter will discuss the unique features, complications, and limitations of each device including the results of some of these clinical trials. Furthermore, a new directional atherectomy device, the Omnicath, which is currently undergoing investigative trials, will be discussed briefly.

SIMPSON ATHERECTOMY DEVICE
Device Description

The Simpson peripheral atherectomy catheter (Atherocath; Devices for Vascular Intervention, Redwood City, Calif.) is a semiflexible catheter with a distal housing unit, a cutter, a retrieval chamber, and an opposing balloon. A flexible guidewire attached to the distal tip of the housing unit enables the operator to advance and partially steer the catheter. A battery-powered, cup-shaped cutter excises the atheroma after balloon dilatation, causing the longitudinal side-opening of the housing unit to engulf the atheroma. Conveniently designed with a hand-held motor, the cutter spins at approximately 2000 rpm. As the cutter swirls, it forces the plaque into the collecting chamber in the distal tip. The catheter is available in 7, 8, 9, 10, and 11 Fr sizes. The cutting window has been designed in both 15 and 20 mm lengths. Some models include an ultrasound chip in the cutting window for precise alignment with the lesion before and after a cut is made for evaluation. Also available is an extended flexible collecting chamber unit that allows multiple cuts.

Techniques

The Simpson atherectomy procedure is illustrated in Fig. 1. First, the atherectomy catheter is advanced past the stenotic lesion. Under fluoroscopic guidance, the catheter is positioned with the cutting window directly facing the plaque. The balloon is inflated to 20 to 40 psi to push the open chamber against the arterial lesion, thereby wedging the atheroma into the window. Then the motor drive of the cutter is activated with the rotating circular blade cutting

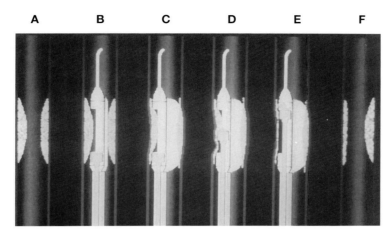

Fig. 1 Simpson atherectomy procedure. **A,** The lesion before atherectomy. **B,** The atherectomy catheter in position across the lesion. **C,** The balloon support is inflated. **D,** The cutter is advanced. **E,** The specimen is trapped in the housing. **F,** The balloon is deflated and the catheter is removed. (From Hinohara T, Robertson GC, Selmon MR, Simpson JB. Transluminal atherectomy: The Simpson atherectomy catheter. In Moore WS, Ahn SS, eds. Endovascular Surgery. Philadelphia: WB Saunders, 1989, p 312.)

Table 1 Applications of atherectomy devices

Device	Amenable lesions	Arterial site	Complications/limitations
Simpson	Stenoses 　Short (<5 cm) 　Eccentric atheroma 　Ulcerative plaque 　Intimal hyperplasia	Iliac Superficial femoral Popliteal	Bulky/stiff catheter Lengthy procedure Hematoma Restenosis
TEC	Stenoses 　Short (<5 cm) 　Concentric atheroma	Superficial femoral Popliteal	Lumen produced too small Restenosis/reocclusion
Trac-Wright	Occlusions 　Short (<5 cm) Stenoses 　Focal	Superficial femoral Popliteal	Dissection Embolization Perforation Reocclusion
Auth Rotablator	Stenoses 　Long or short 　Calcified 　Eccentric or concentric atheroma	Iliac Superficial femoral Popliteal Tibial	Restenosis/reocclusion Thrombosis Microemboli

the selected atheroma and pushing it into the distal collecting chamber. Multiple cuts and passages are required for complete extirpative atherectomy. Once the collecting chamber is full, the catheter is withdrawn and the atheromatous material is removed from the chamber. This entire process is repeated until the diseased vessel is completely recanalized.

Indications

The Simpson atherectomy device is best suited for treatment of short, discrete, and eccentrically placed atheroma (Table 1). With a wide range of catheter sizes available, the Simpson Atherocath is the only atherectomy device with an expansion ratio similar to that of conventional PTA. Thus stenotic, intimal hyperplastic, and ulcerative atherosclerotic lesions are amenable to treatment. However, heavily calcified and occlusive lesions can pose difficulties for the cutter. This atherectomy device can also be used as an adjunct to PTA in treating calcific eccentric stenoses that are nonreceptive to dilatation.

Table 2 Simpson atherectomy

Year	Study	No. of patients	No. of lesions	Initial success (%)	Clinical patency (%)			
					2 mo	6 mo	12 mo	24 mo
1988	Simpson et al.[11]	61	136	87	87	69	—	—
1990	Polnitz et al.[12]	60	94	82	—	99	72	—
1990	Hinohara et al.[13]	100	195	90	—	83	—	—
1990	Graor and Whitlow[14]	106	106	100/93*	—	—	93/86†	—
1991	Dorros et al.[15]	126	213	99	—	45	—	—
1992	Kim et al.[16]	77‡	85	92	—	—	92§	84§
1993	Lugmayr et al.[17]	94	132	95	—	—	69	42
1995	Vroegindewij et al.[18]	38	38	92	—	84	42	35

*100% for lesions ≤5 cm; 93% for lesions >5 cm.
†93% for lesions ≤5 cm; 86% for lesions >5 cm.
‡Adjunctive PTA was performed in 17 (22%) of 77 patients.
§Calculated probability patencies of lesions treated with atherectomy alone were determined using the Kaplan-Meier technique.

Results

Several institutions have reported their experience with the Simpson atherectomy device since its development (Table 2).[11-18] All of these studies have reported impressively high initial success rates varying from 82% to 100%. In spite of these excellent initial success rates, follow-up has been relatively short until recently. The most impressive intermediate results were reported by Graor and Whitlow[14] with a patency rate of 93% for lesions ≤5 cm and 86% for lesions >5 cm at 1 year. Unlike other series in which initial success rates were defined as stenosis <30% to 50% after atherectomy, Graor and Whitlow achieved <20% stenosis among the initially successful patients. However, the long-term patency results of 42% and 35% at 2 years reported by Lugmayr et al.[17] and Vroegindewij et al.,[18] respectively, were disappointing compared to the 95% and 92% initial success rates, respectively. These long-term results clearly are no better than those of PTA.

In an attempt to compare the outcome of Simpson atherectomy with that of PTA, Kim et al.[16] evaluated the patients who underwent atherectomy alone separately from those who underwent combined atherectomy and PTA. They reported calculated probability patencies of 92%, 84%, and 84% at 1, 2, and 3 years, respectively, for lesions (n = 68) treated with the Simpson atherectomy alone and 78%, 67%, and 57%, respectively, for lesions (n = 17) treated with atherectomy and PTA. Conversely, Vroegindewij et al.[18] reported a cumulative 2-year patency rate of 35% in lesions (n = 38) treated with the Simpson atherectomy device alone and 56% in lesions (n = 35) treated with PTA alone. These inconsistencies in reporting endovascular procedures raise serious concerns regarding the proper evaluation of a device, its efficacy, and comparison of different treatment modalities.

Complications and Limitations

Complications related to the Simpson Atherocath have been relatively manageable[11-14,16,18] except for one death reported by Graor and Whitlow[14] (Table 3). They reported an acute myocardial infarction as a result of cardiogenic shock in a patient with a complex lesion of >5 cm occlusion. Major complications include hematoma caused by bleeding at the atherectomy entry site, pseudoaneurysm, and distal embolization. Graor and Whitlow[14] also reported seven cases of hematoma that required major intervention including one patient who also had a pseudoaneurysm. Kim et al.[16] attributed the 11 cases of hematoma in their study to the larger 7 to 12 Fr arterial sheaths used and reported three cases of pseudoaneurysm that required surgical repair. A few cases of distal embolization were also noted,[11-13,16] which required surgical repair in severe cases, urokinase infusion, or no treatment if clinically insignificant.

Simpson et al.[11] developed the concept of directional atherectomy to debulk atheromatous material without dissections or flaps, leaving a smooth luminal wall, along with the expectation of reducing the restenosis rate. The restenosis results reported are still widely disparate.[11-18] Simpson et al.[11] reported a restenosis rate of 36% at 6 months, and Polnitz et al.[12] reported rates of 24% and 11% at 6 months for concentric and

Table 3 Complications of the Simpson atherectomy device

Complications	Simpson et al.[11]	Polnitz et al.[12]	Hinohara et al.[13]	Graor and Whitlow[14]	Kim et al.[16]	Vroegindewij et al.[18]
Cardiorespiratory	—	—	—	1/106 (1%)	—	—
Dissection	3/61 (5%)	—	—	—	—	2/38 (5%)
Embolization	1/61 (2%)	1/60 (2%)	2/100 (2%)	—	3/77 (4%)	—
Hematoma	—	2/60 (3%)	1/100 (1%)	7/106 (7%)	11/77 (14%)	—
Pseudoaneurysm	—	—	—	1/106 (1%)	3/77 (4%)	—
Retroperitoneal bleeding	—	—	—	—	1/77 (1%)	—
Thrombosis	1/61 (2%)	—	1/100 (1%)	—	—	1/38 (3%)

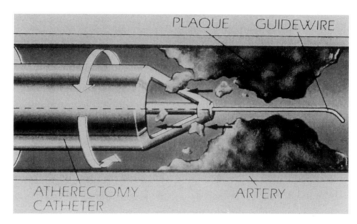

Fig. 2 Cartoon depiction of atherectomy with the transluminal extraction catheter. See text for description.

eccentric lesions, respectively. In contrast, Dorros et al.[15] obtained a 55% recurrence rate at 6 months.

Early studies with the Simpson Atherocath claim that it is relatively ineffective in treating long, diffusely diseased lesions and long, occluded lesions. Polnitz et al.[12] reported a 7.1% restenosis rate at 12 months in patients with simple (≤5 cm) lesions and a 14% rate in patients with complex (>5 cm) occlusion. Vroegindewij et al.,[18] on the other hand, recently reported that their patency rate at 1 year for lesions ≥2 cm treated with the Simpson atherectomy device alone was significantly lower (14%) than that for lesions <2 cm (50%). Furthermore, their patency rate at 1 year for lesions ≥2 cm treated with PTA alone was 66% and 72% for lesions <2 cm.

TRANSLUMINAL EXTRACTION CATHETER
Device Description

The transluminal extraction catheter (TEC) (Interventional Technologies, San Diego, Calif.) is a semiflexible, torque-controlled, hollow catheter. The catheter is available in 5, 7, 9, and 11 Fr sizes. The rotating cone-shaped cutter tracks over the central guidewire (Fig. 2). The cutter rotates at approximately 700 rpm and leaves relatively large-sized (1 mm) particles. Suction, applied from the proximal port, aspirates atheroma particles through the hollow catheter into a separate collecting vacuum bottle (125 ml), making embolic complications unlikely. To maintain efficiency in the aspiration of particles, continuous heparin irrigation is required through the introducer sheath.

Technique

The procedure is generally performed percutaneously, although it can be done intraoperatively. An introducer sheath of appropriate size is placed in the artery, and a guidewire is passed through the obstructive lesion placing it in position. A 4 or 5 Fr polyethylene exchange catheter is inserted into the artery and a 0.014-inch TEC wire is positioned to replace the initial

Table 4 Transluminal extraction catheter

Year	Study	No. of lesions	No. of adjunct PTAs	Technical success (%)	Immediate clinical success (%)	Clinical patency (%) 6 mo	Clinical patency (%) 12 mo
1989	Wholey and Jarmalowski[19]	126	46	92	90	—	—
1994	Myers et al.[20]	144*	109	86	78.8	67	51

*Adjunctive stenting was performed in 17 lesions.

guidewire. The exchange catheter is removed, and the TEC catheter is passed over the TEC guidewire until the catheter meets resistance at the obstructive lesion. The motorized rotating drive unit is activated while suction is applied. The rotating cutter is passed gently over the guidewire until the occluded section is traversed. Fluoroscopy documents the progress of atherectomy and shows the final stage of the lumen. If there is significant residual stenosis, standard balloon angioplasty is performed to dilate the artery to a satisfactory final size.

Indications

Previous clinical trials have used the TEC device primarily to treat total occlusions and long, stenotic lesions.[19,20] However, the treatment of such lesions usually required adjunctive techniques such as PTA to facilitate and/or complete the recanalization of a lesion (Table 4). Thus the currently available TEC atherectomy device is recommended for use only in short, stenotic lesions with eccentrically placed atheroma (see Table 1).

Results

In spite of the appealing concept of directly removing and aspirating the atheroma from circulation, few clinical investigators[19,20] have reported their results of TEC peripheral atherectomy in a reasonably large number of patients. Furthermore, most of these investigators have used adjunctive PTA to obtain a satisfactory lumen: Wholey and Jarmolowski[19] performed adjunctive PTA in 46(37%) of 126 lesions and Myers et al.[20] in 109(76%) of 144 lesions. Again it is difficult to evaluate the efficacy of a device when it is combined with another treatment modality.

Although the initial technical success and immediate clinical success rates reported seem promising, follow-up results have been either lacking[19] or relatively limited[20] (see Table 4). Wholey and Jarmolowski[19] reported an impressive 92% technical success rate and a 90% clinical success rate, even though 60 of their first 95 patients had severe claudication and 30 had one or more significant risk factors. However, only 50 patients had a 6-month follow-up evaluation, 16 of whom underwent repeat angiography. Myers et al.[20] obtained an initial technical success rate of 86% and a clinical success rate of 74% in treating 55 lesions (24 stenoses and 31 occlusions) <5 cm and 70 lesions (11 stenoses and 59 occlusions) between 5 and 10 cm, and 19 lesions (4 stenoses and 15 occlusions) >10 cm. Primary patency rates at 6 months were 80% for lesions ≤5 cm and 64% for lesions >5 cm.

Table 5 Complications of the transluminal extraction catheter

Complications	Wholey and Jarmalowski[19]	Myers et al.[20]
Bleeding	—	3/144 (2%)
Catheter fracture	—	2/144 (1%)
Death	—	2/144 (1%)
Embolization	—	—
Thrombosis	2/126 (2%)	2/144 (1%)

Complications and Limitations

Reports of complications of the TEC device have been scant (Table 5). Of the 126 lesions, Wholey and Jarmolowski[19] reported only two (2%) thrombotic complications in which patency was restored by intra-arterial urokinase administration. Myers et al.[20] reported two deaths (1%) in patients with critical ischemia, fracture of catheters requiring removal and replacement in two (1%), thromboembolism in two (1%), and bleeding at the puncture site in three (2%) within 30 days.

Restenosis and reocclusion are the primary constraints of the TEC device (see Table 1). Of the 16 patients who underwent angiography during the follow-up study, Wholey and Jar-

Table 6 Trac-Wright catheter

Year	Study	No. of lesions	Lesion length (cm) Mean	Lesion length (cm) Range	Technical success (%)	Immediate clinical success (%)	Clinical patency (%) 6 mo	Clinical patency (%) 12 mo	Clinical patency (%) 24 mo
1989	Wholey et al.[21]	12	—	15-40	100	67	—	—	—
1990	Desbrosses et al.[22]	46*	9.8	2-24	87	76	51	40	—
1991	Cull et al.[23]	46*	7.2	1-20	67	59	43	38	37.5
1992	Snyder et al.[24]	46	7.15	2-20	67	59	60	37.5	—
1992	Lukes et al.[25]	12*	—	6-20	58	33	25	25	—
1992	Triller et al.[26]	25*	8	5-15	80	76	59	38	—
1992	Dyet[27]	22*	10.7	3-25	86	80	68	45	—
1993	Meloni et al.[28]	15*	6	—	87	—	51	51	51

*Adjunctive PTA was performed in all cases.

molowski[19] reported restenosis in four patients at 3 months (two of whom underwent combined atherectomy and PTA) and reocclusion in four patients whose lesions were >8 cm in length. At 6 months, Myers et al.[20] reported restenosis in 26 lesions (18%) and reocclusion in 51(35%).

TRAC-WRIGHT CATHETER
Device Description

First known as the Kensey atherectomy device and then as the Theratek catheter, the Trac-Wright catheter (Dow-Corning-Wright, Arlington, Tenn.) is a flexible, ablative atherectomy device with a distal, blunt-nosed cam attached to a central drive shaft (Fig. 3). The rotating cam revolves at 100,000 rpm and seeks the path of least resistance. A high-pressure irrigating system dilates the diseased artery while the rotating cam pulverizes the atherosclerotic intima. The rotating tip selectively micropulverizes fibrous or firm atheromatous tissue while leaving viscoelastic tissue uninjured. The catheter was initially available only in an 8 Fr size and thus required adjunctive balloon angioplasty to create an adequate arterial lumen. The catheter is now also available in 5 and 10 Fr sizes.

Technique

Ablative atherectomy with the Trac-Wright catheter can be performed percutaneously or through a small arteriotomy in the common femoral artery. A 9 Fr introducer sheath is first placed and the catheter is passed through it into the diseased artery. Under fluoroscopic guidance, the catheter tip is positioned directly against the occluded site in the artery. Contrast dye mixed with urokinase, dextran, and heparin is infused at a rate of 30 ml/min. The rotating cam is activated at 100,000 rpm and the catheter is advanced slowly and gently in a to-and-fro manner under direct fluoroscopic control, allowing time for the rotating cam to adequately micropulverize the atheroma. After the recanalization of the occlusive lesion, standard PTA is required to dilate any residual stenosis.

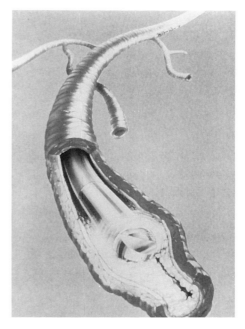

Fig. 3 Trac-Wright catheter is available in 5 and 8 Fr calibers. (From Whittemore AD. The Kensey atherectomy catheter: Indications, technique, results, and complications. In Moore WS, Ahn SS, eds. Endovascular Surgery. Philadelphia: WB Saunders, 1989, p 324.)

Indications

An examination of the clinical investigations of the Trac-Wright catheter (Table 6) indicates that its application has been relatively limited to the treatment of long occlusive lesions[21-28] requiring adjunctive PTA in most of these cases. However, the initial success rates reported are widely disparate, patency rates are poor (see Table 6), and complication rates are high (Table 7). Thus the Trac-Wright catheter appears to be suitable for use in treating short occlusive lesions and focal stenotic lesions (see Table 1).

Results

In most of the clinical trials reported in this series (see Table 6), atherectomy was performed with adjunctive PTA to obtain an adequately large arterial lumen[22,23,25-28] because the Trac-Wright catheter has no expansion ratio. As mentioned earlier, the outcome of such a combination of treatment modalities is confusing in that it is difficult to distinguish the effects and influence of each modality.

The reported initial technical success rates have varied widely from 58% to 100% and clinical success rates from 33% to 80% (see Table 6).[21-28] Overall, patency rates reported at 6 and 12 months have been most disappointing.

Complications and Limitations

Severe complications associated with the Trac-Wright catheter include perforation, dissection, and embolization (see Tables 1 and 7). Perforation induced by the rotating cam occurred mostly in heavily calcified lesions (see Table 7).[22-24,28] These perforations may have been due to the catheter's tendency to follow the path of least resistance, which is often away from hard, calcified plaque. Failure to recanalize occlusive lesions because of plaque dissection is also an immediate complication in some of the reported series (see Table 7).[23,26-28]

In spite of the ablative, micropulverizing ability of the Trac-Wright catheter, some investigators have reported that the atherectomized plaques are not always micropulverized into small particles the size of red blood cells. In studying the distribution and size of atheromatous debris after atherectomy with the Trac-Wright catheter in human cadaveric arteries, Moellmann et al.[29] reported their findings that nearly 80% of all particles ranged from 5 to 15 µm (approximately the size of red blood cells), >20% of particles were >15 µm, and 2% were >100 µm. Indeed, distal embolizations have been documented by some investigators[21,22,26] (see Table 7).

In addition to the complications discussed previously, reocclusion limits the applicability of this device. Wholey et al.[21] reported 4 (33%) of 12 early reocclusions, Desbrosses et al.[22] reported 5 (11%) of 46 reocclusions within 48 hours, and Lukes et al.[25] reported 2 (17%) of 12 reocclusions. Furthermore, Moellmann et al.[29] reported a 50% restenosis/reocclusion rate between 2 weeks and 10 months in treating seven patients with occlusion and three with stenoses.

AUTH ROTABLATOR
Device Description

The Auth Rotablator (Heart Technology, Inc., Bellevue, Wash.) is a flexible, catheter-deliverable, ablative atherectomy device with a variable-sized, football-shaped metal burr on the distal tip (Fig. 4). Multiple diamond chips measuring 22 to 45 µm are embedded in the burr to function as microblades. The burr is available in various sizes ranging from 1.25 to 6.0 mm in diameter. Progressively larger burrs are used during the recanalization process until an adequate arterial lumen is obtained. Rotating at 100,000 to 200,000 rpm, the burr tracks along a central guidewire that must first traverse the lesion before rotational atherectomy can proceed.

The high-speed rotation allows the diamond microchips to attack hard, calcified atheroma preferentially while leaving the surrounding viscoelastic tissue of normal arterial wall intact. The Auth Rotablator leaves a smooth, polished intraluminal surface without intimal flaps (Figs. 5 and 6). The pulverized particles are left in the circulation, with the theoretical assumption that the particles are smaller than red blood cells and thus pass harmlessly through the reticuloendothelial system.

Technique

Atherectomy with the Auth Rotablator is performed preferentially through an open arteriotomy rather than percutaneously. A 9, 12, or 14 Fr introducer sheath is inserted into the artery through the arteriotomy. Using angioscopic or fluoroscopic guidance, a small atraumatic guidewire is passed through the lesion followed by an exchange guiding catheter, a 0.009-inch atherectomy guidewire that is stiffer and more rigid than other standard guidewires. A small burr is passed over the stiff atherectomy guidewire to the site of obstructive lesion. The turbine drive is activated to a rotating speed of

Table 7 Complications of the Trac-Wright catheter

Complications	Wholey et al.[21]	Desbrosses et al.[22]	Cull et al.[23]	Snyder et al.[24]	Lukes et al.[25]	Triller et al.[26]	Dyet[27]	Meloni et al.[28]
Dissection	—	—	2/46 (4%)	—	—	5/25 (20%)	5/22 (23%)	1/15 (7%)
Embolization	1/12 (8%)	3/46 (7%)	—	3/46 (7%)	—	5/25 (20%)	—	—
Hematoma	—	—	2/46 (4%)	3/46 (7%)	1/12 (8%)	—	—	—
Lymphocele	—	—	1/46 (2%)	—	—	—	—	—
Perforation	—	4/46 (9%)	11/46 (24%)	11/46 (24%)	—	—	—	1/15 (7%)
Thrombosis	1/12 (8%)	—	—	—	—	—	—	—

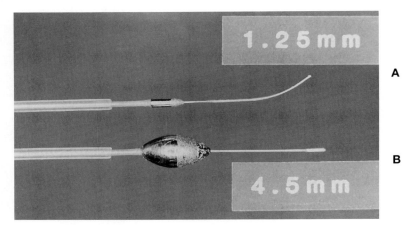

Fig. 4 Rotablator atherectomy burr and guidewire. Burrs shown are 1.25 **(A)** and 4.5 mm **(B)** in diameter. Note the diamond microchips embedded in the distal half of the burr. Also, note the coaxial spring tip **(A)** and semirigid guidewires **(B)**. (From Ahn SS, Auth D, Marcus DR, Moore WS. Removal of focal atheromatous lesions by angioscopically guided high-speed rotary atherectomy: Preliminary experimental observations. J Vasc Surg 7:292-300, 1988.)

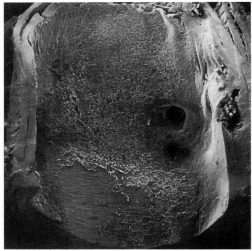

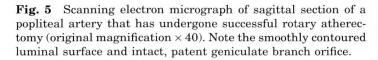

Fig. 5 Scanning electron micrograph of sagittal section of a popliteal artery that has undergone successful rotary atherectomy (original magnification × 40). Note the smoothly contoured luminal surface and intact, patent geniculate branch orifice.

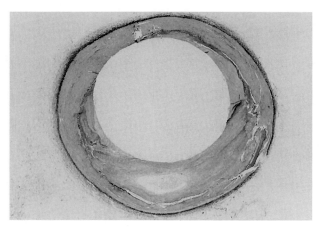

Fig. 6 Cross section of a popliteal artery that has undergone successful rotary atherectomy (Verhoeff's-Giemsa stain; original magnification × 40). Note the smoothly contoured lumen and the essentially intact elastin fibers of the outer media and adventitia.

Table 8 Auth Rotablator

Year	Study	No. of patients	No. of lesions	Technical success (%)	Immediate clinical success (%)	Clinical patency (%) 6 mo	Clinical patency (%) 12 mo	Clinical patency (%) 24 mo
1991	Dorros et al.[30]	43	82	95	88	—	—	—
1993	White et al.[31]	17	18	94	94	82	—	—
1994	CRAG[32]	72	107*	89	77	47	31	18.6
1995	Henry et al.[33]	150	212	97	85	58†	—	—
1995	Myers and Denton[34]	34	36	94	92	68	60.7	—

*107 lesions from 79 limbs.
†At 4 months, 163 lesions were available for evaluation.

100,000 to 200,000 rpm and the burr is advanced slowly over the guidewire in a vibrato-like to-and-fro manner. After the initial atherectomy, the burr is removed and the guidewire is left in place. Then the next size burr is inserted and atherectomy is repeated with progressively larger burrs until an adequate arterial lumen is obtained.

Anticoagulation therapy is administered to the patient during the first 24 hours postoperatively to prevent early thrombosis. Aspirin therapy is administered during long-term follow-up.

Indications

The Auth Rotablator is designed for treating hard, calcified atheroma, especially in diabetic patients who have disabling claudication or limb-threatening ischemia. Long or short, diffusely stenotic lesions also appear uniquely suitable for treatment with the Auth device because these lesions can be readily traversed by a central guidewire (see Table 1). Total occlusions can be treated with the Auth Rotablator only if the central guidewire can traverse the lesion. Eccentric atheroma can be treated quite satisfactorily, since the ablative device preferentially attacks hard, atherosclerotic plaque.

Results

Peripheral atherectomy with the Auth Rotablator has achieved promising initial technical and clinical success rates in several clinical trials (Table 8).[30-34] Most of the series reported only a short follow-up of 6 months and patencies during this time interval were poor, ranging from 47% to 82%.[31-34] Furthermore, patencies at 1 year were worse: the Collaborative Rotablator Atherectomy Group (CRAG) reported a disappointing rate of 31% because of significant early failures and complications in a multicenter trial[32]; Myers and Denton[34] reported a 61% patency rate in a small series of patients.

The CRAG series was the only one in which a long-term study was conducted on the efficacy of the Auth Rotablator.[32] A most disappointing patency rate of 18.6% at 2 years was achieved. Furthermore, these findings revealed that the length of the lesion, indications for atherectomy, use of heparin, and/or the type of lesion (stenosis vs. occlusion) did not significantly influence patency rates.

Complications and Limitations

Peripheral atherectomy with the Auth Rotablator currently has limited application because of its poor long-term results and wide array of complications (Table 9). Significant early thromboses have been reported by the CRAG[32] and Henry et al.[33] Of the nine (11%) thromboses studied by the CRAG, four had an associated hypercoagulable state. Henry et al. attributed the 12 (8%) thromboses in their series to a number of factors including residual stenosis, intimal flaps, elastic recoil, dissection, lengthy lesion, or vasospasm. Arterial spasm has been a frequent complication encountered by Dorros et al.[30] (23%) and Henry et al.[33] (11%) (see Table 9). These arterial spasms occurred mostly in small distal arteries and were attributed to the use of a large burr, long rotation sequences, or the rotation speed.

Gross hemoglobinuria with no clinical sequelae was found in 63% by Dorros et al.[30] and in 13% by the CRAG.[32] These cases were transient and developed in long lesions that required long rotary sequences. Both series also reported cases of groin hematoma that required no surgical intervention (see Table 9). Dorros et al.[30] corre-

Table 9 Complications of the Auth Rotablator

Complications	Dorros et al.[30]	White et al.[31]	CRAG[32]	Henry et al.[33]	Myers and Denton[34]*
Bleeding	—	—	10/79 (13%)	—	1/34 (3%)
Cardiorespiratory	—	1/17 (6%)	—	—	—
Dissection	—	—	5/79 (6%)	3/150 (2%)	—
Embolization	—	—	8/79 (10%)	2/150 (1%)	—
Hematoma	10/43 (23%)	1/17 (6%)	4/79 (5%)	—	—
Hemoglobinuria	27/43 (63%)	—	10/79 (13%)	—	—
Infection	—	—	1/79 (1%)	—	—
Limb loss (device-related)	—	—	2/79 (3%)	—	—
Perforation	2/43 (5%)	—	3/79 (4%)	1/150 (0.7%)	—
Pseudoaneurysm	—	—	1/79 (1%)	—	—
Spasm	10/43 (23%)	—	—	17/150 (11%)	—
Arterial tear	2/43 (5%)	—	—	—	—
Thrombosis	1/43 (2%)	1/17 (6%)	9/79 (11%)	12/150 (8%)	—

*Number of patients who had asymptomatic chemical or macroscopic hemoglobinuria but no change in renal function test results was not reported.

lated the occurrence of hematoma with removal of the sheath immediately after the procedure without reversal of anticoagulation.

Contrary to findings in previous canine studies,[35] the CRAG[32] and Henry et al.[33] demonstrated that some of the atherectomized particles generated by the Auth Rotablator can cause embolic complications (see Table 9). Among the eight embolic events reported by the CRAG, three resulted in cutaneous necrosis and one in toe amputation. Furthermore, in contradistinction to previous studies,[35-37] the perforations and dissections encountered by some of the investigators[30,32,33] (see Table 9) suggest that the arterial wall did not always remain intact. Rapid advancement of the burr may have caused these complications.

In addition to all of the complications previously discussed, late restenoses and reocclusions are significant limiting factors of the Auth Rotablator. Late restenoses and reocclusions occurred in 32 limbs during a follow-up period of 15 to 41 months by the CRAG.[32] Furthermore, arteriographic, angioscopic, or surgical findings in 13 of these lesions suggested intimal hyperplasia. After a follow-up of ≥4 months, Henry et al.[33] reported a 24% restenosis rate. Furthermore, restenosis was more frequent in lesions ≥7 cm.

OMNICATH
Device Description

The Omnicath (American BioMed Inc., The Woodlands, Texas) is a new directional atherectomy device still currently under clinical investigation. This device is comprised of a radiopaque, torque-controlled catheter with a cylindrical housing at the distal end, a longitudinal window on one side, and a nontraumatizing, anchoring deflector wire configuration on the opposite side.[38] This is a unique catheter that has a nonballoon anchoring system, which regulates the depth of cut and provides directional control and distal perfusion. It continuously aspirates the debris and all potential embolic material through a suction port from the operative site.

Technique

The following procedural outline is described in detail by Mazur et al.[38] based on their preliminary animal experiments. The Omnicath is advanced transluminally over a 0.014- or 0.018-inch guidewire. Under fluoroscopic guidance, the cutting window is positioned over the lesion by a radiopaque marker dot on the housing unit distal to the cutting window. The anchoring wire pad is adjusted to the desired depth and stabilized by a gentle tug on the catheter. The cutter is then activated and passed across the lesion while suction is initiated. Additional cuts can be made after repositioning the cutting window.

Indication

The Omnicath atherectomy device is designed for treating concentric and eccentric lesions.[38] The anchoring system has been created to minimize vessel wall injury and perforation and to reduce restenosis. Pending clinical trials will reveal whether the Omnicath can uphold these expectations.

Results

The only preliminary animal data available for the Omnicath were recently reported by Mazur et al.[38] Concentric and eccentric lesions were induced in the bilateral external iliac arteries of 10 miniature swine; this was followed by atherectomy with the Omnicath. Five swine were killed 3 days after atherectomy and the other five at 6 weeks postoperatively. Histologic sections of the 3-day animals revealed depth of cuts ranging from partial plaque removal to near full luminal thickness of the artery. Histologic sections of the 6-week animals showed a minimal healing response. Furthermore, there was no evidence of vessel wall injury or significant neointimal proliferation at the anchoring wire deployment sites. Angiography revealed only one restenosis (20% luminal narrowing) at 6 weeks.

Complications

Postoperative angiography revealed spasm at the atherectomy site in most of the animals. The Omnicath also caused dissection in one lesion. There was no evidence of vessel perforation.

DISCUSSION

Each atherectomy device has been designed to address restenosis/reocclusion and other problems that frequently plague PTA. Each one has utilized remarkable technology to produce the aesthetic result of a smooth lumen without flaps, dissections, perforations, or other abnormalities and consequently reduce the likelihood of thromboembolization and restenosis/reocclusion. Examples of this advanced technology are as follows: the Simpson Atherocath has a retrieval chamber to collect the excised plaque; the TEC uses suction to aspirate the debris; the Trac-Wright catheter has a high-speed rotating cam to micropulverize atheroma without damaging the arterial wall; the Auth Rotablator uses a high-speed rotating burr to micropulverize hard calcified atheroma; and the OmniCath uses an anchoring deflector wire pad to prevent vessel wall injury and neointimal proliferation.

A review of the clinical investigations in which atherectomy devices were used clearly establishes the feasibility of peripheral atherectomy in the treatment of arterial occlusive disease. However, in spite of the impressive and appealing technology associated with these devices, the efficacy of atherectomy remains questionable. Obviously none of the devices can completely fulfill the aforementioned expectations without any complications, but some investigators persist in using these devices as a primary or secondary procedure to minimize the complications commonly associated with PTA alone. Furthermore, although the initial technical and clinical patencies are optimistic, intermediate and long-term patencies are either equivocal or perhaps even worse than those of PTA.

Inconsistencies in reporting endovascular procedures plague most of the clinical data available in the literature. Discrepancies in reporting clinical and hemodynamic assessments, descriptions of lesions, various criteria in reporting early and continued success (short vs. intermediate vs. long-term follow-up), complications, and comparison of different treatment modalities make it difficult if not impossible to precisely evaluate the efficacy of atherectomy devices. Furthermore, any comparison between these inaccurate results and those of other treatment modalities such as PTA is invalid. In reporting endovascular procedures, clinical investigators should refer to and follow the guidelines detailed by the Ad Hoc Subcommittee on Reporting Standards for Endovascular Procedures.[39]

Peripheral atherectomy currently has limited applications in the treatment of arterial occlusive disease. The problem of restenosis/reocclusion and other complications must be solved before atherectomy devices can be widely used as an alternative to standard vascular reconstruction procedures or PTA. In addressing these problems, one should not only attempt to resolve these issues from a technologic perspective but also from the standpoint of their fundamental, scientific causes or origins.

REFERENCES

1. Gardiner GA, Meyerovitz MF, Harrington DP, et al. Dissection complicating angioplasty. Am J Radiol 145: 627-631, 1985.
2. Bredlau CE, Roubin GS, Leimgruber PP, et al. In hospital morbidity and mortality in patients undergoing elective coronary angioplasty. Circulation 62:1044-1052, 1985.
3. Cowley MJ, Dorros G, Kelsey SF, et al. Acute coronary events associated with percutaneous transluminal coronary angioplasty. Am J Cardiol 53:12C-16C, 1984.
4. Ellis SG, Rubin GS, King SB, et al. Angiographic and clinical predictor of acute closure after native vessel coronary angioplasty. Circulation 77:372-379, 1988.
5. Mosley JG, Gulati SM, Raphael M, Marston A. The role of percutaneous transluminal angioplasty for atherosclerotic angioplasty for atherosclerotic disease of the lower extremities. Ann R Coll Surg Engl 67:83-86, 1985.

6. Johnston KW, Rae M, Hogg-Johnston SA, et al. Five-year results of a prospective study of percutaneous transluminal angioplasty. Ann Surg 206:403-413, 1987.
7. Hewes RC, White RI, Murray RR, et al. Long-term results of superficial femoral artery angioplasty. Am J Radiol 146:1025-1029, 1986.
8. Blackshear JL, O'Callaghan WG, Califf RM. Medical approaches to prevention of restenosis after coronary angioplasty. J Am Coll Cardiol 9:834-848, 1987.
9. Leimgruber PP, Roubin GS, Hollman J, et al. Restenosis after successful coronary angioplasty in patients with single-vessel disease. Circulation 73:710-717, 1986.
10. Holmes DR, Vlietstra RE, Smith HC, et al. Restenosis after percutaneous transluminal coronary angioplasty: A report from the PTCA Registry of the National Heart, Lung, and Blood Institute. Am J Cardiol (Suppl)53:77C-81C, 1984.
11. Simpson JB, Selman MR, Robertson GC, et al. Transluminal atherectomy for occlusive peripheral vascular disease. Am J Cardiol 61:96G-101G, 1988.
12. Polnitz A, Nerlich A, Berger H, Hofling B. Percutaneous peripheral atherectomy. J Am Coll Cardiol 15:682-688, 1990.
13. Hinohara T, Selmon MR, Robertson GC, Braden L, Simpson JS. Directional atherectomy: New approaches for treatment of obstructive coronary and peripheral vascular disease. Circulation 81(Suppl IV):IV-79–IV-91, 1990.
14. Graor RA, Whitlow PL. Transluminal atherectomy for occlusive peripheral vascular disease. J Am Coll Cardiol 15:1551-1558, 1990.
15. Dorros G, Iyer S, Lewin R, Zaitoun R, Mathiak L, Olson K. Angiographic follow-up and clinical outcome of 126 patients after percutaneous directional atherectomy (Simpson Atherocath) for occlusive peripheral vascular disease. Cathet Cardiovasc Diagn 22:79-84, 1991.
16. Kim D, Gianturco LE, Porter DA, et al. Peripheral directional atherectomy: Four-year experience. Radiology 183:773-778, 1992.
17. Lugmayr H, Pachinger O, Deutsch M. Long term results of percutaneous atherectomy in peripheral arterial occlusive disease. Rofo Fortschr Geb Rontgenstr Neuen Bildgeb Verfahr 158:532-535, 1993.
18. Vroegindewij D, Tielbeek AV, Buth J, Schol FPG, Hop WCJ, Landman GH. Directional atherectomy versus balloon angioplasty in segmental femoropopliteal artery disease: Two-year follow-up with color-flow duplex scanning. J Vasc Surg 21:255-269, 1995.
19. Wholey MH, Jarmolowski CR. New reperfusion devices: The Kensey catheter, the atherolytic reperfusion wire device, and the transluminal extraction catheter. Radiology 172:947-952, 1989.
20. Myers KA, Denton MJ, Devine TJ. Infrainguinal atherectomy using the transluminal endarterectomy catheter: Patency rates and clinical success for 144 procedures. J Endovasc Surg 1:61-70, 1994.
21. Wholey MH, Smith JAM, Godlewski P, Nagurka M. Recanalization of total arterial occlusions with the Kensey dynamic angioplasty catheter. Radiology 172:95-98, 1989.
22. Desbrosses D, Petit H, Torres E, Barrionuevo D, Figueroa A, Wenger JJ, Ramenah B, Kieny R. Percutaneous atherectomy with the Kensey catheter: Early and midterm results in femoropopliteal occlusions unsuitable for conventional angioplasty. Ann Vasc Surg 4:550-552, 1990.
23. Cull DL, Feinberg RL, Wheeler JR, Snyder SO, Gregory RT, Gayle RG, Parent FN. Experience with laser-assisted balloon angioplasty and a rotary angioplasty instrument: Lessons learned. J Vasc Surg 14:332-339, 1991.
24. Snyder SO, Wheeler JR, Gregory RT, Gayle RG, Parent FN. The Trac-Wright atherectomy device. In Ahn SS, Moore WS, eds. Endovascular Surgery. Philadelphia: WB Saunders, 1992, pp 287-294.
25. Lukes P, Wihed A, Tidebrant G, Risberg B, Ortenwall P, Seeman T. Combined angioplasty with the Kensey catheter and balloon angioplasty in occlusive arterial disease. Acta Radiol 33:230-233, 1992.
26. Triller J, Do DD, Maddern G, Mahler F. Femoropopliteal artery occlusion: Clinical experience with the Kensey catheter. Radiology 182:257-261, 1992.
27. Dyet JF. High-speed rotational angioplasty in occluded peripheral arteries. J Intervent Radiol 7:1-5, 1992.
28. Meloni T, Carbonnato P, Mistretta L, Palombo D, Peinetti F, Porta C. Arterial recanalization with the Kensey catheter. Radiol Med 86:509-512, 1993.
29. Moellmann D, Kuhn FP, Bomer D. Distribution and size of particles after dynamic angioplasty in cadaveric arteries with the Kensey catheter system: A comparison with clinical experience. Cardiovasc Intervent Radiol 15:201-204, 1992.
30. Dorros G, Iyer S, Zaitoun R, Lewin R, Cooley R, Olson K. Acute angiographic and clinical outcome of high-speed percutaneous rotational atherectomy (Rotablator). Cathet Cardiovasc Diagn 22:157-166, 1991.
31. White CJ, Ramee SR, Escobar A, Jain S, Collins TJ. High-speed rotational ablation (Rotablator) for unfavorable lesions in peripheral arteries. Cathet Cardiovasc Diagn 30:115-119, 1993.
32. The Collaborative Rotablator Atherectomy Group (CRAG). Peripheral atherectomy with the Rotablator: A multicenter report. J Vasc Surg 19:509-515, 1994.
33. Henry M, Amor M, Ethevenot G, Henry I, Allaoui M. Percutaneous peripheral atherectomy using the Rotablator: A single center experience. J Endovasc Surg 2:51-66, 1995.
34. Myers KA, Denton MJ. Infrainguinal atherectomy using the Auth Rotablator: Patency rates and clinical success for 36 procedures. J Endovasc Surg 2:67-73, 1995.
35. Ahn SS, Auth D, Marcus D, Moore WS. Removal of focal atheromatous lesions by angioscopically guided high-speed rotary atherectomy: Preliminary experimental observations. J Vasc Surg 7:292-300, 1988.
36. Ahn SS, Arca M, Marcus D, Moore WS. Histologic and morphologic effects of rotary atherectomy on human cadaver arteries. Ann Vasc Surg 4:563-569, 1990.
37. Ahn SS, Yeatman LR, Deutsch LS, Eton D, Moore WS. Intraoperative peripheral rotary atherectomy: Early and late clinical results. Ann Vasc Surg 6:272-280, 1992.
38. Mazur W, Ali NM, Rodgers GP, Schulz DG, French BA, Raizner AE. Directional atherectomy with the Omnicath: A unique new catheter system. Cathet Cardiovasc Diagn 31:79-84, 1994.
39. Ahn SS, Rutherford RB, Becker GJ, Comerota AJ, Johnston KW, McClean GK, Seeger JM, String ST, White RA, Whittemore AD, Zarins CK. Reporting standards for lower extremity arterial endovascular procedures. J Vasc Surg 17:1103-1107, 1993.

11

Outcome of Femoropopliteal and Femorotibial Bypass After Failed Balloon Angioplasty: Is It a Reason to Avoid PTA in Some Patients?

DIETER RAITHEL, M.D., Ph.D.

Without a doubt percutaneous transluminal balloon angioplasty (PTA) represents a broadening of the angiotherapeutic spectrum. Advances in instrumentation and technique as well as differentiated pre- and postoperative treatment have led to improved early and long-term results. In light of the good results achieved with lower extremity PTA, along with the steady decrease in complications, the indications for PTA have been expanded. In the peripheral region not only are radiologists now performing risk interventions further down in the popliteal and tibial segments, but they are also using stents more frequently in all vascular segments, both unilocularly and multilocularly.[1]

Unfortunately this diversification of the radiologic therapeutic protocol has resulted in a higher rate of complications, especially when less experienced radiologists and physicians in other specialties attempt to perform interventions at levels where dilatation is difficult. This is especially problematic when these interventional procedures are attempted without the benefit of consultation with a vascular surgeon. This may explain why a patient who was unable to walk a distance of more than two blocks without pain because of an occluded femoral artery was treated with dilatation, after which radiologists recommended "redo" PTA with stent implantation (Fig. 1, *A* and *B*). In addition, three stents were implanted and after a new occlusion was detected, the patient was referred to our department of radiology where dilatation was repeated and another three stents were implanted for a total of six stents at the femoropopliteal level. These stents were then treated with radiation therapy to reduce the rate of reocclusion, after which local and systemic lysis was performed. However, control angiograms showed complete occlusion from the femoral bifurcation to the midcalf level. A bypass to the posterior tibial artery with autologous saphenous vein was not possible, so a ringed 6 mm Gore-Tex (W.L. Gore & Associates, Inc., Flagstaff, Ariz.) polytetrafluoroethylene (PTFE) prosthesis was implanted with tibial anastomosis by means of a Taylor patch (Fig. 2). The total cost of this treatment including hospitalization, stents, and other related charges was $15,000; the cost of the operation alone and the hospital stay would have been $2500.

This is one example of how radiologists overestimate not only the technical feasibility of a procedure but their skill as well, especially when they do not discuss with a vascular surgeon the possibility that vascular reconstruction may be a more suitable alternative. However, we do want to acknowledge the fact that especially in patients with limb-threatening disease, in those considered high risk, and in those with a limited life expectancy, durable limb salvage can be achieved with little discomfort by intervention with PTA without the need for an open surgical procedure.

Clinical experience also indicates that PTA is performed much more frequently in patients with claudication and in those who are completely asymptomatic. Often there are no comparable indications for reconstructive surgery because vascular surgeons are more conservative in their approach. Therefore we must stress the importance of a cooperative effort among angiologists, radiologists, and vascular surgeons to identify possibly ineffective treatment and to avoid possible complications. Too often when there is uncertainty surrounding the indications for PTA, complications and reocclusions can occur, often resulting in the need for subsequent

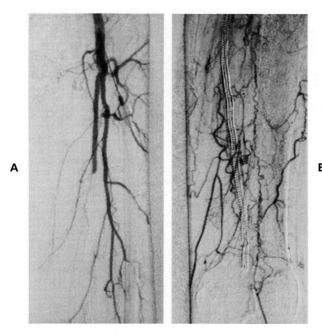

Fig. 1 A, Reocclusion after PTA of the femoral artery. **B,** Repeat PTA with three stents implanted.

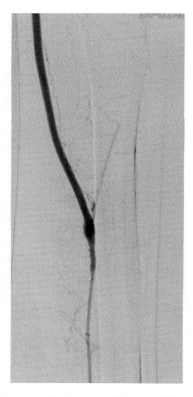

Fig. 2 Same patient as in Fig. 1 with reocclusion after "redo" PTA with three additional stents and PTFE bypass to posterior tibial artery.

Table 1 Complications in 1401 lower extremity PTAs

	No. of cases	Percent
Reocclusion	64	4.6
Distal embolism	47	3.4
Bleeding	37	2.6
Aneurysm	10	0.7
Artery perforation	5	0.3
Operated	35	2.5

From Zeitler E, Ernsting M, Richter E, Seyferth W. Komplikationen nach PTA femoraler und iliacaler Obstruktionen. Vasa 11:270-275, 1982.

vascular reconstruction. After analyzing my own clinical experience I would like to discuss some of the circumstances under which a failed PTA influences the outcome of reconstructive surgery.

COMPLICATIONS OF PERCUTANEOUS TRANSLUMINAL ANGIOPLASTY

Table 1 lists the vascular complications associated with lower extremity PTA as reported in 1982 by Zeitler et al.[2] In this collective review a total of 163 complications occurred in 1401 attempted PTAs of femoropopliteal and tibial vessels. In 35 of them (2.5%) surgery became necessary. The most feared complication was thromboembolism, which occurred in 8% (thrombosis in 4.6% and peripheral embolization in 3.4%). Zeitler (personal communication), in his own series of more than 1500 angioplasties for femoral artery occlusion, showed that the complication rate was dependent on both preoperative symptoms and the length of the occlusion (Tables 2 and 3). The most frequent complications in that series were thrombosis and distal embolization. In the literature, distal embolism represents 1% to 5% of reported PTA complications, yet it is observed clinically in less than 2% of attempted PTAs.[3-5]

Regarding the indications for reintervention, we believe that in cases of reocclusion reintervention should not be performed right away if the patient is in stage II (claudication). In stages III and IV (i.e., rest pain or necrosis) the indications for reintervention are broader. It is known that the rate of infection after previous PTA is much higher, especially if the patient has no suitable saphenous vein and a prosthesis must be implanted. However, in patients with bleeding, perforation, or dissection, as well as in reocclusion with peripheral embolization and subacute or acute ischemia, surgery is clearly indicated.

Table 2 Early complications in lower extremity PTA for claudication

	No. of cases	Percent
SFA stenosis	512	0.4
SFA occlusion <12 cm	273	1.8
SFA occlusion >12 cm	82	2.4

Radiol. Dept. Nbg./Prof. Zeitler (1970-1980).
SFA = superficial femoral artery.

Table 3 Early complications in lower extremity PTA for limb salvage

	No. of cases	Percent
SFA stenosis	349	0.9
SFA occlusion <12 cm	142	2.1
SFA occlusion >12 cm	91	4.3

Radiol. Dept. Nbg./Prof. Zeitler (1970-1980).

Table 4 Complications of lower extremity PTAs in 145 patients

Vessel thrombosis	61
Distal embolism	36
Dissection	15
Bleeding/hematoma	22
Artery perforation	10
Aneurysm/arteriovenous fistula	9
Subintimal wire dislocation	5
Infection	8
Acute ischemia	34

Two thirds of the patients presented within the first 2 months.

CLINICAL FINDINGS IN THE PRESENT STUDY

There were 145 patients who required surgery as a result of complications of PTA. Because of the large area from which these patients were referred to us, this population was not representative of the complications typically encountered in a radiology clinic such as ours with broad experience in PTA. Sixty-one patients had vessel thrombosis, 36 had a distal embolism, 15 had subintimal wire passage with dissection, 10 had a perforated artery, and 22 had bleeding or a hematoma (Table 4). Nine patients had a punctiform aneurysm or arteriovenous-fistula and five had catheter dislocation. Thirty-four patients had emergency surgery for subacute deterioration after PTA. Eight patients showed signs of infection. Additional complications were observed in some patients (i.e., dissection, vessel thrombosis, or distal embolization). More than two thirds of the patients were seen within the first 2 months after PTA for vascular surgical treatment.

OPERATIVE RECONSTRUCTION AFTER PTA

In any evaluation of reocclusion after PTA, with or without peripheral embolization, the indications for operative treatment should be closely examined. If the extremity is determined to have good compensation, caution is advised in considering reintervention, especially if the angiogram shows sufficient runoff. On the other hand, poor compensation and extensively thrombotic peripheral vessels are definite indications for immediate reintervention.

Ten patients required aortofemoral reconstruction, six underwent femorofemoral bypass, and three underwent axillofemoral bypass (Table 5). In other words, in 19 patients reconstruction of the aortoiliac segment alone was sufficient for elimination of ischemia and for limb salvage.

Sixty-one patients had femoropopliteal and 39 had femorotibial reconstructions. Six patients required amputation because of total ischemia or an irreversibly damaged extremity (Table 6). In another two patients lumbar sympathectomy was performed because of insufficient runoff. In 10 patients a spinal cord stimulator was implanted. Eight patients underwent exploration of the popliteal or tibial arteries, but no vessel suitable for vascular reconstruction was found.

RESULTS

Follow-up was carried out in 88 femoropopliteal or femorotibial reconstructions; in 56 the occlusion rate within the first 12 months was particularly high. Cumulative patency rates were 85% after 1 month, 62% after 6 months, and 43% after 1 year (Table 7). After 2, 3, and 5 years, patency rates were 39%, 37%, and 34%, respectively.

Analysis of above- and below-knee reconstructions demonstrated the following: cumulative patency for above-knee reconstructions was 92% after 1 month, 57% after 1 year, and 53% after 5 years; for below-knee reconstructions cumulative patency rates were 73% after 4 weeks, 33% after 6 months, and only 26% after 1 year.

Table 5 Vascular reconstruction after failed PTA

Bypass	No. of cases
Aortofemoral	10
Femorofemoral	6
Axillofemoral	3
Femoropopliteal	61
Femorotibial	39
	119

Table 6 Operations after failed PTA or PTA complications

	No.
Amputation	6
Sympathectomy	2
Spinal cord stimulation	10
Vessel exploration	8

Table 7 Patency rates for infrainguinal reconstruction after failed PTA (1980-1993)

	4 wk (%)	1 yr (%)	3 yr (%)	5 yr (%)
All reconstructions	85	43	37	34
Above-knee	92	57	54	53
Below-knee	73	26		
Tibial	67	28		

Further analysis of the late results showed that the unfavorable findings were primarily due to embolization into the tibial vessels and the pedal arch. We detected embolization into the tibial segment and the pedal arch in 36 patients whose occlusions were treated with a bypass. At follow-up 31 of these reconstructions were already occluded.

DISCUSSION

As stated previously, because of the relatively large area from which these patients were referred, this patient population represents an extremely poor selection of PTA complications. In addition, some of our colleagues were in the "learning phase," and the selection criteria for PTA were often liberal. Particularly problematic from our point of view is the fact that all too often angioplasty is performed in patients with claudication, but patients with peripheral embolization are not referred to a vascular surgeon in time for corrective reconstruction (lysis or extraction). These peripheral embolizations lead to worsening of runoff at the tibial level and as a result peripheral vascular resistance is increased, which has a negative influence on long-term prognosis.

The frequency of distal embolism in lower extremity angioplasty is reported to be 1% to 5%.[1-5] Reliable information on the frequency of so-called clinical asymptomatic microembolization in larger series, however, is not available. These embolisms are frequently asymptomatic if they do not lead to acute worsening of the runoff, especially in those patients for whom PTA of the proximal segment leads to successful recanalization. In the case of subsequent reocclusion, however, these embolic occlusions are significant because they limit peripheral runoff and therefore raise doubts concerning the validity of the success rates for reconstruction in long-term follow-up.

Angiographic documentation of the runoff, particularly in the pedal arch, is mandatory before and after PTA. Only immediate angiography of the runoff after PTA can document peripheral embolisms and thrombotic complications, and the patient can possibly be treated by lysis or clot extraction. This would also lead to improved PTA results.

In our own clinical observations following PTA, we found an occluded or partially occluded pedal arch in 44% of the patients. Based on angiographic evidence, previous embolization was suspected. In our own clinical experience, as well as reports in the literature, there is clear evidence that peripheral embolisms occurring after PTA have an enormously negative influence on the outcome after a bypass.[5] Among our reconstructions after PTA without peripheral embolism, graft occlusion occurred in 32%. In patients with peripheral embolisms following PTA, however, we noted a reocclusion rate of 76% among our subsequent vascular reconstructions. These results clearly show that peripheral embolization during PTA leads to worsening of the runoff (via increasing vascular resistance) and thus to unfavorable long-term results after reconstruction. Furthermore, the length of the occluded segment before PTA has a direct influence on the frequency of peripheral embolization during PTA. We found that short occluded segments (<5 cm) had an embolization rate of 28%,

Table 8 Correlation between lesion characteristics and frequency of embolism in PTA

Lesion	Embolism
<5 cm	28%
5-10 cm	32%
>10 cm	67%

Table 9 Correlation between lesion characteristics in PTA and indications for vascular reconstruction

Lesion characteristics (pre-PTA)	Indications for reconstruction
<5 cm	21%
5-10 cm	30%
>10 cm	49%

longer segments (5 to 10 cm) had a rate of 32%, and in patients with the longest segments (>10 cm) the rate was 67% (Table 8). Based on these results, we recommend dilatation for occlusions greater than 10 cm only under extreme circumstances.

We were also able to prove that the most frequently occurring complication necessitating surgery after PTA was long-segment occlusion. Reconstruction was indicated in 21% of short (<5 cm) occlusions, in 30% of occlusions ranging from 5 to 10 cm, and in 49% of long-segment (>10 cm) occlusions (Table 9).

Along these same lines, it was also particularly noteworthy that not only was dilatation of long-segment occlusions much more difficult, but all too often treatment included the liberal use of stents. These stents appear to function in a manner similar to grafts. From our point of view they are only suitable for arteries with a wider lumen. We believe that in small-vessel segments early reocclusion occurs as a result of intimal hyperplasia.

Further analysis of our data shows significant worsening of patients who had undergone dilatation. Thus 60 patients were in stage I/II (claudication) before PTA as compared to only 12 patients after PTA. Of the 85 patients who had been in stage III/IV (i.e., those who had undergone dilatation for limb salvage), 83 were still in stage III/IV after PTA. Particularly noteworthy was the change in the angiographic pattern before PTA as compared to the pattern before peripheral reconstruction. Before PTA, we found one or more stenoses in 82 patients; after PTA, the number dropped to 39. In 63 patients occlusion of the femoral or popliteal segment was noted before PTA, but in 106 patients occlusion occurred after PTA (before reconstruction). An open pedal arch was observed in 112 patients before PTA but in only 81 after PTA.

This clear worsening of the angiographic pattern as well as the stage of the disease definitely leads to poorer results after reconstruction with a cumulative patency of only 34% after 5 years. Particularly evident was the high rate of reocclusion in below-knee reconstructions. These results are not at all comparable to other femoropopliteal/tibial results in our clinical experience, but they can be attributed to the complications of PTA.

Radiologists have been known to achieve excellent primary results but these were never compared with outcome after vascular reconstruction. Blair et al.[6] compared their PTA findings with results of femoropopliteal and infrapopliteal reconstruction for limb salvage; after 2 years the cumulative patency for PTA was only 18% compared to 68% for femoropopliteal and 47% for femorotibial reconstructions. These results are in no way comparable to previously published findings; in those reports PTA performed for claudication (stage II) showed patency rates ranging from 50% to 80%.[2,7] Only a prospective randomized series could produce results that would help to determine which patients are suitable candidates for bypass or PTA and which are not.

From my perspective as a vascular surgeon and in view of my own clinical experience, I would state that PTA should be avoided in patients with claudication, especially in those with long, diffuse arteriosclerotic disease of the femoral and/or popliteal artery. Furthermore, in the presence of claudication a clear differentiation between conservative and operative treatment is mandatory. PTA should also be avoided in patients with stenosis at the origin of the superficial femoral artery, in those with stenosis or occlusion of the common femoral artery, and in those with diffuse obliteration of the femoropopliteal segment (Fig. 3). Moreover, it must be emphasized that patients with trifurcation stenosis should not be treated by angioplasty. Last but not least, reocclusion, especially after stent implantation, is not an indication for PTA.

We recommend that the indications for PTA be

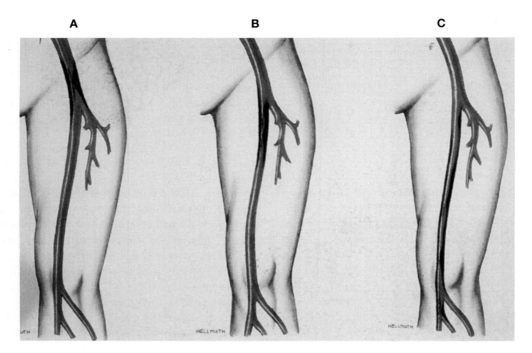

Fig. 3 PTA should be avoided in patients with stenosis at the origin of the superficial femoral artery (**A**), stenoses of the common femoral artery (**B**), and diffuse obliteration of the femoropopliteal segment (**C**).

discussed with a vascular surgeon in all cases.[6,7] This increases the likelihood of a favorable outcome. Patients with borderline indications for therapy would definitely be excluded from consideration for PTA based on our previous recommendations, but they could undergo reconstruction for limb salvage if necessary. These would include patients with no suitable vein as well as those who develop overlying soft tissue infection after prosthetic bypass.

REFERENCES

1. Richter GM, Nöldge G, Roeren T. Intraluminale vaskuläre Endoprothesen. In Maurer PC, Dörrler J, Somoggy S, eds. Gefäßchirurgie im Fortschritt. Stuttgart: Thieme, 1990, pp 266-281.
2. Zeitler E, Ernsting M, Richter E, Seyferth W. Komplikationen nach PTA femoraler und iliacaler Obstruktionen. Vasa 11:270-275, 1982.
3. Bergquist BK, Jonsson K, Weibull H. Complications after percutaneous transluminal angioplasty of peripheral and renal arteries. Acta Radiol 28:3-11, 1987.
4. Lamerton A. Percutaneous transluminal angioplasty. Br J Surg 73:91-97, 1986.
5. Schweiger H. Arterienrekonstruktion als Zweiteingriff nach peripherer PTA. In Maurer PC, Dörrler J, Somoggy S, eds. Gefäßchirurgie im Fortschritt. Stuttgart: Thieme, 1990, pp 215-222.
6. Blair JM, Gewertz BC, Moosa H, Lu C-T, Zarins CK. Percutaneous transluminal angioplasty versus surgery for limb-threatening ischemia. J Vasc Surg 9:698-703, 1989.
7. Raithel D. Chirurgische Maßnahmen nach PTA-Indikationsstellung und Ergebnisse. Langenbecks Arch Chir (Suppl 1)529-533, 1991.

12

Value and Limitations of Angioscopy and Intravascular Ultrasound

RODNEY A. WHITE, M.D., F.R.A.C.S., GEORGE E. KOPCHOK, B.S., and CARLOS DONAYRE, M.D.

Angioscopy and intravascular ultrasound (IVUS) are rapidly evolving catheter-based endovascular imaging techniques. The two methods are complementary with angioscopy providing a three-dimensional view of the luminal morphology of a vessel and IVUS displaying the transmural anatomy of the vessel wall and adjacent structures. Angioscopy requires that blood be cleared from the vessel before visualization is possible, whereas IVUS imaging is easily accomplished through liquid media and soft tissue but is attenuated by air and calcified portions of an artery. This chapter discusses the evolving role of these methods in endovascular therapy, emphasizing both the complementary and individually unique properties of each technology.

ANGIOSCOPY

Angioscopy, the endoscopic examination of the luminal anatomy of blood vessels, is being used to establish the diagnosis and etiology of vascular diseases, to evaluate the technical accuracy of vascular reconstructions, and to visualize intraluminal instrumentation. Available devices range from 0.5 to 3.3 mm diameter and have high-quality fiberoptic imaging systems and light sources that enable intraluminal inspection.

Percutaneous Angioscopy

To provide access to the vessel being evaluated, the Seldinger technique is used to enable insertion of the angioscope via hemostatic introducer sheaths. Several problems exist that make it difficult to obtain good images with percutaneous angioscopes. Some currently available systems are relatively stiff, which makes control and centering of the devices difficult. To aid in manipulation of the tip of the scope, a steering mechanism in at least one plane is desirable. Control of proximal blood flow in the area being examined can be achieved by inflation of a balloon on the tip of the catheter. A rapid flow of irrigating solution through the delivery catheter is then required to control blood flow from collateral vessels. "Backbleeding" from the distal circulation can also be limited by having an assistant apply a tourniquet around the distal point of an extremity.

Percutaneous angioscopy is currently being used to inspect the vessel lumen before endovascular procedures and to define the mechanisms and accuracy of interventions. In these procedures angioscopy is performed before an angioplasty device is inserted. Using the percutaneous technique, the angioscope and delivery catheter must be removed during an intervention, since the angioscope and angioplasty device will not both fit simultaneously through the percutaneous introducer. Following completion of angioplasty performed under fluoroscopic control, the angioscope is then reinserted to inspect the treated vessel. Small intimal flaps, mural thrombus, or other forms of damage to the vessel wall are easily visualized if blood can be adequately cleared from the arterial lumen (Fig. 1).

Intraoperative Angioscopy

Angioscopy can be performed intraoperatively within a relatively brief interval through an opening in the vessel. To perform the intraluminal inspection, vascular occlusion is achieved by conventional operative means or by placing a balloon on the end of the angioscope. Infusion of saline solution under approximately 300 mm Hg of pressure (30 to 75 ml/min) through an irrigation channel in the angioscope or by a coaxial catheter clears the intraluminal blood and enables visualization in approximately 80% to 90% of cases.

APPLICATIONS OF ANGIOSCOPY

Several investigators have reported that angioscopy provides clinically important information that is not revealed by extraluminal inspec-

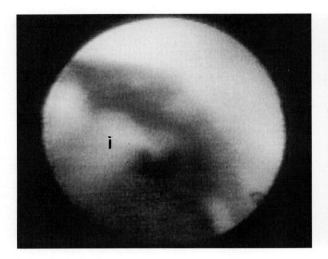

Fig. 1 Intimal flaps (*i*) that remain following balloon angioplasty of a superficial femoral artery lesion.

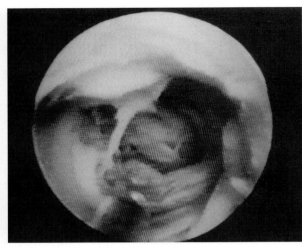

Fig. 2 Angioscopic inspection of a partially thrombectomized superficial femoral artery demonstrating residual thrombosis and complete distal occlusion of the lumen.

tion, probing, or angiography in 15% to 30% of vascular procedures.[1-3] The angioscopic findings alter the surgical protocol in a significant number of these cases. In our prospective evaluations angioscopic findings differed significantly from preoperative or intraoperative angiograms in approximately 25% of cases, resulting in a change in the form of therapy used in a significant number of procedures.[3]

Angioscopic Thrombectomy

Embolectomy and thrombectomy of peripheral vessels are enhanced by angioscopy.[4] Unless the entire length of the vessel is occluded, the angioscope may initially be introduced through an arteriotomy to inspect the lumen and define the exact site and extent of thrombosis or embolism, and to determine whether there is preexisting atherosclerotic disease. Thrombectomy catheters may then be passed alongside the angioscope if the arterial lumen is large enough to accommodate both devices. Balloon inflation and detachment and removal of thrombus and debris can then be visually monitored (Fig. 2).

Frequently balloon catheters do not completely remove all of the thrombus that is adherent to the wall, leaving large fragments that may or may not be removed with repeated passes of the catheter and are frequently not adequately demonstrated on completion arteriograms. When adherent thrombus is observed, further attempts at retrieval may be made by positioning the balloon just distal to the clot and then oscillating the balloon back and forth over the site. If this is not successful, a decision must be made as to whether extraction attempts by other instruments are warranted, such as flexible grasping forceps, rotary atherectomy devices, vascular brushes, or newer thrombectomy extraction devices. An additional possible alternative is the intraoperative use of fibrinolytic agents.

When thromboembolectomy is considered complete, a final angioscopic inspection of the entire artery is performed. Angiographic examination of the smaller runoff vessels may be performed by injection of contrast medium through the fluid channel of the angioscope before the scope is withdrawn and the arteriotomy is closed. One of the advantages afforded by angioscopy is that it allows correction of complications and technical errors such as retained thrombus or intimal flaps before blood flow is restored. The angiogram usually fails to demonstrate the smaller irregularities of the wall caused by intimal flaps or adherent thrombus and may underestimate larger lesions as well. These aspects are easily demonstrated with the three-dimensional intraluminal view provided by the angioscope. In prosthetic grafts neointimal hyperplasia may be difficult to differentiate from chronic thrombus. Twists or kinks of the graft can also be identified by angioscopic inspection.

In a preliminary series we reported that residual thrombus was identified angioscopically within arteries and vascular prostheses after standard thromboembolectomy procedures in approximately 80% of cases.[4] The direct view obtained provided significantly more information regarding luminal compromise than did contrast radiologic imaging. Additional experience in more than 60 cases of thromboembolectomy revealed some residual thrombus after passage of a balloon in almost every treated vessel or graft. This was an unexpected finding since angiograms of the site often appeared normal. In many cases the additional retrieved thrombus was quite small and probably would not significantly jeopardize outcome. In some instances the balloon catheter had been observed to pass between the vessel wall and thrombus without dislodging it.

With residual thrombus, especially nonobstructing mural thrombus, it is often difficult to judge whether further attempts at removal are indicated. It is likely that many minor defects would normally be resolved by the natural fibrinolytic and healing processes. The physician must remember that mural thrombus may simulate spasm on angiograms and that good backflow does not necessarily correlate with a satisfactory result. In some cases angioscopy identifies severe dissections or atherosclerotic stenosis or occlusion that cannot be treated. In this situation angioscopic inspection provides information that leads immediately to vascular bypass rather than persistent unproductive attempts at thrombectomy. During angioscopic inspection the infusion of the irrigating fluid simulates blood flow and helps demonstrate potential flaps and loose debris.

Angioscopy-Assisted In Situ Vein Bypasses

Observing the completeness of valvulotomy in in situ vein bypasses has improved the technical accuracy of the procedure and reduced the operative time by assuring complete incompetence of valve cusps. The valvulotome is inserted through a side branch of the upper segment of the saphenous vein or through the vein lumen at

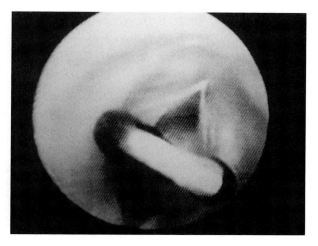

Fig. 3 Division of the valve cusps using a Mills valvulotome. The valve cusp and valvulotome are clearly visible. (From White RA, White GH. Angioscopy. In Color Atlas of Endovascular Surgery. London: Chapman & Hall, 1990, p 108.)

the distal end. The valulotome is passed proximally from the distal vein through the most proximal valve, and the angioscope is inserted proximally and passed distally until the valvulotome can be visualized at the valve site. We prefer to perform the valvulotomy using a low-profile valvulotome because this type of device can be easily visualized and controlled by angioscopic inspection and does not obstruct the field of vision. Incompetence of valve cusps is easily tested under direct vision by distending the vein by infusion of saline solution and compressing the vein lumen by external pressure (Fig. 3). As valve cusps are serially disrupted, the valvulotome and angioscope are advanced distally to the next valve.

Intraluminal identification of tributary veins during the procedure helps limit dissection and isolation of the vein and prevents tears in the vein caused by hooking a side branch with the valvulotome. Microinstruments that can be passed through a lumen in an angioscope or coaxial to the scope to enhance accurate and expedient valvulotomy under direct vision are also available. New catheters combine the valvulotomy device and the angioscope to expedite the procedure. At all times extreme care must be taken to prevent damage to the vein by the intraluminal instruments. Angioscopes too small to pass easily through the lumen can produce severe trauma.

Angioscopic Monitoring of Angioplasty Procedures

Angioscopy has an appealing theoretical advantage over arteriography for monitoring angioplasty procedures in that it helps reduce the hazards of radiation exposure and contrast reactions and allows immediate detection and correction of technical complications. Arteriography tends to underestimate wall irregularities and stenoses. Angioscopic inspection under magnification and video control has enabled placement of the intraluminal devices without deviation into collateral vessels. Proximal stenotic lesions or tapering of the vessel near the site of an occlusion limits angioscopic inspection and prevents clear visualization of the occlusion. Angioscopy following angioplasty has been extremely helpful in determining the adequacy of recanalizations, inspecting the surface for fragments, and helping to determine the mechanism of action of recanalization devices.

Another benefit of angioscopy is that the examination can be conducted before blood flow is restored and may help prevent embolization of fragments of arterial wall or thrombus. Angioscopic examinations are limited in that assessment of distal smaller vessels is usually not possible because of the angioscope diameters. Examination of normal vessels beyond the treated segment may cause intimal lesions or induce spasm. Angiography of the distal vasculature can be performed by injecting contrast medium through an ancillary channel in the scope. This allows direct correlation of the angiogram with angioscopic image.

We have found angioscopy to be of limited value during the angioplasty procedure itself, since in most cases the device is not visible once it has entered an occlusion. Angioscopy has therefore been of limited value in preventing perforations. This experience parallels that of Abela et al.,[5] who found that when angioscopy was used to control the position of the laser fiber, perforation was still a frequent occurrence in early cases but was avoided in later patients as the improved techniques were developed. An obvious limitation of current angioscopic equipment is that it does not provide a means to determine vessel wall thickness or concentricity of lesions. In the future, combining angioscopy with intraluminal ultrasound imaging may provide a complete perspective of vessel wall morphology.

OVERVIEW OF THE UTILITY OF ANGIOSCOPY

At present, angioscopy is an alternative to angiography with the advantage of providing repeatable three-dimensional intraluminal views before blood flow is restored. Potential complications of angioscopy include vessel perforation and fluid overload from excessive administration of irrigant fluid, producing intimal trauma and embolization. Fluid overload can be averted by occluding both the vessel being inspected and its collateral branches, or by performing the procedures with a tourniquet on the extremity. Inspecting vessels that approximate or are smaller than the diameter of the angioscope can produce spasm and possible thrombosis. The clarity of angioscopic images is usually excellent, but adequate cleaning of blood flow from collateral and distal vessels by fluid infusion and centering of the device for examinations requires an initial learning curve. These are frequently the factors that limit visualization, although adequate examinations can be performed in approximately 85% of cases.

INTRAVASCULAR ULTRASOUND IMAGING

IVUS has developed rapidly within the past few years. By providing an accurate luminal and transmural image of vascular structures, IVUS displays vascular abnormalities and illustrates immediate results of interventions. In addition to obvious diagnostic applications, the potential significance of IVUS has become even more apparent because of the simultaneous development of minimally invasive catheter-based therapeutic techniques including balloon angioplasty, atherectomy, laser angioplasty, and intravascular stents. The thrust of current development is to incorporate IVUS as an adjunct to peripheral and coronary angioplasty procedures. IVUS will likely become a critical component of future interventional devices, and an understanding of the technique will be essential for individuals involved in the management of patients with cardiovascular disease.

INTRAVASCULAR ULTRASOUND IMAGING TECHNIQUES

IVUS catheters can be introduced either percutaneously through standard arterial access sheaths (5 to 9 Fr) or through an opening in a vessel during a surgical procedure. If large vessels proximal to the arteriotomy are to be imaged (e.g., iliac artery imaging via a femoral cutdown), a hemostatic access device should be used to reduce blood loss and prevent catheter damage during insertion. Most devices can be passed over a guidewire, which allows more controlled maneuvering of the device within the lumen of the vessel from a remote introduction site, particularly in tortuous or tightly stenotic vessels.

It is important to orient the IVUS catheter within the vessel so that anteroposterior accuracy can be achieved. The best methods for maintaining orientation are use of the image artifact produced by the transducer connecting wires and/or establishment of correct initial alignment at the point of catheter insertion. For example, when imaging the aortoiliac segments via a femoral puncture site, rotational alignment can be confirmed by the relative position of anatomic landmarks such as the aortic and iliac bifurcation. Because the catheters are rotationally rigid there is very limited loss of orientation with torquing and manipulation during imaging. Careful positioning of the catheter tip within the vessel and appropriate size matching of the device to the caliber of the artery is essential to optimize visualization. Image quality is best when the catheter is parallel to the vessel wall, that is, the ultrasound beam is directed at 90 degrees to the luminal surface, whereas minor angulations may affect the luminal shape and dimensional accuracy. Eccentric positioning causes the vessel wall nearer the imaging chamber to appear more echogenic than the distant wall, producing an artifactual difference in wall thicknesses. Positioning the catheter in the center of the lumen is especially difficult in tortuous vessels and is often best achieved as the catheter is withdrawn rather than during advancement. Luminal flushing with saline solution or radiographic contrast agent has been reported to improve delineation of acoustic interfaces in small and medium-sized vessels.[6,7]

CLINICAL UTILITY OF INTRAVASCULAR ULTRASOUND
Disease Distribution and Characterization

Several studies have reported that IVUS is accurate in determining the luminal and vessel wall morphology of normal or minimally diseased arteries both in vitro and in vivo.[7-13] In muscular arteries distinct sonographic layers are visible with the media appearing as an echolucent layer sandwiched between the more echodense intima and adventitia. The precise correlation between the ultrasound image and the microscopic anatomy of the muscular artery wall is still uncertain. The internal and external elastic laminae and adventitia are considered to be the backscatter substrates for the inner and outer echodense zones.[8,14] Precise measurements of the adventitia may be difficult to obtain unless the vessel is surrounded by tissues of differing echogenicity (e.g., echolucent fat). Even small intimal lesions such as flaps or intimal tears are well visualized because of their high fibrous tissue content and the difference in echoic properties of these structures in comparison to surrounding blood. The three-layer appearance of muscular arteries is not readily seen in larger vessels (e.g., aorta) because of the increased elastin content in the media.

IVUS devices are sensitive in differentiating calcified and noncalcified vascular lesions (Fig. 4). Because the ultrasound energy is strongly reflected by calcific plaque, it appears as a bright image with dense acoustic shadowing behind it. For this reason the exact location of the media and adventitia cannot be seen in segments of vessels containing heavy calcific disease, and dimensions must be estimated by interpolation using adjacent vessel wall measurements.

Numerous investigations have compared angiography and IVUS for determining luminal and transmural dimensions of normal and moderately atherosclerotic human arteries.[13,15,16] The cross-sectional areas calculated from biplanar angiograms and measured from IVUS images correlate well for normal or minimally diseased peripheral arteries in vivo. Most studies reveal that IVUS and angiography also correlate well when used to image mildly elliptical lumens, but when used to derive dimensions from severely diseased vessels, the angiogram tends to underestimate the severity of disease. By offering a method to define the luminal and transmural morphology and dimensions, IVUS provides a new perspective from which to investigate arterial disease.

Recent studies have compared two- and three-dimensional (2D and 3D) IVUS to angiography, CT, and 3D CT for imaging abdominal aortic aneurysms.[17] Each modality provides unique information regarding the anatomy of the aorta

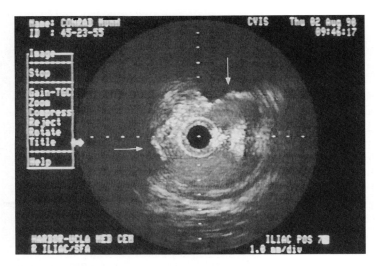

Fig. 4 IVUS image of human iliac artery. Note calcific plaque *(arrows)* with complete attenuation of the signal beyond the lesion. (From Tabbara MR, White RA, Cavaye DM, Kopchok GE, et al. In vivo comparison of intravascular ultrasonography and angiography. J Vasc Surg 14:496-504, 1994.)

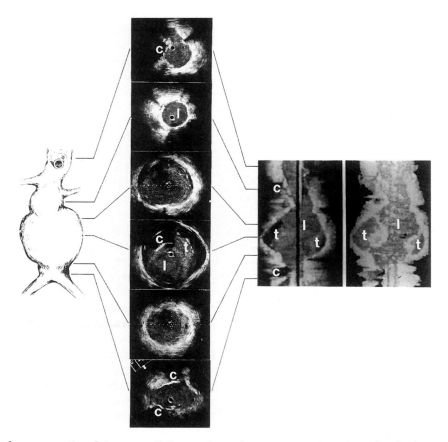

Fig. 5 Selected cross-sectional images of the aorta and aneurysm at various levels (center) compared to schematic diagram of the lesion (left) and longitudinal gray scale and 3D IVUS images (right) of the aneurysm. Note evidence of thrombus *(t)* and calcification *(c)* at several levels throughout the length of the vessel; l = lumen. (From White RA, Scoccianti M, Back M, Kopchok G, Donayre C. Innovations in vascular imaging: Arteriography, three-dimensional CT scans, and two- and three-dimensional intravascular ultrasound evaluation of an abdominal aortic aneurysm. Ann Vasc Surg 8:285-289, 1994.)

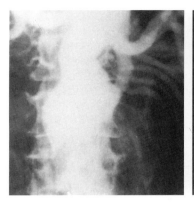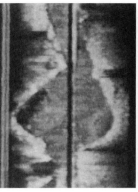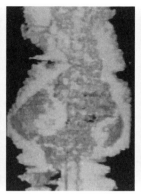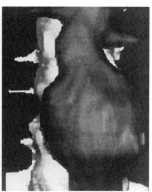

Fig. 6 Left to right: Aortogram, longitudinal gray scale IVUS, surface-rendered 3D IVUS, and 3D CT of the external surface of the aortic aneurysm. Images are of comparable lengths of aorta with similar magnification to enable comparison of methods. (From White RA, Scoccianti M, Back M, Kopchok G, Donayre C. Innovations in vascular imaging: Arteriography, three-dimensional CT scans, and two- and three-dimensional intravascular ultrasound evaluation of an abdominal aortic aneurysm. Ann Vasc Surg 8:285-289, 1994.)

and the distribution of components of the aneurysm (Figs. 5 and 6). In the case that is illustrated, the aortogram confirmed that the aneurysm was confined to the infrarenal aorta and documented the patency of adjacent branch arteries. The luminal morphology imaged on the angiogram underestimated the size of the aneurysm, although displacement of the right ureter suggested a larger dimension. In addition, the angiogram did not provide precise cross-sectional and volumetric data regarding the dimensions of the neck of the aneurysm such as quantity of thrombus and aortic wall characteristics which were apparent on CT and IVUS.

Tomographic views of cross sections of the aneurysm acquired by CT and IVUS enabled accurate sizing of luminal and wall dimensions and correlated closely at various levels along the aorta. Surrounding anatomic structures and characteristics of the vessel wall were highlighted using each method. The IVUS images demonstrated the origin of visceral vessels (superior mesenteric and renal arteries) in relation to the aneurysm and displayed areas of calcification compared to thrombus and fibrous wall components. Calcification was clearly identified by IVUS as hyperechoic areas with shadowing beyond the lesion. Calcification of the wall of the aorta was more readily apparent on IVUS images compared to angiograms and CT scans. Although the 2D cross-sectional CT and IVUS images corresponded closely for determining the luminal and vessel wall dimensions, 3D IVUS reconstructions demonstrated some variation in the shape and topography of the wall surface along the longitudinal axis of the aneurysm compared to 3D CT. Three-dimensional CT outlined the external surface of the aorta, whereas IVUS visualized the lumen and transmural wall characteristics. Development of future interventional methods such as intravascular graft deployment will utilize specific applications of each method to enhance the precision of endovascular repairs. In particular, IVUS is being used to size and assess the characteristics of the aortic wall and aneurysm prior to deployment, to precisely place the device during the procedure, and to assess the accuracy of graft positioning.

Conventional angiography has been unable to provide adequately sensitive data regarding the effects of endovascular therapies. For meaningful critical assessment of these new methods, plaque consistency and distribution of residual lesions following intervention must be known. IVUS provides the ability to accurately measure percentages of stenoses produced by comparing luminal dimensions to normal-appearing adjacent reference vessels. This is due in part to the restrictions of single or biplanar arteriography and also to the fact that an angiogram is a luminal silhouette rather than a transmural image.

Three-dimensional IVUS can be used to demonstrate atherosclerotic lesion volume, distribution, and tissue characteristics and is particularly relevant to investigation of the natural history of atherosclerotic disease and to the development volumetric plaque studies before and after endovascular interventions.[18] Lesion volume can be measured using 3D IVUS imaging but data regarding its accuracy are not currently available. Estimation of plaque volume is based on the concept of differing cylindrical volumes, where the inner (smaller) cylinder is represented by the vessel lumen and the outer (larger) cylinder is confined by the adventitia. By creating a surface-rendered luminal image and a complete cylindrical adventitial reconstruction of a vascular segment, these two volumes can be displayed. The difference between the two cylinders represents the "volume" occupied by the arterial wall elements, either normal or pathologic. If this volume is measured before and after intervention (e.g., atherectomy), the difference in the volumes represents the amount of actual lesion removed. This information is required to delineate the mechanisms of angioplasty failure, since the roles of residual stenosis and recurrent stenosis have not been adequately defined using currently available angiographically determined data.

IVUS provides essential information in the investigation of arterial wall dissections by determining the size, location, and extent of intimal flaps. Because IVUS imaging is a dynamic, real-time imaging modality, the movement of arterial flaps with systolic-diastolic blood flow can be seen. The precise location and orientation of the flap is important since it may determine the need for excision and grafting, stenting, or repair. IVUS has been used to identify the location and severity of dissections and flaps and may enable endovascular assessment and treatment alone.[19-22] Three-dimensional IVUS imaging is especially useful in this role because aortic dissection commonly results in a spiral or complex-shaped flap that is difficult to appreciate in three dimensions using alternative imaging modalities. Three-dimensional reconstructions allow identification of the dissection entry site, extent of the flap, and relation of the false lumen to major visceral branches and plays a vital role in experimental endoluminal stenting of aortic dissections.

IVUS as an Adjunct to Endovascular Interventions

Recent studies have indicated that percutaneous transluminal balloon angioplasty balloon size is often underestimated when selection is made using quantitative angiography, and that optimal balloon size is more accurately determined by IVUS.[23] Additional findings suggest that angiographic success of balloon angioplasty is more likely when hard lesions are disrupted, with dissections extending into the media of the vessel, whereas angiographic failure is seen in lesions that are nondisplaceable or when circumferential dissections or intimal flaps occur.[24] Angiographic success in soft lesions is associated with superficial fissures or fractures of the luminal surface, whereas vessel recoil and luminal disruption or thrombosis at sites of plaque rupture lead to failure. IVUS is capable of imaging all of these features and may be invaluable in providing information that will be used to select lesions suitable for balloon therapy. By combining information about plaque and vessel wall consistency with data on lesion location, such as eccentricity, and by quantitating residual stenosis and dissections, IVUS is ideally suited to act as a screening and guidance method for improving results of balloon angioplasty.[25,26] The balloon ultrasound imaging catheter (BUIC, Boston Scientific, Watertown, Mass.) has been used clinically with promising results. It has been confirmed that single-plane images can be obtained through the midsection of the angioplasty balloon at all times during the course of the angioplasty procedure, and preinflation, inflation, and postinflation luminal features such as plaque fracture and elastic recoil can be monitored with real-time IVUS.[27,28] Peripheral balloon angioplasty has been monitored with IVUS and has been especially useful in identifying and assessing the effect of intimal flaps.

Preliminary studies have used IVUS to locate and treat coarctation of the aorta both experimentally and clinically.[29] IVUS clearly shows the coarctation and accurately measures the adjacent normal aortic lumen for balloon sizing. Following dilatation, IVUS displays the appearance of the dilatation including documentation of dissections.

IVUS has been used as a method for studying the mechanism of action and function of atherectomy devices, lasers, and stents.[30-34] For each type of interventional device, the combination of the guidance and lesion assessment capabilities of IVUS and an interventional technique may produce specific benefits for a particular type of approach.

IVUS provides a method to guide deployment and assess the effect of intravascular stents in peripheral vessels. It allows selection of the correct stent size for a particular vessel and is useful in identifying the most appropriate site for stenting. Two- and three-dimensional IVUS is ideally suited to assessing vascular segments before and after stent deployment. In addition, unique information regarding adequacy of deployment and changes in morphology produced by the stent can be seen.

Real-Time IVUS Assessment of Intravascular Graft Deployment

Candidates for surgical repair of vascular lesions are selected on the basis of physical examination, transcutaneous ultrasound, angiography, CT, and MRI to characterize the size and extent of the lesion and to plan operative strategy. New intraluminal approaches to deploy vascular prostheses additionally require accurate assessment of factors such as the diameter of the proximal and distal neck of aneurysms, the length of the lesions, the position and volume of thrombus in relation to adjacent arteries, the characteristics of the vessel wall, and other variables. For these reasons multiple diagnostic modalities are required to properly select patients and ensure adequate imaging and precise device deployment during the intervention.

Comparison of various imaging modalities demonstrates that each provides information that may be useful for preinterventional selection of patients, for sizing of the vessel lumen and ensuring accurate deployment of devices during interventions, and for follow-up assessments. Some information is complementary to that acquired by other methods and some is unique to a particular modality. Angiography is useful for defining the continuity and morphology of vascular anatomy and for determining the presence of associated vascular abnormalities. Two- and 3D CT scans and MRI are useful for determining both luminal and wall characteristics in a noninvasive manner in addition to providing anatomic information on the location of surrounding structures. CT and MRI examinations are limited to pre- and postintervention studies and cannot be used intraoperatively. They are especially important for selecting patients for whom a particular device is appropriate and for determining vessel lumen dimensions of proximal and distal fixation sites.

IVUS enables catheter-based interrogation of vascular segments during interventional angiographic or operative procedures and provides unique information regarding luminal and vessel wall cross-sectional dimensions and the distribution of arterial disease in the vessel wall. IVUS is useful for detecting the presence of calcium and for inspecting the morphology and distribution of intraluminal thrombus. IVUS is particularly helpful in assessing the relationship of branch artery ostia as well as determining the total length and diameters along the lesion.

Experimental laboratory studies have shown that IVUS is useful for choosing the site of graft deployment and for determining the appropriate-sized device by accurately measuring the luminal dimensions of the aorta.[17] IVUS interrogation of the aortic lumen before device deployment enables accurate identification of the branch arteries and selection of the appropriate site for proximal stent placement. During placement of an intraluminal graft, IVUS is the most accurate means to determine full stent expansion and to obtain information regarding the continuity and alignment of the graft material in the aortic lumen. With the use of certain devices it is possible to place prostheses by IVUS guidance alone. Although cinefluoroscopy and IVUS are complementary in enabling expedient placement of intraluminal grafts, an additional important aspect supporting the use of IVUS in this application is that the time required for fluoroscopy can be significantly reduced during the procedures, thereby minimizing exposure of both personnel and the patient.

In approximately 20% of graft deployments in an experimental series, incomplete proximal stent expansion was determined by IVUS when there was no apparent abnormality on the angiogram.[34] This is an important observation because it averted potential migration of the devices by enabling further expansion of the stent before the procedure was completed. The implications of secure proximal stent positioning are obvious. The improved accuracy of IVUS in determining stent deployment has been confirmed by other investigators who documented that IVUS examination leads to repositioning of intravascular stent devices in approximately 20% to 30% of cases when results of cinefluoroscopy suggest that the deployment is adequate.[35] The implications of these observations for the development of future deployment devices and the effect that IVUS will have on the success of procedures is yet to be determined.

DEVELOPING APPLICATIONS FOR INTRAVASCULAR ULTRASOUND

Intravascular ultrasound is an invasive technique requiring intravascular puncture and catheter insertion. The diagnostic applications are useful when combined with invasive studies such as peripheral angiography or cardiac catheterization, or as a guidance method during therapeutic procedures including angioplasty stent deployment and intraluminal graft placement. Developing potentials of this method range from improved localization of vascular tumors before surgery[36] or imaging the long-term function of vena caval filters[37] to possible application as the primary guidance method for laser angioplasty.[38]

A priority in the development of IVUS technology is the need for further miniaturization and cost-effective manufacturing. Current devices are relatively expensive, and if the technique is to be of clinical benefit as a component of a disposable catheter system for diagnostic or therapeutic intervention, the cost of individual units must be justified by the benefits of IVUS imaging.

Future angioplasty guidance devices may combine the benefits of angioscopy and IVUS in a single delivery system suitable for incorporating mechanical or laser ablation devices. Angioscopy would allow visual inspection of the lumen with ultrasound determining the vessel wall characteristics and dimensions. An added benefit of this type of guidance device would be the ability to select an appropriate ablation method for particular plaque types or volumes. Tissue characterization by analysis of the raw radiofrequency ultrasound signal shows promise for differentiating plaque types.

IVUS also provides exciting opportunities for vascular research including investigation of blood vessel compliance, dynamic changes in the vascular wall caused by disease or pharmacologic intervention, and the natural history of atherosclerosis.

REFERENCES

1. Towne JB, Bernhard VM. Vascular endoscopy: Useful tool or interesting toy. Surgery 82:415-419, 1977.
2. Grundfest WS, Litvack F, Sherman CT, et al. Delineation of peripheral and coronary detail by intraoperative angioscopy. Ann Surg 202:394-400, 1985.
3. White GH, White RA, Kopchok GE. Intraoperative video angioscopy compared to arteriography during peripheral vascular operations. J Vasc Surg 6:488-495, 1987.
4. White GH, White RA, Kopchok GE, Wilson SE. Angioscopic thromboembolectomy: Preliminary observations with a recent technique. J Vasc Surg 7:318-325, 1988.
5. Abela GS, Seegar JM, Barbieri E, Franzini D, Fenech A, Pepine CJ, Conti CR. Laser angioplasty with angioscopic guidance in humans. J Am Coll Cardiol 8:184-192, 1986.
6. van Urk H, Gussenhoven WJ, Gerritsen GP, et al. Assessment of arterial disease and arterial reconstructions by intravascular ultrasound. Int J Card Imaging 6:157-164, 1991.
7. Burns PN, Goldberg BB. Ultrasound contrast agents for vascular imaging. In Cavaye DM, White RA, eds. Arterial Imaging: Modern and Developing Technologies. London: Chapman & Hall, 1993, pp 61-67.
8. Gussenhoven WJ, Essed CE, Lancee CT. Arterial wall characteristics determined by intravascular ultrasound imaging: An in-vitro study. J Am Coll Cardiol 14:947-952, 1989.
9. Kopchok GE, White RA, Guthrie C, et al. Intraluminal vascular ultrasound: Preliminary report of dimensional and morphologic accuracy. Ann Vasc Surg 4:291-296, 1990.
10. Kopchok GE, White RA, White G. Intravascular ultrasound: A new potential modality for angioplasty guidance. Angiology 41:785-792, 1990.
11. Mallery JA, Tobis JM, Griffith J, et al. Assessment of normal and atherosclerotic arterial wall thickness with an intravascular ultrasound imaging catheter. Am Heart J 119:1392-1400, 1990.
12. Nissen SE, Grines CL, Gurley JC, et al. Application of new phased-array ultrasound imaging catheter in the assessment of vascular dimensions. Circulation 81:660-666, 1990.
13. Nissen SE, Gurley JC, Grines CL, et al. Intravascular ultrasound assessing of lumen size and wall morphology in normal subjects and patients with coronary artery disease. Circulation 87:1087-1099, 1993.
14. Gussenhoven WJ, Essed CE, Frietman P, et al. Intravascular echographic assessment of vessel wall characteristics: A correlation with histology. Int J Card Imaging 4:105-116, 1989.
15. Tabbara MR, White RA, Cavaye DM, Kopchok GE. In vivo human comparison of intravascular ultrasound and angiography. J Vasc Surg 14:496-504, 1991.
16. Tobis JM, Mahon D, Lehmann K, et al. The sensitivity of ultrasound imaging compared to angiography for diagnosing coronary atherosclerosis [abst]. Circulation 82(Suppl III):439, 1990.
17. White RA, Scoccianti M, Back M, Kopchok G, Donayre C. Innovations in vascular imaging: Arteriography, three-dimensional CT scans and two- and three-dimensional intravascular ultrasound evaluation of an abdominal aortic aneurysm. Ann Vasc Surg 8:285-289, 1994.
18. Cavaye DM, White RA. Intravascular Ultrasound Imaging. New York: Raven Press, 1993.

19. Cavaye DM, French WJ, White RA, et al. Intravascular ultrasound imaging of an acute dissecting aortic aneurysm: A case report. J Vasc Surg 13:510-512, 1991.
20. Pandian NG, Fries A, Broadway B, et al. Intravascular high-frequency two-dimension detection of arterial dissection and intimal flaps. Am J Cardiol 65:1278-1280, 1990.
21. Neville RF, Yasuhara H, Watanabe BI, et al. Endovascular management of arterial intimal defects: An experimental comparison by arteriography, angioscopy and intravascular ultrasonography. J Vasc Surg 13:496-502, 1991.
22. Cavaye DM, White RA, Lerman RD, et al. Usefulness of intravascular ultrasound for detecting experimentally induced aortic dissection in dogs and for determining the effectiveness of endoluminal stenting. Am J Cardiol 69:705-707, 1992.
23. Cacchione J, Nair R, Hodson J. Intracoronary ultrasound is better than conventional methods for determining optimal PTCA balloon size [abst]. J Am Coll Cardiol 17:112A, 1991.
24. Leon M, Keren G, Pichard A, et al. Intravascular ultrasound assessment of plaque responses to PTCA helps to explain angiographic findings [abst]. J Am Coll Cardiol 17:47A, 1991.
25. Davidson CJ, Sheikh KH, Kisslo K, et al. Intracoronary ultrasound evaluation of interventional procedures [abst]. Circulation 82(Suppl III):440, 1990.
26. Gurley J, Nissen S, Grines C, et al. Comparison of intravascular ultrasound following percutaneous transluminal coronary angioplasty [abst]. Circulation 82:90, 1990.
27. Crowley RJ, Hamm MA, Joshi SH, et al. Ultrasound guided therapeutic catheters: Recent developments and clinical results. Int J Card Imaging 6:145-156, 1991.
28. Isner JM, Rosenfield K, Losordo DW, et al. Combination balloon-ultrasound imaging catheter for percutaneous transluminal angioplasty. Circulation 84:739-754, 1991.
29. Sanzobrino B, Gillam L, McKay R, et al. A direct clinical role for intravascular ultrasound: Utility in the assessment of coarctation of the aorta [abst]. J Am Coll Cardiol 17:68A, 1991.
30. Smucker ML, Scherb DE, Howard PF. Intracoronary ultrasound: How much "angioplasty effect" in atherectomy? [abst]. Circulation 82(Suppl):676, 1990.
31. Mintz G, Potkin B, Keren G, et al. Intravascular ultrasound evaluation of the effect of rotational atherectomy in obstructive athereroscleortic coronary disease. Circulation 86:1383-1393, 1992.
32. Cavaye DM, Tabbara MR, Kopchok GE, et al. Intravascular ultrasound assessment of vascular stent deployment. Ann Vasc Surg 5:241-246, 1991.
33. Cavaye DM, Diethrich EB, Santiago OJ, Kopchok GE, Laas T, White RA. Intravascular imaging: An essential component of angioplasty assessment and vascular stent deployment. Int Angiol 12:212-220, 1993.
34. Katzen BT, Benenati JF, Becker GJ, Zemel G. Role of intravascular ultrasound in peripheral atherectomy and stent deployment. Circulation 84(Suppl II):2152, 1991.
35. White RA, Verbin C, Scoccianti M, Kopchok G, Donayre C. Role of cinefluoroscopy and intravascular ultrasound in the deployment and healing of endoluminal vascular prostheses in normal canine aortas. J Vasc Surg 21:365-374, 1995.
36. Barone GW, Kahn MB, Cook JM, et al. Recurrent intracaval renal cell carcinoma: The role of intravascular ultrasonography. J Vasc Surg 13:506-509, 1990.
37. Greenfield LJ, Tauscher JR, Marx V. Evaluation of a new percutaneous stainless steel Greenfield filter by intravascular ultrasonography. Surgery 109:722-729, 1991.
38. White RA, Kopchok GE, Tabbara MR, Cavaye DM, Cormier F. Intravascular ultrasound guided Holmium: YAG laser recanalization of occluded arteries. Lasers Surg Med 12:239-245, 1992.

13

Surgery vs. Thrombolysis for Lower Extremity Ischemia: Updates on STILE and TOPAS Randomized Studies

KENNETH OURIEL, M.D.

Lower extremity peripheral arterial occlusion is responsible for a wide variety of complications culminating in limb loss or death. Native artery occlusions usually occur in the setting of severe atherosclerotic stenoses; alternatively, an artery may become occluded when an embolus becomes dislodged from a proximal source and is trapped at the site of a peripheral arterial bifurcation. Bypass graft occlusions generally occur following reductions in graft flow from a stenotic lesion within the conduit, compromised outflow, or reduced inflow. The exception to this caveat is the prosthetic graft where thrombosis may develop in the absence of a causative anatomic lesion.[1]

Over the past four decades, operative methods have been the mainstay of treatment for peripheral arterial occlusion.[2] Chronic occlusions are safely and efficiently treated with surgical bypass procedures or endarterectomy. Patients presenting with acute symptoms can be managed in a similar manner, employing open techniques to restore patency. Operative intervention for acute limb ischemia, however, has been associated with limb salvage at the cost of an alarmingly high mortality rate.[3-5]

Thrombolytic agents have been clinically employed since the mid-1950s,[6,7] providing an attractive alternative to surgery. Proponents of thrombolysis have addressed potential benefits such as relief of the arterial obstruction through a less invasive treatment modality, recanalization of small vessels without the mechanical trauma associated with balloon catheter thrombectomy, and identification of the causative lesion underlying the occlusive event.[8-11] Despite widespread use of thrombolytic agents for peripheral arterial occlusion, there was a dearth of objective data critically comparing thrombolysis with surgery. Prospective randomized comparisons were few, and what studies did exist were small[12] and lacking in statistical power.[13] Recently, however, two large randomized clinical trials were completed, each comprising a head-to-head comparison of thrombolysis with surgery in the setting of lower extremity arterial occlusion. A discussion of these trials forms the basis of this report.

Table 1 Eligibility criteria for the STILE trial

Inclusion criteria	Absolute exclusion criteria
Native artery or bypass graft occlusion	Age <18 years or >90 years
Symptoms of <6 months' duration	Embolic occlusions
Thrombotic occlusions	History of TIA, CVA, or cerebral neoplasm
No contraindications to surgery or lytic therapy	Severe hemorrhagic diathesis
	Known or suspected pregnancy
	Ophthalmic surgery within 3 months
	Puncture of vessel within 10 days

TIA = transient ischemic attack; CVA = cerebrovascular accident.

THE STILE TRIAL

In the late 1980s Drs. Anthony Comerota and Robert Graor met informally and discussed the prospect of conducting an investigation comparing urokinase, recombinant tissue plasminogen activator (rt-PA), and surgery in the treatment of peripheral arterial occlusion. A multicenter trial was designed and funding was obtained from Genentech Corporation. This study was termed the **S**urgery or **T**hrombolysis for the **I**schemic **L**ower **E**xtremity (STILE) trial.[14] Overall, 31 centers within North America participated.

The eligibility criteria for the STILE trial are listed in Table 1 and identified patients with lower extremity symptomatic native artery bypass graft occlusions of less than 6 months'

Table 2 Thrombolytic protocols in the STILE trial

Group	Bolus dose	Initial infusion	Subsequent infusion	Maximum duration (hr)
rt-PA	None	0.05 mg/kg/hr	Same	12
Urokinase	250,000 IU	4000 IU/min, 4 hr	2000 IU/min	36

rt-PA = recombinant tissue plasminogen activator.

Table 3 Outcome variables in the STILE trial

Primary end point (composite index, tabulated at 30 days of follow-up)
  Ongoing or recurrent ischemia
  Death
  Major amputation
  Life-threatening hemorrhage
  Major periprocedural complications
  Renal failure requiring dialysis
  Vascular complications requiring surgical repair

Secondary end points
  Reduction in the magnitude of required surgical procedures
  Clinical improvement

duration. Patients with embolic occlusions were specifically excluded from randomization. The mean duration of symptoms was 50.3 days. Threatened limb loss was present in 69% of patients, with symptoms of claudication alone in the remaining 31%.

Patients were randomized to one of three treatment groups: urokinase, rt-PA, or immediate surgical intervention. All thrombolytic infusions were administered through an intra-arterial, catheter-directed approach. The dosages of urokinase and rt-PA are summarized in Table 2. It should be noted that the dosage of rt-PA was 0.1 mg/kg/hr during the initial months of the study but it was decreased to 0.05 mg/kg/hr after clinical information became available that suggested the lower dosage was equally effective and was associated with a lower incidence of hemorrhagic complications. In all instances the goal of thrombolysis was to uncover any causative arterial lesion that might be present and be responsible for the thrombotic event. Thus in many cases successful thrombolytic therapy would be expected to be followed by a directed endovascular procedure or open operative intervention.

The primary end-point was a composite outcome variable that was triggered by the development of any one of a variety of untoward events at 30 days, as listed in Table 3. The secondary end-points included improvement in the patients' clinical status and a reduction in the magnitude of the required surgical intervention. Patient acquisition was begun and by 1993 a total of 393 patients had been enrolled. The trial was terminated prematurely at that point because significant differences in the primary end-point had been detected between the surgical and thrombolytic groups. Notably, technical problems accounted for many of the thrombolytic failures. The angiographer was unable to place the infusion catheter into the thrombus in 41% of patients with occluded bypass grafts and in 22% of patients with occluded native arteries.

On an intent-to-treat basis the primary outcome variable occurred with greater frequency in the thrombolytic group: 61.7% vs. 36.1% ($p < .001$). Further analysis revealed that the major differences did not involve the end-points of death, limb loss, or major morbidity. Rather the difference in the composite outcome occurred primarily as a result of an increase in the frequency of ongoing or recurrent ischemia in the thrombolytic patients: 54.0% vs. 25.7% ($p < .001$). Thus the study was not terminated as a result of differences in limb loss or mortality; rather termination was elected because of the failure of thrombolysis to improve limb perfusion, as judged by the investigators.

Although not entirely based on sound statistical principles, the STILE subgroup analyses were nevertheless interesting. Assessed at 6 months of follow-up, patients presenting within 14 days of the occlusive event had a lower risk of amputation when treated with thrombolysis (Table 4, $p = .02$). In contrast, patients with more chronic symptoms had a lower amputation rate with surgical treatment ($p = .01$). These results suggest that thrombolytic therapy may be most appropriate for patients with acutely ischemic extremities, whereas surgery may be best for patients with subacute or chronic symptoms.

Table 4 Subgroup analysis in the STILE trial: Intent-to-treat analysis

Group	Acute ischemia (0-14 days)		Subacute ischemia (15-180 days)	
	Amputation (%)	Mortality (%)	Amputation (%)	Mortality (%)
Thrombolysis	11.1*	5.6	12.1	6.9
Surgery	30.0	10.0	3.0†	7.9

*p = .02.
†p = .01.

One of the factors analyzed in the STILE trial was the relationship between the plasma fibrinogen concentration and the risk of bleeding complications. Previously there had been much controversy in this regard.[15] The fibrinogen concentration was significantly lower in the STILE patients with major hemorrhagic complications—188 mg/dl vs. 310 mg/dl in patients without bleeding. The activated partial thromboplastin time appeared higher in the patients with hemorrhage—114 seconds vs. 58 seconds—but this difference did not reach statistical significance.

Although economic factors were not specifically tabulated in the STILE trial, the length of hospitalization was compared in the subgroups. Patients with symptoms of 14 days' duration or less had a mean hospital stay of 14.3 days in the surgical group compared to only 9.7 days in the thrombolytic patients ($p = .04$). No such differences were evident in patients with symptoms of longer duration.

THE TOPAS TRIAL

The **T**hrombolysis **O**r **P**eripheral **A**rterial **S**urgery (TOPAS) trial was begun in 1993. The study, funded by Abbott Laboratories, was modeled after a study performed at the University of Rochester.[12] In contrast to the Rochester study, recombinant urokinase was used instead of the clinically available tissue culture urokinase and patients in general manifested a less severe degree of ischemia than was common in the Rochester series. Patients were eligible for inclusion in the TOPAS trial if they had lower extremity symptoms of 14 days' duration or less. The occlusive process could involve either a native artery or a bypass graft, and both thrombotic and embolic etiologies were included. In general, patients had severe but reversible limb ischemia and fell within Rutherford class II.[16] Urokinase infusions were intra-arterial and catheter directed. The major study end-points were patient survival and limb salvage. Secondary end-points included the frequency and magnitude of invasive interventions in the two treatment groups.

The TOPAS study was designed as a multicenter, international trial with two phases. Phase I was a dose-ranging study that sought to randomize approximately 200 patients into one of four treatment groups: three urokinase groups of increasing dosages and one surgical group. Phase II was a direct comparison between (1) the optimum urokinase dose, chosen after review of the phase I data, and (2) immediate surgical intervention. The goal of 550 patients in phase II was achieved in December 1994 and patient acquisition was terminated.

Three dosages of urokinase were evaluated in phase I.[17] The initial 4-hour infusion dose was either 2000, 4000, or 6000 IU/min. The subsequent infusion dose was 2000 IU/min in all three thrombolytic groups, continued to a maximum of 48 hours of total therapy. A dose of 4000 IU/min was chosen by the executive and safety committees after a review of the phase I data. This dosage appeared to maximize thrombolytic efficacy, balancing the untoward effects of hemorrhage and fibrinogenolysis.

As of this writing the phase II TOPAS data are not complete, since all of the patients in the study have not reached the 6-month follow-up point. It is expected that the data will be available in early 1996.

REFERENCES

1. Ouriel K, Shortell CK, Green RM, DeWeese JA. Differential mechanisms of late failure of autogenous and prosthetic bypass conduits. Cardiovasc Dis 3:469-473, 1995.
2. Veith FJ, Gupta SK, Ascer E, et al. Six-year prospective multicenter randomized comparison of autologous saphenous vein and expanded polytetrafluoroethylene grafts in infrainguinal arterial reconstructions. J Vasc Surg 3:104-114, 1992.

3. Blaisdell FW, Steele M, Allen RE. Management of acute lower extremity arterial ischemia due to embolism and thrombosis. Surgery 84:822-834, 1978.
4. Jivegard L, Holm, J, Schersten T. Acute limb ischemia due to arterial embolism or thrombosis: Influence of limb ischemia versus pre-existing cardiac disease on postoperative mortality rate. J Cardiovasc Surg 29:32-36, 1988.
5. Yeager RA, Moneta GL, Taylor LM Jr, Hamre DW, McConnell DB, Porter JM. Surgical management of severe acute lower extremity ischemia. J Vasc Surg 15:385-393, 1992.
6. Cliffton EE. The use of plasmin in humans. Ann NY Acad Sci 68:209-229, 1957.
7. Tillett WS, Johnson AJ, McCarty WR. The intravenous infusion of the streptococcal fibrinolytic principle (streptokinase) into patients. J Clin Invest 34:169-185, 1955.
8. Hess H, Ingrisch H, Mietaschk A, Rath H. Local low-dose thrombolytic therapy of peripheral arterial occlusions. N Engl J Med 307:1627-1630, 1982.
9. Horvath L, Illes I, Molnar Z, Bohm K, Schanzl A, Fendler K, et al. The combined use of transluminal angioplasty and selective clot lysis. Int Angiol 4:111-116, 1985.
10. Gardiner GA Jr, Sullivan KL. Catheter-directed thrombolysis for the failed lower extremity bypass graft. Semin Vasc Surg 5:99-103, 1992.
11. Graor RA, Risius B, Denny KM, Young JR, Beven EG, Hertzer NR, et al. Local thrombolysis in the treatment of thrombosed arteries, bypass grafts, and arteriovenous fistulas. J Vasc Surg 2:406-414, 1985.
12. Ouriel K, Shortell CK, DeWeese JA, et al. A comparison of thrombolytic therapy with operative revascularization in the treatment of acute peripheral arterial ischemia. J Vasc Surg 19:1021-1030, 1994.
13. Nilsson L, Albrechtsson U, Jonung T, Ribbe E, Thorvinger B, Thorne J, et al. Surgical treatment versus thrombolysis in acute arterial occlusion: A randomised controlled study. Eur J Vasc Surg 6:189-193, 1992.
14. The STILE investigators. Results of a prospective randomized trial evaluating surgery versus thrombolysis for ischemia of the lower extremity. The STILE trial. Ann Surg 220:251-268, 1994.
15. Marder VJ. The use of thrombolytic agents: Choice of patient, drug administration, laboratory monitoring. Ann Intern Med 90:802-812, 1979.
16. Rutherford RB, Flanigan DP, Gupta SK, et al. Suggested standards for reports dealing with lower extremity ischemia. J Vasc Surg 4:80-94, 1986.
17. Ouriel K. The TOPAS trial: Phase I results. Abstract presented at the Annual Meeting of the North American Chapter of the International Society for Cardiovascular Surgery. New Orleans, La., June, 1995.

SECTION II

Endovascular Treatment of Aneurysms

This section features an update on the various endovascular graft devices that can be used in the treatment of aortic and other arterial aneurysms. It also describes early experimental and clinical experience with laparoscopically assisted abdominal aortic aneurysm repair. Several chapters highlight specific problems that have occurred with these new techniques.

14

Aortic Aneurysm Morphology for Planning Endovascular Aortic Grafts

HUGH G. BEEBE, M.D., TONYA L. JACKSON, B.A., and JOHN P. PIGOTT, M.D.

Surgeons alter operative procedures as necessary when repairing abdominal aortic aneurysms by conventional techniques. There is no need for preoperative definition of precise infrarenal aneurysm morphology in such procedures because intraoperative decisions regarding the dimensions of grafts and placement of anastomoses are made without difficulty by the experienced surgeon. In fact, it is the opinion of many authors that routine preoperative aortography is unnecessary for managing ordinary aortic aneurysms.[1,2]

In contrast, endovascular grafting for treatment of abdominal aortic aneurysms has profoundly increased the need for accurate definition of aneurysm morphology when planning such procedures. Endovascular surgery requires information not ordinarily considered important in evaluating indications for surgery or operative strategies. For example, the length and diameter of a proximal segment of normal aorta between the lower renal artery and the aneurysm become critically important in deciding whether to attempt endovascular repair. A comparison of the diameters of the aorta above and below the aneurysm, the length of the infrarenal aortic segment, and the degree of curvature of iliac vessels emerge as important considerations when contemplating endovascular grafting but are of little consequence when preparing to repair an aortic aneurysm by means of conventional surgery. This chapter describes abdominal aortic aneurysm dimensions and also discusses the limitations and difficulties involved in using conventional imaging methods for planning endovascular graft procedures.

CONVENTIONAL IMAGING METHODS AND MEASUREMENTS

We collected data from conventional CT and cut-film contrast angiography (CA) in 50 consecutive patients, all of whom underwent both examinations preoperatively.[3] The mean interval between the two imaging studies was 26 days in these 41 men and nine women (mean age 65 years). Aneurysms varied in size from 3.3 to 9.1 cm with a relatively uniform distribution. In several patients with smaller aneurysms, the indication for surgery was aortoiliac occlusive disease symptoms.

Aortography was performed after retrograde catheterization for contrast injection using a standard cut-film technique with a 100 cm focal point to film distance. Digital computerized images were not used. Magnification error was estimated to be within 20% to 30% depending on body habitus. Since the precise magnification artifact for each patient could not be ascertained, we chose to record raw arteriographic data with no interpolation for it. Dimensions obtained by aortography were measured at right angles to a line drawn tangential to the viewed lumen. Common iliac artery measurements represent the maximum diameter or greatest angle along that segment. Lengths were measured between lines drawn perpendicular to the aorta.

Occasionally the infrarenal aorta above an infrarenal aneurysm is slightly cone shaped rather than cylindrical. When such is the case the proximal "neck" is defined as the distance from the lowest renal artery border to the point at which the aorta is more than 1.2 times greater than the immediate infrarenal diameter. Tortuosity represents measurement of angular change from a straight axis direction of the aorta. Two methods were used to describe aneurysm tortuosity: (1) the difference between axial length measured centrally along the aortic lumen following its course and straight length between the lower renal artery and the aortic bifurcation, and (2) direct measurement of aortic angles.

CT scans with contrast injection of the abdomen and pelvis were obtained using contiguous 8 mm slices describing vessel diameter, estimated lengths, and calculations. CT length measurements were approximate since they were obtained by multiplying the number of images showing the measured segment with a standard error of 16 mm. The presence of a distal cuff was noted if there was at least one slice above the aortic bifurcation that was not aneurysmal. Common iliac artery diameters were taken from the first CT slice in which these arteries were identified.

Dimensions are expressed as mean ± standard deviation. Measurements of length were best obtained from CA images; however, the error induced by magnification could not be accurately defined on an individual basis. The term "neck" refers to the segment of normal aorta between the lower renal artery and the aneurysm; "cuff" refers to a normal-sized aortic segment distal to the aneurysm above the bifurcation.

Neck and Cuff Length and Diameter

Proximal neck length above the aneurysm was 2.7 cm (±1.8) by CA and 2.1 cm (±1.2) by CT in 42 patients, which is not significantly different if a magnification artifact of 25% is assumed. In eight patients, measurements of neck length were problematic by either method because of angulation error on CT and poor contrast filling on CA. Neck length was estimated with a difference of >2 cm between CA and CT in 16 cases. It was overestimated by CA in 11 of 42 patients because of the effects of luminal thrombus, whereas CT neck length error in five occurred when the exact renal artery location could not be clearly defined.

Using measurements obtained from CT slices at the immediate infrarenal aorta for neck diameter and the slice immediately proximal to the aortic bifurcation for cuff diameter, apparent differences of >4 mm were noted in 28 patients (56%). It was not possible to control for artifacts caused by CT slices not perpendicular to the axis of an angled aorta at a particular location; thus such differences may be more apparent than real. In general, cuff diameter appeared larger than neck diameter and tended to correlate with aneurysm diameter (Figs. 1 and 2).

Infrarenal Aortic Tortuosity and Length

Although exceptions are not uncommon, larger aortic aneurysms tend to be more tortuous than those less than 5.5 cm. Angulation measured from the axis of the suprarenal aorta and

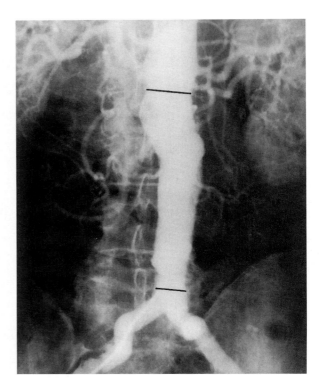

Fig. 1 Aortogram showing unequal neck and cuff diameters (black lines) as judged by contrast lumen. Since luminal thrombus may cause inaccuracy, such diameters are better judged by CT scans.

more distal relative to this second axis are shown in Table 1. The length of the infrarenal aorta including the neck, aneurysm, and cuff, was determined by CT when the lowermost renal artery could be identified and by CA when sufficient contrast was present for measurement regardless of luminal diameter. The mean difference between axial and straight lengths was 0.99 cm (±1.37) for all patients. There was a significant difference in the axial–straight length dimension for aneurysms less than 5.5 cm in diameter, 0.65 cm (±0.98), compared to those greater than 5.5 cm, 1.42 cm (±1.64) ($p = .05$, Student's t-test) (Figs. 3 and 4).

Aortic Bifurcation Angle and Iliac Artery Dimensions

The mean bifurcation angle was 56 degrees (±23.7) for all aneurysms, with a range from 13 to 127 degrees. This was no different from the bifurcation angle of 57.9 degrees (±26.1) for aneurysms greater than 5.5 cm in diameter.

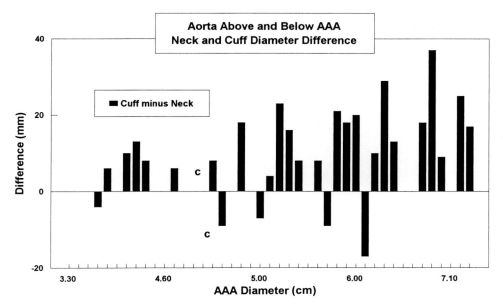

Fig. 2 Graph showing differences between cuff and neck diameters in 28 patients relative to aneurysm size. Neck diameter is subtracted from the usually larger cuff diameter (differences are in millimeters). (From Beebe HG, Jackson T, Pigott JP. Aortic aneurysm morphology for planning endovascular grafts: Limitations of conventional methods. J Endovasc Surg 2:139-148, 1955.)

Table 1 CA and CT measurements by source

	Mean (cm/degrees)	Minimum	Maximum	SD
CA data				
L3 diameter	6.42	3.0	8.1	0.79
Suprarenal diameter	2.8	2.1	3.6	0.38
Infrarenal diameter	2.6	0.2	3.8	0.56
Neck length	3.16	0.0	13.8	2.77
Maximum aneurysm diameter	4.54	1.7	9.0	1.27
Bifurcation diameter	2.84	0.9	6.9	1.06
Left iliac diameter	1.59	0.2	3.8	0.63
Right iliac diameter	1.74	0.9	3.2	0.55
Axial length	15.56	11.5	20.5	2.38
Straight length	14.46	11.0	18.5	1.9
Tortuosity No. 1	26.4	0.0	65.0	18.79
Tortuosity No. 2	25.12	0.0	37.0	50.24
Left iliac tortuosity	55.46	0.0	121.0	30.4
Right iliac tortuosity	38.72	2.0	90.0	20.1
Bifurcation angle	54.24	0.0	127.0	25.53
CT data				
Suprarenal diameter	2.81	2.1	3.8	0.36
Infrarenal diameter	2.92	2.1	5.5	0.7
Neck length	2.16	0.0	5.6	1.32
Maximum aneurysm diameter	5.62	3.3	9.1	1.31
Bifurcation diameter	3.54	0.7	6.6	1.19
Maximum clot	1.79	0.0	4.9	1.23
Left iliac diameter	1.92	1.2	4.4	0.6
Right iliac diameter	2.01	1.0	5.3	0.72

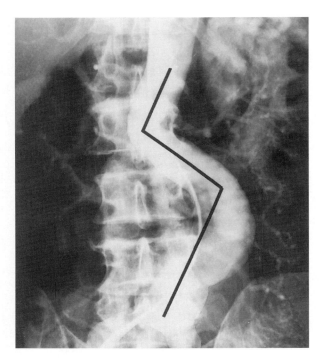

Fig. 3 Frontal aortogram showing the axial lumen as traced (black line) to determine axial length-straight length difference as a measure of tortuosity. Straight length is a line from the lowest renal artery to the aortic bifurcation (see text). (From Beebe HG, Jackson T, and Pigott JP. Aortic aneurysm morphology for planning endovascular grafts: Limitations of conventional methods. J Endovasc Surg 2:139-148, 1955.)

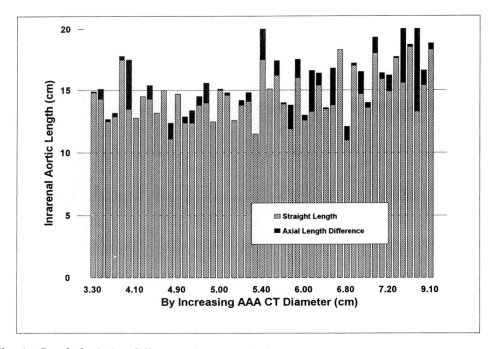

Fig. 4 Graph depicting differences between the length of the infrarenal aorta in a straight line from the lower renal artery to the aortic bifurcation and the axial length following the center of the lumen. With few exceptions, larger aneurysms are more tortuous and thus have greater differences in these two measurements.

Common iliac artery angulation was generally greater on the left side than on the right, and more so in association with larger aneurysms. The mean right common iliac angle was 37.8 degrees (±19.3), whereas the left angle was 55.6 degrees (±30.3). However, when the aortic aneurysm diameter was greater than 5.5 cm, left common iliac artery angulation averaged 67.3 (±31.2) with a total range of 16 to 121 degrees. Eight right iliac arteries had maximum angulation greater than 60 degrees, whereas this amount of tortuosity was present in 18 (37%) on the left. Thirteen patients had one or both common iliac arteries with a diameter greater than 2 cm by CT that was not shown by CA. Table 1 lists CA and CT measurements by source.

MAKING USE OF CONVENTIONAL IMAGING DATA

It is very difficult to obtain accurate measurements of aortic morphology by conventional imaging techniques. This fact is generally unappreciated by vascular surgeons who have not begun to think in terms of endovascular grafting. The obvious truth is that most surgeons who are experienced in repair of aortic aneurysms easily make adjustments as circumstances require when they observe and touch the involved anatomy. When that direct information is no longer available and when simple maneuvers such as holding the graft next to the vessel cannot be used, it becomes necessary to substitute indirect imaging information. Furthermore, decisions need to be made regarding size, length, and placement of endovascular grafts before the procedure can be undertaken. This transition from dimensional data limited to defining only the greatest diameter and the extent of the aneurysmal segment to an extensive and detailed definition of diameters, lengths of adjacent normal segments, degree of tortuosity, patterns of thrombus, iliac artery angulation and size, and the like is an awakening for even the most experienced surgeons. There is a need for extensive information when planning endovascular procedures, and this is more difficult to acquire with any degree of accuracy by means of conventional CA and CT studies than one might suppose before attempting it.

If only CT data are available, it is difficult to interpret the artifact of the radiographic plane intersecting an angled aorta creating an appearance of increased diameter. CT and CA data can be used together to achieve a far greater understanding of aortic morphology than can be attained by using either test alone, and accuracy is increased because aberrant images or artifacts are identified. Indeed, no patient in this series could be completely evaluated in terms of all the dimensions necessary for endovascular graft planning by either test alone.

It is well known that luminal size is often falsely represented because thrombus prevents contrast circulation throughout the full extent of an aneurysmal segment. However, the impact of this artifact in predicting neck or cuff length is far greater when planning endovascular grafting as compared to conventional open aortic graft surgery. Similarly, iliac aneurysms cannot be excluded with confidence by arteriography either, when the lumen is nearly filled with thrombus. This illustrates how multiple imaging modalities may be required to supply sufficient detail for endovascular surgery.

Defining tortuosity or the degree of angulation in the aorta and iliac arteries is important in the design of endovascular devices and in planning their use in endovascular surgery. It may be that extremes of aortic aneurysm tortuosity correlate with difficulty in judging the length of remotely inserted prosthetic grafts or with risk of embolism from a disturbed aortic thrombus during the procedure. A system for standardizing the measurement and describing vessel tortuosity such as the one suggested here permits assessment of its influence on outcome and level of risk. The difference between axial and straight lengths results in a single number that increases with greater degrees of angulation. However, it is subject to operator error in taking the measurements and requires large volumes of radiopaque contrast material in large aneurysms, which are apt to have the most significant tortuosity.

Experience with endovascular devices crossing iliac arteries to reach the aorta has created increased interest in common iliac artery tortuosity.[4] Those with greater than 60-degree tortuosity may present technical difficulties because of the frictional forces that are exerted, particularly when larger diameter delivery devices are used. When a choice of unilateral access is available, the less angled side may be desirable. Severe iliac artery or aneurysm tortuosity may complicate endovascular procedures by causing delivery devices to be directed toward aortic aneurysm thrombus. Therefore knowledge of large-vessel tortuosity is necessary before endovascular aortic surgery is performed.

Conventional angiography does provide useful information concerning lateral tortuosity of the common iliac artery, the most variable angulation in the iliac segment. However, it does not accurately demonstrate iliac arteries for length measurements because of the curvature of these vessels in the anteroposterior plane as they transit the true pelvis. Although common iliac artery angulation usually varies as a function of aneurysm size, and thus presumably changes as the aneurysmal segment enlarges, angulation of the aortic bifurcation does not correlate with aneurysm size. Thus this angle appears to be a function of body habitus. At the extremes of angulation, bifurcations that diverge by as much as 100 degrees or more may represent a challenge for endovascular prosthesis design.

Others have emphasized the relationship between larger, more angulated aortic aneurysms and iliac artery conditions that complicate an endovascular approach to treatment such as tortuosity, stenosis, or associated aneurysm.[5] Obtaining ideal information for endovascular surgery by conventional CA and CT may be very difficult in aneurysms that have progressed beyond the earliest simple stage. The advent of three-dimensional reconstruction imaging using spiral CT or MRI may offer greater assistance in the future.[6] If so, this will impose a requirement for sophisticated software with which to obtain dimensional measurements, since this cannot then be accomplished by use of simple tools and two-dimensional images.

REFERENCES

1. Couch NP, O'Mahoney J, McIrvine A, et al. The place of abdominal aortography in abdominal aortic aneurysm resection. Arch Surg 118:1029-1034, 1983.
2. Gaspar MR, Campbell JJ, Bell DD. Role of arteriography in assessment of abdominal aortic aneurysm. In Ernst CB, Stanley JC, eds. Current Surgical Therapy. Philadelphia: BC Decker, 1991, pp 251-255.
3. Jackson T, Pigott JP, Beebe HG. Aortic aneurysm morphology for planning endovascular grafts: Limitations of conventional imaging methods. J Endovasc Surg 2:139-148, 1995.
4. Chuter TAM, Green RM, Ouriel K, et al. Infrarenal aortic aneurysm structure: Implications for transfemoral repair. J Vasc Surg 20:44-50, 1994.
5. White GH, Weiyun Y, May J, et al. A new nonstented balloon-expandable graft for straight or bifurcated endoluminal bypass. J Endovasc Surg 1:16-24, 1994.
6. Rubin GD, Walker PJ, Dake MD, et al. Three-dimensional spiral computed tomographic angiography: An alternative imaging modality for the abdominal aorta and its branches. J Vasc Surg 18:656-664, 1993.

15

Endovascular Treatment of Arterial Aneurysms

AMIT V. PATEL, M.D., MICHAEL L. MARIN, M.D., and FRANK J. VEITH, M.D.

Advances in the technology of prosthetic grafts and vascular stents, along with interventional angiographic techniques, have led to the introduction of newer, less invasive alternatives for the treatment of arterial aneurysms. The current standard surgical treatment for aneurysms requires exclusion and bypass of the diseased vessel. During the 1950s surgeons introduced the technique of endoaneurysmorrhaphy, in which the proximal and distal vessels are clamped and the dilated aneurysmal sac is opened but not excised. A prosthetic graft is then sutured from within to effectively exclude the diseased artery. Flow is then restored and the aorta is closed over the graft. Additionally, branch vessels such as the inferior mesenteric artery can be revascularized if necessary.[1]

Endovascular repair of aneurysms accomplishes the same goal by entering the arterial system at a remote site, advancing to the diseased area, and deploying an intraluminal prosthesis to exclude the aneurysm. This approach has the advantage of being less invasive and should result in lower morbidity, mortality, and ultimately, lower cost. Most devices have an attachment system at each end that secures them to the arterial wall and an intervening graft to exclude the aneurysm (Fig. 1). Radiographic imaging is essential for accurate placement and evaluation of results. Device systems consist of three basic components: the prosthetic graft, attachment devices, and a delivery system. Numerous devices are now in various stages of development and clinical evaluation. They are designed to function as a single unit as opposed to separate components.

Successful endovascular repair of aortic, iliac, popliteal, brachiocephalic, and traumatic aneurysms has been reported by numerous investigators using various devices.[2-5] The basic techniques are similar for all of them. Preoperative evaluation using a combination of angiography and CT scanning provides essential information regarding proximal and distal vessel size as well as the length of the lesion. Equally important is the confirmation of the caliber and the quality of the approach vessels. Then, usually in the operating room, an arteriotomy is performed in a distal vessel and, under fluoroscopic guidance, a guidewire is advanced to traverse the aneurysm. The abdominal aorta is usually approached from one of the femoral vessels and sometimes requires bilateral catheterization. An arteriogram is then obtained to mark the anticipated deployment site and im-

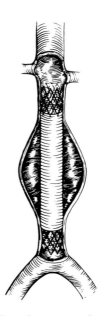

Fig. 1 Straight Parodi stent graft. Palmaz stents are used as proximal and distal attachment devices. The weft-knitted Dacron graft is sutured to the Palmaz stents. (From Parodi JC, Palmaz JC, Barone HD. Transfemoral intraluminal graft implantation for abdominal aortic aneurysms. Ann Vasc Surg 5:491-499, 1991.)

portant branch vessels such as the renal arteries. Once this has been accomplished, the device is advanced and positioned using "over-the-wire" techniques. Contrast material is then injected to confirm positioning before deployment of the device. The final result is then examined with an intraoperative arteriogram.

BASIC DEVICE DESIGN

The ideal device system has a low profile, is very flexible, and includes a system that permits secure attachment to the native vessel. Also, it must be relatively simple to deploy and have some ability to adapt to different anatomic requirements. The three basic components—attachment devices, grafts, and delivery systems—can be discussed individually but must function as a unit and in some of the newer devices the separations between them are not readily apparent.

The ideal graft material must be thin but must still have sufficient strength to protect the aneurysm from further stresses. The prosthetic grafts currently being used are modifications of existing Dacron and polytetrafluoroethylene (PTFE) technology. Existing Dacron grafts are thin and long-term results in stress changes are known, but to further reduce the profile of the fabric, variables such as thickness and porosity must be modified. PTFE is unique in its ability to expand, but the long-term implications of implanting such a material are not known. This theoretically allows the introduction of a small-diameter graft, with subsequent expansion at the site. Other materials such as polyurethane and polyolefin, as well as different weave patterns for Dacron and PTFE, are being studied.

Attachment devices are needed to securely fix the entire device to the proximal and distal vessels. Ideally this will prevent late complications such as migration, pseudoaneurysm formation, leaks, and subsequent rupture of the aneurysm. Currently, attachment devices can be broadly classified as those that are self-expanding and those that are balloon expandable (Fig. 2). A common self-expanding device is the modified Gianturco Z stent (Cook, Inc., Bloomington, Ind.). This stent is made of a stainless steel wire that is formed into a circular zigzag pattern and most commonly has hooks welded onto it for greater attachment. Another self-expanding stent is the Wallstent (Schneider Stent, Minneapolis, Minn.), which is composed of multiple helical wires that are woven into a tubular device and when deployed shorten as the diameter enlarges. This stent is very flexible in both the longitudinal and radial directions. Both of these stents exert a continuous radial force on the vessel and can probably expand further if necessary. This may be advantageous, but the long-term implications are not known and theoretically erosion and perforation may occur, as well as stress fractures from metal fatigue. The most common balloon-expandable stent in use, and the only one approved by the U.S. Food and Drug Administration (FDA) for occlusive disease is the Palmaz stent. This stent is a small slotted stainless steel tube, which when expanded changes into a diamond-shaped porous tube. The fixation of the stent is completed at initial deployment by imbedding the mesh structure into the arterial wall. The Strecker stent (Boston Scientific, Boston, Mass.) is a balloon-expandable stent composed of a single tantalum wire, which is knitted into a series of loose loops that are expandable. This stent is also very flexible in the longitudinal and radial directions. Different configurations are required for varying diameters, and a balloon of appropriate diameter is necessary for all balloon-expandable devices. An inherent problem is the possibility of balloon rupture from the metallic stent, thereby resulting in failure of the system. Other materials such as nitinol are being investigated along with different configurations with excellent initial results.

Delivery systems are tailored specifically to each device and constitute a very important part of this entire concept. They must work smoothly and precisely and must be relatively simple to use (Fig. 3). A variety of catheters, wires, and balloons are necessary and further innovations in this field will result in improvements to the entire device.

CLINICAL APPLICATIONS
Aortic Aneurysms

In the early 1980s Volodos et al.,[6] in the former Soviet Union, began using a device that was composed of Gianturco Z stents and Dacron grafts for the treatment of aortic aneurysms. In 1990 Palmaz et al.[7] reported one of the first clinical applications of an endovascular device for repair of an abdominal aortic aneurysm. Their work was based on a system developed through the use of existing endovascular stents combined with a Dacron prosthetic graft. Since these initial reports, at least nine additional devices have been clinically tested. The remainder of this chapter will outline the significant

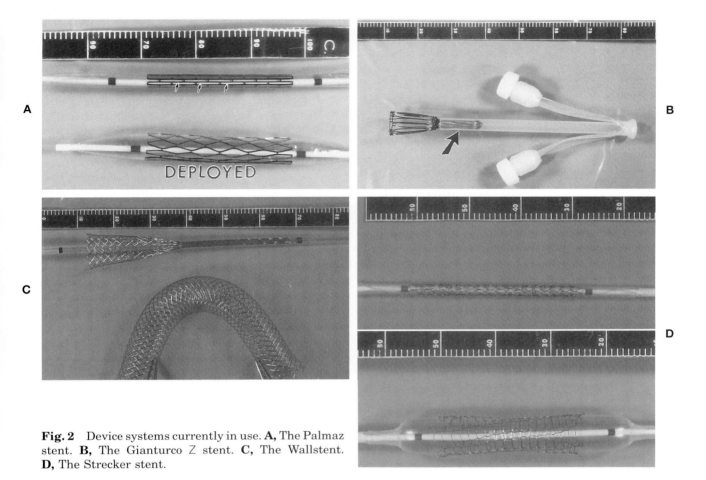

Fig. 2 Device systems currently in use. **A,** The Palmaz stent. **B,** The Gianturco Z stent. **C,** The Wallstent. **D,** The Strecker stent.

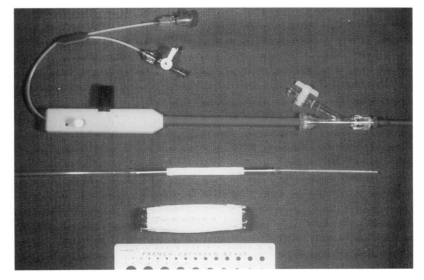

Fig. 3 The "bullet" endovascular grafting system. Note the handle portion of the catheter delivery system, which permits capsule manipulation for graft deployment. The capsule itself is also shown, demonstrating the graft within the capsule and covered by the outer jacket. (From Moore WS. Transfemoral endovascular repair of abdominal aortic aneurysm: Feasibility study of the EGS system. In Parodi JC, Veith FJ, Marin ML, eds. Endovascular Grafting Techniques. Baltimore: Williams & Wilkins, in press.)

features of these devices and the results obtained thus far.

The Parodi device uses Palmaz-type balloon-expandable stents for attachment at each end and a special weft-knitted Dacron graft, the ends of which are radially expandable. A sheath containing the stent-graft device is introduced through an open femoral artery and then advanced under fluoroscopic guidance into the infrarenal aorta.[2] Using this type of device, 65 patients with abdominal aortic aneurysm have been treated in Argentina, 14 in New York, and 10 in Australia. Overall the results have been encouraging, and although significant problems have occurred, the frequency of these complications is declining as investigators gain experience with the use of this device.

In Parodi's series, 45 of these patients had an aortoaortic procedure, whereas the remaining 20 had an aortoiliac graft accompanied by a subsequent femorofemoral bypass for aneurysms involving the aortic bifurcation. In the latter group the contralateral common iliac artery was occluded with an occluding stent (Fig. 4). The longest follow-up was 57 months. Initial success was achieved in 84% of aortoaortic and 75% of aortoiliac procedures. There were four procedure-related deaths (6%): one after conversion to an open repair, two resulting from massive microembolization, and one from mesenteric embolization. Follow-up at 12 months revealed success rates of 78% for aortoaortic and 90% for aortoiliac procedures. Causes of late failure include distal aortic dilatation and anastomotic leaks (12%). Parodi[3] has recently reported the rupture of an aneurysm following endovascular repair, which when treated had a proximal leak that had thrombosed. All of these patients were followed with CT scans and color duplex ultrasonography.

Other investigators have described the use of similar endovascular grafting systems. These systems incorporate a Gianturco-type Z stent at each end with a Dacron graft. The first one to receive FDA approval for clinical trials is the Endograft (Endovascular Technologies, Inc., Menlo Park, Calif.). This device consists of two Gianturco Z stents with hooks and a Dacron graft (Fig. 5). The attachment mechanism makes use of the self-expanding effect of the Gianturco stent but also has hooks that are imbedded into the arterial wall using an expandable balloon (Fig. 6). It is deployed in a manner similar to Parodi's from one of the femoral vessels by means

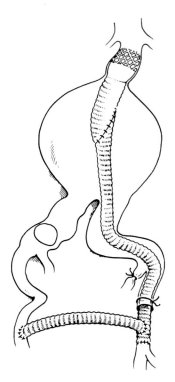

Fig. 4 Modified Parodi device. The tapered aortoiliac graft is used in conjunction with a femorofemoral bypass and occlusion of the contralateral iliac artery with a detachable balloon. Note that the left internal and external iliac arteries are ligated. (From May J, White G, Waugh R, et al. Treatment of complex abdominal aortic aneurysms by a combination of endoluminal and extraluminal aortofemoral grafts. J Vasc Surg 19:824-833, 1994.)

of a 27 Fr sheath. Currently only a straight aortoaortic graft configuration is being studied but a bifurcated design is under development.[8]

The EVT Endograft device was tested in an FDA-approved phase I clinical trial at three centers and until recently was undergoing phase II trials. In January 1995 enrollment of patients in clinical trials of the device was voluntarily suspended. Worldwide data at that time were available for 102 treated patients. Deployment was successful in 91 patients (90%). Inability to deploy the device, requiring conversion to an open procedure, was a frequent problem in the early experience and has occurred in 10 patients (10%). Other complications reported in the United States include anastomotic leaks (9 of 42 patients) and access vessel trauma (5 of 42 patients). These trials were suspended because fractures of the attachment system were de-

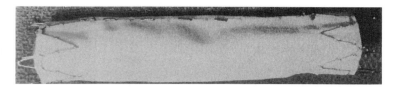

Fig. 5 The Endograft stent delivery system. This is a typical straight endovascular graft consisting of a thin-walled woven Dacron prosthesis with self-expanding stents incorporated at each orifice. The stent fixation pins are set at 80- and 85-degree angles to the prosthesis. The pins engage the aorta and provide intimate fixation. (From Moore WS. Endovascular grafting technique. In Yao JST, Pearce WH, eds. Aneurysms: New Findings and Treatments. Norwalk, Conn.: Appleton & Lange, 1994, pp 333-340.)

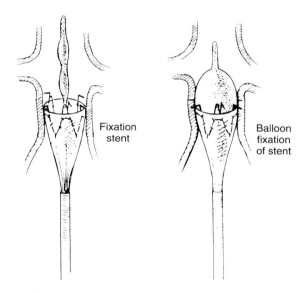

Fig. 6 Deployment of the proximal fixation device. Artist's rendering shows self-expansion of the stent followed by expansion of the balloon to drive the fixation pins into the wall of the aorta. (From Moore WS. Endovascular grafting technique. In Yao JST, Pearce WH, eds. Aneurysms: New Findings and Treatments. Norwalk, Conn.: Appleton & Lange, 1994, pp 333-340.)

tected in 23 of the 91 patients evaluated beyond 30 days after the procedure. The manufacturer is now in the process of redesigning the system to eliminate this problem. The details of these fractures and any clinical significance has not yet been reported. As with any new device and technology, there are many undetermined factors that contribute to the ultimate outcome of the patients treated. This trail is an example of why carefully controlled trials must be conducted, especially when proved surgical alternatives are bypassed for newer less invasive treatment modalities in "good" risk patients.

A similar device that uses Gianturco Z–type barbed stents, a thin Dacron graft in the bifurcated configuration, and a system for stent deployment has been developed by Chuter et al.[10] A stone retrieval basket and a cross-femoral catheter with a guidewire are used to deploy the contralateral distal limb of the bifurcated graft (Figs. 7 and 8). Thus far at least 27 patients have been treated with the Chuter device in Europe and Australia. Technical difficulties were more prevalent early in the clinical experience and improved results have been seen more recently. Conversion to an open repair was required in four patients (14%)—two because of deployment failure and two because of kinking and

120 Endovascular Treatment of Aneurysms

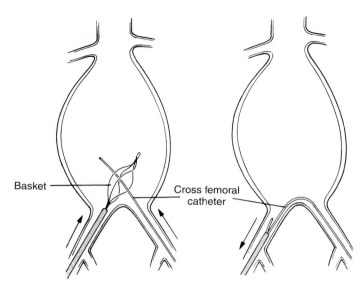

Fig. 7 The stone retrieval basket is used to pass the cross-femoral catheter from one side to the other. (From Chuter TA, Nowygrod R. Bifurcated endovascular grafts for aortic aneurysm repair. In Parodi JC, Veith FJ, Marin ML, eds. Endovascular Grafting Techniques. Baltimore: Williams & Wilkins, in press.)

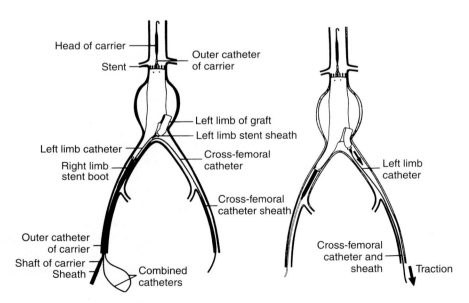

Fig. 8 The cross-femoral catheter is used to translocate and position the contralateral limb. (From Chuter TA, Nowygrod R. Bifurcated endovascular grafts for aortic aneurysm repair. In Parodi JC, Veith FJ, Marin ML, eds. Endovascular Grafting Techniques. Baltimore: Williams & Wilkins, in press.)

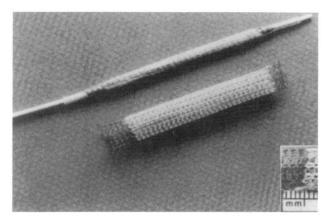

Fig. 9 The balloon-expandable endoluminal prosthesis is shown mounted on a balloon catheter, then expanded. Inset: Closeup of the expanded stent with scale. (From Piquet P, Rolland P-H, Bartoli J-M, Tranier P, Moulin G, Mercier C. Tantalum-Dacron coknit stent for endovascular treatment of aortic aneurysms: A preliminary experimental study. J Vasc Surg 19:698-706, 1994.)

thrombosis of the graft. Kinking occurred in two additional patients and was corrected by means of endovascular placement of a Wallstent within each graft limb. Three patients had perianastomotic leaks, one of whom had subsequent rupture of the aneurysm. Overall the device was successful in 18 patients (67%).[11]

The Sydney device was developed at the University of Sydney and the Royal Prince Alfred Hospital. This device incorporates Gianturco Z-type stents along the entire length of the graft and a thin Dacron graft. Various configurations have been used including 19 straight aortoaortic, three bifurcated, 10 aortoiliac, and six ilioiliac grafts. This system has been used in 38 patients with successful deployment in 34. It is significant that the bifurcated graft failed to deploy satisfactorily in all cases. Four patients (9%) required open repair and three patients experienced self-limited perianastomotic leaks. There were no procedure-related deaths.[12,13]

At Stanford University 25 grafts have been placed in the thoracic aorta with immediate technical success. These devices are similar to the others in that they consist of a Dacron graft and multiple Gianturco Z stents, which are advanced from one of the femoral vessels into the thoracic aorta. The only complication was paraplegia, which developed in one patient.[14]

In terms of newer experimental devices, there are several that use novel materials such as nitinol wire and different stent designs such as the Strecker and Wallstent. One such device that has been used in Europe is a tantalum-Dacron coknit device, which is a modification of the Strecker stent (Fig. 9). It is introduced from a femoral approach and requires balloon dilatation for deployment. Various questions remain regarding its long-term success including the ultimate porosity of the device, which is much greater than that of any other system.[15] Other devices use woven materials over Wallstent-type stents and these may be suitable for aortic aneurysms but they are still in the developmental stage.

Other Aneurysms

Other aneurysms elsewhere in the body have been treated similarly with excellent results. The most commonly used device is one that contains Palmaz stent attachments at each end with an expanded PTFE graft. These devices are delivered to the affected site via a remote distal arteriotomy and then deployed. Isolated iliac aneurysms have been treated using the Parodi device,[3] the Sydney device,[12] the tantalum-Dacron coknit stent graft,[16] and the Wallstents.[17] At Montefiore Medical Center 15 iliac aneurysms as well as six subclavian and two popliteal aneurysms have been treated this way.[4,5] The immediate results are excellent for the iliac lesions and to date there have been no postoperative complications. One of the two patients with a popliteal aneurysm developed an

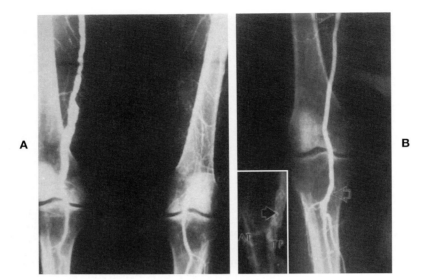

Fig. 10 A, Bifemoral arteriogram from a patient with a popliteal artery aneurysm. Occlusion of the left above-knee popliteal artery is seen with reconstitution of the popliteal artery below the knee. The right popliteal artery is patent, tortuous, and aneurysmal. **B,** Completion angiogram after placement of a PTFE stent-graft device shows exclusion of the aneurysm and graft patency (arrow = stent). Inset shows detail of the stent in the distal popliteal artery. (TP = tibioperoneal trunk; AT = anterior tibial artery.) (From Marin ML, Veith FJ, Panetta TF, et al. Transfemoral endoluminal stented graft repair of a popliteal artery aneurysm. J Vasc Surg 19:754-757, 1994.)

immediate postoperative thrombosis and required open surgical repair (Fig. 10). The subclavian aneurysms were approached from the ipsilateral brachial artery and all were successfully repaired. The Montefiore group has also treated nine patients with traumatic pseudoaneurysms using single Palmaz stents that are covered with expanded PTFE. Immediate success was achieved in all of these patients and there have been no reports of short-term complications.

CONCLUSION

It has clearly been shown that arterial aneurysms can be treated using endovascular techniques. The current devices have limited applicability, which will probably be overcome as newer designs are introduced. The results thus far are encouraging and as more experience is gained, complications will decrease. Current limitations include inaccessibility, inadequate proximal and distal vessel necks, and lack of experience in deployment techniques. Many questions remain regarding the long-range significance of clinical findings such as small leaks that thrombose, porosity and stability of the device materials, and long-term patency and protection from rupture. As these devices gain wider clinical acceptance, many other observations will be reported leading to refinements and ultimately the development of an ideal device.

REFERENCES

1. Dubost C, Allary M, Oeconomos N. Resection of aneurysm of abdominal aorta: Reestablishment of continuity by preserved human arterial graft, with result after five months. Arch Surg 64:405-408, 1952.
2. Parodi JC, Palmaz JC, Barone HD. Transfemoral intraluminal graft implantation for abdominal aortic aneurysms. Ann Vasc Surg 5:491-499, 1991.
3. Parodi JC. Endovascular repair of abdominal aortic aneurysms and other arterial lesions. J Vasc Surg (in press).
4. Marin ML, Veith FJ, Panetta TF, et al. Transfemoral endoluminal stented graft repair of a popliteal artery aneurysm. J Vasc Surg 19:754-757, 1994.
5. Marin ML, Veith FJ, Panetta TF, et al. Transluminally placed endovascular stented graft repair for arterial trauma. J Vasc Surg 20:61-69, 1994.
6. Volodos NL, Shekhanin VE, Karpovich IP, et al. Self-fixing synthetic prosthesis for endoprosthetics of the vessels. Vestn Khir (Russia) 11:123-125, 1986.
7. Palmaz JC, Parodi JC, Barone HD, et al. Transluminal bypass of experimental abdominal aortic aneurysm. Proceedings of the Seventy-Sixth Scientific Assembly

and Annual Meeting of the Radiological Society of North merica. Chicago, Ill., November 25-30, 1990.
8. Moore WS. Endovascular grafting technique. In Yao JST, Pearce WH, eds. Aneurysms: New Findings and Treatments. Norwalk, Conn.: Appleton & Lange, pp 333-340, (in press).
9. Moore WS, Vescera CL. Repair of abdominal aortic aneurysm by transfemoral endovascular graft placement. Ann Surg 220:331-341, 1994.
10. Chuter TAM, Green RM, Ouriel K, et al. Transfemoral endovascular aortic graft placement. J Vasc Surg 18:185-197, 1993.
11. Chuter TA, Nowygrod R. Bifurcated endovascular grafts for aortic aneurysm repair. In Parodi JC, Veith FJ, Marin ML, eds. Endovascular Grafting Techniques. Baltimore: Williams & Wilkins (in press).
12. May J, White G, Waugh R, et al. Treatment of complex abdominal aortic aneurysms by a combination of endoluminal and extraluminal aortofemoral grafts. J Vasc Surg 19:824-833, 1994.
13. White GH, May J, Yu W. Development of a clinical program of endoluminal aneurysm grafting: Experience in 60 patients. In Parodi JC, Veith FJ, Marin ML, eds. Endovascular Grafting Techniques. Baltimore: Williams & Wilkins (in press).
14. Fogarty TJ. Stanford Experience with Stented Graft Repair of Thoracic Aortic Aneurysms. Twenty-First Annual Symposium on Current Critical Problems in Vascular Surgery. New York, November 17, 1994.
15. Strecker EP, Berg G, Schneider B, et al. A new vascular balloon-expandable prosthesis: Experimental studies and first clinical results. J Intervent Radiol 3:59-62, 1988.
16. Piquet P, Rolland P-H, Bartoli J-M, Tranier P, Moulin G, Mercier C. Tantalum-Dacron coknit stent for endovascular treatment of aortic aneurysms: A preliminary experimental study. J Vasc Surg 19:698-706, 1994.
17. Vorwerk D, Gunther RW, Wendt G, et al. Ulcerated plaques and focal aneurysms of iliac arteries: Treatment with noncovered, self-expanding stents. Am J Radiol 162:1421-1424, 1994.

16

Problems Encountered With EVT Devices (Tube and Bifurcated) for Treatment of Abdominal Aortic Aneurysms

WESLEY S. MOORE, M.D.

The feasibility of placing a graft within the vascular tree from a remote site was first demonstrated by Dotter[1] in 1969. Since then, a number of experimental studies have evaluated this option and offered several imaginative designs. However, it was not until the report by Parodi et al.[2] documenting their clinical experience with endovascular repair of abdominal aortic aneurysm that surgeons focused considerable interest on this approach. Since Parodi's initial report in 1991, there has been an accelerating interest around the world in studying the efficacy of endovascular repair of abdominal aortic aneurysm (AAA).

Several investigators hold patents on various devices for endovascular repair. During Parodi's experimental phase, Lazarus[3] independently developed a technique for tube graft repair of AAA. This was subsequently developed by Endovascular Technologies, Inc. (Menlo Park, Calif.), who submitted a protocol to the FDA and received permission to begin a clinical trial. The first implantation of this device took place at UCLA Medical Center on February 10, 1993,[4] and since that time there have been nearly 100 implants worldwide.

TECHNIQUE
Tube Graft Repair

The first prosthesis that was developed for implantation was of the tube graft configuration. This device required that patients with AAA have a proximal neck between the renal arteries and the beginning of the aneurysm. That neck should have sufficient length to anchor the proximal portion of the prosthesis as well as a neck between the distal extent of the aneurysm and the aortic bifurcation. Obviously, this limited implantation to relatively few patients. Our own experience suggests that only one of seven patients with AAA would be suitable for this type of implant.[4]

The procedure is done in an operating room with the patient under general anesthesia. The patient's abdomen and the groin areas on both sides are prepared, and the patient, operating room, and team are prepared for conversion to an open repair should that be necessary. One femoral artery is exposed surgically and accessed with a 9 Fr sheath. A marker angiogram catheter and guidewire are advanced through the sheath into the suprarenal position. A repeat angiogram is performed with roadmap imaging to define the anatomy once again. The points of desired deployment in the proximal and distal neck are defined and marked with movable radiopaque cursors as a part of the marker board that the patient is lying on.

Heparin is then administered and the femoral artery clamped proximally and distally. A transverse arteriotomy is made, and the large working sheath is passed over the guidewire up the iliac artery and into the aneurysm. The EVT catheter delivery system is then threaded over the guidewire and passed up the sheath into the appropriate location. The graft within the catheter delivery system has been premeasured and selected for the individual patient. The attachment systems are then positioned appropriately in relation to the radiopaque cursors as previously determined by the angiographic roadmap image. The proximal attachment system is then remotely deployed. Once this has sprung into place, the coaxial balloon is positioned across the proximal attachment system and inflated to drive the pins, which are part of a self-expanding attachment system, into the wall of the aorta for ultimate security. The distal attachment system is then deployed in a similar fashion.

A completion angiogram is obtained to document the position and functioning of the graft and to determine whether there is any evidence of a perigraft leak into the aneurysm sac. The femoral arteriotomy is closed. The patient is taken to the recovery room and then to a regular room. The patient can be discharged from the hospital the next day.

Bifurcation Graft Repair

Endovascular Technologies has also developed a bifurcated graft configuration. This solves the problem with respect to use of the endovascular approach in patients whose AAA does not have a distal neck. A proximal neck is required, as well as the absence of iliac artery aneurysm or significant occlusive disease.

The procedure is similar to that for the tube graft, with the exception that both femoral arteries are exposed. The device is passed up the ipsilateral femoral artery through the large working sheath. However, a secondary sheath is placed in the contralateral femoral artery so that the contralateral graft limb can be manipulated. After the preinsertion angiogram and roadmap image is obtained, a stiff Amplatz guidewire is left in position. A pullwire, which is a part of the device, is then inserted up the ipsilateral sheath, and at the same time an Amplatz snare is passed up the contralateral sheath. The snare is opened at the level of the aortic bifurcation and the pullwire is passed through the snare. The snare is then pulled tight, and the pullwire is drawn across the aortic bifurcation down the contralateral limb. This provides contralateral access to the contralateral limb of the graft that is at the moment within the sheath of the capsule. Next the whole device is passed up into a suprarenal position. The jacket is retracted, which allows both graft limbs to become free, but their individual attachment systems are still collapsed. The graft is then brought back down the aorta and positioned so that the proximal attachment system is immediately below the renal arteries and the ipsilateral and contralateral iliac limbs are within the respective iliac arteries. Radiopaque marking permits the appropriate orientation so that twisting does not occur.

The proximal graft attachment system is initially deployed as with the tube graft. The contralateral attachment system is deployed at the contralateral iliac artery, and then the iliac attachment system in the ipsilateral limb is deployed. All three attachment systems are seated with balloon catheters. They are self-expanding but also have pins around the circumference that provide ultimate security. A completion angiogram is then obtained and the femoral arteriotomies and incision sites closed.

FDA THREE-PHASE PROTOCOL

The endovascular tube and bifurcated prostheses are currently the only devices that are approved by the FDA for clinical investigation. The protocol involves a three-phase trial. Phase 1 involves a series of implantations of either the tube or bifurcated graft to determine safety and efficacy. Phase 1 of the tube graft configuration is complete, and phase 1 of the bifurcated graft configuration had just begun. The phase 2 protocol is designed to compare endovascular prosthetic grafts with conventional open operation. Initially this was designed to be a prospective randomized trial but has been subsequently modified. The tube graft is currently in phase 2, and all patients who are candidates for a tube graft endovascular prosthesis will receive that graft. Patients whose AAAs have an inadequate distal neck for endovascular repair but who are clearly candidates for a tube graft repair using a conventional open technique will serve as concurrent controls. The objective will be to compare morbidity, mortality, and cost between the two techniques. Phase 3 is designed to be a long-term follow-up of patients who have undergone endovascular repair of AAA to determine whether the repair achieves the objective of preventing aneurysm enlargement and rupture and to assess the durability of the prosthetic device itself.

CLINICAL EXPERIENCE

Phase 1 of the tube graft implantations has been completed, and a manuscript has been submitted for publication describing the experience with 46 patients who have undergone tube graft repair in North America.[5] In our own institution we have implanted 16 tube grafts. Two of these required open conversion, and 14 functioned well. Thirteen of these 14 patients are alive and well; one patient died approximately 6 months after implantation from respiratory failure. That patient underwent the procedure on a compassionate basis because he was disabled as a result of severe repiratory problems.

The initial phase 1 implants of the bifurcated graft were carried out at UCLA Medical Center on September 21, 1994. Two patients underwent successful implantation, and a third implant was performed approximately 1 month later. Currently these three patients are being followed.

PROBLEMS

Major problems associated with endovascular repair, to date, fall into three major categories:

(1) difficulty with access and deployment, (2) perigraft leaking into the aneurysm sac, and (3) fractures of the attachment system components.

Problems with deployment occurred early on and represented difficulties associated with the surgeon's learning curve. Problems with perigraft leakage also occurred relatively early and reflected difficulties with judging graft size appropriate for the patient. There was a tendency to match the diameter of the graft close to the diameter of the available aneurysm neck. We now know the importance of oversizing graft diameter to maintain a total contact seal between the circumference of the graft and the aneurysm neck.

The most recent problem identified was a pin fracture within the attachment system. Once that was noted, an immediate report was made to the FDA, and the trial was placed on hold. This required an engineering reevaluation of the forces associated with implantation and function to assess the reason for pin fracture and correct it. Those changes have now been completed and bench testing has been successful. At the time of this writing, the FDA has approved the resumption of investigations of both the tube and bifurcation grafts.

REFERENCES

1. Dotter CT. Transluminally-placed coilspring endarterial tube grafts. Long-term patency in canine popliteal artery. Invest Radiol 4:329-332, 1969.
2. Parodi JC, Palmaz JC, Barone HD. Transfemoral intraluminal graft implantation for abdominal aortic aneurysms. Ann Vasc Surg 5:491-499, 1991.
3. Lararus HM. Endovascular grafting for the treatment of abdominal aortic aneurysms. Surg Clin North Am 72:959-968, 1992.
4. Moore WS, Vescera CL. Repair of abdominal aortic aneurysm by transfemoral endovascular graft placement. Ann Surg 220:331-341, 1994.
5. Moore WS, Rutherford RB, for the EVT Investigators. Transfemoral endovascular repair of abdominal aortic aneurysm: Results of the North American EVT phase 1 trial. J Vasc Surg (in press).

17

Endovascular Bifurcated Graft Insertion for Abdominal Aortic Aneurysm Repair

TIMOTHY A.M. CHUTER, M.D., and ROMAN NOWYGROD, M.D.

The main advantage of abdominal aortic aneurysm (AAA) repair by insertion of an endovascular stent-graft combination is the avoidance of an abdominal operation.[1] The main limitation has been the frequent lack of a suitable implantation site in the aorta distal to the aneurysm.[2] Therefore we have focused on the development of a bifurcated endovascular graft, for which the distal implantation site is the common iliac artery.

PATIENTS AND METHODS
Patient Selection

Preoperative imaging is used for patient selection and graft sizing. The imaging modalities include conventional sectional CT, conventional contrast arteriography, spiral CT, MRI, and magnetic resonance angiography. Angiography is used mainly as a means of assessing the configuration of the aneurysm neck and iliac arteries. Angiography can be used to obtain arterial dimensions but CT scanning of one kind or another is more reliable. Spiral CT scanning is particularly useful in this regard because it permits the reformatting necessary for accurate measurement of tortuous vessels.

The anatomic criteria depend on the patient's health. The current exclusion criteria for low-risk patients are:

1. Aneurysm neck shorter than 10 mm, wider than 25 mm, angulated relative to the suprarenal aorta by more than 75 degrees, or highly irregular or lined with thrombus
2. Inhomogeneity or multiple lumens within the mural thrombus of the aneurysm
3. External iliac artery internal diameter less than 6 mm following balloon dilatation
4. Common iliac artery internal diameter less than 8 mm following balloon dilatation or greater than 14 mm
5. Bilateral iliac artery aneurysm
6. Patent inferior mesenteric artery, which appears indispensable for intestinal perfusion

Procedure

All procedures are performed in the operating room under general anesthesia. The patient is positioned on a radiolucent operating table to permit fluoroscopic examination up to the level of the xyphoid process. The patient's abdomen, groin, and thighs are prepared and draped as for standard aortobifemoral bypass. Broad-spectrum intravenous antibiotics are administered at the start of the procedure. Both common femoral arteries are exposed using standard surgical technique and encircled with hemostatic loops. Heparin (10,000 units) is administered intravenously 3 minutes before clamping. The arteries are opened transversely. The technique of prosthesis insertion varies according to the anatomy of the infrarenal aorta and iliac arteries, but in all cases the procedure involves the following basic maneuvers:

1. Cross-femoral catheter placement using a stone retrieval basket in the aneurysm to pull a catheter from one side to the other (Fig. 1)
2. Insertion of a guidewire into the proximal aorta through one lumen of a double-lumen dilator, while the cross-femoral catheter occupies the other lumen to prevent twisting of the guidewire and cross-femoral catheter
3. Insertion of an angiographic catheter into the proximal aorta from the left femoral arteriotomy
4. Angiography to locate the renal arteries
5. Insertion of the delivery system over the right femoral guidewire
6. Repeat angiography before and during graft deployment to confirm the exact location of the renal arteries

128 Endovascular Treatment of Aneurysms

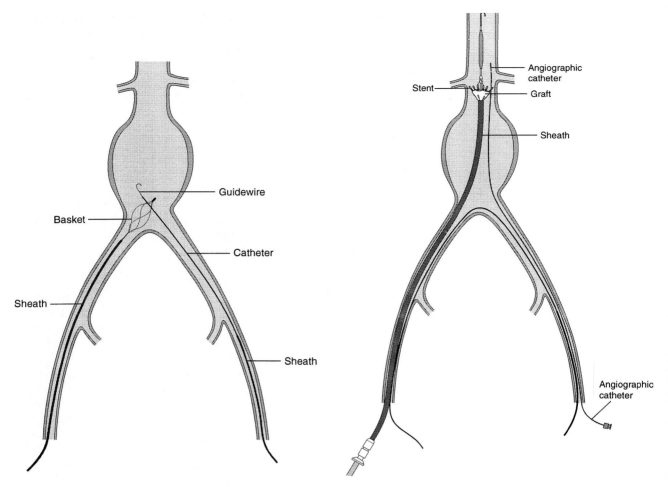

Fig. 1 Use of a stone retrieval basket for cross-femoral placement.

Fig. 2 Graft extrusion.

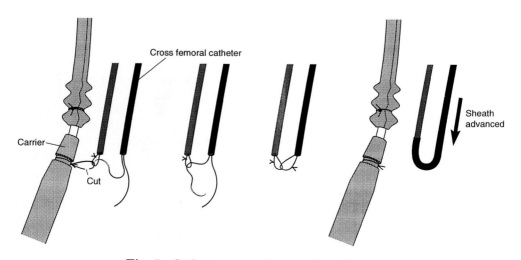

Fig. 3 Catheter connections at the right groin.

7. Graft deployment by removal of the sheath of the delivery system (Fig. 2)
8. Connection of the small catheters at the right groin (Fig. 3)
9. Traction on the combined catheter at the left groin to unwind the large loop in the right iliac artery and then pulling the left limb of the graft into the left common iliac artery (Fig. 4)
10. Release of the graft from the delivery system by removal of a central catheter
11. Deployment of the right limb stent by withdrawal of the right limb sheath and removal of the delivery system (Fig. 5)
12. Deployment of the left limb stent by severing the catheter and the suture that holds the stent within its sheath, then removing the catheter with the attached sheath (Fig. 6)
13. Deployment of Wallstents within the limbs of the graft to prevent kinking
14. Completion angiography
15. Flushing of blood from the femoral arteries onto pads

Follow-up

Follow-up includes serial abdominal radiographs to detect graft migration and serial CT and duplex scans to detect aneurysm growth or perigraft leakage.

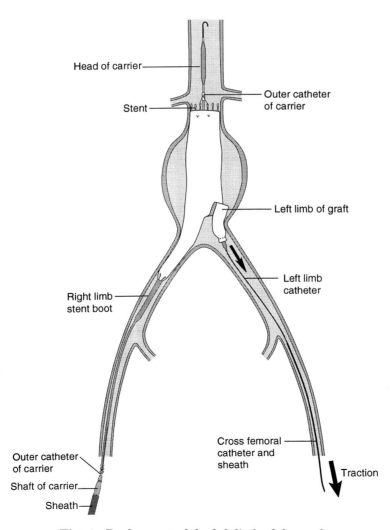

Fig. 4 Deployment of the left limb of the graft.

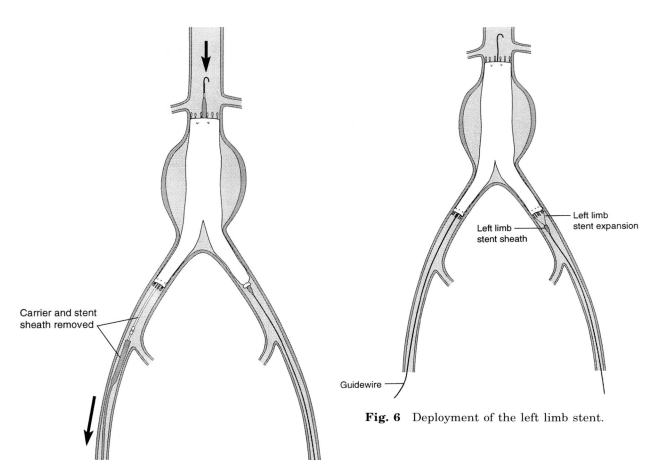

Fig. 5 Removal of the delivery system with deployment of the right limb stent.

Fig. 6 Deployment of the left limb stent.

RESULTS

AAAs were treated by insertion of a bifurcated endovascular graft in 27 patients between October 1993 and August 1994. It is instructive to consider results in three separate groups (early, middle, and late) of nine patients each. In the early group there were four cases of graft limb thrombosis (two requiring graft removal), two failed insertions, one proximal perigraft leak, and one wound infection. In the middle group there was one case of graft limb thrombosis and two cases of retrograde perigraft leakage (apparent on completion angiography). One of these leaks resolved, whereas the other was followed by aneurysm rupture on postoperative day 3, leading to the only death in the series. The late group included one failed insertion. There were no instances of embolism or graft migration. The three groups also differed with regard to patient selection. The first nine patients were all low risk with relatively favorable arterial anatomy. The last 18 included high-risk patients and those with more challenging findings. These included necks as short as 10 mm (Fig. 7, *A* and *B*), angulated necks, and iliac arteries affected by aneurysm, stenosis, or tortuosity (Fig. 8).

DISCUSSION

The first insertions were plaqued by kinking of the graft limbs followed by thrombosis. Whatever the cause—iliac angulation or stiffness of the graft material—the treatment was placement of a Wallstent. The problem was so common that Wallstent insertion became routine. Since then 16 insertions have been performed with no signs of kinking or thrombosis.

Another problem in the early part of the series was failure of the left limb stent to release from

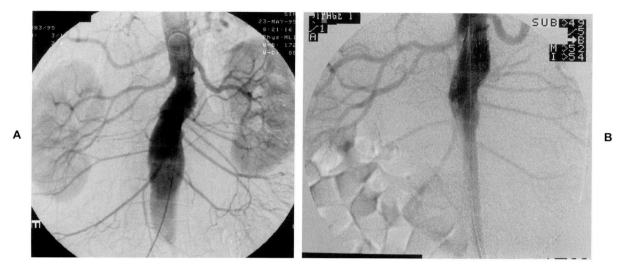

Fig. 7 A, Preoperative angiogram showing a low right renal artery and short (10 mm) aneurysm neck. **B,** Completion angiogram showing the Gianturco Z stent implanted immediately below the renal arteries.

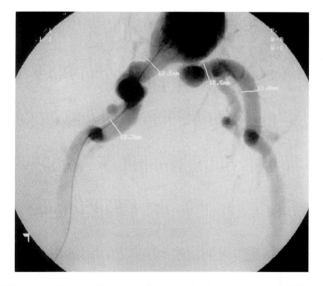

Fig. 8 Preoperative angiogram showing tortuous common iliac arteries.

its sheath, leading to failed deployment. This problem has not recurred since the size of the sheath was increased. The only unsuccessful deployment occurred in a patient whose proximal neck consisted of a ridge between a bulge, at the level of the renal arteries, and the main body of the aneurysm. The proximal stent could not be implanted securely at this site—hence the present stipulation that the neck be free of major irregularities.

The case of distal perigraft leakage in which the aneurysm ruptured on postoperative day 3 illustrates the following two points: (1) it is important to assess the iliac arterial implantation sites as carefully as the aneurysm neck and (2) distal perigraft leakage is not benign.

CONCLUSION

The declining complication rate reflects a steady improvement in our understanding of the method. It is now possible to isolate an aortic aneurysm from the circulation by transfemoral insertion of an endovascular bifurcated graft in a wide variety of cases. Whether this translates into long-term protection against rupture remains to be seen.

REFERENCES
1. Parodi JC, Palmaz JC, Barone HD. Transfemoral intraluminal graft implantation for abdominal aortic aneurysms. Ann Vasc Surg 5:491-499, 1991.
2. Chuter TAM, Green RM, Ouriel K, DeWeese JA. Infrarenal aortic aneurysm morphology: Implications for transfemoral repair. J Vasc Surg 20:44-50, 1994.

18

Laparoscopically Assisted Abdominal Aortic Aneurysm Repair: Technique and Early Clinical Experience

JON R. COHEN, M.D., MARIE H.M. CHEN, M.D., EUGENE A. MURPHY, M.D., and ANTHONY J. D'ANGELO, M.D.

Investigation of alternative minimally invasive approaches to aneurysm surgery originated in the animal laboratory with a feasibility study to determine whether laparoscopic dissection and replacement of the intra-abdominal porcine aorta was possible. Although the aorta was not calcified or aneurysmal, initial studies revealed that laparoscopic dissection of the aorta was feasible but was associated with a significant learning curve. Twenty-one pigs underwent laparoscopic dissection of the abdominal aorta by a transabdominal approach and two pigs by a retroperitoneal approach. Fifteen grafts were successfully placed in the transabdominal group and one in the retroperitoneal group. Complications included injuries to the bladder, ureter, renal vein, inferior vena cava (IVC), aorta, and lumbar vessels. Operative time decreased from 6 to 2 hours, blood loss from 1 L to 150 ml, and cross-clamp time from 60 to 20 minutes by the conclusion of the study.[1]

Based on the initial encouraging results of this feasibility study, a survival study was undertaken to compare the hemodynamic and postoperative results of pigs undergoing an open versus laparoscopic replacement of the abdominal aorta.[2] Twenty pigs were divided into four groups. Aortic replacement was accomplished by (1) open hand-sewn graft, (2) open insertion of a cuffed graft, (3) laparoscopically assisted hand-sewn graft, or (4) total laparoscopic insertion of a cuffed graft. The cuffed graft is similar in concept to the grafts used for the treatment of thoracic aortic dissection.

The aorta was replaced in all animals, with no intraoperative deaths. There were no differences between groups in blood loss, fluid requirement, temperature, and urine output. Except for cardiac index, there were no differences in systemic and pulmonary hemodynamics. The two laparoscopic groups maintained a higher cardiac index during cross-clamping of the aorta. Cross-clamp time was the longest in the laparoscopic-assisted group in which the graft was sewn in through a small minilaparotomy. Operative time for the laparoscopic group was longer than for the open control group. However, the longer operative time did not result in a more profound hypothermia, most likely because of the use of a heated insufflator and smaller incisions.

Information learned in the animal laboratory was brought into the human arena for laparoscopically assisted human abdominal aortic aneurysm (AAA) repair.[3] Under institutional review board approval, patients with infrarenal AAA requiring a tube graft and with no contraindications to laparoscopy were carefully selected.

The operative goals were to laparoscopically dissect the neck of the aneurysm and both iliac arteries and then, through a minilaparotomy, to cross clamp the aorta and repair the aneurysm using a conventional open Creech technique.[4] To date, a preliminary study of 10 patients has been completed.[5] In nine patients the dissection was successfully completed laparoscopically; in the first patient conversion to a standard open incision was necessary because the neck of the aneurysm could not be completely dissected laparoscopically.

In the animal studies, the dissection ports were placed in the lower abdomen. While these port positions were ideal for the iliac dissection, they were too low to get over the hump of the aneurysm and reach the neck. Modifications in the trocar location resulted in successful laparoscopic dissection of the neck of the aorta and the iliac vessels in the next nine patients.

There were no deaths in this study. Three minor complications, unrelated to laparoscopy, occurred in 10 patients. One patient developed a mild case of rhabdomyolysis following emboli from an iliac cross clamp. Another patient underwent a pericardial window following a coronary artery bypass graft, which was performed 10 days before the aneurysm repair. The third complication was a superficial wound infection requiring additional days of antibiotic therapy. Operative times averaged 4.48 ± 0.72 hours, longer than the standard times of 3 to 3.5 hours for open approaches. The initial average laparoscopy time was 1.68 ± 0.43 hours, accounting for about 40% of the total operative time. With experience, this operative time has been decreased to less than 1 hour. The average length of hospital stay was 5.8 ± 1 days, which is not significantly different from that for open AAA repair. The average length of stay in the intensive care unit was 2.1 ± 0.78 days. The data from this feasibility study of laparoscopically assisted abdominal aortic aneurysm repair are preliminary, and prospective randomized trials are needed to clearly define the advantages and disadvantages of laparoscopically assisted in comparison to open repair of AAA.

CONCLUSION

Laparoscopically assisted AAA is the first step to total laparoscopic AAA repair. At the present time the major obstacles to be overcome are laparoscopic control of the lumbar vessels and laparoscopic intracorporeal sewing of the graft.

REFERENCES

1. Chen MHM, Murphy EA, Levison J, Cohen JR. Laparoscopic aortic replacement in the porcine model: A feasibility study in preparation for laparoscopically assisted abdominal aortic aneurysm repair in humans. J Am Coll Surg (accepted for publication).
2. D'Angelo AJ, Chen MHM, Murphy EA, Rivera L, Spector R, Nathan R, Marini C, Cohen JR. Comparison of laparoscopic and open abdominal aortic replacement in the porcine model [abst]. Surg Endosc (accepted for publication).
3. Chen MHM, Murphy EA, Halpern V, Faust GR, Cosgrove JM, Cohen JR. Laparoscopic-assisted abdominal aortic aneurysm repair. Surg Endosc 9:905-907, 1995.
4. Creech O Jr. Endoaneurysmorrhaphy and treatment of aortic aneurysm. Ann Surg 164:935-946, 1966.
5. Chen MHM, Murphy EA, D'Angelo AJ, Halpern V, Marini CP, Cohen JR. Laparoscopically assisted abdominal aortic aneurysm repair: A report of ten cases [abst]. Surg Endosc (accepted for publication).

19

Stanford Experience With Stent-Graft Repair of Thoracic Aortic Aneurysms

MICHAEL D. DAKE, M.D., D. CRAIG MILLER, M.D., CHARLES SEMBA, M.D.,
R. SCOTT MITCHELL, M.D., CHRISTOPHER K. ZARINS, M.D., and
THOMAS J. FOGARTY, M.D.

There is no disease more conducive to clinical humility than aneurysm of the aorta.

This quote by Sir William Osler still holds true today. Surgical repair of thoracic aneurysms is associated with high mortality and morbidity. Mortality rates range from 5% to an alarming 35%. The major morbidity, paraplegia, occurs in 10% to 25% of patients who undergo standard surgical interventions to repair this type of aneurysm.

An alternative to major operative procedures, with their attendant high mortality rates and frequent complications, is welcomed by even the most aggressive surgeon. From the perspective of every clinician who has ever treated these aneurysms, endoluminal thoracic stent grafting represents an attractive approach. Patients too, when faced with the prospect of a major operation associated with significant mortality and morbidity, immediately accept and embrace a less-invasive alternative.

INDICATIONS

Indications for aortic stent-graft repair in the Stanford series of patients include extreme debility, renal and pulmonary insufficiency, and severely compromised myocardial function. Pathologic and anatomic indications include prior aneurysm surgery with aneurysms at the anastomotic site. Additional indications include prior dissection, with or without repair, and continued diffuse and/or discrete enlargement. Twenty-five percent of the patients had discrete excavating ulcerations leading to blisterlike aneurysms.

Graft

The thoracic stent graft is a custom device approved by the Stanford Investigational Review Board for compassionate use only. The graft consists of a self-expanding stainless steel Z-shaped stent covered by thin, uncrimped Teflon or Dacron. The graft material covering is sutured to the stent at multiple points (Fig. 1). The stents are contiguous and line the entire linear length of the graft material. The graft is loaded into a 24 Fr delivery system that is guidewire compatible (Fig. 2).

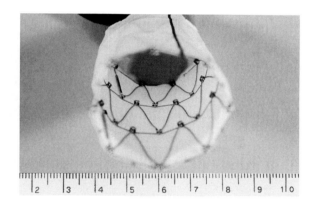

Fig. 1 Cross-sectional view of cloth-covered Z stent used in the Stanford series.

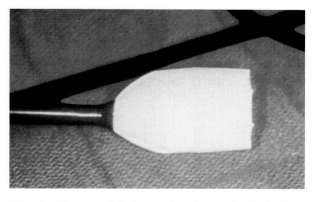

Fig. 2 Stent graft being loaded into a 24 Fr loading capsule.

OPERATIVE PROCEDURE

Procedures are performed in the operating room under general anesthesia with standby cardiopulmonary bypass. The patient is positioned so that C-arm fluoroscopy with road mapping can be used for visualization from the takeoff of the transverse arch to the diaphragm. Transesophageal echocardiography is a useful aid for visualization and provides critical placement benchmarks.

CLINICAL DATA

This report details a series of 25 men and five women in the Stanford study, which is ongoing. The mean age was 63.5 years (range, 35 to 83 years), and the mean diameter of the aneurysms treated was 6.1 cm (range, 5 to 9 cm). The longest graft used was 28 cm and the shortest was 5 cm.

The cause of aneurysm was atherosclerosis in 24 patients, dissection in three, trauma in two, and surgery in one. Access was achieved by direct cutdown in all patients. Femoral exposure provided access in 17 patients and retroperitoneal aortic exposure was used in 13 patients. Eight patients underwent standard simultaneous surgical repair of an abdominal aortic aneurysm at the time of thoracic stent-graft placement. Three patients had a previously placed aortic bifemoral graft for aneurysm and access was directly through the graft body.

RESULTS AND COMPLICATIONS

There were two postoperative deaths. One patient, an 83-year-old man, died 48 hours after surgery as a result of continued progression of multisystem organ failure. The second death occurred in a 66-year-old man who had an abdominal aortic aneurysm involving the visceral vessels. Simultaneous surgical abdominal and endovascular thoracic repair was attempted. The patient developed a coagulopathy at the time of surgery and died 18 hours after the operation. Additional complications included paraplegia in one patient, device misplacement in one, pleuritis in four, incomplete thrombosis in two, and distal embolus in one.

The device misplacement in one patient was handled by a subclavian carotid transposition. The second patient required an additional distal stent-graft placement 6 days after the first procedure. There were no conversions to surgery, no strokes, and no infections in the series.

CONCLUSION

A preliminary study of thoracic stent-graft placement was successfully performed in 30 selected patients with advanced aortic disease. The mortality and morbidity in these patients compared quite favorably with outcomes reported for standard surgical interventions. Continued clinical evaluation is justified. Long-term follow-up of endovascular repair is mandatory to validate this minimally invasive interventional technique.

20

Sydney Experience With Endovascular Stent-Graft Repair of Abdominal Aortic Aneurysms: New Findings and Limitations

JAMES MAY, M.S., F.R.A.C.S., and GEOFFREY H. WHITE, M.D., F.R.A.C.S.

Between May 1992 and November 1995 we undertook endoluminal repair of aneurysms at the Royal Prince Alfred Hospital on 111 patients (Table 1). The aneurysm was situated in the abdominal aorta in 94 patients. We will report on this group of patients, and we will discuss new findings on the fate of aneurysms following endoluminal repair and the limitations of the endoluminal method of repair in our experience.

Of the 94 patients, 88 were men and six were women. The mean age was 70 years. The procedures were performed in the operating room with the patient prepared for an open operation in the event that endoluminal repair failed. We have described the techniques used in previous reports.[1-6] The configuration of the grafts was tubular in 51 patients, tapered aortoiliac/aortofemoral in 21, and bifurcated in 22. The devices used were a modification of the Parodi graft in 10 patients, the Sydney endograft (White-Yu) in 61, the Endovascular Technologies (EVT) graft in 12, the Stentor in 10, and the Chuter in one. Comorbid conditions were present in 40 patients, the most common being poor left ventricular function. The other causes are listed in Table 2.

RESULTS

There were 12 failures in which the endoluminal repair had to be abandoned in favor of an open repair. The causes of failure leading to open repair are shown in Table 3. Local/vascular complications were seen in 20 patients. Damage to the femoral artery requiring repair occurred in three patients. In an additional two patients perforation of the iliac artery occurred. In both cases the iliac artery was repaired without requiring conversion of the endoluminal repair to an open one. Graft stenosis occurred in two endoluminal aortofemoral grafts; one was corrected by balloon dilatation and the other by

Table 2 Comorbid conditions

Poor left ventricular function (with renal impairment in three)	23
Renal failure	1
Chronic obstructive airway disease	6
Bilateral thoracoplasties	1
Chronic hepatitis	3
Hostile abdomen	6
TOTAL	40

Table 1 Endoluminal repair of aneurysms at Royal Prince Alfred Hospital, May 1992 to November 1995

Abdominal aortic	94
Thoracic aortic	2
Iliac	12
Femoral	1
Popliteal	1
Subclavian	1
TOTAL	111

Table 3 Causes of failure leading to open repair

Access problems	2
Balloon-related	
Malfunction	1
Aortic rupture	1
Stent-related	
Dislodgement	3
Graft thrombosis	1
Inability to deploy bifurcated graft	4
TOTAL	12

surgery. Occlusion of the common iliac artery occurred in three patients. Two were corrected by balloon dilatation and stent deployment; the third was treated with a femorofemoral crossover graft. An endoluminal leak occurred in five patients; two were corrected by secondary endoluminal repair and two required conversion to open repair. The fifth patient is awaiting a secondary endoluminal repair. Bleeding in the postoperative period occurred in two patients, one of which required return to the operating room. Wound problems comprising infection and lymph fistula were seen in four patients. In addition to the two patients with paragraft flow who required later conversion to open operation, there were another two patients whose endografts covered the renal arteries and required conversion to open repair at a second operation.

Systemic or remote complications occurred in 18 patients. These are detailed in Table 4. There were five deaths within 30 days of operation (5.3%); three were cardiac and two were renal in origin and all were procedure related. There have been six later deaths, three cardiac, two hepatic, and one from ruptured esophagus. None of the late deaths was procedure related.

NEW FINDINGS
Fate of AAA Following Endoluminal Repair

Several centers have now confirmed the experience of Parodi et al.[7] and demonstrated that it is possible to exclude an aneurysmal sac from the general circulation by means of a transluminary placed graft. It was not known, however, whether the natural history of continued expansion of an abdominal aortic aneurysm (AAA) is prevented by such repair. We recently studied this potential problem with a prospective analysis of early changes in morphology and dimensions of AAAs following endoluminal grafting.[8,9] Forty-two patients who had endoluminal repairs before the end of May 1994 were potentially available for follow-up at 6 months or more following operation. Excluded were patients with failed endoluminal repairs leading to open operation (n = 8), patients who died within 6 months of operation (n = 3), and patients with anastomotic aortic aneurysms (n = 1). This left 30 patients in these study groups.

All patients underwent contrast-enhanced CT examination of the abdominal aorta and iliac arteries before operation, within 10 days after operation, and at 6 and 12 months after operation. The maximum transverse diameter of the

Table 4 Endoluminal repair of AAA: Systemic remote complications

Renal insufficiency	
Obstructive	2
Contrast media induced	5
Cardiac	
Congestive failure	2
Myocardial infarction	4
Cardiac arrhythmia	2
Stroke/transient ischemic attack	3
TOTAL	18

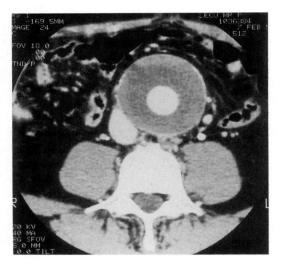

Fig. 1 Postoperative CT scan demonstrating contrast within the endograft and exclusion of the aneurysmal sac (group I).

AAA and the appearance of any contrast within the aneurysmal sac were noted.

On the basis of postoperative CT evaluation, patients were divided into two groups: those with no extravasation of contrast medium into the aneurysmal sac (group I, n = 26) (Fig. 1) and those in which contrast was seen in the aneurysmal sac (group II, n = 4) (Fig. 2). The mean maximum diameter of AAAs in group I progressively decreased, whereas those in group II progressively increased (Table 5). Twenty-three patients (88%) in group I had decreased AAA diameters (Fig. 3). All patients with a documented endoluminal leak of contrast medium into the aneurysmal sac had a progressive increase in AAA diameter. Patients who had an increase in AAA diameter had a significantly higher incidence of endoluminal leakage com-

Table 5 Mean maximum transverse diameter of AAAs in groups I and II before and after endoluminal repair

	Group I (cm)	Group II (cm)
Preoperative	5.18	6.46
Postoperative		
6 mo	4.97	7.28
12 mo	4.25	7.75

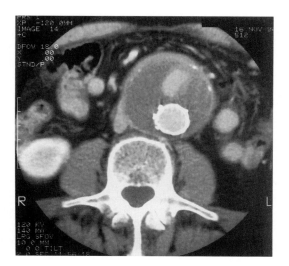

Fig. 2 Postoperative CT scan demonstrating extravasation of contrast medium into the aneurysmal sac (group II).

pared with those who had a decrease in diameter ($p = .001$). Although these early findings are encouraging in that the majority of AAAs appear to diminish in size after successful endoluminal repair, it is clear that continued careful follow-up is required to determine the long-term outcome.

Trombone Technique

We recently reported the advantages of endoluminal repair of AAAs using the double-tube endograft or "trombone" technique.[4] In those type 1 aneurysms[5] that have both a proximal and a distal neck and are thus suitable for endoluminal tube graft repair, one of the critically important parts of the operation is the estimation of the length of the graft. If the graft if too long, it will end up in the common iliac artery. If it is too short, a communication will remain between the lumen of the aorta and the aneurysmal sac at the lower end of the graft. Several methods have been devised to assist in the estimation of the length of graft required for endoluminal tube graft repair of AAA. A calibrated angiographic pigtail catheter with metallic bands at 1 cm intervals can be used for minimizing errors of measurement because of magnification. These are not foolproof, however, since the catheter will usually take the shortest course in the presence of aortic angulation. The markers may also be closer together than 1 cm if the catheter is curved in the same plane to that

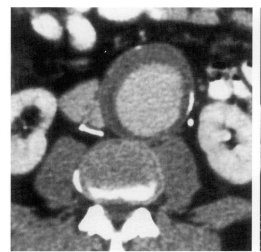 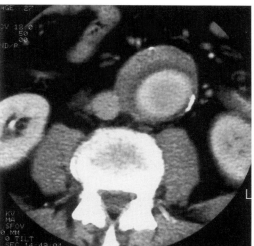

Fig. 3 **A,** Preoperative CT scan demonstrating AAA with a maximum transverse diameter of 7.0 cm. **B,** CT scan 12 months after endoluminal repair of AAA; the maximum transverse diameter is now 5.4 cm. (From May J, White GH, Yu W, et al. A prospective study of changes in morphology and dimensions of abdominal aortic aneurysms following endoluminal repair: A preliminary report. J Endovasc Surg 2:343-347, 1995.)

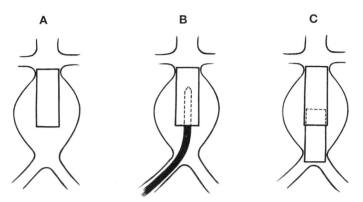

Fig. 4 A, The first endograft has been deployed immediately below the renal arteries. **B,** The introducing sheath with its mandrel has been reintroduced and lies within the first endograft. **C,** The mandrel is removed and the second endograft delivered through the introducing sheath to lie within and overlapping the first endograft. (From Yu W, White GW, May J, et al. Endoluminal repair of abdominal aortic aneurysms using the double tube endograft or "trombone" technique. Asian J Surg 19:37-40, 1996.)

in which the aortogram is filmed. Parodi (Personal communication, 1995) has developed a computerized system for plotting the position of the lumen within the thrombus relative to the aneurysmal sac. This assists in avoiding underestimating the length of graft required as a result of the tortuousity of the lumen. Until a foolproof method emerges, however, the trombone technique minimizes the risk of failure from an error in estimating the length of the graft required.

The technique involves the deployment of the first of two endografts immediately inferior to the renal arteries (Fig. 4). The introducing sheath is reintroduced so that it lies within the first endograft. The second endograft is delivered through this sheath and deployed in such a manner that it is within and overlapping the first endograft. The advantages of this system result from the fact that it is easier to deploy the superior end of the first endograft immediately below the renal arteries when one does not have to worry about the position of the distal end. Similarly, it is easier to deploy the inferior end of the second endograft accurately at the aortic bifurcation when one does not have to worry about the position of the proximal end. The area of overlap is not critical provided there is a minimum of 2 cm.

The trombone technique also lends itself to repair of more complex AAA. We have used the technique in the aortoiliac configuration, with

Table 6 Morphology of AAA in 26 of 53 patients who were unsuitable for endoluminal repair

Proximal neck too short or absent	16
Excessive angulation of AAA	3
Tortuous iliac arteries	3
Small-diameter iliac arteries	2
Accessory renal artery	1
Presence of renal transplant	1
TOTAL	26

the endograft comprising two components and the bifurcated configuration with the endograft comprising three components.

LIMITATIONS

The limitations of endoluminal grafting fall into two categories: unfavorable morphology that precludes the endoluminal method and complications that militate against use of the method.

In studying the first category we retrospectively reviewed aortograms and CT scans from 53 patients who had undergone conventional open repair of AAA in the year preceding the commencement of the endoluminal program at our institution (1992). In this review we found that 27 of 53 patients would have been suitable for endoluminal repair. The reasons that the remaining 26 were unsuitable are listed in Table 6. The major limiting factor is an inadequate proximal neck, which accounted for 64% of the patients being unsuitable for endoluminal repair. The number of patients excluded from endoluminal repair for this reason may be reduced in a number of ways. Operating on the AAA at an earlier stage, while the proximal neck is suitable and before it is absorbed into the aneurysmal process, would solve the majority of problems. However, this approach will have to wait until the safety of endoluminal grafting of small aneurysms has been established and the long-term outcome is known. Alternatively, endografts are now available with attachment devices designed to be deliberately placed above the renal arteries without obstructing them. Such devices should allow endografts to be successfully deployed in AAA with short proximal necks. Another option in selected cases would be to undertake preliminary renal revascularization by either splenorenal anastomosis or autotransplantation to the iliac fossa.

With the enthusiasm that accompanies any new technology there is a tendency for the risks to be downplayed. With this in mind we recently analyzed our experience of endoluminal AAA repair with special emphasis on complications.[10] Between May 1992 and August 1994, endoluminal repair of AAA was undertaken in 53 patients. Successful endoluminal repair was achieved in 43 patients (81%). In the remaining 10 patients endoluminal repair was abandoned in favor of an open repair. There were 17 local vascular complications (32%) and 13 systemic remote complications (25%). The sum of these complications occurring in successful endoluminal repairs and those complications leading to failure of endoluminal repair was 40 (75%). There were two cardiac deaths within 30 days, both procedure related. Endoluminal repair of AAA in this study was therefore shown to have a low perioperative (less than 30 days) mortality rate (3.7%) but a high morbidity rate (75%). We believe it is important to obtain a clear picture of the true morbidity of endoluminal repair by combining those complications that lead to failure of endoluminal repair and conversion to open operation with the local vascular complications occurring in patients with successful endoluminal repairs. When this was done it could be seen that half the patients developed surgical complications directly related to the endoluminal technique. This minimally invasive method clearly has many advantages, but these come at a price—that of a high complication rate.

REFERENCES

1. May J, White G, Yu W, et al. Treatment of complex abdominal aneurysms by a combination of endoluminal and extraluminal aortofemoral grafts. J Vasc Surg 19:924-933, 1994.
2. White GH, Yu W, May J, et al. A new non-stented endoluminal graft for straight or bifurcated endoluminal bypass. J Endovasc Surg 1:16-24, 1994.
3. White GH, May J, Yu W. Stented and non-stented grafts for aneurysmal disease: The Sydney experience. In Chuter T, Donayre C, White R, eds. Endoluminal Vascular Prostheses. Boston: Little, Brown, 1995, pp 107-152.
4. Yu W, White GH, May J, et al. Endoluminal repair of abdominal aortic aneurysms using the double tube endograft or "trombone" technique. Asian J Surg 19:37-40, 1996.
5. May J, White G, Yu W, et al. Results of endoluminal grafting of abdominal aortic aneurysms are dependent on aneurysm morphology. Ann Vasc Surg 10:254-261, 1996.
6. White GH, May J, McGerhan T, et al. Historical control comparison of outcome for matched groups of patients undergoing endoluminal versus open repair of abdominal aortic aneurysms. J Vasc Surg (in press).
7. Parodi JC, Palmaz JC, Barone HD. Transfemoral intraluminal graft implantation abdominal aortic aneurysms. Ann Vasc Surg 5:491-499, 1991.
8. May J, White GH, Yu W, et al. A prospective study of changes in morphology and dimensions of abdominal aortic aneurysms following endoluminal repair: A preliminary report. J Endovasc Surg 2:343-347, 1995.
9. May J, White GH, Yu W, et al. A prospective study of anatomico-pathological changes in abdominal aortic aneurysms following endoluminal repair: Is the aneurysmal process reversed? Eur J Vasc Endovasc Surg (in press).
10. May J, White GH, Yu W, et al. Surgical management of complications following endoluminal grafting of abdominal aortic aneurysms. Eur J Vasc Endovasc Surg 10:51-59, 1995.

SECTION III

Surgery of Aneurysms, the Aorta, and Its Visceral Branches

This section offers new and updated information on aortic aneurysms and other procedures involving the aorta and its visceral branches. Chapters are included that discuss factors associated with the growth of abdominal aortic aneurysms, statewide variations in the prevalence of aneurysms, and the operative mortality for aneurysm repairs. The topic of nonoperative management of thoracoabdominal aortic aneurysms is explored along with unusual methods for treating abdominal aortic aneurysms. Several interesting aspects of renal artery surgery are examined, and a variety of techniques for approaching the renal arteries are described. Chapters on the management of aortoenteric fistulas and late complications following aortic aneurysm resection are also included.

21

Factors Associated With the Growth of Abdominal Aortic Aneurysm: The Importance of Smoking

JANET T. POWELL, M.D., Ph.D., SHANE T.R. MacSWEENEY, F.R.C.S., NEIL R. POULTER, M.R.C.P., and ROGER MALCOLM GREENHALGH, M.A., M.D., M.Chir., F.R.C.S.

Most patients with abdominal aortic aneurysm (AAA) have been smokers. The first clear association between smoking and AAA was provided by the Framingham study.[1] More recently the Whitehall study has indicated that death from AAA is four times more common in smokers than in nonsmokers and death from AAA is 14 times more common in smokers of hand-rolled cigarettes than in nonsmokers.[2]

During the past two decades there has been an apparent increase in the incidence of AAA in the United Kingdom, the United States, and Australia.[3-5] This apparent increase in incidence follows some 35 to 40 years after the increase in popularity of smoking earlier this century (Fig. 1). AAAs appear to be much more common in men than in women, and approximately 15 years ago surgeons would have reported operating on only one woman for every 11 men. Recently, more women have presented with AAA, and currently approximately 20% of our new referrals with AAA are women. This change in referral patterns between the sexes may also reflect the change in smoking habits. Men started smoking in large numbers before World War II, whereas the emancipation of women, and during World War II the movement of women into the workplace, marked the rise of smoking among women from the late 1940s onward. If a long history of smoking promotes the formation of AAA, we may be seeing many more such aneurysms in women in the near future.

During the past two or three decades, where the age-standardized rates for death from AAA have been increasing, there has been a marked change in the composition of manufactured cigarettes, with a reduction of 50% or more in the tar yield and a corresponding reduction in nicotine yield. There is little evidence to indicate which specific aspects of the smoking habit might favor the development of an AAA, although a review of historical data would indicate that the tar yield of cigarettes might not be a significant factor. Recently we attempted to determine what aspects of smoking favor the development of AAAs and whether such aneurysms grow more rapidly in those who continue to smoke.

We approached the first issue—what specific aspects of smoking favor the development of AAA—in the framework of a case-control study. In this study both cases and control subjects were current smokers. The cases were patients who were still smoking and newly referred to the Vascular Surgical Service at Charing Cross Hospital with AAAs ranging in diameter from 5 to 10 cm. Between 1989 and the end of 1992 we recruited 44 such patients. The demographic

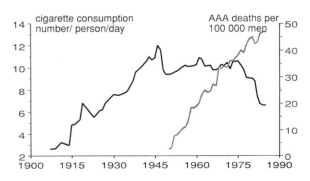

Fig. 1 Cigarette consumption and death from abdominal aortic aneurysm. There is a lag interval of approximately 40 years between increasing consumption of cigarettes and increasing deaths from abdominal aortic aneurysm in England and Wales. Data for cigarette consumption are from the U.K. Tobacco Advisory Council and the age-standardized mortality figures are taken from Fowkes, MacIntyre, and Ruckley.[3]

details of these patients were recorded, and the patients were interviewed concerning their medical and social history and asked to complete a detailed questionnaire about their smoking habits, both present and past. Patients were asked when they had first started smoking, how many cigarettes per day or how many ounces of tobacco per day they smoked during each decade of their lives, and whether they inhaled into the mouth, to the back of the throat, moderately into the lungs, or very deeply into the lungs. More detailed information was collected regarding current tobacco usage so that the tar and nicotine yields could be calculated. From the cumulative history of smoking, a pack-year estimate of smoking was calculated. We also identified 244 age- and sex-matched control subjects who were attending outpatient clinics in the Departments of Orthopaedics, Dermatology, or Urology. The controls had no history of cardiovascular disease and no evidence of AAA on clinical examination. The controls completed a Rose questionnaire to provide further evidence that they had neither angina nor intermittent claudication. The control subjects completed the same detailed questionnaire concerning their medical and social history, in addition to providing information on their smoking habits, as the patients with AAA.

The baseline demographic data for the cases and control subjects are shown in Table 1. Cases and controls were well matched in terms of height, body mass index, and pack-year history of smoking. The control group contained the greater proportion with diabetes, whereas the patients with AAA reported a higher incidence of hypertension. This latter reporting of hypertension is in keeping with the higher blood pressure measurements in the patients with AAA compared with the control subjects. The data were analyzed using conditional logistic regression analysis.

The median cumulative tobacco exposure of the patients with AAA was calculated as 49 pack-years (range, 38 to 72 pack-years) and was not significantly different from that of the control group (median, 43 pack-years; range, 30 to 61 pack-years; $p = .113$) (Table 2). For this analysis, as for the other analyses in Table 2, the 288 subjects (44 cases and 244 controls) have been split into tertiles, and the odds ratio of developing AAA was calculated for each tertile. There was no apparent association between the tar yield of the cigarettes currently smoked and the risk of developing AAA. However, there was a strong association between the number of cigarettes currently smoked and the risk of developing AAA. The odds ratio increased to 3.03 for those who smoked 11 to 20 cigarettes/day and was 1.99 for those who smoked 21 or more cigarettes/day ($p = .008$). The risk of developing AAA also appeared to increase with the depth of inhalation, with those who inhaled into the lungs being at much greater risk of developing an aneurysm than those who only inhaled into the mouth or the back of the throat. The odds ratio was highest in those subjects who inhaled deeply into the lungs, these subjects having a three- to fourfold increase in the risk of developing an aneurysm ($p = .027$). These results indicate that continued heavy smoking, particularly with deep inhalation, increases the risk of developing an AAA.

Continuation of the smoking habit may also result in a predisposition toward more rapid aneurysmal growth.[6] Previously we reported the high yield of aneurysms detected by ultrasound screening of patients with peripheral arterial disease.[7] Consecutive patients with peripheral arterial disease attending the Regional Vascular Service at Charing Cross Hospital between 1989 and 1991 were screened for the presence of AAA by ultrasonography. An aneurysm with a maximum anterior/posterior diameter equal to or greater than 3 cm was found to be present in 53 (9.4%) of 561 patients. Of those aneurysms

Table 1 General characteristics of abdominal aortic aneurysm cases and controls

	Cases	Controls
No.	44	244
Mean age (yrs)	69.8	70.7
Male (%)	84	83
Mean height (m)	1.73	1.72
Body mass index (kg/m^2)	228	238
History of hypertension	30%	19%
Diabetes	2%	7%
History of smoking (median pack-years)	49	43
Median systolic pressure (mm Hg)	156	137
Median diastolic pressure (mm Hg)	87	80

Table 2 Smoking habits and risk of developing AAA

		Odds ratio	95% CI	p Value
History of smoking (pack-years)	<35	1.0		
	35-55	2.23	(1.05-4.74)	.113
	56+	1.39	(0.60-3.23)	
Currently smoking (cigarettes/day)	0-10	1.0		
	11-20	3.03	(1.29-7.10)	.008
	21+	1.99	(0.97-5.64)	
Tar yield of current cigarette (mg)	0-8	1.0		
	9-13	1.04	(0.39-2.79)	.495
	14+	0.62	(0.25-1.56)	
Depth of inhalation	Mouth	1.0		
	Throat	1.0	(0.27-3.80)	
	Lungs, moderate	2.55	(0.92-7.09)	.027
	Lungs, deep	3.93	(1.33-11.60)	

detected at screening, only five were equal to or greater than 5.5 cm and hence considered for immediate elective surgery. Some patients 60 to 76 years of age with aneurysm diameters between 4 and 5.5 cm have been randomized within the U.K. Small Aneurysm Trial.[8] The remaining 42 patients with small aneurysms, 3.0 to 5.5 cm in diameter, and one patient who had a large aneurysm but was not a candidate for surgery because of a coexistent tumor were followed up using annual ultrasound surveillance for 3 years. At entry the median age of these patients was 72 years (range, 68 to 78 years), and there were 33 men and 10 women. The median follow-up time was 2 years (range, 1 to 4 years). Serial ultrasonography was performed with an Aloka SSD-500 scanner equipped with a 3.5 MHz probe and with the observer being blind to the previous aortic diameter. At the first follow-up visit, blood pressure, height, and weight were recorded and a fasting blood sample was obtained for analysis of serum cholesterol and triglyceride values and the smoking marker cotinine. Serum cotinine was assayed using gas-liquid chromatography and a concentration of 200 nmol/L or higher was considered indicative of current smoking.

The growth rate of these small aneurysms appears to be slow and the mean annual change in aneurysm diameter during follow-up, as a function of initial diameter, is shown in Fig. 2. The median growth rate was 0.13 cm/yr. Some of the aneurysms appeared to decrease in diameter, which reflects the variability in ultrasound as a

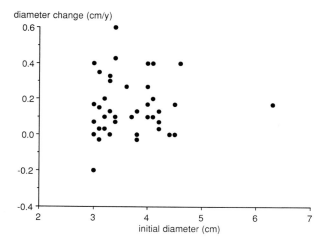

Fig. 2 Aneurysm growth rate according to initial aneurysm diameter.

technique.[9] There were no associations observed between growth rate and initial diameter, systolic or diastolic blood pressure, or serum cholesterol or triglyceride concentrations. The median systolic blood pressure was 160 mm Hg, the median diastolic pressure was 86 mm Hg, the median serum cholesterol concentration was 6.6 mmol/L, and the median triglyceride concentration was 1.6 mmol/L. Approximately half of the patients, 20 of 43 (47%), admitted to being current smokers. However, serum cotinine concentrations indicative of current smoking were

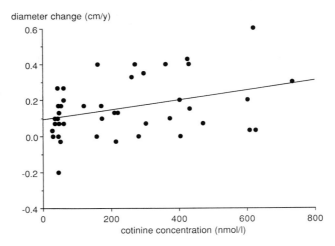

Fig. 3 Aneurysm growth rate according to serum cotinine concentration. Serum cotinine concentrations greater than 200 nmol/L are used to identify current smokers.

observed in 23 patients (54%). The serum cotinine concentration was used to categorize persons who continued to smoke and those who no longer smoked. The median aneurysm growth rate in the smokers was 0.16 cm/yr compared to 0.09 cm/yr in those who no longer smoked (Mann-Whitney U test, $p = .038$). Moreover, the serum cotinine concentration was significantly correlated with the aneurysm growth rate ($r = .36$, $p = .04$; Fig. 3). During the study 12 patients died, but none of these deaths was attributed to the aortic lesion.

In Britain a national screening program to detect abdominal aortic aneurysms has been proposed.[10] Most aneurysms detected on screening are too small to justify early surgical repair, but if we could identify measures to prevent or reduce further aneurysm growth, screening might be of increased value. Smoking appears to be one such factor, since here we have shown that continued smoking is associated with more rapid growth of small AAAs. However, the patients we studied were selected from a group of patients with peripheral arterial disease, which is also closely associated with smoking. A study of a larger number of patients selected with a different referral pattern will be needed to confirm our observations pertaining to smoking and aneurysm growth rates. Our other data from the case-control study also would support a connection between smoking and aneurysm growth rates. The aspect of smoking that was most closely associated with the risk of developing AAA was current tobacco consumption. It is always difficult to persuade a patient to stop smoking. To those who cannot stop smoking we might be able to offer some counseling on the depth of inhalation, since deep inhalation appears to be a much greater risk factor in the development of abdominal aortic aneurysm than inhalation into the mouth and throat. In contrast, changing to a cigarette with a lower tar content does not appear to confer any advantages.

It is particularly important to clearly establish whether smoking contributes to more rapid growth of all aneurysms. If this proves to be the case, the emphasis of aneurysm screening may change from identification of large aneurysms for elective surgical repair to detection of small aneurysms. Since an effective therapeutic intervention (i.e., stopping smoking) would be available for small aneurysms, patients might be able to prevent their aneurysms from reaching a size at which surgery would be considered.

We thank the Tobacco Products Research Trust for support and Peter Franks for help with data analysis.

REFERENCES

1. Hammond EC, Garfinkel L. Coronary heart disease, stroke and abdominal aortic aneurysm. Factors in the etiology. Arch Environ Health 19:167-182, 1967.
2. Strachan DP. Predictors of death from aortic aneurysm among middle-aged men: The Whitehall study. Br J Surg 78:401-404, 1991.

3. Fowkes FGR, MacIntyre CCA, Ruckley CV. Increasing incidence of aortic aneurysms in England and Wales. Br Med J 298:33-35, 1989.
4. Melton LJ, Bickerstaff LK, Hollier LH, van Peenen HJ, Lie JT, Pairolero PC, Cherry KJ, O'Fallon WM. Changing incidence of abdominal aortic aneurysms: A population-based study. Am J Epidemiol 120:379-386, 1984.
5. Castleden WM, Mercer JC, Members of the West Australian Vascular Service. Abdominal aortic aneurysms in Western Australia: Descriptive epidemiology patterns of rupture. Br J Surg 72:109-112, 1985.
6. MacSweeney STR, Ellis M, Worrell PC, Greenhalgh RM, Powell JT. Smoking and growth rate of small abdominal aortic aneurysms. Lancet 344:651-652, 1994.
7. MacSweeney STR, O'Meara M, Alexander C, Powell JT, Greenhalgh RM. High prevalence of unsuspected abdominal aortic aneurysm in patients with confirmed symptomatic peripheral or cerebral arterial disease. Br J Surg 80:582-584, 1993.
8. The UK Small Aneurysm Trial Participants. The UK Small Aneurysm Trial: Design, methods and progress. Eur J Vasc Surg 9:42-48, 1995.
9. Ellis M, Powell JT, Greenhalgh RM. The limitations of ultrasound for the surveillance of abdominal aortic aneurysms. Br J Surg 78:614-616, 1991.
10. Harris PL. Reducing the mortality from abdominal aortic aneurysms: Need for national screening programme. Br Med J 305:697-699, 1992.

22

Abdominal Aortic Aneurysm Surgery: Statewide Variations in Prevalence and Operative Mortality

DOLORES J. KATZ, Ph.D., JAMES C. STANLEY, M.D., and GERALD B. ZELENOCK, M.D.

Population-based mortality associated with the surgical treatment of an abdominal aortic aneurysm (AAA) remains ill defined. Many published series since 1980, most reflecting large referral practices, have reported operative mortality rates below 4% for the treatment of intact AAAs.[1-6] The few U.S. and Canadian studies that have attempted population-based estimates have reported mortality rates ranging from 4.6% to 7.6%.[7-11] However, relating these studies to the general population is problematic because they have been based on select populations, include relatively few cases, or covered brief periods of time, thus preventing identification of long-term trends.

A recent investigation of AAAs in Michigan (1) defined the operative mortality rates for intact and ruptured AAAs, (2) documented time trends over 11 years, and (3) identified factors associated with operative mortality.[12] This experience, herein referred to as the Michigan study, represents the largest reported series of AAA operations and is the basis for this chapter.

MICHIGAN STUDY DATA BASE

The Michigan Inpatient Data Base (Michigan Health Data Corporation, Lansing, Mich.) has maintained records on all patients admitted to Michigan acute care hospitals since 1980. Information extracted for the Michigan study included age, gender, race, length of stay, discharge status, codes from the International Classification of Diseases (ICD-9-CM) for primary diagnoses and up to six secondary diagnoses, and ICD-9-CM codes for primary procedures and up to six secondary procedures.

Data were analyzed for 47,739 admissions from 1980 to 1990 having (1) any mention of intact or ruptured AAA (ICD-9-CM 441.4 and 441.3, respectively), (2) any mention of intact or ruptured aortic aneurysm of unspecified site (441.9 and 441.5, respectively), or (3) any mention of resection of the aorta with replacement (ICD-9-CM 38.44). The given hospital's annual surgical volume was also obtained for each admission for intact AAAs (classified as follows: none, 1 to 10, 11 to 20, and 21 or more) and for ruptured AAAs (classified as follows: none, 1 to 4, and 5 or more). Individual surgeon caseload information was not available for analysis in this study.

Principal mortality analysis in the Michigan study included only admissions with a primary diagnosis of AAA and a primary procedure of resection of the aorta with replacement (ICD-9-CM 38.44). This provided consistency in the analysis over the 11-year study period. The effect of excluding other procedure codes in the primary mortality analysis was assessed using two secondary mortality analyses. One secondary analysis used procedure codes ICD-9-CM 38.44 and 38.34 (resection of aorta with anastomosis), and the second analysis used the two former codes and 13 others that also might have indicated a AAA repair (ICD-9-CM 38.36, 38.40, 38.46, 38.60, 38.64, 38.66, 38.84, 39.24, 39.25, 39.26, 39.52, 39.56, and 39.57). Mortality rates and trends in both secondary analyses were similar to those in the principal analysis. All 15 procedure codes were used in calculating the percent of AAAs repaired during each of the 11 years of the Michigan study.

Additional variables investigated for their effect on surgical mortality included the frequency of ICD-9 comorbidities (number of secondary diagnoses, excluding ICD-9 codes associated with postoperative complications) and selected comorbidities. Comorbidities analyzed included diabetes mellitus (ICD-9-CM 250.0-250.9), hypertension (ICD-9-CM 401.0-405.9), preoperative renal failure (ICD-9-CM 584.0-586.0 and 403.0-403.9), chronic obstructive pulmonary disease (ICD-9-CM 490.0-496.0), ischemic heart disease (ICD-9-CM 410.0-414.9), cerebrovascular disease (ICD-9-CM 430.0-438.0), and arterial occlusive disease (ICD-9-CM 440.0-440.9 and 443.0-443.9).

Data were initially analyzed by plotting variables of interest against mortality rates, with time trends analyzed using chi-square tests and logistic regression. Categoric variables that appeared associated with mortality were tested with chi-square tests, as were continuous variables after division into categories. The latter were also evaluated with t-tests. Those variables having significant associations with mortality ($p < .05$) were analyzed further by stepwise logistic regression to control for confounding among variables. Variables were entered into this stepwise regression model if they were associated with mortality at a significance level of $p < .05$, and they were removed from the model if their association dropped below the $p < .05$ level as new variables were added. Preliminary analysis showed age to be associated with mortality in a curvilinear fashion, and thus age-squared was also included in the model.[13] To reduce the strong correlation between age and its squared value, age was calculated as the true value minus the mean age of all cases.[14]

Michigan's age 50 and older population remained stable over the 11-year period of study, ranging from a low of 2.26 million in 1980 to a high of 2.34 million in 1988. Among the 6,474,429 admissions of patients 50 years of age and older from 1980 to 1990, 39,040 (0.6%) had a primary or secondary diagnosis of intact AAA, and 3401 (0.05%) had a primary diagnosis of ruptured AAA. Among the 16,618 patients with a primary diagnosis of intact AAA, 11,529 (69.4%) were treated surgically, as were 2576 (75.7%) with a primary diagnosis of ruptured AAA. Admissions for intact AAA as a primary diagnosis increased significantly over the 11 years ($p = .005$), but admissions for a primary diagnosis of ruptured AAA did not (Fig. 1). The proportion of all admissions with a diagnosis of AAA increased from 0.19% to 0.40% during the study period. The total number of hospital admissions decreased during this time. From 1980 to 1990 the proportion of intact AAAs treated operatively increased from 58.3% to 82% ($p < .001$) and the proportion of ruptured AAAs treated operatively increased from 72% to 80% ($p = .003$).

Hospitals performing 21 or more operations annually for intact AAAs accounted for 10.2% of

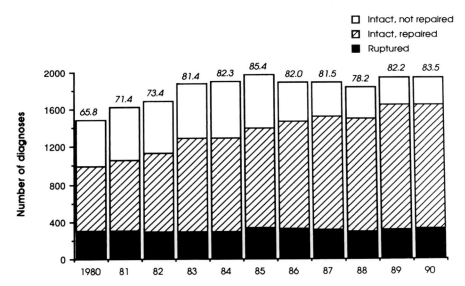

Fig. 1 AAA as principal diagnosis among patients admitted to Michigan hospitals, 1980-1990. Proportion of intact AAAs repaired rose from 58.3% in 1980 to 82% in 1990. (From Katz DJ, Stanley JC, Zelenock GB. Operative mortality rates for intact and ruptured abdominal aortic aneurysms in Michigan: An eleven-year statewide experience. J Vasc Surg 19:804-817, 1994.)

all repairs in 1980 and 52.5% in 1990 ($p <.001$). However, when the data were examined regarding the relative volume of AAA repairs, hospitals in the top quartile accounted for a near identical proportion of all repairs in 1980 (70.4%) as compared with 1990 (70.8%). During the same time period the number of acute care hospitals in Michigan dropped from 205 to 176, primarily as a result of small hospital closures and mergers.

OPERATIVE MORTALITY FOR INTACT AAA

Men accounted for 82% and women for 18% of the 8185 admissions in the Michigan study with a primary diagnosis of intact AAA and a primary procedure of resection of aorta with replacement. The mean age at operation was 69.6 ± 7.7 years ($\bar{x} \pm 1$ SD). Mean age at operation increased slightly, but significantly, over the 11 years, from 68.8 years in 1980 to 69.9 years in 1990 ($p = .001$). Men underwent surgical treatment of AAA at a significantly ($p <.001$) younger mean age (69.1 years) than women (72.1 years). The proportion of surgical admissions with four or more reported comorbidities increased from 23% in 1980 to 53.2% in 1990 ($p <.001$). Among the 8185 admissions for intact AAAs undergoing aortic resection and replacement, there were 614 hospital deaths, for an overall mortality rate of 7.5% (Fig. 2). The mortality for intact AAA repair improved during the 11 years, decreasing from 13.6% in 1980 to 5.6% in 1990. This improvement occurred at the same time that patients' risk factor profiles worsened.

Although the Michigan study demonstrates an impressive improvement in survival over time, it nevertheless reaffirms the observation that intact AAA repair is a formidable surgical procedure associated with an overall mortality higher than reported for nonrandomly selected patients from referral practices.[15] It is evident that selection bias is important. In the Michigan study, the 11-year mortality rate was only 1.3% for men under age 70 who had no more than one comorbidity and were treated at hospitals with high volumes of AAA surgery. Unfortunately, such patients represented only 5.5% of admissions for repair of intact AAAs. Most other patients with AAAs were at much higher risk.

Mortality decreased significantly in all risk categories examined in the Michigan study (Figs. 3 through 8). However, certain individual risk factors were more likely to be associated with in-hospital death, including older age, female

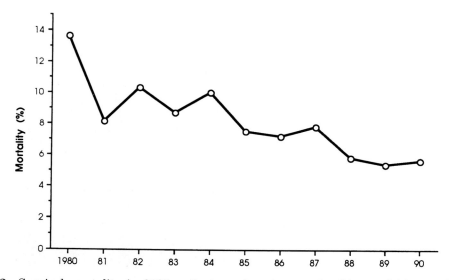

Fig. 2 Surgical mortality in 8185 patients undergoing repair of intact AAAs, Michigan, 1980-1990. Mortality dropped from 13.6% in 1980 to 5.6% in 1990. (From Katz DJ, Stanley JC, Zelenock GB. Operative mortality rates for intact and ruptured abdominal aortic aneurysms in Michigan: An eleven-year statewide experience. J Vasc Surg 19:804-817, 1994.)

Variations in Outcome of AAA Surgery **153**

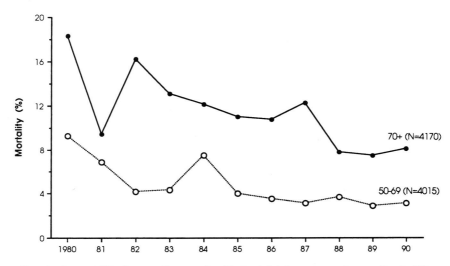

Fig. 3 Surgical mortality by age for repair of intact AAAs, comparing patients 70 years and older with those 50 to 69 years of age. (From Katz DJ, Stanley JC, Zelenock GB. Operative mortality rates for intact and ruptured abdominal aortic aneurysms in Michigan: An eleven-year statewide experience. J Vasc Surg 19:804-817, 1994.)

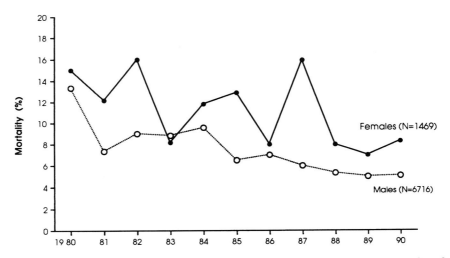

Fig. 4 Surgical mortality by gender for repair of intact AAAs. (From Katz DJ, Stanley JC, Zelenock GB. Operative mortality rates for intact and ruptured abdominal aortic aneurysms in Michigan: An eleven-year statewide experience. J Vasc Surg 19:804-817, 1994.)

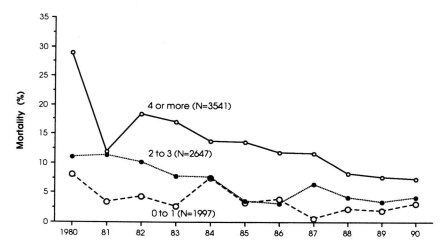

Fig. 5 Surgical mortality by number of comorbidities for repair of intact AAAs, comparing 0 to 1, 2 to 3, and 4 or more. (From Katz DJ, Stanley JC, Zelenock GB. Operative mortality rates for intact and ruptured abdominal aortic aneurysms in Michigan: An eleven-year statewide experience. J Vasc Surg 19:804-817, 1994.)

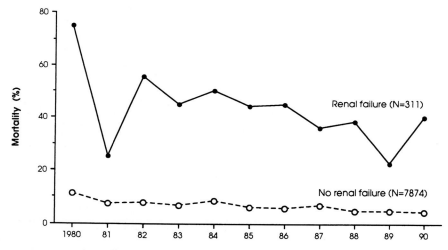

Fig. 6 Surgical mortality by presence or absence of renal failure for repair of intact AAAs. (From Katz DJ, Stanley JC, Zelenock GB. Operative mortality rates for intact and ruptured abdominal aortic aneurysms in Michigan: An eleven-year statewide experience. J Vasc Surg 19:804-817, 1994.)

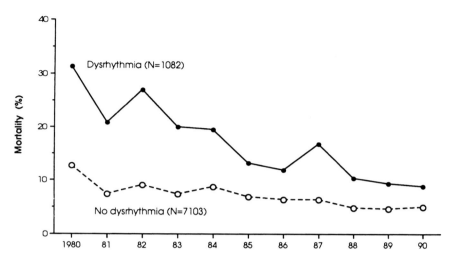

Fig. 7 Surgical mortality by presence or absence of cardiac dysrhythmia for repair of intact AAAs. (From Katz DJ, Stanley JC, Zelenock GB. Operative mortality rates for intact and ruptured abdominal aortic aneurysms in Michigan: An eleven-year statewide experience. J Vasc Surg 19:804-817, 1994.)

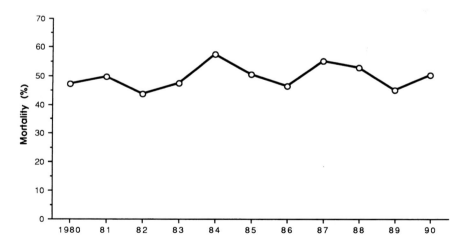

Fig. 8 Surgical mortality in 1829 patients with ruptured AAAs. (From Katz DJ, Stanley JC, Zelenock GB. Operative mortality rates for intact and ruptured abdominal aortic aneurysms in Michigan: An eleven-year statewide experience. J Vasc Surg 19:804-817, 1994.)

gender, multiple comorbidities, preoperative renal failure, dysrhythmia, ischemic heart disease early in the study period, and treatment in a hospital that reported fewer than 21 intact AAA repairs (Table 1). Diabetes mellitus, chronic obstructive pulmonary disease, cerebrovascular disease, and peripheral arterial occlusive disease were not associated with increased mortality rates.

Logistic regression analysis identified renal failure as the strongest predictor of operative mortality for AAAs, followed by number of comorbidities, older age, dysrhythmia, female gender, and higher hospital surgical volume (Table 2). Mortality rates in the Michigan study averaged 10.7% in patients 70 years or older, which supports several previous reports that older patients face higher operative mortality risks.[7,16,17] The Canadian study suggested that age was not an independent predictor of operative mortality when more detailed information regarding clinical risk factors was available, but it did not provide sufficient data to document this conclusion or show the relative importance of risk factors other than age.[9]

Gender differences were apparent in the Michigan study, which documented an average mortality of 10.7% in women and 6.8% in men ($p < .001$). Previous studies had not found significantly higher mortality for women undergoing intact AAA repair. However, most studies included relatively few women. An earlier Canadian study of 666 patients, which included only 133 women, did not identify statistically significant gender differences.[18] Although a West Virginia study reported a fourfold increase in mortality for women, the series included only 76 women and 253 men and the difference was not statistically significant.[1] Similarly, a New York State study, which included 778 women, reported a 15% increased risk for women that also was not statistically significant.[7]

Women have been reported to have higher mortality rates for other types of cardiovascular surgery. For coronary artery bypass and heart transplantation, their relative risks compared with men were 1.5 and 1.6, respectively, suggest-

Table 1 Operative mortality associated with specific patient and hospital characteristics in 8185 operations for intact AAAs

Characteristic	No. of patients	Mortality (%)	p Value
Gender			
Female	1469	10.6	
Male	6716	6.8	.001
Age			
70 years or older	4170	10.7	
50 to 69 years	4015	4.2	.001
Comorbidities			
0 to 1	1997	3.7	
2 to 3	2647	5.7	
4 or more	3541	11.0	.001
Renal failure			
Renal failure	311	41.2	.001
No renal failure	7874	6.2	
Dysrhythmia			
Present	1082	13.6	
Absent	7103	6.6	.001
Hospital AAA surgery volume			
1 to 20/year	3967	8.9	
21 or more/year	4218	6.2	.001

Table 2 Predictors of operative mortality in 8185 operations for intact AAAs

Variable	Regression coefficient	Odds ratio	95% Confidence interval	p Value
Gender	0.34	1.4	1.1-1.7	.002
Age	0.05*	2.0†	1.9-2.6	.0001
Comorbidities	0.79	2.3‡	1.8-2.8	.0001
Renal failure	2.2	9.0	6.7-11.4	.001
Dysrhythmia	0.57	1.8	1.4-2.2	.0001
Hospital AAA surgical volume	0.22	1.2	1.03-1.5	.02

NOTE: Variables significant ($p < .05$) in the final model by stepwise logistic regression analysis were as follows: years of surgery numbered 1 (1980) to 11 (1990); comorbidities—0 = 3 or fewer, 1 = 4 or more; gender—0 = male, 1 = female; hospital volume—0 = 21 or more/year, 1 = 20 or fewer/year; renal failure and dysplasia—0 = no, 1 = yes.
*Coefficient for age squared = .00174. Model sets mean age to zero and measures risk by number of years above or below the mean.
†Comparing age 79 years to age 69 years.
‡Comparing four or more to none or one.

ing 50% and 60% increases in risk of mortality for women undergoing these procedures.[19-22] These risks are very similar to the odds ratio of 1.4 for AAA repair in the Michigan study, which suggests a 40% increase in the risk of mortality among women. The basis for higher mortality rates among women is unknown but may reflect both biologic and practice pattern differences.

Preexisting renal failure in the Michigan study was associated with an average overall mortality rate of 41.2% as compared with 6.2% without this comorbidity. The role of renal failure in contributing to mortality associated with treatment of AAAs has been recognized by others.[7,9] Dysrhythmia increased mortality rates from 6.6% to 13.6%. The presence of ischemic heart disease was associated with higher surgical mortality from 1980 to 1983 ($p < .001$) but not afterward ($p = .3$). The latter may reflect both the increasing use of myocardial revascularization before AAA repair and more intensive management of intraoperative cardiac dysfunction.[6,23,24]

The finding of lower operative survival among admissions to hospitals that perform fewer operations for AAA is consistent with many other studies.[7] Although the Michigan study did not assess the effect of surgeon volume on mortality, a recent study evaluating effect of both surgeon and hospital volumes on AAA surgical mortality found little effect of surgeon volume once hospital volume was taken into account.[4]

Race was not associated with mortality in the Michigan study, as it was in the only other study to report mortality by race.[7] However, both reports had so few nonwhites (168 in the New York State study, 345 in the Michigan study) that only large differences would have been evident.

OPERATIVE MORTALITY FOR RUPTURED AAA

The Michigan study counted 3401 admissions with a primary diagnosis of ruptured AAA, including 1829 with a primary procedure code of aortic resection with replacement. Overall surgical mortality for the 11 years was 49.8%; annual variations ranged from 43.5% to 57.5%, with no apparent trend over time (Fig. 8). Many risk factors associated with increased operative mortality for intact AAAs were also associated with higher operative mortality for ruptured AAAs. Female gender was associated with a 61.6% average mortality as compared with 47.4% for males ($p = .0006$). Patients 70 years of age and older had an average mortality rate of 58.3% as compared with 37.7% for patients 50 to 69 years of age ($p = .0001$). Preoperative renal failure was associated with a 70.2% mortality rate as compared with 45.1% for patients without renal failure ($p = .0001$). Patients with dysrhythmia had a 61.2% mortality rate as compared with 47.3% for patients without dysrhythmia ($p = .0001$). Treatment in a hospital with a surgical volume for ruptured AAAs of fewer than five procedures a year was associated with a 53.6% mortality rate as compared with 45.7% for repairs in hospitals with five or more procedures a year ($p = .0026$).

Certain peculiarities in the Michigan study appear to be related to the nature of the data base. For example, in the years after 1984 patients with four or more comorbidities had a mortality rate of 45% as compared with 56% for patients with fewer comorbidities ($p = .0002$). Similar findings were noted in the New York study.[7] This apparent anomaly may have been related to changes in Medicare reimbursement formulas after 1984, which stimulated more thorough documentation of comorbidities. It is also possible that patients who survived were more likely to have their comorbidities documented during hospitalization because physicians were required to treat these conditions. In addition, physicians simply had more time to document comorbidities in patients who survived to discharge. Survivors had a mean hospital stay of 20 days as compared with 8.3 days for patients who died.

COMMENT

The Michigan study had a number of limitations. It was based on admissions, not patients, and therefore could not identify multiple admissions of the same patient. This may have inflated AAA prevalence estimates, particularly in the early part of the study period when patients were more likely to be admitted twice, first for a diagnostic workup and second for operation. Reliance on admission data may also have resulted in an underestimate of elective AAA mortality because a patient discharged after operation and readmitted a few days later with a fatal myocardial infarction would not be classified as a surgical fatality.

The Michigan data base had no information on AAA size. One recent report has related greater size to increased operative mortality,[25] an association attributed to postponement of surgery in patients with prohibitive risk factors.[15] The

Michigan data base also lacked information on whether the admission was urgent or elective, which in some studies has been strongly associated with mortality.[26] Finally, ICD-9-CM comorbidity codes provide only limited information about severity of disease.

The documented increase over time in the prevalence of comorbidities among patients raises the possibility that creep from diagnosis-related groups (DRGs) influenced many of the associations found in the Michigan study. However, a recent Rand Corporation study of national Medicare data found that although some of the change could be attributed to efforts to increase reimbursement, most of the increases in comorbidities were the result of an actual worsening of the patient profile.[27] Moreover, the prevalence of comorbidities in the Michigan study increased selectively, not uniformly as would be expected if DRG creep was a dominant factor in the observed trends. Finally, even if DRG creep accounted for all increases in comorbidities, the associations between comorbidities and mortality would still remain valid. In fact, the effect of DRG creep would be to reduce mortality differences between patients with and without a particular comorbidity and thus mortality differences noted in the Michigan study would represent the minimum effect of the comorbidity.

The marked improvement in survival of patients undergoing elective AAA repair in the Michigan study should not overshadow the continued dismal outcomes of operations for ruptured AAAs. Mortality rates for surgical treatment of ruptured AAAs remained close to 50% over the entire study period. It is relevant that one statewide experience with ruptured AAAs documented that 40% of patients were known to have AAAs prior to rupture.[10] The lethal nature of this disease would be diminished by more timely elective interventions for intact AAAs.

REFERENCES

1. AbuRahma AF, Robinson PA, Boland JP, et al. Elective resection of 332 abdominal aortic aneurysms in a southern West Virginia community during a recent five-year period. Surgery 109:244-251, 1991.
2. Bernstein EF, Dilley RB, Randolph HF III. The improving long-term outlook for patients over 70 years of age with abdominal aortic aneurysms. Ann Surg 207:318-322, 1988.
3. Ernst CB. Abdominal aortic aneurysm. N Engl J Med 328:1167-1172, 1993.
4. Golden MA, Whittemore AD, Donaldson MC, Mannick JA. Selective evaluation and management of coronary artery disease in patients undergoing repair of abdominal aortic aneurysms. Ann Surg 212:415-423, 1990.
5. Perry MO, Calcagnos D. Abdominal aortic aneurysm surgery: The basic evaluation of cardiac risk. Ann Surg 208:738-742, 1988.
6. Reigel MM, Hollier LH, Kazmier FJ, et al. Late survival in abdominal aortic aneurysm patients: The role of selective myocardial revascularization on the basis of clinic symptoms. J Vasc Surg 5:222-227, 1987.
7. Hannan EL, Kilburn H Jr, O'Donnell JF, et al. A longitudinal analysis of the relationship between in-hospital mortality in New York State and the volume of abdominal aortic aneurysm surgeries performed. Health Serv Res 27:517-542, 1992.
8. Hertzer NR, Avellone JC, Farrell CJ, et al. The risk of vascular surgery in a metropolitan community with observations on surgeon experience and hospital size. J Vasc Surg 1:13-21, 1984.
9. Johnston KW, Scobie TK. Multicenter prospective study of nonruptured abdominal aortic aneurysms. I. Population and operative management. J Vasc Surg 7:69-81, 1988.
10. Richardson JD, Main KA. Repair of abdominal aortic aneurysms: A statewide experience. Arch Surg 126:614-616, 1991.
11. Roger VL, Ballard DJ, Hallett JW Jr, Osmundson PJ, Puetz PA, Gersh BJ. Influence of coronary artery disease on morbidity and mortality following abdominal aortic aneurysmectomy: A population-based study, 1971-87. J Am Coll Cardiol 14:1245-1252, 1989.
12. Katz DJ, Stanley JC, Zelenock GB. Operative mortality rates for intact and ruptured abdominal aortic aneurysms in Michigan: An eleven-year statewide experience. J Vasc Surg 19:804-817, 1994.
13. Hosmer DW, Lemshow S. Applied Logistic Regression. New York: Wiley, 1989, pp 15, 88-90.
14. Breslow NE, Day NE. Statistical Methods in Cancer Research. The Analysis of Case-Control Studies. Lyons: International Agency for Research on Cancer (IARC Scientific Publications No. 32), 1980 p 235.
15. Ballard DJ, Etchason JA, Hilborne LH, et al. Abdominal aortic aneurysm surgery: A literature review and ratings of appropriateness and necessity. Santa Monica, Calif.: Rand Corporation, 1992.
16. Diehl JT, Call RF, Hertzer NR, Beven EG. Complications of abdominal aortic reconstruction: An analysis of perioperative risk factors in 557 patients. Arch Surg 197:49-56, 1983.
17. Goldman L. Cardiac risks and complications of noncardiac surgery. Ann Intern Med 98:504-513, 1983.
18. Johnston KW. Influence of sex on the results of abdominal aortic aneurysm repair. J Vasc Surg 20:914-926, 1994.
19. Hannan EL, Bernard HR, Kilburn HC Jr, O'Donnell JF. Gender differences in mortality rates for coronary artery bypass surgery. Am Heart J 123:866-872, 1992.
20. Kennedy JW, Kaiser GC, Gischer LD, et al. Clinical and angiographic predictors of operative mortality from the collaborative study of coronary artery surgery (CASS). Circulation 63:793-802, 1981.

21. Khan SS, Nessim S, Gray R, Czer LS, Chaux A, Matloff J. Increased mortality of women in coronary artery bypass surgery: Evidence for referral bias. Ann Intern Med 112:561-567, 1990.
22. Laffel GL, Barnett AI, Finkelstein S, Kaye MP. The relation between experience and outcome in heart transplantation. N Engl J Med 327:1220-1225, 1992.
23. Acinapure AJ, Rose DM, Kramer MD, Jacobowitz IJ, Cunningham JN Jr. Role of coronary angiography and coronary artery bypass surgery prior to abdominal aortic aneurysmectomy. J Cardiovasc Surg 28:552-557, 1987.
24. Elmore JR, Hallett JW, Gibboins RJ, et al. Myocardial revascularization before abdominal aortic aneurysmorrhaphy: Effect of coronary angioplasty. Mayo Clin Proc 68:637-641, 1993.
25. Amundsen S, Skjaerven R, Trippestad A, et al. Abdominal aortic aneurysms—A study of factors influencing postoperative mortality. Eur J Vasc Surg 3:405-409, 1989.
26. Sullivan CA, Rohrer MJ, Cutler BS. Clinical management of symptomatic but unruptured abdominal aortic aneurysm. J Vasc Surg 11:799-803, 1990.
27. Carter GM, Newhouse JP, Relles DA. How much change in the case mix index is DRG creep? J Health Econ 9:411-428, 1990.

23

Mortality After Elective Aortic Reconstruction

JAMES M. SEEGER, M.D., and THOMAS S. HUBER, M.D., Ph.D.

Initial reports on abdominal aortic aneurysm repair demonstrated complications of coronary artery disease (myocardial infarction, fatal arrhythmias, congestive heart failure) to be the leading cause of postoperative death.[1-4] Furthermore, Hertzer et al.[5] found that only 8% of 1000 patients undergoing all types of peripheral vascular surgical procedures had normal coronary arteries, whereas 60% had severe coronary disease (stenosis of >70% in at least one coronary artery). As a result of these findings, significant emphasis has been placed on preoperative cardiac testing in an attempt to identify patients in whom correction of coronary artery disease would decrease the risk of postoperative cardiac complications. However, Taylor et al.[6] and Seeger et al.[7] recently reported low (<1%) cardiac mortality rates in patients undergoing elective vascular reconstruction (without the use of extensive preoperative cardiac testing), whereas recently reported mortality rates after aortic reconstruction still range from 3% to 6%.[8-11] This suggests either that the low cardiac-related mortality rates achieved by Taylor et al.[6] and Seeger et al.[7] are not widespread or, more likely, that in many series, postoperative complications other than cardiac events now account for the majority of deaths after aortic reconstruction.

Apart from intraoperative technical problems, morbidity and mortality after aortic reconstruction depend largely on a balance between the stress of the surgical procedure and the patient's response to that stress. Procedure stress includes the trauma of surgery, the ischemia/reperfusion injury associated with aortic clamping, and any postoperative complications (e.g., infection or bleeding). The patient's response to these stresses is influenced by his or her comorbid diseases, immune system, and nutritional status. Current techniques of intensive care can support patients with single or multiple organ failure after aortic reconstruction, but recovery still depends on the patient's response to the stress of such complications. The age of patients requiring vascular reconstruction appears to be increasing, and improvements in anesthetic and operative techniques allow more complex vascular reconstructions to be undertaken. Thus changes in the incidence and types of postoperative complications after elective aortic reconstruction should be expected.

RISK AND CAUSE OF DEATH AFTER AORTIC RECONSTRUCTION

As previously noted, early studies of results of repair of abdominal aortic aneurysm (AAA) demonstrated complications of cardiac disease to be the primary cause of postoperative death in most series. DeBakey et al.[1] reviewed results from 1449 patients undergoing AAA repair and found a 30-day mortality rate of 9%[2] (Table 1). Seventy-seven percent of these deaths were the result of complications of atherosclerosis (mostly cardiac atherosclerosis), whereas 21% were caused by complications of the operation. Szilagyi et al.[2] studied 401 patients undergoing repair of asymptomatic or expanding AAAs and reported a postoperative mortality rate of 14.7%. Coronary artery disease accounted for 47.5% of these postoperative deaths (cardiac mortality rate, 7%), whereas noncardiac causes (e.g.,

Table 1 Risk and causes of death after aortic reconstruction: Early studies

	Mortality (%)		
Author	Overall	Cardiac	Noncardiac
DeBakey et al. (1964)[1]	9	Majority	
Szilagyi et al. (1966)[2]	14.7	7	7.7
Thompson et al. (1975)[3]	5.5	4.6	0.9
Crawford et al. (1981)[4]	4.8	2.5	2.3

renal failure, hemorrhage, pulmonary failure, or peritonitis) accounted for 52.5%. Subsequently Thompson et al.[3] reviewed 108 patients undergoing AAA repair and reported a mortality rate of 5.5%, with five of six deaths resulting from heart-related causes (cardiac mortality rate, 4.6%), whereas Crawford et al.[4] reported results from 860 patients undergoing repair of AAA and found an operative mortality of 4.8%, a cardiac mortality of 2.5%, and a noncardiac mortality of 2.3%.

More recent reports have demonstrated improvement in postoperative mortality after aortic reconstruction and have no longer consistently found cardiac complications to be the primary cause of death after such procedures (Table 2). Johnston[12] found an operative mortality of 4.8%, a cardiac mortality of 3.3%, and a noncardiac mortality of 1.5% in a prospective multicenter study of 666 patients undergoing repair of nonruptured AAAs. Similarly, Golden et al.[13] found a 1.5% operative mortality and a 1.2% cardiac mortality in 500 patients undergoing AAA repair, whereas Lachapelle et al.[14] reported a 4.8% postoperative mortality rate and a 3.4% cardiac mortality rate in 146 patients undergoing similar procedures. In contrast, Taylor et al.[6] reported a 0.8% cardiac mortality and a 1.6% noncardiac mortality (overall mortality rate 2.4%) in 491 patients undergoing various vascular reconstructive procedures and Cambria et al.[15] found a 0.5% cardiac mortality and a 1.5% noncardiac mortality (2.0% overall mortality) in 202 patients undergoing aortic reconstructive procedures. Baron et al.[16] also reported that only half of the deaths in their series resulted from cardiac causes (cardiac mortality, 2.2%; overall mortality, 4.4%) in 457 consecutive AAA repairs, and Seeger et al.[7] found a cardiac mortality of 0.6% and a noncardiac mortality of 2.9% (overall mortality 3.5%) in a selected group of 318 patients undergoing elective aortic reconstruction in whom the value of aggressive preoperative cardiac assessment was evaluated. Multisystem organ failure (MSOF) was the cause of death in the other half of patients who died in the study of Baron et al.[16] and of 11% of the patients who died in the study of Seeger et al.[7]

In 1995, Huber et al.[17] reviewed all of the 722 aortic reconstructions done at the University of Florida between January 1982 and June 1994 and reported an overall operative mortality of 6.1%. This mortality rate did not vary with the indication for the aortic reconstruction (aneurysmal disease, 6.3%; occlusive disease, 5.7%) but was significantly influenced by whether additional vascular procedures were performed in conjunction with the aortic reconstruction. Patients undergoing aortic reconstruction alone had a postoperative mortality rate of only 4.9%, whereas the addition of a renal artery bypass increased the mortality rate to 8.9%, and the addition of a lower extremity procedure increased the mortality rate to 15.8%. The addition of repair of an inferior mesenteric artery or internal iliac artery in conjunction with aortic reconstruction did not change the postoperative mortality rate. MSOF was the leading cause of death in these patients, accounting for 25 of the 44 deaths (56.8%); cardiac complications were the second leading cause of death (11 patients [25%]). MSOF was the cause of 50% of deaths after aortic reconstruction alone, 55.6% of deaths after aortic reconstruction plus lower extremity vascular procedures, and 80% of deaths after aortic reconstruction and renal artery bypass.

Thus it appears that cardiac mortality after aortic reconstruction has decreased significantly during the past decade and that overall mortality has also decreased, but not to the same degree as cardiac mortality. Pulmonary complications, renal failure, postoperative hemorrhage, and mesenteric infarction were reported by Szilagyi et al.[2] in 1966 to account for more than half of deaths after aortic reconstruction, and as the incidence of cardiac complications has declined, these problems now account for the majority of deaths after aortic surgery in many recent studies. In addition, MSOF appears to be an increasingly common cause of death after aortic reconstruction, probably because of the increasing recognition of this problem as well as the ability of improved intensive care techniques to

Table 2 Risk and cause of death after aortic reconstruction: Recent studies

Author	Mortality (%)		
	Overall	Cardiac	Noncardiac
Johnston (1989)[12]	4.8	3.3	1.5
Golden et al. (1990)[13]	1.6	1.2	0.4
Lachapelle et al. (1992)[14]	4.8	3.4	1.4
Taylor et al. (1991)[6]	2.4	0.8	1.6
Cambria et al. (1992)[15]	2.0	0.5	1.5
Baron et al. (1994)[16]	4.4	2.2	2.2
Seeger et al. (1994)[7]	3.5	0.6	2.9

prolong but not necessarily overcome life-threatening organ failure. Unfortunately, progressive MSOF is generally unresponsive to current therapy, and death occurs in 60% to 95% of patients who develop this problem, depending on the number of organ systems involved.[18]

CAUSES OF MSOF AFTER AORTIC RECONSTRUCTION

Visceral organ dysfunction was the most common cause of MSOF in the Huber et al. review[17] of 722 aortic reconstruction done at the University of Florida, occurring in 14 patients. The initiating event for MSOF was liver failure in six, bowel infarction in four, pancreatitis in two, perforated sigmoid diverticulitis in one, and upper gastrointestinal bleeding in one. In the remaining patients, postoperative pneumonia was the cause of MSOF in nine, aortoenteric fistula in one, and severe extremity ischemia in one. Sepsis was the initiating event in 66% of patients developing MSOF, whereas 33% developed MSOF without an initial identifiable septic episode. Seventy-four percent of patients who died of MSOF required at least one reoperative procedure for treatment of a complication.

Patient age, the severity of disease, and a diagnosis of sepsis at the time of admission to the intensive care unit have previously been identified as risk factors for development of MSOF.[18]

Mean age and incidence of preexisting renal disease were significantly higher in patients in Huber's study[17] who died after aortic reconstruction compared to patients who survived (Table 3). In addition, both a history of heart disease as indicated by a history of myocardial infarction, angina or congestive heart failure and/or a left ventricular ejection fraction of less than 55% were more common in patients who died. Patients who died also underwent longer operations with a higher incidence of additional vascular procedures than patients who survived. Surprisingly, the incidence of smoking and preoperative pulmonary dysfunction were similar in both survivors and in patients who died. Similar findings were seen when patients who developed MSOF were compared with those who did not. Thus the overall mortality rate and high incidence of MSOF in our series of aortic reconstructions appear to have been primarily the result of performing complex procedures in older, sicker patients.

Other studies of the results of aortic reconstruction have not specifically investigated the influence of preoperative and intraoperative risk factors on mortality and cause of death after aortic surgery. However, Katz et al.[10] in a statewide review did report renal failure to be the strongest predictor of mortality after aortic aneurysm repair. In addition, in several other

Table 3 Comparison of preoperative and operative parameters in patients undergoing elective aortic reconstruction

Preoperative/operative parameter	Survivors	Nonsurvivors	p Value
Age	64.7 ± 8.1	69.0 ± 9.1	<.01
Noncardiac			
Hypertension	60.1%	75.0%	.06
Renal insufficiency	17.7%	53.7%	<.01
Diabetes mellitus	11.6%	20.5%	.11
Smoking	89.0%	93.2%	.78
Abnormal PFT	61.5%	65.4%	.72
Cardiac			
Myocardial infarction	26.3%	47.7%	<.01
Angina	10.5%	25.0%	<.01
Congestive heart failure	5.6%	25.0%	<.01
Ejection fraction <55%	22.8%	53.6%	<.01
Operative			
Duration of procedure	5.7 ± 2.0	7.7 ± 2.8	<.01
Additional procedure	15.5%	31.8%	<.01
Aortic cross-clamp time	70.0 ± 32.2	80.3 ± 38.8	<.23
Estimated blood loss	1908 ± 1444	2262 ± 1638	.17

From Huber TS, Harward TRS, Flynn TC, Albright JL, Seeger JM. Operative mortality rates after elective infrarenal aortic reconstruction. J Vasc Surg 22:287-294, 1995.
PFT = pulmonary function test.

series, the incidence of MSOF as a cause of postoperative death appears to be directly related to the percentage of patients undergoing other vascular procedures in addition to aortic reconstruction. Lachapelle et al.[14] and Johnston[12] found MSOF to be an uncommon cause of death after aortic surgery in patients who had few additional vascular procedures (3.4% in Lachapelle's series, 3.8% in Johnston's series) (Table 4). In contrast, Baron et al.[16] reported MSOF accounted for 50% of deaths in their patients, 38.5% of whom underwent vascular procedures in addition to aortic reconstruction and Harward et al.[19] found that MSOF was the cause of death in 50% of patients undergoing aortic plus lower extremity reconstruction. Cambria et al.[15] also reported that prolonged surgical morbidity in patients undergoing aortic reconstruction was associated with an operating time of more than 5 hours and more complex procedures in patients undergoing aortic reconstruction. Furthermore, Atnip et al.[20] reported that all three operative deaths after aortic reconstruction and visceral revascularization were caused by MSOF, and Brothers et al.[21] found MSOF to be the cause of death in 53% of patients undergoing renal revascularization, with the risk of MSOF increasing as the complexity of the reconstruction increased.

Development of MSOF was initially believed to be a response to sepsis. However, it is now recognized that although sepsis is the most common cause of MSOF, this problem can be associated with severe trauma, pancreatitis, cardiopulmonary bypass, and multiple other problems in patients without evidence of infection. The term "systemic inflammatory response syndrome" (SIRS) has recently been developed to describe a clinical presentation consistent with sepsis[22] (with or without documented infection).

SIRS can progress to severe sepsis, septic shock, and MSOF without an identified septic source. The underlying mechanism for SIRS appears to be mediated through macrophage-derived cytokines, presumably activated by bacterial endotoxin lipopolysaccharide products.[22-24] Alternatively, skeletal muscle and visceral ischemia/reperfusion have been shown to activate macrophages, leading to cytokine release, and animal studies have shown that distant organ dysfunction, particularly pulmonary injury, can occur after lower torso or mesenteric ischemia/reperfusion.[25,26] Harward et al.[27] also recently reported that multiorgan dysfunction after thoracoabdominal aneurysm repair in humans (with its obligatory period of mesenteric ischemia) appears to be directly related to the level of circulating tumor necrosis factor–alpha in the first few hours after reperfusion of the acutely ischemic bowel. Whether postoperative splanchnic ischemia contributes to the development of MSOF in patients undergoing infrarenal aortic reconstruction remains speculative, but inadequate gut perfusion (potentially caused by cardiac failure) could lead to bowel ischemia, breakdown of the gut mucosal barrier, and release of bacterial endotoxin and significant amounts of proinflammatory cytokines into the circulation.

CONCLUSION

Recognition of cardiac complications as the primary cause of death in early seminal series of aortic reconstruction led to improved intraoperative and postoperative cardiac care, resulting in significant reductions in the risk of cardiac complications and mortality after aortic surgery. However, other problems, particularly MSOF, continue to pose substantial risk to patients undergoing elective aortic reconstruction. Unfortunately, further significant reductions in postoperative mortality after aortic surgery may be difficult to achieve, because the causes of MSOF after aortic reconstruction are diverse (and thus difficult to prevent) and because MSOF is a complex problem that has defied successful treatment since its recognition. Anticytokine therapy has recently been shown to be promising in reducing mortality associated with severe sepsis,[28] but such therapy is extremely expensive. In addition, it is unknown whether modulation of the inflammatory response will affect or reverse the course of MSOF once it is established. Until MSOF can be effectively treated, recognition of the association between complex

Table 4 Risk of additional/complex procedures with aortic reconstruction

Author	Additional/complex procedures (%)	MSOF (%)
Johnston (1989)[12]	3.8	3.0
Lachapelle et al. (1992)[14]	3.4	14.0
Baron et al. (1994)[16]	38.5	50.0
Harward et al. (1995)[19]	35.2	50.0
Brothers et al. (1995)[21]	62.9	53.3

arterial reconstructions (additional or prolonged procedures) and significant comorbid diseases (particularly renal and cardiac failure) and an increased risk of mortality from MSOF can at least aid in patient selection for elective aortic surgical procedures.

REFERENCES

1. DeBakey ME, Crawford ES, Cooley DA, Morris GC Jr, Royster TS, Abbott WP. Aneurysm of abdominal aorta: Analysis of results of graft replacement therapy one to eleven years after operation. Ann Surg 160:622-639, 1964.
2. Szilagyi DE, Smith RF, DeRusso FJ, Elliott JP, Sherrin FW. Contribution of abdominal aortic aneursymectomy to prolongation of life. Ann Surg 164:679-699, 1966.
3. Thompson JE, Hollier LH, Patman RD, Persson AV. Surgical management of abdominal aortic aneurysms: Factors influencing mortality and morbidity—a 20-year experience. Ann Surg 181:654-661, 1975.
4. Crawford ES, Salwa SA, Babb JW, et al. Infrarenal-abdominal aortic aneurysm. Ann Surg 193:699-709, 1981.
5. Hertzer NR, Beven EG, Young JR, et al. Coronary artery disease in peripheral vascular patients: A classification of 1000 coronary angiograms and results of surgical management. Ann Surg 199:223-233, 1984.
6. Taylor LM, Yeager RA, Moneta GL, McConnell DB, Porter JM. The incidence of perioperative myocardial infarction in general vascular surgery. J Vasc Surg 15:52-61, 1991.
7. Seeger JM, Rosenthal GR, Self SB, Flynn TC, Limacher MC, Harward TRS. Does routine stress-thallium cardiac scanning reduce postoperative cardiac complications? Ann Surg 219:654-663, 1994.
8. Whittemore AD, Clowes AW, Hechtman HB, et al. Aortic aneurysm repair reduced operative mortality associated with maintenance of optimal cardiac performance. Ann Surg 120:414-421, 1980.
9. Hertzer NR. Myocardial ischemia. Surgery 93:97-101, 1983.
10. Katz DJ, Stanley JC, Zelenock GB. Operative mortality rates for intact and ruptured abdominal aortic aneurysms in Michigan: An eleven-year statewide experience. J Vasc Surg 19:804-817, 1994.
11. Veith FJ, Goldsmith J, Leather RP, Hannan EL. The need for quality assurance in vascular surgery. J Vasc Surg 13:523-526, 1991.
12. Johnston KW. Multicenter prospective study of nonruptured abdominal aortic aneurysm. Part II. Variables predicting morbidity and mortality. J Vasc Surg 9:437-447, 1989.
13. Golden MA, Whittemore AD, Donaldson MC, Mannick JA. Selective evaluation and management of coronary artery disease in patients undergoing repair of abdominal aortic aneurysms. Ann Surg 212:415-423, 1990.
14. Lachapelle K, Graham AM, Symes JF. Does the clinical evaluation of the cardiac status predict outcome in patients with abdominal aortic aneurysms. J Vasc Surg 15:964-971, 1992.
15. Cambria RP, Brewster DC, Abbott WM, et al. The impact of selective use of dipyridamole-thallium scans and surgical factors on the current morbidity of aortic surgery. J Vasc Surg 15:43-51, 1992.
16. Baron JF, Mundler O, Bertrand M, et al. Dipyridamole-thallium scintigraphy and gated radionuclide angiography to assess cardiac risk before abdominal aortic surgery. N Engl J Med 330:663-669, 1994.
17. Huber TS, Harward TRS, Flynn TC, Albright JL, Seeger JM. Operative mortality rates after elective infrarenal aortic reconstructions. J Vasc Surg 22:287-294, 1995.
18. Knaus WA, Wagner DP. Multiple systems organ failure: Epidemiology and prognosis. In Pinsky MR, Matuschak GM, eds. Critical Care Clinics. Philadelphia: WB Saunders, 1989, pp 221-232.
19. Harward TRS, Ingegno MD, Carlton L, Flynn TC, Seeger JM. Limb-threatening ischemia due to multilevel arterial occlusive disease. Ann Surg 221:498-506, 1995.
20. Atnip RG, Neumyer MM, Healy DA, Thiele BL. Combined aortic and visceral arterial reconstruction: Risks and results. J Vasc Surg 12:714-715, 1990.
21. Brothers TE, Elliott BM, Robison JG, Rajagopalan PR. Stratification of mortality risks for renal artery surgery. Am Surg 61:45-51, 1995.
22. American College of Chest Physicians–Society of Critical Care Medicine Consensus Conference. Definitions of sepsis and organ failure and guidelines for the use of innovative therapies in sepsis. Crit Care Med 20:864-875, 1992.
23. Parrillo JE. Pathogenetic mechanisms of septic shock. N Engl J Med 328:1471-1477, 1993.
24. Nathan CF. Secretory macrophages. J Clin Invest 79:319-326, 1987.
25. Seekamp A, Warren JS, Remick DG, Till GO, Ward PA. Requirements for tumor necrosis factor-α and interleukin-1 in limb ischemia/reperfusion injury and associated lung injury. Am J Pathol 143:453-463, 1993.
26. Caty MG, Guice KS, Oldham KT, Remick DG, Kunkel SI. Evidence for tumor necrosis factor-induced pulmonary microvascular injury after intestinal ischemia/reperfusion injury. Ann Surg 212:694-700, 1990.
27. Harward TRS, Martin TD, Welborn MB III, et al. Tumor necrosis factor-α, interleukin-1β and interleukin-8 are released following thoracoabdominal aneurysm repair and TNF-α levels are related to patient outcome. Surg Forum 46:360-362, 1995.
28. Abraham E, Wunderink R, Silverman H, et al. Efficacy and safety of monoclonal antibody to human tumor necrosis factor-α in patients with sepsis syndrome. JAMA 273:934-941, 1995.

24

Prognosis for Thoracoabdominal Aortic Aneurysms Managed Nonoperatively

ROBERT A. CAMBRIA, M.D., JOHN W. HALLETT, Jr., M.D., W. ANTHONY STANSON, M.D., and PETER GLOVICZKI, M.D.

The indications for repair of a large abdominal aortic aneurysm (AAA) have become well defined. The classic study of Szilagyi et al.[1] illustrated the prolongation of survival following repair of these aneurysms, and continued improvement in results of aneurysm repair have supported the application of this technique to smaller aneurysms. However, a survival benefit must be inherent to the application of these procedures. This has been most clearly stated by Katz et al.,[2] who wrote: "[The optimal] strategy minimizes the risk of AAA rupture while avoiding unnecessary surgery in patients who would have died from other causes before AAA rupture." Ongoing clinical trials are seeking to define which patients with small AAAs would benefit from repair and which can be successfully managed nonoperatively.

Thoracoabdominal aortic aneurysms (TAAAs) are less common than infrarenal aneurysms.[3] Although repair of these complex aneurysms is technically feasible, several factors contribute to a significantly greater risk of morbidity and mortality following their repair. Visceral, renal, and spinal ischemia associated with aortic reconstruction can lead to coagulopathy, renal failure or paralysis even following a rapid and proficient repair. In addition, the scarcity of these aneurysms dictates that surgeons are less familiar with these procedures than with other types of aortic reconstruction. Results in the literature highlight these considerations. Even the extraordinary experience of Svensson et al.[4] in over 1500 thoracoabdominal aortic reconstructions was associated with a 10% in-hospital mortality, a 16% risk of neurologic dysfunction, and a 9% risk of dialysis.

In order to recommend surgical repair of a TAAA with its inherent risks, we must define the outcome of nonoperative management in these patients. We have recently compiled a retrospective review of TAAAs treated nonoperatively,[5] the results of which will be presented in this chapter. Before our report, Crawford and DeNatale[6] had the only paper in the literature addressing this issue. They noted an extremely poor prognosis among those patients observed with TAAA, reporting a two year survival of only 24%, with half of the deaths resulting from aneurysm rupture. These two studies will be contrasted and a logical algorithm for the evaluation and treatment of these patients suggested.

SCOPE OF THE PROBLEM

The true incidence of thoracoabdominal aortic aneurysms is difficult to determine. In a population-based study from our institution, the incidence of *any* type of thoracic aneurysm was 5.3 patients per 100,000 person-years.[3] Only five of the 72 aneurysms in this study were TAAAs, demonstrating the rarity of these extensive aneurysms. Although the abdominal aorta is more commonly involved by aneurysmal disease than the thoracoabdominal aorta, patients with AAA may harbor more proximal aneurysms. Up to 20% of patients in some series of AAAs have proximal extension into the chest.[7] However, only five of 49 true aneurysms detected among 1112 patients who were followed after repair of an AAA involved the thoracoabdominal aorta.[8] Consequently, repair of TAAA remains an infrequent procedure. Although Crawford et al.[9] reported performing more than 200 of these procedures in a 13-month period, recent review of our experience over 14 years at the Mayo Clinic demonstrated an average rate of 14 TAAA repairs per year (unpublished data); and at the Cleveland Clinic over a recent 4-year period an average of 10 TAAA repairs per year were performed.[10]

PATIENTS MANAGED NONOPERATIVELY

We recently completed a retrospective review of 57 patients identified by CT scan to have aneurysmal dilatation of their thoracoabdominal aortic segment.[5] Patients with evidence of aortic dissection or rupture or those who proceeded directly to aneurysm repair following diagnosis were excluded from this study. All CT scans were reviewed for each patient, and the aorta was carefully measured. Reasons for deferral of aneurysm repair were recorded as follows: any aneurysm of 5 cm or less in diameter was deferred because of small size. Aneurysms larger than 5 cm in patients over the age of 75 or with a history of significant cardiac, pulmonary, or renal disease were deferred because of increased surgical risk. Surgery was deferred in some patients because of a more urgent problem requiring medical management or surgical correction, such as a larger aneurysm of the ascending aorta or coronary artery disease. Several patients refused operation. Reasons for nonoperative management are listed in Table 1.

Thirty-three (58%) men and 24 (42%) women with a mean age of 72 years were included in our series. Coexistent risk factors in our patients were typical of any series of aneurysm patients and included hypertension in 44 (77%) patients, tobacco use in 43 (75%), history of coronary artery disease in 24 (44%), and chronic obstructive pulmonary disease in 23 (40%). The mean follow-up among this cohort was 37 months (range, 6 days to 82 months). Follow-up was complete in 52 of the 57 patients (91%). Information was obtained by review of the medical record, solicitation of death certificates from the patients' home county, and by brief questionnaire sent to the patient and their referring physician designed only to confirm continued survival, date of last contact, and cause of death.

The Crawford classification of aneurysmal disease[9] among our patients was as follows: 20 type I (35%), eight type II (14%), 22 type III (39%), and seven type IV (12%). The median diameter of the aneurysms at the time of diagnosis was 5.0 cm (range, 3.4 to 7.8 cm). Thirty-five patients had 38 aneurysms of aortic segments distinct from their TAAA, including 13 aneurysms of the ascending aorta, one of the aortic arch, two of the descending thoracic aorta, and 22 of the infrarenal aorta. Eighteen aneurysms in 16 patients had been repaired previously, an average of 10 years before presentation (range, 1.5 to 20 years), involving the ascending aorta in two patients, descending thoracic aorta in one, and the infrarenal abdominal aorta in 13. Four patients (7%) had a history of peripheral arterial aneurysms: popliteal and femoral in two, and popliteal alone in two.

SURVIVAL

Life-table analysis demonstrated an overall 2- and 5-year survival of 69% and 39%, respectively (Fig. 1). Actuarial 2- and 5-year *repair-free* survival was 52% and 17%, respectively (see Fig. 1). More than half of the patients surviving 5 years had undergone eventual TAAA repair. Excluding patients who eventually underwent aneurysm repair (n = 15), actuarial survival rates were 58% and 23% at 2 and 5 years, respectively. Thirty-four of the 57 patients (60%) died over the follow-up period, three of whom had undergone repair of their TAAA. The cause of death in the 34 patients is listed in Table 2.

RISK OF RUPTURE

Eight of the 57 patients (14%) suffered a ruptured TAAA, and subsequently died. Ruptured TAAA was the second most frequent cause of death in our series. Actuarial risk of rupture among the 42 patients managed nonoperatively throughout follow-up was 12% at 2 years and 32% at 4 years (Fig. 2). When stratified by aneurysm size, patients with aneurysms of greater than 5 cm in diameter were at significantly increased risk of rupture (18% vs. 7% at 2 years; see Fig. 2).

Clinical data from the eight patients with ruptured TAAAs are presented in Table 3. At last measurement, the median size of the aneurysms that ruptured was 5.8 cm, and all ruptures occurred in aneurysms of greater than 5 cm. However, five of the eight ruptures occurred in aneurysms whose last measured diameter was 6.0 cm or less, and four of these had been imaged within the preceding 4 months. Both chronic obstructive pulmonary disease and chronic renal insufficiency were associated with aneurysm

Table 1 Reasons for nonoperative management among 57 patients with thoracoabdominal aneurysms

	No. of patients	Percent
Small aneurysm (<5 cm)	28	49
Increased surgical risk	18	32
Other illness requiring treatment	8	14
Patient preference	3	5

Table 2 Cause of death in 34 of 57 patients with thoracoabdominal aneurysms

Cause of death	Nonoperative management (n = 42) (%)	Operation following nonoperative management* (n = 15) (%)	Total (n = 57) (%)
Cardiopulmonary disease	10 (24)	2 (13)	12 (21)
Thoracoabdominal aneurysm rupture	8 (19)	—	8 (14)
Carcinoma	5 (12)	—	5 (9)
Cerebrovascular disease	3 (7)	—	3 (5)
Other causes	3 (7)	1 (7)	4 (7)
Unknown	2 (5)	—	2 (4)
TOTAL	31 (74)	3 (20)	34 (60)

*Includes one early and two late deaths.

Table 3 Data from eight patients with ruptured thoracoabdominal aortic aneurysms

Initial diameter (cm)	Last measured diameter (cm)	Time since last CT scan (mo)	Expansion rate (cm/yr)	Reasons for nonoperative management
5.3	6.5	1	0.36	Increased risk
4.3	5.4	3	0.40	Small aneurysm size
5.0	5.7	<1	0.20	Small aneurysm size
5.0	5.2	4	0.13	Increased risk
—	6.0	<1	—	Small aneurysm size
—	6.4	1	—	Colostomy repair
—	5.5	41	—	Increased risk
7.0	9.0	12	0.71	Patient preference

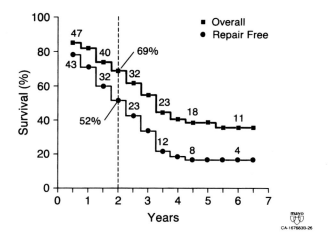

Fig. 1 Survival of patients with thoracoabdominal aortic aneurysms initially managed nonoperatively. Numbers of patients are depicted above each line, and standard error of the means are less than 10% for both lines. Cumulative survival rates in all patients (■) at 2 and 5 years were 69% and 39%, respectively. Survival rates free of TAAA repair (•) were 52% at 2 years (dashed line) and 17% at 5 years.

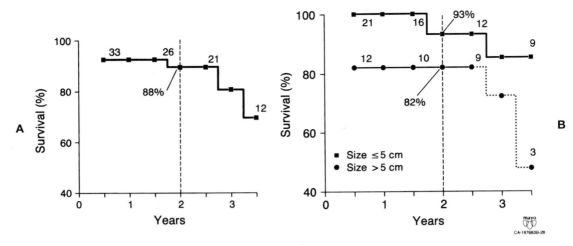

Fig. 2 A, Rupture-free survival of patients with thoracoabdominal aortic aneurysms, excluding those who eventually had repair. Numbers of patients are depicted above each line, and standard error of the mean is less than 10% throughout. Cumulative 2-year risk of rupture was 12%. **B,** Rupture-free survival of patients without eventual repair is stratified by aneurysm size. Patients with aneurysms 5 cm or less in diameter (■) had a significantly higher rupture-free survival ($p < .05$, log rank statistic) than those with aneurysms larger than 5 cm (●). Two-year rupture-free survival risks in both groups are noted at the dashed line. Dotted line indicates a standard error of the mean greater than 10%.

rupture ($p = .06$ for both), but no association with hypertension or smoking could be demonstrated.

REPAIR FOLLOWING NONOPERATIVE MANAGEMENT

Fifteen of the 57 (26%) patients underwent repair of their TAAA after a median of 24 months of initial nonoperative management (range, 2 to 110 months). Aneurysmal enlargement prompted operation in nine patients; in six patients the operation was delayed for surgical or medical therapy of concomitant illness. One of the 15 patients (7%) died during attempted TAAA repair; another became paraplegic after the operation.

RATE OF EXPANSION

Serial CT scans separated by more than 1 month were available in 29 of our 57 patients (51%). The mean interval between the initial and final scan was 2.4 years (range, 2 months to 8.7 years). The calculated median annual expansion rate was 0.2 cm/year (range, 0 to 1.4 cm/year). In six of the 29 patients (21%), the aneurysm enlarged at a rate of 0.4 cm/year or greater. Rate of expansion was unrelated to aneurysm size at diagnosis (Fig. 3). Among 15 patients with four or more CT scans, the rate of aneurysm expansion between their first and second scan (mean aneurysm diameter, 4.8 cm) was not different than between their third and fourth scan (mean diameter, 5.1 cm; average interval between both groups of scans, 1 year).

Chronic obstructive pulmonary disease was associated with an increased expansion rate; hypertension, chronic renal insufficiency, and smoking were not. Expansion rate did not appear to be related to rupture. The median rate of enlargement was 0.36 cm/year in patients with ruptures (see Table 3), but this was not statistically different from the expansion rate of aneurysms that did not rupture. Notably, two of the ruptures occurred in aneurysms with expansion rates of less than 0.2 cm/year.

DISCUSSION

Data on the outcome of nonoperative management of TAAAs are scarce. Crawford and DeNatale[6] reported a 2-year survival of only 24% in a group of 94 patients; 38% of the group died from aneurysm rupture. This seems at odds with the 2-year repair-free survival of 52% and 2-year

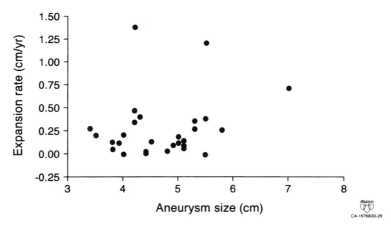

Fig. 3 Calculated annual expansion rate of 29 thoracoabdominal aneurysms determined by serial CT examinations, as related to aneurysm size at initial diagnosis. Note the lack of correlation between aneurysm size and expansion rate and the propensity of aneurysms to expand at a rate of less than 0.4 cm/year, regardless of their size.

rupture rate of only 12% in our group; however, these differences can be explained by the patient population and subsequent management in these two series. Dissections, which have been associated with a poorer prognosis in multiple studies, were included in the series from Crawford but were excluded in our series because we specifically wished to address the prognosis of degenerative aneurysms. Many patients in the series of Crawford were symptomatic, whereas our patients were asymptomatic. This is most likely the result of the method of entry into the study: Crawford's patients were admitted for evaluation for surgical repair of their aneurysm, which was then withheld, whereas the aneurysms in our patients were largely discovered incidentally. For the same reasons, the aneurysms in our series were most likely smaller than those in Crawford's cohort, although aneurysm size was not reported. Finally, once denied surgery in Crawford's series, patients were simply observed to the end points of death or rupture, whereas patients in our series crossed over to surgical repair if this was recommended by their surgeon.

An interesting finding from our series, which seems to be supported by other series in the literature, is the gender distribution of patients with thoracoabdominal aneurysms. More than 40% of our patients were women, and an even higher percentage of women were reported in the series of both Crawford and DeNatale[6] and Bickerstaff et al.[3] The latter study represents a population-based analysis, which is more likely to be an accurate representation of the true incidence in the general population. In any event, the predilection for the development of infrarenal aortic aneurysms in men[11] is less apparent in the thoracoabdominal aortic segment.

We have documented an expansion rate of 0.2 cm/year in TAAAs, which is in concurrence with much of the previous literature on abdominal aortic aneurysms. Nevitt et al.[12] found a similar expansion rate in a population-based analysis of more than 100 AAAs from our institution. In addition, they found a similar distribution of expansion rates, with approximately 25% of the aneurysms enlarging at a rate of 0.4 cm/year or greater. Dapunt et al.[13] examined a series of thoracic aneurysms including both dissections and aneurysms of the ascending aorta. Although they documented an expansion rate of 0.4 cm/year, the follow-up was short and the aneurysms were heterogeneous. These factors may lead to an overestimation of expansion rate in aneurysms of the thoracoabdominal aortic segment.

Expansion rate was not associated with aneurysmal diameter in our series; however, there is some dispute in the literature with regard to this point. Cronenwett et al.[14] found no association between expansion rates and initial aneurysm size in a series of 73 AAAs followed for more than 3 years. Conversely, Guirguis and Barber[15] noted an increase in expansion rate, with increasing aneurysmal diameter among 300 patients also followed for 3 years. Multifactorial analysis of the series of Dapunt et al.[13] of thoracic aneurysms indicated that initial aneurysm diameter of greater than 5 cm was the only independent risk factor for accelerated expansion. Perhaps the most convincing data relating expansion rate to aneurysm diameter are derived from following the same aneurysm over time and determining whether the rate of expansion for that aneurysm changes as it enlarges. Although we were unable to document an increase in expansion rate as an aneurysm enlarges in the current series, Nevitt et al.[12] did show an increased expansion rate as the aneurysm became larger.

Even less clear is the association of expansion rates to risk of rupture. We were unable to demonstrate any relation between expansion rate and risk of rupture. Although we had limited data to analyze, others have also failed to demonstrate this association.[12,16] While it seems intuitive that aneurysms that enlarge at a more rapid rate are more likely to rupture, it is noteworthy that two of the eight ruptures in our series occurred in aneurysms with expansion rates of 0.2 cm/year or less, and others[16] have also noted the potential for slowly enlarging aneurysms to rupture. Finally, we and others[16] have found chronic obstructive pulmonary disease to be associated with an increased expansion rate and risk of rupture.

CONCLUSION

The management of TAAAs remains a challenge. Crawford et al.[17] recommended operative repair of aneurysms greater than 5 cm in diameter in good-risk patients, symptomatic TAAAs, and most larger TAAAs based on their excellent surgical results. Our series of patients managed nonoperatively supports these recommendations. Our 5-year survival following repair of TAAA is 50% (unpublished data), compared with 23% in this series of patients managed nonoperatively. No aneurysms less than 5 cm in diameter ruptured in our series, and our data support nonoperative management of these patients. Patients who are otherwise healthy, have a prolonged life expectancy, and aneurysms of greater than 5 cm in diameter should be considered for repair. In those who are aged or are at increased surgical risk, with asymptomatic aneurysms of greater than 5 cm, the 2-year rupture risk of 18% must be weighed against the operative morbidity and mortality. This rupture risk is probably understated if the aneurysm is much larger, is symptomatic, or is associated with an aortic dissection.

REFERENCES

1. Szilagyi DE, Smith RF, DeRusso FJ, et al. Contribution of abdominal aortic aneurysmectomy to prolongation of life. Ann Surg 164:678-699, 1966.
2. Katz DA, Littenberg B, Cronenwett JL. Management of small abdominal aortic aneurysms: Early surgery vs watchful waiting. JAMA 268:2678-2686, 1992.
3. Bickerstaff LK, Pairolero PC, Hollier LH, et al. Thoracic aortic aneurysms: A population-based study. Surgery 92:1103-1108, 1982.
4. Svensson LG, Crawford ES, Hess KR, et al. Experience with 1509 patients undergoing thoracoabdominal aortic operations. J Vasc Surg 17:357-370, 1993.
5. Cambria RA, Gloviczki P, Stanson AW, et al. Outcome and expansion rate of 57 thoracoabdominal aortic aneurysms managed nonoperatively. Am J Surg 170:213-217, 1995.
6. Crawford ES, DeNatale RW. Thoracoabdominal aortic aneurysm: Observations regarding the natural course of the disease. J Vasc Surg 3:578-582, 1986.
7. Qvarfordt PG, Stoney RJ, Reilly LM, et al. Management of pararenal aneurysms of the abdominal aorta. J Vasc Surg 3:84-93, 1986.
8. Plate G, Hollier LA, O'Brien P, et al. Recurrent aneurysms and late vascular complications following repair of abdominal aortic aneurysms. Arch Surg 120:590-594, 1985.
9. Crawford ES, Svensson LG, Hess KR, et al. A prospective randomized study of cerebrospinal fluid drainage to prevent paraplegia after high risk surgery on the thoracoabdominal aorta. J Vasc Surg 13:36-46, 1990.
10. Cox GS, O'Hara PJ, Hertzer NR, et al. Thoracoabdominal aneurysm repair: A representative experience. J Vasc Surg 15:780-788, 1992.
11. Bickerstaff LK, Hollier LH, VanPeenen HJ, et al. Abdominal aortic aneurysms: The changing natural history. J Vasc Surg 1:6-12, 1984.
12. Nevitt MP, Ballard DJ, Hallett JW. Prognosis of abdominal aortic aneurysms: A population-based study. N Engl J Med 321:1009-1014, 1989.
13. Dapunt OE, Galla JD, Sadeghi AM, et al. The natural history of thoracic aortic aneurysms. J Thorac Cardiovasc Surg 107:1323-1333, 1994.
14. Cronenwett JL, Sargent SK, Wall MH, et al. Variables that affect the expansion rate and outcome of small abdominal aortic aneurysms. J Vasc Surg 11:260-269, 1990.

15. Guirguis EM, Barber GG. The natural history of abdominal aortic aneurysms. Am J Surg 162:481-483, 1991.
16. Cronenwett JL, Murphy TF, Zelenock GB, et al. Actuarial analysis of variables associated with rupture of small abdominal aortic aneurysms. Surgery 98:472-483, 1985.
17. Crawford ES, Hess KR, Cohen ES, et al. Ruptured aneurysms of the descending thoracic and thoracoabdominal aorta: Analysis according to size and treatment. Ann Surg 213:417-426, 1991.

25

Use of Ligation Treatment for Abdominal Aortic Aneurysms

WILLIAM C. PEVEC, M.D., JAMES W. HOLCROFT, M.D., and F. WILLIAM BLAISDELL, M.D.

Almost all abdominal aortic aneurysms are treatable by conventional surgical techniques. However, there is an occasional patient in whom the risk of standard operation is unacceptable, such as one with chronic obstructive pulmonary disease, overt respiratory failure, acute or chronic cardiac disease, renal failure, or associated abdominal conditions such as active diverticulitis or previous high-dose radiation therapy. In these circumstances the use of extra-anatomic bypass combined with proximal and distal aneurysm ligation may offer an acceptable alternative.

BACKGROUND

Our experience with abdominal aortic ligation dates to 1963.[1] A patient who had been gassed in World War I was admitted with acute respiratory failure, with severe back pain and abdominal tenderness secondary to what was perceived to be a rupturing abdominal aortic aneurysm. The patient could not lie down for an examination and had to be anesthetized in a sitting position. The first stage of the operation consisted of an axillofemoral bypass. At a second procedure the aneurysm was ligated between the renal arteries and the neck of the aneurysm, followed by ligation of both common iliac arteries, completely isolating the aneurysm. Because of the patient's inanition, the total intra-abdominal portion of the procedure took 10 minutes. The patient tolerated the procedure well: he survived, left the hospital, and was still alive 6 months later at the time of that initial report.

CLINICAL EXPERIENCE

Subsequent to that experience we used this operation perhaps once a year in equivalent high-risk patients. However, because of the high incidence of referrals of complex cases to our medical center, we have carried out 26 such operations between March 1980 and September 1992.[2]

A decision to perform extra-anatomic bypass and aortic exclusion, as opposed to direct aortic reconstruction, was based on the presence of conditions that significantly increased the predicted operative risk. These included history of myocardial infarction or of congestive heart failure, severe pulmonary disease, complex anatomic conditions, and morbid obesity. Most patients had more than one factor that increased surgical risk.

In 69% of patients the aneurysms were symptomatic, making deferral of treatment an unacceptable option. Aneurysm diameter averaged 7.0 ± 1.5 cm (range, 4.7 to 9.5 cm); seven aneurysms were ≥8 cm in diameter. One or both iliac arteries were aneurysmal in 42%. Average age was 71 ± 7 years. Ninety-six percent of patients had a history of smoking.

In each case an axillobifemoral bypass was constructed first. The infrarenal aorta was ligated in 62% of the patients. In the remainder, because of anatomic factors or severe cardiopulmonary disease that precluded aortic ligation, some combination of iliac and/or femoral artery ligation was performed without ligation of the infrarenal aorta.

TECHNIQUE

The bypass in almost all instances should be axillobifemoral. Our standard technique for bypass is to carry out end-to-side axillofemoral bypass on or near the femoral artery bifurcation. The external iliac artery is then divided at the inguinal ligament, and the proximal end on the ipsilateral side is oversewn. The divided distal end is then used for the proximal anastomosis of the femorofemoral bypass (Fig. 1). If bilateral common iliac artery ligation has been done, then the distal anastomosis of the femorofemoral bypass is carried out end to side. If no common iliac artery ligation has been done, to avoid back pressure on the iliac or aortic aneurysm, the distal anastomosis is carried out end to end, dividing and oversewing the contralateral external iliac artery, as was done on the ipsilateral axillofemoral side. If an ipsilateral femoral aneurysm requires resection, a side-to-end anastomosis is carried out and the graft is curved medially to the opposite groin (Fig. 2).

Depending on the nature of the patient's associated disease, we have carried out proximal ligation alone, distal ligation alone, and proximal and distal ligation. The optimal technique consists of complete isolation of the aneurysm, with proximal aortic ligature and bilateral common iliac ligation (Fig. 3).

Our approach for proximal ligation is to use a right subcostal incision followed by a Kocher maneuver to mobilize the duodenum. This permits exposure of the neck of the aneurysm at the level of the renal arteries. The periaortic plane is exposed by gentle dissection, and the neck of the aneurysm is encircled below the renal arteries with two umbilical tapes. The aorta is then briefly cross clamped above the renal arteries and the most proximal tape is tied down gently just below the renal arteries. The second tape is then tied down forcefully to ensure occlusion of the aorta, ideally 1 cm or more below the first tape.

One of the risks of the procedure is that dense calcification may result in the aorta fracturing at the site of the ligature if it is tied down too forcefully. By ensuring proximal control with the first ligature, the second ligature can be tied more tightly with less risk. Before tying the ligature, the area to be enclosed by the ties should be carefully palpated to determine compressibility. If the vessel is calcified, there are three alternatives. The first consists of dividing the aorta and oversewing the proximal and distal ends with or without bolster reinforcement. When the cuff between the renal arteries and the aneurysm is not adequate for ligature, mattress

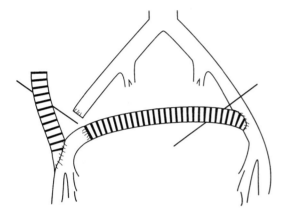

Fig. 1 Our standard technique for axillobifemoral bypass, which uses the double-outflow principle from the axillofemoral graft.

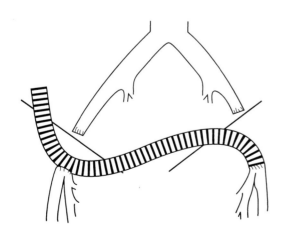

Fig. 2 The same principle applied when common femoral artery aneurysms require resection. The distal anastomosis is preferably made end-to-side to a left femoral replacement graft when the abdominal aortic aneurysm is to be ligated.

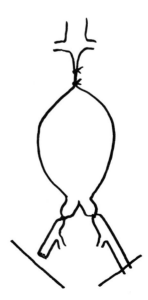

Fig. 3 Optimal technique for aneurysm ligation. The first umbilical tape is tied down lightly on the proximal aortic cuff. The second distal umbilical tape is tied down firmly.

sutures placed through the aorta and tied over fabric bolsters may be the optimal method of treatment. The third possibility is to carry out distal ligation only, encouraging the aneurysm to thrombose proximally.

Distal control is usually carried out by ligation of the common iliac arteries. On occasion, if there is marked aneurysmal degeneration of the vessels, ligation of the internal iliac and external iliac arteries on one side may be more easily and safely done.

RESULTS

There were two postoperative deaths for an operative mortality rate of 7.7%. There was one acute axillofemorofemoral graft occlusion; patency was restored with thrombectomy and common iliac artery ligation. There was one episode each of myocardial infarction, pneumonia, and renal insufficiency.

Follow-up ranged from 0 to 42 months and averaged 11.2 ± 10.3 months. Survival by the Kaplan-Meier life-table method was 59% at 1 year and 38% at 2 years. There were three deaths from ruptured abdominal aortic aneurysm; the infrarenal aorta had not been ligated in two of these. The remaining deaths were the result of comorbid conditions. Late graft occlusion occurred in five patients, but no limbs were lost.

DISCUSSION

Repair of abdominal aortic aneurysm has become a fairly safe procedure with an operative mortality rate of less than 5% in most series.[3-11] However, in some groups of patients the mortality of abdominal aortic aneurysm repair can be expected to be much greater than 5%. This includes patients with profound cardiac dysfunction or ischemia and debilitating pulmonary disease, and patients with technical risk factors such as a potentially contaminated peritoneal cavity or retroperitoneum or simultaneous intraabdominal inflammation.

An alternative to direct aortic repair is extra-anatomic reconstruction with an axillobifemoral bypass and ligation of the aortic outflow, with or without ligation of the infrarenal aorta. Such an approach has several attractive qualities. Most of the dissection occurs in the subcutaneous space, leading to less physiologic insult and smaller fluid shifts. The aorta is not clamped until after an effective bypass circuit is in place, avoiding the deleterious effects on the heart of aortic cross-clamping with the associated acute rise in outflow resistance. The risk of distal embolization is decreased, since the aorta is not cross clamped until after the iliac or femoral arteries are ligated. No prosthetic device is placed in the abdomen; this is advantageous, since potential contamination is an issue. Furthermore, the operation can be performed in stages if the patient does not tolerate the axillofemorofemoral bypass operation well.

However, the approach of extra-anatomic bypass and aortic occlusion has several disadvantages as well. Long-term patency of aortoiliac and aortofemoral grafts may be superior to that of axillobifemoral grafts. The data on patency of axillobifemoral grafts placed in conjunction with primary exclusion of the abdominal aortic aneurysm are restricted to three series. Kwaan et al.[12] reported two thrombectomies in 15 patients who were followed for 6 months to 3.5 years. Karmody et al.[13] reported 18 thrombectomies in 15 patients of 56 surviving patients; the length of follow-up is not mentioned. In our series five of 24 surviving patients required thrombectomy during a follow-up that averaged 11.2 ± 10.3 months.[2] It can therefore be expected that at least 15% to 30% of patients will at some time need thrombectomy if an axillobifemoral bypass is used in the treatment of abdominal aortic aneurysm.

Of greater concern is the fact that patients treated with axillobifemoral bypass and aortic occlusion are still at risk for aortic rupture. At least 33 incidents of abdominal aortic aneurysm rupture after axillobifemoral bypass and aortic exclusion have been reported.[12-20] In only four of these had the proximal aorta been ligated. In the reported series the incidence of aortic aneurysm rupture after extra-anatomic bypass with infrarenal aortic ligation varies from 0% to 6%[2,12,14] vs. 5% to 40% after extra-anatomic bypass without infrarenal aortic ligation.[2,13-15,19,20]

Long-term survival is poor for patients undergoing extra-anatomic bypass and aortic exclusion for the treatment of aortic aneurysm. In a series of 13 patients Schwartz et al.[15] reported a 31% 6-month survival. Karmody et al.[13] reported a 50% survival at 2.5 years in a series of 60 patients. Our patients had a 1-year survival of 59% and a 2-year survival of 38%.[2] The poor survival after axillobifemoral bypass and aortic exclusion is best attributed to patient selection. These patients are selected to undergo extra-anatomic reconstruction because of severe comorbid conditions. The majority do not die of aneurysm rupture but of their associated diseases.

We do not advocate ligation of an aortic aneurysm in a patient who can tolerate conventional aneurysm resection. However, when patients are symptomatic or have large aneurysms with a high risk of rupture and an operative mortality in excess of 10% is anticipated, abdominal aortic ligation offers an alternative that has less immediate morbidity and mortality. It permits the operation to be staged rather than carried out all at once, and we have demonstrated that it is well tolerated in high-risk patients.

REFERENCES

1. Blaisdell FW, Hall AD, Thomas AN. Ligation treatment of an abdominal aortic aneurysm. Am J Surg 109:560-565, 1965.
2. Pevec WC, Holcroft JW, Blaisdell FW. Ligation and extra-anatomic arterial reconstruction for the treatment of aneurysms of the abdominal aorta. J Vasc Surg 20:629-636, 1994.
3. Crawford ES, Saleh SA, Babb JW III, Glaeser DH, Vaccaro PS, Silvers A. Infrarenal abdominal aortic aneurysm: Factors influencing survival after operation performed over a 25-year period. Ann Surg 193:699-709, 1981.
4. Hollier LH, Plate G, O'Brien PC, et al. Late survival after abdominal aortic aneurysm repair: Influence of coronary artery disease. J Vasc Surg 1:290-299, 1984.
5. Whittemore AD, Clowes AW, Hechtman HB, Mannick JA. Aortic aneurysm repair. Reduced operative mortality associated with maintenance of optimal cardiac performance. Ann Surg 192:414-421, 1980.
6. Brown OW, Hollier LH, Pairolero PC, Kazmier FJ, McCready RA. Abdominal aortic aneurysm and coronary artery disease. Arch Surg 116:1484-1488, 1981.
7. Yeager RA, Weigel RM, Murphy ES, McConnell DB, Sasaki TM, Vetto RM. Application of clinically valid cardiac risk factors to aortic aneurysm surgery. Arch Surg 121:278-281, 1986.
8. White GH, Advani SM, Williams RA, Wilson SE. Cardiac risk index as a predictor of long-term survival after repair of abdominal aortic aneurysm. Am J Surg 156:103-107, 1988.
9. Blombery PA, Ferguson IA, Rosengarten DS, et al. The role of coronary artery disease in complications of abdominal aortic aneurysm surgery. Surgery 101:150-155, 1987.
10. Olsen PS, Schroeder T, Agerskov K, et al. Surgery for abdominal aortic aneurysms. A survey of 656 patients. J Cardiovasc Surg 32:636-642, 1991.
11. Balas P, Xeromeritis N, Massouridou E, Ioannou N. Ruptured abdominal aortic aneurysms. Clinical and surgical considerations. Int Angiol 9:243-245, 1990.
12. Kwaan JHM, Khan RJ, Connolly JE. Total exclusion technique for the management of abdominal aortic aneurysms. Am J Surg 146:93-97, 1983.
13. Karmody AM, Leather RP, Goldman M, Corson JD, Shah DM. The current position of nonresective treatment for abdominal aortic aneurysm. Surgery 94:591-597, 1983.
14. Lynch K, Kohler T, Johansen K. Nonresective therapy for aortic aneurysm: Results of a survey. J Vasc Surg 4:469-472, 1986.
15. Schwartz RA, Nichols WK, Silver D. Is thrombosis of the infrarenal abdominal aortic aneurysm an acceptable alternative? J Vasc Surg 3:448-455, 1986.
16. Schanzer H, Papa MC, Miller CM. Rupture of surgically thrombosed abdominal aortic aneurysm. J Vasc Surg 2:278-280, 1985.
17. Ricotta JJ, Kirshner RL. Case report: Late rupture of a thrombosed abdominal aortic aneurysm. Surgery 95:753-755, 1984.
18. Kwaan JH, Dahl RK. Fatal rupture after successful surgical thrombosis of an abdominal aortic aneurysm. Surgery 95:235-237, 1984.
19. Savarese RP, Rosenfeld JC, DeLaurentis DA. Alternatives in the treatment of abdominal aortic aneurysms. Am J Surg 142:226-230, 1981.
20. Cho SI, Johnson WC, Bush HL Jr, Widrich WC, Huse JB, Nabseth DC. Lethal complications associated with nonrestrictive treatment of abdominal aortic aneurysms. Arch Surg 117:1214-1217, 1982.

26

Late Complications of Standard Aortic Aneurysm Resection: What Is the Ultimate Fate of the Graft and of the Patient Based on a 35-Year Experience?

JAMES A. DeWEESE, M.D.

Abdominal aortic aneurysms (AAAs) are usually found in patients over the age of 50 years and it is estimated that by the age of 80 they occur in 5% of patients. Because of the risk of rupture, elective resection has become a standard operation for aneurysms of significant size in otherwise reasonably healthy patients.

Early and late morbidity and mortality may, of course, follow even the most successful of operations. We performed 506 operations on nonruptured abdominal aneurysms between 1959 and 1994. The operative mortality rate was 4.7%, which is similar to the 4.5% reported in a combined series of more than 500 patients, each recorded by Ernst.[1]

The cumulative survival rates at 5, 10, 15, and 20 years were 68%, 41%, 19%, and 6%, respectively. Five-, 10-, and 15-year survival rates in a combined series were 67%, 40%, and 18%, respectively.[1] The causes of death in our series were cardiac (33.0%), cancer (17.0%), stroke (11.0%), renal (4.0%), late operative complications (3.6%), and arterial aneurysms (3.4%). These results are very similar to those reported by Crawford et al.[2] and Hollier et al.[3]

The long term results of AAA resections also include morbidity and mortality related to (1) late operative complications such as para-anastomotic aneurysms, aortoenteric fistulas, and infection, (2) Late graft complications such as thrombosis and dilatation, and (3) Remote aneurysms occurring in the thoracic aorta, iliac arteries, and peripheral arteries.

LATE OPERATIVE COMPLICATIONS
Para-anastomotic Aneurysms

Aneurysms may develop at or adjacent to anastomoses performed at operations for any type of aneurysm. The new aneurysm may be a false aneurysm secondary to disruption of the suture line, which appears as a localized outpouching of the lumen proximal and distal to the anastomosis, or a true aneurysm, which appears as a dilatation of the artery beginning at the suture line.

The incidence of intra-abdominal para-anastomotic aneurysms following operations for AAA was considered to be quite low—29 cases (8%)—in earlier clinical series.[4] Recent operative series using postoperative ultrasound surveillance suggest that the incidence may be much higher.[5] We have recognized this complication in 1.2% (6 of 506) of our patients.

Possible reasons for the development of false aneurysms include deterioration of sutures such as silk, dilatation of grafts, compliance mismatch, and periprosthetic infection. The etiology of a true aneurysm may merely be an intrinsic defect in the arterial wall with continued degeneration with age. In some instances the original aneurysm may have been inadequately resected, for example, when only the distal half of an infrarenal dumbbell-shaped aneurysm was removed.

Complications of para-anastomotic aneurysms include expansion, aortoenteric fistulas, thrombus formation, and rupture. Symptoms may therefore include chronic pain, gastrointestinal bleeding, peripheral emboli, claudication and acute pain, and shock. Rupture and aortoenteric fistulas are the most dreaded of the complications and result in death if left untreated.[6] Even if surgery is possible, the mortality rate for ruptured intra-abdominal para-anastomotic aneurysms is 67% to 100%.[4,7,8] On the other hand, elective operative mortality rates have been reported to be less than 16%.[4,7,8]

In the absence of an aortoenteric fistula or infection, the operation consists of excision of the para-anastomotic aneurysm with insertion of an interposition graft. If a true aneurysm involves the visceral and thoracic aorta, a more extensive operation is required.

Because of the significantly better survival rate if operations are performed on intra-abdominal aneurysms before they rupture, close surveillance of postoperative AAAs by means of ultrasound or CT scans has been recommended. Further studies are needed before the benefit of such surveillance can be justified. There are concerns about the cost of such routine testing and the possible overtreatment of lesions the natural history of which is unknown.[4]

Aortoenteric Fistulas

Aortoenteric fistulas are said to occur in approximately 2% of patients following abdominal aortic operations.[9] We have seen only two (0.4%) of 506 in our series. Fistulas most often occur between the proximal aortic anastomosis or anastomotic pseudoaneurysm and the duodenum. Erosion of the jejunum, ileum, and colon occurs at the iliac anastomosis or from any portion of the graft to which the intestine adheres.

A modest "herald" bleed later followed by a severe bleed usually occurs from the anastomotic defect. Chronic slow bleeding occurs when intestine adherent to the graft becomes eroded. Intestinal enzymes and bacteria then digest the surrounding tissue allowing bleeding through the interstices of the graft and progression of infection along the graft.

Gastrointestinal bleeding in a patient with an aortic graft should be presumed to be secondary to an aortoenteric fistula until proven otherwise. Fiberoptic endoscopy should be the initial diagnostic procedure to identify the site of bleeding. CT scans can identify false aneurysms or perigraft fluid. Aortography may occasionally demonstrate false aneurysms or extravasation of dye. Barium contrast studies are rarely helpful. Laparotomy may be required to make the diagnosis and should not be unnecessarily delayed.

Operative management of the fistula may require simple transverse closure or segmental resection of the bowel with an end-to-end anastomosis. Satisfactory control of the fistula and prevention of continued vascular infection requires the removal of any of the foreign graft material that is possibly infected and any surrounding infected aortic or necrotic tissue. Usually this means removing the entire graft and a portion of the aortic stump. The wound is then thoroughly irrigated with antibiotic solution, the aortic stump is oversewn with monofilament suture, and the stump is covered by an omental flap. Revascularization of the lower extremity can be accomplished with extra-anatomic bypasses.[9-11] If there is no visible infection and necrotic tissue is away from the fistula, reconstruction may be achieved by means of a new in situ graft with omental coverage.[10,12,13] In rare instances only a portion of the graft need be replaced.[12] The overall mortality rate for cases treated with axillofemoral bypasses was 38% and for those treated using in situ techniques was 56% in Bunt's[14] review of 1983. Walker et al.[13] reported a 22% mortality rate in 23 patients for the in situ technique, but an additional two patients (9%) died within 3 months of rupture of the proximal anastomosis.

Graft Infection

Graft infection occurs following approximately 2% of all operations for AAA. It occurs more frequently when groin incisions are necessary.

Staphylococcus epidermidis is the most common offending organism followed by gram-negative bacteria, *Staphylococcus aureus,* and mixed gram-negative bacteria.[15] The infection may remain localized for a short time but then progresses along the graft and when it reaches an anastomosis a false aneurysm and or aortoenteric fistula may develop.

Graft infection may occur in the early postoperative period but may also occur several years after operation. It must be suspected in the presence of a groin infection or unexplained malaise, fever, and elevated white blood cell count. Back pain may be associated with an anastomotic aneurysm or bleeding may occur in the presence of an associated aortoenteric fistula.

The diagnosis may be suggested by perigraft fluid seen with ultrasonography or preferably on CT scan. CT scan can also identify associated false aneurysms, perigraft air, loss of tissue planes, and aortoenteric fistulas. Indium- or gallium-labeled leukocyte nuclear scans have been particularly helpful in determining the extent of spread of the infection. The diagnosis can be established by CT-directed needle aspiration of perigraft fluid. Cultures and sensitivities can be obtained making appropriate antibiotic treatment possible.

Surgical treatment for infected grafts has varied. Patients with graft infections that appear to be localized to a portion of the graft have in some instances been successfully managed by means of irrigation of antibacterial solutions with or without removal of a portion of the graft, but persisting infection with late complications is common.[15] The usual treatment has been complete removal of the graft and infected tissue with either in situ replacement of a new graft or an extra-anatomic bypass. In situ replacement has been advocated for patients with very localized infection or infection resulting from a low-virulence bacteria such as *Staphylococcus epidermidis*.[16] Extra-anatomic bypasses have been the preferred method for restoring distal blood flow. We and others have performed a staged procedure consisting of unilateral or bifemoral placement of a graft a few days before or just prior to removal of the graft.[11,17] The staged approach decreased the postoperative amputation rate from 41% to 7% in one series.[18] Aortic anastomotic or stump rupture is the most frequent serious complication following any method of management. To prevent this the infected aorta must be adequately debrided, monofilament suture must be used for closure, and autogenous material may be used as a patch but coverage of the aorta with an omental flap is a very important step in the operation. The use of long-term antibiotics is also very important. Reported mortality rates following treatment of aortic graft infections prior to 1983 were 37% to 75%. Since 1983 they have been 14% to 44%.[15]

GRAFT COMPLICATIONS
Graft Thrombosis

Reconstruction in a personal series of 506 AAA operations consisted of 213 tube grafts, 212 aortoiliac grafts, and 81 aortofemoral grafts. One woven Dacron tube graft occluded 5 years after operation and despite thrombosis of axillofemoral bypass grafts collateral circulation preserved his limbs until his death 5 years later. One aortoiliac woven Dacron tube graft occluded 14 years after operation and the limbs were preserved with axillobifemoral bypass grafts for 6 years despite the need for thrombectomy on two occasions. One limb of another aortoiliac woven Dacron graft occluded 6 years after operation and was successfully lysed with urokinase. One aortofemoral bypass graft occluded 8 years after operation, and the patient was admitted in extremis and died. One limb of another aortobifemoral graft occluded 1 year after operation, and a femorofemoral bypass graft preserved the limb for the remaining year of the patient's life.

Thrombosis of aortic grafts for aneurysmal disease is very rare and is not even mentioned in other reports of long-term results of such operations.[1,2,5,7]

Graft Aneurysms

Two types of postoperative alterations in graft materials have been described. The first is localized disruption of fibers secondary to structural failure resulting in holes in the prosthetic wall. Either bleeding or a false aneurysm ensues. An emergency or elective operation is required. The involved portion or the entire graft must be replaced. This complication has been said to occur in all types of synthetic prostheses.[19]

The second type of change is a dilatation of the entire graft, which is presumably initiated by stretching and followed by chemical and/or mechanical deterioration of the yarn over time. Nunn et al.[20] described its occurrence in several types of knitted Dacron bifurcation grafts. In retrospective studies CT scanning was performed to measure the diameter of the graft. There were 32 patients followed for an average of 175 months. The maximum diameter of the dilatation ranged from 26% to 267% with a mean of 94%. At least one part of the graft was dilated 100% or more in 12 patients. There were three aortic anastomotic aneurysms. Blumenberg et al.[21] followed knitted double-velour prostheses with ultrasound. Graft diameter increased by a mean of 23% during a mean follow-up of 25 months. The occurrence of anastomotic aneurysms did not relate to the degree of aneurysmal dilatation. Dilatation of woven Dacron grafts has not been reported.

REMOTE ANEURYSMS
Common Iliac Artery Aneurysms

The use of tube grafts whenever possible rather than bifurcation grafts has become the preferred treatment. The operation is easier and faster to perform and probably is associated with less morbidity. In a personal series of 506 aneurysm operations, however, bifurcation grafts were performed in 31% (157 of 506) of patients because of the presence of common iliac artery aneurysms. If tube grafts are used, the risk of developing a common iliac aneurysm is increased. Plate et al.[7] described the development of six new iliac artery aneurysms, three of which occurred in patients with tube grafts and two of which ruptured. On the other hand, Calcagno et al.[22] reported 39 patients with an average follow-up of 6 years who did not develop iliac artery aneurysms following tube grafts. Provan et al.[23] reported no dilatation of common iliac arteries as determined by postoperative CT scans 3 to 5 years following insertion of tube grafts. Crawford et al.[2] reported that common iliac artery aneurysm operations were not required in any of their patients with tube grafts. Among our 506 elective aneurysm patients, three had progression of a common iliac aneurysm, which was demonstrated by CT scan in one, angiography in the second, and rupture in the third. Two of the aneurysms were seen in patients with tube grafts and the third was distal to a proximal iliac artery anastomosis.

Thoracic Aneurysms

Crawford et al.[2] followed 860 patients undergoing elective infrarenal AAA operations. Rupture of the thoracic aorta was the cause of death in six of 41 patients who died in the hospital following AAA operations. Rupture of 16 other aneurysms including some thoracic aortic aneurysms was the cause of death in 26 of 348 patients who died late. Plate et al.[7] followed 1112 patients who underwent AAA repair. Thoracic aortic aneurysms (TAAs) were identified in 24 (2.2%) of these patients and caused death in 20 of them. Among the 506 elective AAA resections we performed, one patient died in the hospital and two patients died later of a ruptured TAA. Another six patients required operations for symptomatic TAAs.

Femoral Artery Aneurysms

Plate et al.[7] detected seven true femoral artery aneurysms in 1112 patients who had undergone AAA repair. Operations were performed by us on five true femoral aneurysms in four patients following 506 elective AAA operations. One aneurysm had thrombosed. Femoral artery aneurysms rarely rupture and the success rate for elective repair is quite high.

Popliteal Artery Aneurysms

Plate et al.[7] detected four popliteal artery aneurysms in three (0.3%) of the 1112 patients who underwent AAA repair. We have operated on six popliteal artery aneurysms in five patients following elective resection of 506 AAAs. Significant popliteal and femoral aneurysms are only rarely found in patients with AAA. Surgery is currently advised for patients with thrombosis or rupture or when an aneurysm becomes larger than 2 cm in diameter.[24]

REFERENCES

1. Ernst CB. Abdominal aortic aneurysm. N Engl J Med 328:1167-1172, 1993.
2. Crawford ES, Salehy SA, Babb JW III, et al. Infrarenal abdominal aortic aneurysm. Ann Surg 193:699-709, 1981.
3. Hollier LH, Plate G, O'Brien PC, et al. Late survival after abdominal aortic aneurysm repair: Influence of coronary artery disease. J Vasc Surg 1:290-299, 1984.
4. Curl GR, Faggioli GL, Ricotta JJ. Proximal paraanastomotic aortic aneurysms. In Veith FJ., ed. Current Critical Problems in Vascular Surgery, vol 5. St. Louis: Quality Medical Publishing, 1993, pp 240-246.
5. Edwards JM, Teefey SA, Zierler E, et al. Intraabdominal paraanastomotic aneurysms after aortic bypass grafting. J Vasc Surg 15:344-353, 1992.
6. Allen RC, Schneider J, Longenecker L, et al. Paraanastomotic aneurysms of abdominal aorta. J Vasc Surg 18:424-432, 1993.
7. Plate G, Hollier LA, O'Brien P, et al. Recurrent aneurysms and late vascular complications following repair of abdominal aortic aneurysm. Arch Surg. 120:590-594, 1985.
8. Treiman GS, Weaver FA, Cossman DV, et al. Anastomotic false aneurysms of abdominal aorta and the iliac arteries. J Vasc Surg 8:268-273, 1988.
9. Bernhard VM. Aortoenteric fistulas. In Rutherford R, ed. Vascular Surgery, ed 3. Philadelphia: WB Saunders, 1989, pp 528-535.
10. Perdue GD Jr, Smith RB III, Ansley JD, et al. Impending aortoenteric hemorrhage. The effect of early recognition on improved outcome. Ann Surg 192:237-243, 1980.
11. Jamieson GG, DeWeese JA, Rob CG. Infected arterial grafts. Ann Surg 181:840-842, 1975.
12. Vollmar JF, Kogel H. Aorto-enteric fistulas as postoperative complication. J Cardiovasc Surg 28(Suppl):479-484, 1987.
13. Walker EW, Cooley DA, Duncan JM, et al. The management of aortoduodenal fistula by "in situ" replacement of the infected abdominal aortic graft. Ann Surg 205:727-732, 1987.
14. Bunt TJ. Synthetic vascular graft infections. II. Graft-enteric erosions and graft-enteric fistulas. Surgery 94:1-9, 1983.
15. Faggioli GL, Ricotta JJ. Aortic graft infections. In Veith FJ, ed. Current Critical Problems in Vascular Surgery, vol 4. St. Louis: Quality Medical Publishing, 1992, pp 371-380.
16. Bandyk DF. Prosthetic infections due to bacterial biofilms: Clinical and experimental observations. J Vasc Surg 13:757-758, 1991.
17. Reilly LM, Altman H, Lusby RJ. Late results following surgical management of vascular graft infection. J Vasc Surg 1:36-44, 1984.

18. O'Hara PJ, Hertzer NR, Beven EG, et al. Surgical management of infected abdominal aortic grafts: Review of 25-year experience. J Vasc Surg 3:725-731, 1986.
19. Ohta T, Kato R, Kaqui H, et al. Disruption of externally supported knitted Dacron graft three years after implantation—A case report. J Vasc Surg 12:66-69, 1990.
20. Nunn DB, Carter MM, Donohue MT, et al. Postoperative dilation of knitted Dacron aortic bifurcation graft. J Vasc Surg 12:291-297, 1990.
21. Blumenberg RM, Gelfand ML, Barton EA, et al. Clinical significance of aortic graft dilation. J Vasc Surg 14:175-180, 1991.
22. Calcagno D, Hallett JW Jr, Ballard DJ, et al. Late iliac artery aneurysms and occlusive disease after aortic tube grafts for abdominal aortic aneurysm repair. Ann Surg 214:733-736, 1991.
23. Provan JL, Fialkov J, Ameli FM, et al. Is tube repair of aortic aneurysm followed by aneurysmal change in the common iliac arteries? Can J Surg 33:394-397, 1990.
24. Shortell CK, DeWeese JA, Ouriel K, Green RM. Popliteal artery aneurysms: A 25-year surgical experience. J Vasc Surg 14:771-779, 1991.

27

Ischemic Nephropathy and Concomitant Aortic Disease: When Should Renal Artery Repair Be Undertaken?

ELLIOT L. CHAIKOF, M.D., Ph.D., and ROBERT B. SMITH III, M.D.

The premise that occlusive disease of the renal artery is an important and underestimated cause of renal insufficiency is not disputed within the vascular surgical community. Nonetheless, therapeutic strategies remain somewhat ill-defined because of the lack of information regarding the natural history of ischemic nephropathy and, specifically, our ability to alter the long-term course of progressive renal insufficiency by surgical intervention. The risk/benefit ratio is particularly blurred in the patient with concomitant aneurysmal or occlusive disease of the aorta. Should patients be subjected to combined aortic and renal artery reconstruction without a clear-cut test of who will benefit from renal artery reconstruction? In the absence of an accurate predictor of outcome, is there a level of renal insufficiency or anatomic configuration that warrants surgical intervention, particularly if hypertension is well controlled? In the final analysis few studies have adequately addressed, even in a retrospective fashion, how many patients will be spared dialysis and for how long. Nor do we know whether intervention will improve overall survival. *The need for a multi-institutional prospective study is at hand.* However, until such data become available, we are left to compare cohorts of patients who have demonstrated a beneficial response after operative intervention with those who have not. At the very least, such an analysis provides clinical guidelines in the short term and postulates for more rigorous testing in the long term. In this regard we have reviewed our own 10-year experience with surgical intervention for chronic renal insufficiency in patients with concomitant atherosclerotic aortic and renovascular disease at the Emory University Hospital.[1] Particular emphasis in our analysis was directed at characterizing the effect of renal revascularization on the clinically meaningful end points of dialysis and death.

PATHOPHYSIOLOGY

It is remarkable that although the cause of ischemia-induced acute renal failure has been extensively investigated, the mechanisms that contribute to progressive renal dysfunction in the presence of chronic or intermittent ischemia have been little studied or defined. Dean et al.[2] have speculated that there are two mechanisms that may lead to renal dysfunction: a reversible form of chronic ischemia that is related to the presence of a flow-limiting lesion and an irreversible type related to renal microemboli produced by disease in the main renal artery. They have postulated that if left untreated, the former is associated with rapid deterioration but at the same time offers the best opportunity for retrieval of function. The latter is associated with a slower decline in function and may be less affected by surgical intervention. These postulates remain untested, but both are based on the presumption that the natural history of ischemic nephropathy will be altered by improved renal perfusion.

In many forms of renal disease progressive deterioration may occur even in the absence of the initial cause of injury. Apart from continued small-vessel disease, nonhemodynamic mechanisms, including genetic, metabolic, lipid, and coagulation factors, may act synergistically in potentiating and promoting continued glomerular damage.[3] Perhaps ischemia of an undefined duration is an initiating event. Three hypotheses appear plausible. Molitoris[4] has speculated that chronic ischemia may lead to proximal tubular damage, which could reduce the glomerular filtration rate (GFR) by nephron obstruction. Alternatively, changes in oxygen tension or wall shear rates produced by a flow-limiting lesion may activate or directly injure glomerular endothelium, leading to the release of procoagulant, mitogenic, or chemotactic peptides. Potentially, local activation of monocytes or platelets would further accelerate this cascade of events, terminating in glomerular scarring. Finally, ischemia-induced injury of glomerular mesangial or epithelial cells may lead to enhanced extracellular matrix synthesis, producing renal fibrosis as in glomerulosclerosis.[5] Once these events are in play, GFR may continue to decline despite the correction of renal ischemia.

MONITORS OF RENAL FUNCTION

Stenosis of the main renal artery of ≥70% or a gradient of at least 40 mm Hg is typically associated with a reduction of GFR.[6] However, in most studies the assessment of renal revascularization has been limited to the measurement of serum creatinine levels as a substitute for GFR determinations. Changes in muscle mass, meat intake, tubular secretion, and extrarenal metabolism of creatinine are all confounding factors in its use.[7] The failure in a number of studies to demonstrate a direct correlation between serum creatinine level and progression of renal artery stenosis reflects, in part, these limitations.[8,9] Such criticisms apply equally to the use of creatinine clearance, inverse creatinine slopes, and the Cockcroft and Gault[10] estimated GFR (EGFR). We agree, however, with Dean et al.[2] that the EGFR may be a useful approximation when applied to an entire group. The Rolin modification[11] of the Cockcroft and Gault formula is stated as follows:

$$EGFR = \frac{(140 - age)(weight)(1.73)}{(72)(serum\ creatinine)(BSA)}$$

where age is in years, weight in kilograms, and serum creatinine in milligrams per deciliter. BSA is body surface area determined from standard nomograms. The value for females is multiplied by 0.85 to correct for an average lower rate of creatinine synthesis.

PATIENT POPULATION

We undertook a review of all Emory University Hospital patients with renal insufficiency (creatinine level of 1.8 mg/dl or greater) and concomitant atherosclerotic aortic and renovascular disease. Fifty patients underwent both renal revascularization (71 kidneys) and the repair of aneurysmal and/or symptomatic aortic occlusive disease between 1982 and 1992. Hypertension was present in 96%, diabetes in 10%, and 90% of the population had a history of tobacco use. Fifty-two percent were taking three or more antihypertensive medications. The median age was 67 years; 74% were men and 26% were women. The preoperative EGFR was 25.18 ± 8.29 ml/min (creatinine level, 3.1 ± 1.5 mg/dl). Operative management included bilateral renal artery repair (21), unilateral repair alone (17), and unilateral repair with contralateral nephrectomy (12).

EARLY OUTCOME AFTER COMBINED REPAIR

The 30-day operative mortality rate in this review was 2%, which is comparable to that of an earlier review of our experience.[12] Likewise, a number of recent series of combined aortic and renal artery reconstruction have documented operative mortality rates of approximately 3% or less.[13-15] Higher incidences of 10% or greater may reflect sample sizes and heterogeneity with regard to the complexity of operation and underlying medical problems. Although our preference has been to perform bilateral revascularization when needed and not to "stage" the procedures, treatment recommendations should be tempered by the condition of the individual patient. In our review a 14% incidence of nonfatal cardiac morbidity after surgery reinforces the inherent perioperative hazards.

In our own hands revascularization had a short-term beneficial effect in nearly half of the patients when considered in terms of improvement in EGFR (Fig. 1). In contrast to an earlier report from our institution, benefit was observed in patients with both unilateral and bilateral renal artery disease (Table 1).[12] Nor could we detect a statistically significant relationship between early or late outcome and whether a bilateral or unilateral procedure was performed. Dean et al.[2] have failed to observe a statistically significant level of improvement in patients with

Table 1 Site of disease and early functional response

Change in EGFR	Unilateral disease		Bilateral disease	
	No.	Percent	No.	Percent
Improved	3	30	18	45
No change	7	70	20	50
Worsened	0	0	2	5
TOTAL	10		40	

unilateral disease when analyzed as a group. Nonetheless, they noted an increase in EGFR of 20% or greater in 33% of these patients (4 of 12). The small number of patients who fall into the category of unilateral renal artery involvement prevents hard and fast rules at this time. Otherwise, there were no clinical or anatomic variables that clearly predicted short-term outcome, including the level of preoperative renal function. This finding is in contrast to the other reports[12,13,16] in which early functional responses were most notable in patients with higher preoperative serum creatinine levels. As reported by Dean et al.,[2] patients with a slow decline in GFR often demonstrate little, if any, improvement following revascularization. Perhaps in our study there was bias toward this category as a consequence of intervention that was more often triggered by the presence of an aneurysm or aortoiliac occlusive symptoms and not be accelerated hypertension or renal insufficiency. A median decline in preoperative EGFR of 0.79 (ml/min) per month suggests that this may well be the case.

LATE OUTCOME AFTER COMBINED REPAIR
Impact on Survival

Although serum creatinine levels can provide some insight into renal function, the ability to draw reliable conclusions in the absence of isotopically determined serial GFRs ultimately depends on an analysis of clinically meaningful end points—that is, improvement in life span or an impact on quality of life in terms of dialysis-free survival.[7] The potential benefits of combined renal artery and aortic surgery are often weighed against the advanced age and associated medical problems that are characteristic of this population. The overall 5-year survival rate was 62% (95% confidence interval: 0.48, 0.81), similar to 5-year survival rates of approximately 65% reported from both the Cleveland and Mayo Clinics in 1987.[17,18] However, we were somewhat surprised that long-term survival remains compromised among those patients with preoperative serum creatinine levels less than 3.0 mg/dl despite their lower probability of eventual dialysis (Fig. 2). Accelerated mortality rates among patients with renovascular disease receiving dialysis have been reported.[19,20] In contrast, we did note a trend, although not statistically significant, toward better survival rates for patients with relative measures of operative success (an increase in EGFR of 20% or more or a decrease in serum creatinine level of 15% or greater in the early postoperative period). Although dialysis may significantly compromise the life expectancy of a young or middle-aged adult, in the elderly patient with associated comorbid conditions, the effect of dialysis on late survival may be marginal. More patients will be needed to definitely establish the survival impact of renal functional response to surgery.

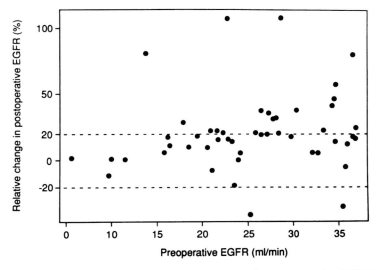

Fig. 1 Relationship between preoperative and postoperative EGFRs.

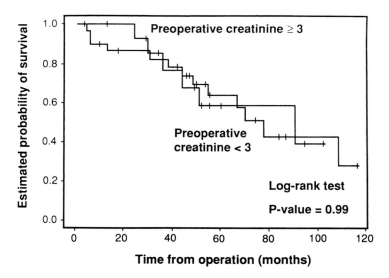

Fig. 2 Kaplan-Meier life-table analysis of subgroups categorized with respect to preoperative serum creatinine levels less than 3.0 mg/dl vs. serum creatinine levels of 3.0 mg/dl or greater.

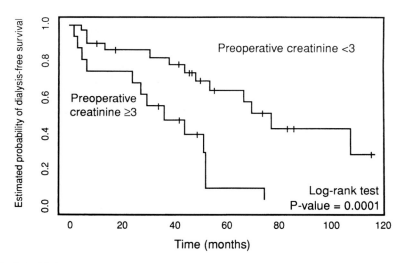

Fig. 3 Kaplan-Meier estimated probability of dialysis-free survival of subgroups categorized with respect to preoperative serum creatinine levels less than 3.0 mg/dl vs. serum creatinine levels of 3.0 mg/dl or greater.

Impact on Quality of Life

Certainly the need for dialysis is a great economic and emotional burden for the patient and society as a whole. However, the reported incidence of late dialysis following revascularization has received comment in only a few reports which reflected somewhat limited study periods. In general, end-stage renal disease (ESRD) has ranged from 4.4% to 14% despite surgery.[2,17,21] In our review the need for eventual dialysis was greatest among patients with an elevated preoperative creatinine level or depressed EGFR and was not predicted by other clinical variables, including the pattern of renal artery occlusive disease (Fig. 3). In fact, the relative risk for eventual dialysis was 3.0 for each 1.0 mg/dl increment in preoperative serum creatinine. Among patients whose preoperative creatinine level was 3.0 mg/dl or greater, the estimated 3-year probability of ESRD was 32% (95% confidence interval: 4%, 51%). In contrast, the incidence of late renal failure was low among our patients with only a moderate degree of preoperative azotemia (serum creatinine level: 1.8 to 3.0 mg/dl). Bredenberg et al.[21] have recently noted a failure to avoid dialysis in five of six patients who had serum creatinine levels above 5.5 mg/dl despite proven graft patency.

The ability to maintain normal blood pressure with minimal or no medication may well affect the rate of progressive renal insufficiency. Untreated malignant or accelerated hypertension can certainly cause ESRD; however, the frequency with which mild to moderate essential hypertension leads to renal failure is unclear.[22] A recent randomized prospective study in Europe found no change in creatinine clearance in elderly patients with untreated hypertension over a 5-year follow-up period.[23] In contrast, a decline in creatinine clearance was observed in those receiving antihypertensives, suggesting that treatment, and not blood pressure per se, is the cause of worsening renal function. Hypertension was cured or improved in approximately 50% of our patients evaluated at late follow-up. This result is in the range of the 53% to 78% noted in other reviews of combined aortic and renal artery reconstruction.[12,13] Poor late blood pressure control was statistically related to high preoperative serum creatinine. Indeed, it is difficult to account with certainty for the contribution of antihypertensives either to the level of renal function noted before surgery or to its decline at late follow-up.

CONCLUSION

It is most noteworthy that our ability to have an impact on the quality of life, as measured by dialysis-free survival, is significantly less among patients with lower preoperative renal reserve. In many, but not all, patients markedly compromised preoperative renal function is a probable marker for likely poor outcome. Thus, in the current absence of prospective data, intervention prior to marked deterioration of renal function remains the best option. This offers the best hope for preserving the patient's quality of life by reducing the decline in renal function and decreasing the need for subsequent dialysis. We would recommend repairing all angiographically significant (>60%) stenoses in patients with associated aortic disease who present with a preoperative serum creatinine level in the range of 1.8 to 3.0 mg/dl. In those who have higher levels of serum creatinine, advocacy for conservative, nonoperative management in the good-risk patient with aortic disease would be premature at this time. In our experience patients in this category can occasionally benefit from revascularization, particularly in the face of recent accelerated functional deterioration. As we begin to understand the basic pathophysiology of chronic ischemia, additional therapeutic options may provide a means of altering the path to renal failure that some of our patients follow despite surgery. Until then, early intervention to minimize the duration of the ischemic insult remains a prudent choice.

REFERENCES

1. Chaikof EL, Smith RB, Salam AA, Dodson TF, Lumsden AB, Kosinski AS, Allen RC. Ischemic nephropathy and concomitant aortic disease: A ten-year experience. J Vasc Surg 18:135-146, 1994.
2. Dean RH, Tribble RW, Hansen KJ, O'Neil E, Craven TE, Redding JF II. Evolution of renal insufficiency in ischemic nephropathy. Ann Surg 213:446-455, 1991.
3. Bourgoignie JJ. Progression of renal disease: Current concepts and therapeutic approaches. Kidney Int 41(Suppl 36):S61-S65, 1992.
4. Molitoris BA. The potential role of ischemia in renal disease progression. Kidney Int 41(Suppl 36):S21-S25, 1992.
5. Meguid E, Nahas A. Growth factors and glomerular sclerosis. Kidney Int 41(Suppl 36):S15-S20, 1992.
6. Jacobson HR. Ischemic renal disease: An overlooked clinical entity? Kidney Int 34:729-743, 1988.
7. Perrone RD. Means of clinical evaluation of renal disease progression. Kidney Int 41(Suppl 36):S26-S32, 1992.
8. Schreiber MJ, Pohl MA, Novick AC. The natural history of atherosclerotic and fibrous renal artery disease. Urol Clin North Am 11:383-392, 1984.
9. Tollefson DF, Ernst CB. Natural history of atherosclerotic renal artery stenosis associated with aortic disease. J Vasc Surg 14:327-331, 1991.
10. Cockcroft DW, Gault MH. Prediction of creatinine clearance from serum creatinine. Nephron 16:31-41, 1976.
11. Rolin HA, Hall PM, Wei R. Inaccuracy of estimated creatinine clearance for prediction of iothalamate glomerular filtration rate. Am J Kidney Dis 4:48-54, 1984.
12. Stewart MT, Smith RB III, Fulenwider JT, Perdue GD, Wells JO. Concomitant renal revascularization in patients undergoing aortic surgery. J Vasc Surg 2:400-405, 1985.
13. O'Mara CS, Maples MD, Kilgore TL Jr, McMullan MH, Tyler HB, Mundinger GH Jr, Kennedy RE. Simultaneous aortic reconstruction and bilateral renal revascularization. Is this a safe and effective procedure? J Vasc Surg 8:357-366, 1988.
14. Barral X, Delorme JM, Favre JP, et al. Lésions artérielles rénales et anéurysmes de l'aorte abdominale sous-rénale. In Keiffer E, ed. Les Anéurysmes de l'Aorte Abdominale Sous-Rénale. Paris: AERCV, 1990, pp 337-348.

15. Branchereau A, Espinoza H, Magnan PE, Rosset E, Castro M. Simultaneous reconstruction of infrarenal abdominal aorta and renal arteries. Ann Vasc Surg 6:232-238, 1992.
16. Dean RH, Englund R, Dupont WD, Meacham PW, Plummer WD Jr, Pierce R, Ezell C. Retrieval of renal function by revascularization: Study of preoperative outcome predictors. Ann Surg 202:367-375, 1985.
17. Hallett JW, Fowl R, O'Brien PC, Bernatz PE, Pairolero PC, Cherry KJ, Hollier LH. Renovascular operations in patients with chronic renal insufficiency: Do the benefits justify the risks? J Vasc Surg 5:622-627, 1987.
18. Tarazi RY, Hertzer NR, Beven EG, O'Hara PJ, Anton GE, Krajewski LP. Simultaneous aortic reconstruction and renal revascularization: Risk factors and results in eighty-nine patients. J Vasc Surg 5:707-714, 1987.
19. Mailloux LU, Bellucci AG, Mossey RT, Napolitano B, Moore T, Wilkes BM, Bluestone PA. Predictors of survival in patients undergoing dialysis. Am J Med 84:855-862, 1988.
20. Novick AC, Textor SC, Bodie B, Khauli RB. Revascularization to preserve renal function in patients with atherosclerotic renovascular disease. Urol Clin North Am 11:477-490, 1984.
21. Bredenberg CE, Sampson LN, Ray FS, Cormier RA, Heintz S, Eldrup JJ. Changing patterns in surgery for chronic renal artery occlusive diseases. J Vasc Surg 15:1018-1023, 1992.
22. Weisstuch JM, Dworkin LD. Does essential hypertension cause end-stage renal disease? Kidney Int 41(Suppl 36):S33-S37, 1992.
23. De Leeuw PW. Renal function in the elderly. Results from the European working party on high blood pressure in the elderly trial. Am J Med 90(Suppl 3A):45S-49S, 1991.

28

Transaortic Renal Endarterectomy: Techniques, Pitfalls, and Results

DANIEL G. CLAIR, M.D., MICHAEL BELKIN, M.D., ANTHONY D. WHITTEMORE, M.D., MAGRUDER C. DONALDSON, M.D., and JOHN A. MANNICK, M.D.

Renal artery disease in patients older than 50 years of age is almost always atherosclerotic in origin and is commonly associated with atherosclerosis of the aortic and iliac arteries and/or with infrarenal abdominal aortic aneurysm.[1] In these patients atherosclerotic renal artery disease not only contributes to hypertension but also is now recognized as an important cause of kidney failure.[2-5] Recent studies of the natural history of renal artery disease strongly suggest that atherosclerotic stenoses progress inexorably to renal artery occlusion.[2,6,7] Thus a relatively aggressive approach toward renal revascularization for hemodynamically significant renal artery disease appears warranted.

In selected circumstances it appears logical to consider combining renal artery revascularization with aortic reconstruction for clinically significant occlusive disease or aneurysms. However, many surgeons have been cautious in performing combined renal and aortic reconstruction in light of past reports indicating increased operative mortality associated with this procedure.[8-11] Because atherosclerotic renal artery disease usually results from an extension of an adjacent aortic plaque into the orifice and proximal part of the renal artery, eversion endarterectomy[12,13] of the adjacent aorta and the renal artery orifices should be a convenient and expeditious technique for combined aortic and renal artery reconstruction. The present study was undertaken to define the safety and efficacy of transaortic renal endarterectomy, particularly when it is used as an adjunct to aortic surgery.

METHODS

Clinical data for consecutive patients who underwent transaortic renal endarterectomy for atherosclerotic disease at the Brigham and Women's Hospital between 1985 and 1994 were compiled by review of a computerized vascular registry, hospital records, and appropriate arteriograms. Preoperative biplane arteriography was performed on all patients with selective oblique views for evaluation of orificial stenoses and associated aortic disease. Renal artery stenosis was considered significant when there was diameter reduction of 60% or more. Lesions extending into the distal half of the renal artery or into branches of the main renal artery were not considered suitable for endarterectomy.

Transaortic renal endarterectomy was performed through midline abdominal or left flank incisions. The left retroperitoneal approach appeared to be advantageous in obese patients or in patients with previous abdominal surgery and allowed easy exposure for aortic clamping at any level below the diaphragm. The midline abdominal approach appeared best in the presence of right renal or right iliac artery disease. This was the more common exposure used in the present series. The perirenal aorta was dissected with wide mobilization of the left renal vein, usually with division of the left gonadal and adrenal branches. The renal arteries were freed up for at least 1 cm beyond the extent of the proximal atherosclerotic disease. The dissection was continued superiorly to the origin of the superior mesenteric artery. In the absence of severe atherosclerotic involvement of the aorta just below the superior mesenteric artery, the aortic clamp was applied at this level. If the inframesenteric aorta appeared inappropriate for clamping, supraceliac aortic exposure was obtained via the gastrohepatic ligament. Distal exposure was determined by the extent of the associated aortic occlusive or aneurysmal disease.

After systemic administration of heparin and infusion of mannitol, the renal arteries were occluded, followed by aortic outflow and suprarenal proximal aortic clamping. For isolated renal endarterectomy (n = 4), the aorta was opened transversely or obliquely between the renal orifices. In the presence of associated aortic disease (n = 39), the aorta was opened longitudinally, extending proximally between the renal arteries. In most instances the presence of continuous aortic plaque required localized endarterectomy of the aorta as well as the renal artery orifices. In some instances endarterectomy was initiated near the renal orifice by incising the aortic wall in a circular manner around each involved artery, freeing a button for traction and gentle eversion, with accompanying dissection with a spatula to allow delivery of the specimen with a tapered end point under direct vision. Gentle probing with a clamp was helpful to retrieve any residual plaque. If any question remained regarding the end point, a balloon catheter was introduced into the renal artery, gently inflated, and then retracted into the aortic lumen, allowing prolapse of the artery into the aorta for further visualization of the end point. In the few instances of isolated renal endarterectomy, the transverse aortotomy was closed primarily. In the combined procedures the aortic prosthesis was tailored to fit into the aortic incision between the renal arteries. The graft was flushed vigorously before release of renal artery clamps to minimize the chance of atheroembolization. Continuous-wave Doppler ultrasonography was routinely used to assess adequacy of flow into the renal arteries, supplemented occasionally with duplex ultrasonography or operative arteriography.

Blood pressure, antihypertensive medications, and serum creatinine were recorded at serial intervals postoperatively. Renal dysfunction was defined as a serum creatinine level of 1.5 mg/dl or greater, and changes of 1 mg/dl or greater were considered significant. Response of hypertension to surgery was classified according to the criteria of Dean et al.,[10] by which "cure" implies diastolic blood pressure less than 95 mm Hg with no medication and "improvement" implies reduction by two antihypertensive medications with adequate (diastolic less than 95 mm Hg) pressure control, reduction by one medication with moderate (diastolic pressure reduction less than 20 mm Hg) decrease in pressure, or a significant (diastolic pressure reduction greater than 20 mm Hg) decrease in pressure with no increase in the number of medications. Postoperative evaluation of renal artery patency was performed selectively as dictated by changes in blood pressure or serum creatinine.

RESULTS

Transaortic renal endarterectomy was performed in 78 arteries in 43 patients in the study period. An additional 56 patients underwent renal artery bypass during the same time interval. Patient characteristics (Table 1) were remarkable for rough gender equivalence and a low prevalence of diabetes. Significant aortic disease was repaired at surgery in 39 of the 43 patients including 30 with infrarenal aortic aneurysms and nine with severely symptomatic aortoiliac occlusive disease. Indications for renal artery revascularization were hypertension or kidney failure in 41 patients (95%), with highly significant but asymptomatic renal artery disease in the remaining two. Mean serum creatinine for the 28 patients with preoperative renal dysfunction was 3.0 mg/dl, and the mean number of antihypertensive medications used by the 38 patients with hypertension was 2.5 per patient. All but three procedures were elective. Two of these patients required urgent surgery because of the rapid onset of dialysis-dependent renal failure. One patient had malignant hypertension requiring intravenous antihypertensive medication.

The operative approach was transabdominal in 32 patients and retroperitoneal in 11. The suprarenal aorta was clamped below the superior mesenteric artery in 37 patients and above the celiac axis in six. Transaortic endarterectomy was performed in 78 renal arteries, 10 of which were totally occluded (Table 2). Thirty of the 43 patients underwent bilateral renal endarterectomy including an involved accessory renal artery in three patients. Nine had unilateral renal endarterectomy. Two of these had unilateral endarterectomy with contralateral bypass to a renal artery distal to an occlusion, and two had unilateral endarterectomy with contralateral

Table 1 Clinical characteristics and surgical indications for 43 patients undergoing transaortic renal endarterectomy between 1985 and 1994

Mean age	68 years (46-81)
Male: female	25:18
Coronary artery disease	25 (58.1%)
Smoking	18 (41.9%)
Diabetes mellitus	2 (4.7%)
Hypertension	13 (30.2%)
Renal insufficiency	3 (7.0%)
Hypertension and renal insufficiency	25 (58.1%)
Aortic disease	39 (90.7%)
Infrarenal aneurysm	30 (69.8%)
Occlusive disease	9 (20.9%)
Isolated atherosclerotic kidney disease	4 (9.3%)

nephrectomy for small kidneys distal to occluded renal arteries. A hilar renal aneurysm was repaired after bilateral renal endarterectomy in one patient. Mean renal ischemia time was 35 minutes (range, 12 to 60 minutes). Five (6.5%) of the 76 renal endarterectomies required intraoperative revision by implantation into the aortic graft (n = 2) or by bypass originating from the aortic graft (n = 3). All revascularized renal arteries were patent by palpation and Doppler ultrasonography at the completion of surgery.

Major postoperative morbidity occurred within 30 days of surgery in six patients (14%) (Table 3). No patient with normal preoperative renal function experienced postoperative renal insufficiency. Among the 26 surviving patients with preoperative renal dysfunction, serum creatinine levels rose to a mean maximum of 3.4 mg/dl within the first 30 postoperative days. Six of these patients (14.6%) experienced postoperative elevation of serum creatinine of one mg/dl or greater above baseline levels, four of whom have remained stable without dialysis at follow-up ranging from 1 to 4 years. Two patients required institution of hemodialysis after operation. In one of these patients dialysis was discontinued after 1 week with recovery of renal function. Serum creatinine in that patient fell to levels below preoperative levels and has remained so. The other patient has required long-term hemodialysis. This individual had a preoperative creatinine level of 10.2 mg/dl. Of the two patients undergoing dialysis preoperatively, dialysis was continued after surgery in one. Of the four patients who required intraoperative revision after renal endarterectomy, only one had significant postoperative serum creatinine elevation without requiring dialysis.

Two deaths (4.75%) occurred within 30 days of surgery. One patient had a fatal cardiac arrest on the first postoperative day after an uneventful operative procedure. The other patient died 1 day after operation of uncontrollable coagulopathy related to intraoperative bleeding after bilateral endarterectomy and repair of an abdominal aortic aneurysm.

At the end of the first 30 postoperative days, 4 (11.1%) of the surviving 36 patients with preoperative hypertension were cured of hypertension, 26 (72.2%) were improved, and six (16.7%) were unchanged according to previously defined criteria (Table 4). The mean number of postoperative antihypertensive medications among patients with preoperative hypertension was 1.3 per

Table 2 Operative procedures performed on 43 patients undergoing transaortic renal endarterectomy

	Patients	Arteries
Isolated transaortic endarterectomy	4	9
Bilateral	3	6
Bilateral plus accessory artery	1	3
Combined with aortic reconstruction	39	69
Bilateral endarterectomy	24	48
Bilateral plus accessory endarterectomy	2	6
Unilateral endarterectomy	9	9
Unilateral plus elective contralateral aortorenal bypass	2	4
Unilateral plus elective contralateral nephrectomy	2	2
TOTAL	43	78

Table 3 Morbidity and mortality rates within 30 days of transaortic renal endarterectomy

	No.	Percent
Major complications	6	14.0
Kidney failure requiring dialysis	2	4.7
Myocardial infarction	2	4.7
Sepsis	1	2.3
Pneumonia	1	2.3
Deaths	2	4.7

Table 4 Early response of hypertension and renal function among 41 survivors after renal revascularization*

Patients with preoperative hypertension	36
Cured	4 (11.1%)
Improved	26 (72.2%)
Unchanged	6 (16.7%)
Patients with preoperative renal insufficiency	26
Creatinine decreased ≥1 mg/dl	5 (19.2%)
Creatinine stable	15 (57.8%)
Creatinine increased ≥1 mg/d	6 (23.1%)

* At time of discharge or 30 days after operation.

patient. Among the 26 surviving patients with preoperative serum creatinine levels of 1.5 mg/dl or greater, five (19.2%) had a reduction in serum creatinine of 1 mg/dl or greater postoperatively.

Eleven patients (26.8% of survivors) underwent postoperative evaluation of 17 renal arteries for increasing antihypertensive requirement or continued elevation of serum creatinine. Renal scintigraphy was performed in six patients (10 arteries), arteriography in four patients (six arteries), and duplex ultrasonography in one patient. All but two arteries studied were widely patent. An occlusion was found at 21 months in a small accessory artery that had been chronically occluded before operation, and a stenosis was found at 8 months by arteriography and corrected with percutaneous angioplasty.

DISCUSSION

Several recent reports have noted the changing patterns of clinical presentation and treatment of renal artery disease.[14-17] With an aging population, an increasing number of patients present with a combination of peripheral vascular disease and renal artery disease. A recent study[1] showed renal artery stenosis of greater than 50% on arteriography in 33% of patients with aortoiliac occlusive disease and 39% of patients with infrainguinal arteriosclerotic disease. Renal artery disease has been found on angiography in 10% to 38% of patients with abdominal aortic aneurysms.[1,18] Despite the high incidence of arteriosclerotic renal artery disease, it has been difficult to be certain about the link between hypertension and renal dysfunction found in these patients and their renal artery disease because atheroembolism, nephrosclerosis, and diabetic nephropathy are also often present.

Nevertheless, information on the natural history of atherosclerotic renal artery disease gives strong support to the idea that this disease is an important cause not only of hypertension but also of progressive kidney failure.[2-5] Retrospective studies have shown progression of atherosclerotic renal artery disease in 44% of arteries with a 15% occlusion rate over a 3- to 72-month interval in one study[2] and 53% of arteries, progressing over 15 months to 23 years of follow-up with a 9% occlusion rate in another study.[6] In both studies, occlusion appeared to be predicted by stenosis greater than 75%. A more recent prospective duplex ultrasonography study has confirmed a progression rate of renal artery atherosclerotic disease of 20% per year with eventual occlusion.[7] In these studies there appears to be no clear association between progression of hypertension and kidney failure.[2,5]

The present study reviews experience with a consecutive series of patients who underwent treatment for atherosclerotic renal artery disease which, in all but four instances, was associated with aorto-iliac disease requiring reconstruction. Renal revascularization was performed therapeutically in 41 of 43 patients with the goal of improving control of hypertension or renal dysfunction. Two patients underwent prophylactic renal endarterectomy in the hope of altering the natural history of disease progression. If indications for aortic surgery had not existed many of these patients would not have been investigated following traditional guidelines. Current understanding of the natural history and pathophysiology supports more liberal criteria for evaluation and intervention for atherosclerotic renal artery disease.

A number of reports verify the safety and efficacy of renal revascularization.[11,14,16,19,20] Because of the high prevalence of combined aortic and renal artery disease, more surgeons are performing renal artery surgery as an adjunct to aortic repair.[13,21-24] Some authors have found increased mortality rates of 8.3% to 24% when combined aortic and renal artery surgery was performed, compared with low rates when either procedure was performed alone.[8-11] More recent series have demonstrated lower mortality rates of 1% to 5.6%.[13,21-24] The risk associated with combined surgery is not likely to be related simply to surgical factors, although the choice of the revascularization technique undoubtedly plays a role in some instances. Most reports of combined aortic and renal reconstruction have used aortorenal bypass as the principal technique. Renal endarterectomy, although first used in 1952,[12] has been preferred less often because of the general success of bypass operations and a relative lack of familiarity with endarterectomy. Because atherosclerotic renal artery disease is so often caused by aortic plaque extending into the renal arteries, endarterectomy should lend itself especially well to safe expeditious renal revascularization, particularly in patients who have bilateral renal artery disease and who require concomitant aortic surgery.

Patient selection and operative technique are critical to optimal outcome. In general, patients with disease that extends beyond the proximal third of the renal artery by arteriography or palpation are probably best treated with bypass rather than endarterectomy. Total renal occlusion is not a contraindication to endarterectomy provided the main renal artery reconstitutes just distal to the proximal plaque and is of reasonable quality and size. Mobilization of the renal artery for at least 1 cm beyond the palpable plaque is essential to the proper circumferential eversion technique critical to securing a good end point. In some instances, circumferential aortic endarterectomy is not necessary and only those portions of aortic plaque contiguous with the renal orifice need be removed. Aortorenal endarterectomy should be avoided in the presence of focally aneurysmal or thin aorta at the renal orifice or when extensive calcification obliterates the normal endarterectomy plane leaving nothing but excessively attenuated intima after the plaque is removed.

In this series the reliability of producing a satisfactory renal artery end point was 96%, as judged by direct visualization, palpation, and ultrasonography. With more sensitive duplex ultrasonography after endarterectomy in a comparable series by Stoney et al.[13] defects were found in 49.3% of 75 arteries. However, only nine of the arteries were involved to a moderate or "large" degree and only three (4%) required operative revision. Early postoperative arteriography in 25 of their 44 patients revealed four or more defects, including a single occlusion that resulted from an unsuccessful attempt to open a chronically occluded artery. With color-assisted duplex ultrasonography, Dougherty et al.[25] found lesions requiring revision in six (10.7%) of 56 renal arteries treated by transaortic endarterectomy and one (12.5%) of eight aortorenal bypass grafts. It appears that transaortic endarterectomy by the methods used in these series is acceptably reliable when applied to patients with proximal atherosclerotic renal artery disease.

Deep endarterectomy around the renal orifices in patients with highly calcific atherosclerotic aortic disease may cause severe thinning of the residual adventitia. One of our patients died in large part because of intraoperative hemorrhage from a weakened aortic wall after aortic and renal endarterectomy for heavily calcified aortorenal plaque. Stoney et al.[13] found it necessary to revise the aortic anastomosis for similar reasons in one of their 44 patients. In retrospect, the hemorrhage in the present series would most likely have been avoided by recognition of the hazards of circumferential calcific aortic plaque including and extending above the renal arteries. Use of bypass instead might have reduced the 30-day operative mortality rate to 2.3%, which is nearly identical to that for elective infrarenal aneurysm surgery at our institution.[26] The 30-day mortality rate was 2.3% in the comparable series of Stoney et al.[13] and 1% in a recent series reported by McNeil et al.,[24] thus indicating that combined aortic and renal artery surgery can be performed in selected patients without incurring substantial added risk.

The early beneficial effect of renal revascularization on hypertension and renal function was comparable to other series recently reported.[5,14,16,17,19] Blood pressure control was improved in 83% of patients, preoperative dialysis was discontinued in one of two patients, and the serum creatinine level was reduced by 1 mg/dl or greater in 19.2% of patients with preoperative renal insufficiency. Transient postoperative deterioration in renal function occurred in 14.6% of our patients, with improvement in all but one patient, who has required long-term dialysis. Documentation of late renal artery patency after endarterectomy was clearly incomplete in this series and is not yet available in the literature. Further investigations will undoubtedly make use of modern duplex ultrasonography for this important purpose.[27]

REFERENCES

1. Olin JW, Meliai M, Young JR, et al. Prevalence of atherosclerotic renal artery stenosis in patients with atherosclerosis elsewhere. Am J Med 88:46N-51N, 1990.
2. Schreiber MJ, Pohl MA, Novick AC. The natural history of atherosclerotic and fibrous renal artery disease. Urol Clin North Am 11:383-392, 1984.
3. Jacobson HR. Ischemic renal disease: An overlooked clinical entity. Kidney Int 34:729-743, 1988.
4. Mailloux LU, Bellucci AG, Mossey RT, et al. Predictors of survival in patients undergoing dialysis. Am J Med 84:855-862, 1988.
5. Dean RF, Tribble RW, Hansen KH, et al. Evolution of renal insufficiency in ischemic nephropathy. Ann Surg 213:446-456, 1991.
6. Tollefson DFJ, Ernst CB. Natural history of atherosclerotic renal artery stenosis associated with aortic disease. J Vasc Surg 14:327-331, 1991.
7. Zierler RE, Bergelin RO, Isaacson JA, et al. Natural history of atherosclerotic renal artery stenosis: A prospective study with duplex ultrasonography. J Vasc Surg 19:250-258, 1994.
8. Shahian DM, Najafi H, Javid H, et al. Simultaneous aortic and renal artery reconstruction. Arch Surg 115:1491-1497, 1980.
9. Diehl JT, Cali RF, Hertzer NR, et al. Complications of abdominal aortic reconstruction. An analysis of perioperative risk factors in 557 patients. Ann Surg 197:49-56, 1983.
10. Dean RH, Keyser JE, DuPont WD, et al. Aortic and renal vascular disease: Factors affecting the value of combined procedures. Ann Surg 200:336-344, 1984.
11. Cambria RP, Brewster DC, L'Italien GJ, et al. The durability of different reconstructive techniques for

atherosclerotic renal artery disease. J Vasc Surg 20:76-87, 1994.
12. Wylie EJ, Perloff DL, Stoney RJ. Autogenous tissue revascularization techniques in surgery for renovascular hypertension. Ann Surg 170:416-428, 1969.
13. Stoney RJ, Messina LM, Goldstone J, et al. Renal endarterectomy through the transsected aorta: A new technique for combined aortorenal atherosclerosis—a preliminary report. J Vasc Surg 9:224-233, 1989.
14. Novick AC, Ziegelbaum M, Vidt DG, et al. Trends in surgical revascularization for renal artery disease— ten years' experience. JAMA 257:498-501, 1987.
15. Libertino JA, Flam TA, Zinman LN, et al. Changing concepts in surgical management of renovascular hypertension. Arch Intern Med 148:357-359, 1988.
16. Bredenberg CE, Sampson LN, Ray FS, et al. Changing patterns in surgery for chronic renal artery occlusive diseases. J Vasc Surg 15:1018-1023, 1992.
17. Stanley JC. The evolution of surgery for renovascular occlusive disease. Cardiovasc Surg 2:195-202, 1994.
18. Couch NP, O'Mahoney J, McIrvine A, et al. The place of abdominal aortography in abdominal aortic aneurysm resection. Arch Surg 118:1029-1034, 1983.
19. Dean RH, Kureger TC, Whiteneck JM, et al. Operative management of renovascular hypertension: Results after a follow-up of fifteen to twenty-three years. J Vasc Surg 1:234-242, 1984.
20. Hallett JW, Fowl R, O'Brien PC, et al. Renovascular operations in patients with chronic renal insufficiency: Do the benefits justify the risks? J Vasc Surg 5:622-627, 1987.
21. O'Mara CS, Maples MD, Kilfore TL, et al. Simultaneous aortic reconstruction and bilateral renal revascularization: Is this a safe and effective procedure? J Vasc Surg 8:357-366, 1988.
22. Chaikof EL, Smith RB, Salam AA, et al. Ischemic nephropathy and concomitant aortic disease: A ten-year experience. J Vasc Surg 19:135-148, 1994.
23. Mason RA, Newton GB, Kvilekval K, et al. Transaortic endarterectomy of renal visceral artery lesions in association with infrarenal aortic surgery. J Vasc Surg 12:697-704, 1990.
24. McNeil JW, String ST, Pfeiffer RB. Concomitant renal endarterectomy and aortic reconstruction. J Vasc Surg 20:331-337, 1994.
25. Dougherty MJ, Hallett JW, Naessens JM, et al. Optimizing technical success of renal revascularization: The impact of intraoperative color-flow duplex ultrasonography. J Vasc Surg, 17:849-857, 1993.
26. Golden MA, Whittemore AD, Donaldson MC, et al. Selective evaluation and management of coronary artery disease in patients undergoing repair of abdominal aortic aneurysms: A 16-year experience. Ann Surg 212:415-423, 1990.
27. Hudspeth DA, Hansen KJ, Reavis SW, et al. Renal duplex sonography after treatment of renovascular disease. J Vasc Surg 18:381-390, 1993.

29

Management of Aortoenteric Fistula

STEVEN M. SANTILLI, M.D., Ph.D., and JERRY GOLDSTONE, M.D.

Development of a fistula between the aorta or its prosthetic replacement and the gastrointestinal tract is a rare late complication of aortic reconstructive surgery. It is among the most devastating and difficult problems to confront a vascular surgeon. The reported incidence is low, varying between 0.36% and 1.6%,[1-3] so most surgeons will treat very few of these lesions. Unfortunately, they are usually encountered under urgent or emergency conditions, which makes transfer of the patients to a tertiary care center hazardous.

An aortoenteric fistula (AEF) is classified as either primary or secondary. *Primary* AEFs are extremely rare and usually caused by the erosion of an abdominal aortic aneurysm into a segment of adjacent inherent intestine, usually the duodenum. Most of these patients present with exsanguinating upper gastrointestinal hemorrhage and require emergent surgical treatment. Repair of the intestinal fistula and in-line prosthetic replacement of the aortic aneurysm is appropriate treatment in this setting.

Secondary AEFs are caused by the erosion of a vascular prosthesis or suture line into a loop of bowel. This results from either infection and/or mechanical erosion of the graft into the bowel, with infection being a factor in most cases. An *anastomotic* AEF is one that occurs when a fistula forms between an aortic suture line (usually an anastomotic false aneurysm) and the previously mobilized, scarred, and fixed duodenum. This most frequently involves the third and fourth portions of the duodenum, but occasionally the cecum or sigmoid colon are the sites of fistula formation. AEFs can also be *periprosthetic,* a form that occurs when a prosthetic graft lies in direct contact with, and erodes into, a loop of bowel at a distance away from a suture line. Anastomotic and periprosthetic AEFs occur with almost equal frequency.[2,4,5]

The treatment of the secondary AEF has been associated with very high morbidity and mortality rates. Reports of mortality rates between 25% and 90% and major amputation rates of 5% to 25% continue to appear in the literature.[6-10] We believe that these rates can be substantially reduced.

We consider secondary AEF to be primarily a manifestation of an infected prosthetic aortic graft. Long intervals, ranging from 3 to more than 6 years, typically elapse between the initial aortic grafting operation and the treatment for the AEF.[2,4,5] The indications for the initial aortic procedure are evenly divided between aneurysmal and occlusive disease.[2] In our most recent series of secondary AEFs, the original aortic operations were aortofemoral in 52% of cases, aortoiliac in 39%, and aortic tubes in 9%.[2] Approximately two thirds of patients with AEF will present with some evidence of gastrointestinal bleeding. Gastrointestinal hemorrhage will be the only clinical manifestation of the AEF in less than one third of patients. Most of the time the bleeding is acute, and in almost one third of the patients in our series the bleeding episodes were recurrent. Most patients stopped bleeding and were hemodynamically stable, making emergency operations necessary in only four of 33 patients. It is important to emphasize that there was no evidence of bleeding in approximately one third of our patients.[2]

Thus the gastrointestinal tract and a prosthetic aortic graft can interact in three ways: (1) fistula formation with bleeding, (2) fistula formation without bleeding, and (3) bleeding without fistula formation. Clinical evidence of infection is common in patients with secondary AEF; approximately two thirds have elevated temperatures and 60% demonstrate leukocytosis.[2] In patients with probable or proven aortic graft infections, the presence of signs and symptoms of frank sepsis strongly suggests the presence of an associated AEF.

DIAGNOSTIC STUDIES

Upper gastrointestinal endoscopy is the only definitive method for establishing the presence of an AEF. This requires visualization of the graft material through the intestinal wall, an uncommon finding (occurring only twice in our series), but other abnormalities will be seen in approximately half the patients.[2] To be complete, the endoscopy must include the third and fourth portions of the duodenum. CT and/or magnetic resonance scans are almost always abnormal in the presence of an AEF but are diagnostic in very few patients. Aortography, extremely helpful in the planning of arterial reconstruction of the lower extremities, is rarely diagnostic of an AEF, although the presence of a proximal anastomotic false aneurysm may be helpful. Overall, the diagnosis of AEF is definitively made in only one third of patients prior to surgical treatment.[2]

SURGICAL TREATMENT

Surgical treatment should be performed as soon as possible after the diagnosis of AEF is either likely or proven. There are two aspects to the treatment: infected graft removal and revascularization of the lower extremities. Most authors believe that the latter can best be accomplished with extracavitary reconstructions, usually involving axillary artery to femoral artery bypass. Our experience suggests that results are best when the treatment is performed in stages, with the lower extremity revascularization performed first and the infected graft removal second.[2] The interval between stages should be kept short, from 3 to 4 days. There are several advantages to the performance of the extracavitary revascularization before transabdominal removal of the infected graft. Lower body ischemia is avoided along with all of its adverse metabolic consequences. This allows for retrograde perfusion of the pelvic arteries with a subsequent lowering of the risk of bowel ischemia. In addition, when the groins are involved in the infected graft process, neither the extracavitary reconstruction nor the infected graft removal can be considered the "easy" part of the treatment. The restoration of blood flow to the lower extremities can be extremely difficult and tedious, requiring unilateral axillary femoral bypass with a prosthetic graft attached to the midprofunda or superficial femoral arteries out of the infected field combined with an autogenous femorofemoral bypass to perfuse the contralateral lower extremity. Patients with secondary AEF seem to do better with two shorter operations than with one very long, extensive procedure. Finally, by placing the extracavitary bypass first, the need for heparinization is eliminated during the infected graft removal portion of the treatment, which results in a reduced need for blood and blood product replacement.

Obviously not all patients are candidates for this type of staged treatment. In patients with active gastrointestinal bleeding that cannot be stopped and is associated with hemodynamic instability, the bleeding must first be controlled. In these situations repair of the fistula, infected graft removal, and the extracavitary reconstruction will be necessary in that order during one long operation. Patients who have had active bleeding with associated hemodynamic instability but in whom the bleeding has stopped should undergo extra-anatomic bypass followed immediately by infected graft removal and repair of the AEF. Patients who have had active bleeding without any hemodynamic instability and patients who have had only occult bleeding are candidates for extracavitary bypass followed by infected graft removal in a staged fashion. Staging intervals should be minimal when there is an associated aortic anastomotic aneurysm. In general, the interval should be as short as the patient's clinical condition will allow.

We prefer to use an externally supported polytetrafluoroethylene graft for the extracavitary arterial reconstruction. When neither groin is involved in the infectious process, a prosthetic femorofemoral bypass is also preferred. Occasionally a direct ilioiliac anastomosis can be performed to accomplish this purpose. When there is contamination of one or both groins, an autogenous conduit is necessary for the crossfemoral reconstruction. Greater saphenous vein, endarterectomized superficial femoral artery (if it was occluded), or superficial femoral veins have been used for this purpose. We have found that autogenous cross-femoral grafts are more likely to fail when the caliber of the conduit is suboptimal.[2,5] For this reason, we now consider cross-femoral grafts with the saphenous vein and the endarterectomized superficial femoral artery to be temporary bridge grafts until it is safe to replace them with a prosthetic conduit.

There are several other important technical aspects to the treatment of secondary AEF. In slightly less than half the patients, either supraceliac or suprarenal aortic cross-clamping will be required.[2,5] This is preferable to performing an inadequate debridement of the infrarenal aortic wall because of the presence of an infrarenal clamp. Aggressive excision and debridement of the retroperitoneum and the aorta are critical components of the treatment. The aortic stump at the site of closure must be healthy. Stump closure should be performed with a double layer of monofilament sutures. Stump reinforcement with omental pedicles or anterior spinous ligaments may be helpful but is no substitute for adequate debridement and a secure tension-free closure. Rarely, one or both renal arteries will need to be revascularized from an alternative source in order to ensure adequate aortic debridement.

The intestinal closure should also be carefully debrided and repaired. Most of the intestinal defects can be closed primarily, but occasionally segmental resection with end-to-end anastomosis is required.

All of the prosthetic graft material must be removed. With adequate surgical debridement retroperitoneal drains are rarely necessary. We have limited their use to situations in which there is a large cavity that cannot be obliterated. Care must be taken in placing the drains away from the aortic and intestinal suture lines.

DISCUSSION

We have recently reported our experience using these principles in the treatment of 33 patients with secondary AEF.[2] Two patients died between the first and second stages of their treatment, one from rupture of a proximal aortic pseudoaneurysm 2 days after extracavitary bypass. The perioperative mortality rate was 18.2%, with amputation and aortic stump disruption rates of 6.1% each. After an average follow-up of 4.4 years, the cumulative "cure" rate for the treatment of these AEFs was 74.5% at 1 year, 70% at 3 years, and has remained constant at this level thereafter. These results represent a 21% reduction in the mortality rate, a 27% reduction in limb loss, and a 19% reduction in the rate of aortic stump disruption compared with our earlier results using different treatment protocols.

There are several factors that have contributed to these improved results. Certainly there have been improvements in preoperative preparation, intraoperative anesthetic management, and postoperative care over the past 15 to 20 years. There is also an increased awareness of the importance of thorough retroperitoneal and aortic debridement. Finally, performing the extracavitary revascularization before the transabdominal infected graft removal has played a major role for the reasons discussed previously.

Other investigators have proposed different treatment modalities in an effort to reduce the morbidity and mortality of a secondary AEF. Among these are in-line aortic replacement with either homografts or antibiotic-impregnated prosthetic grafts. Clagett et al.[11] have recently introduced the use of the superficial femoral vein for in-line reconstruction in the treatment of infected aortic prosthetic grafts, but they report less than favorable results when this method has been applied to the treatment of patients with AEF.

In summary, the optimal treatment for the vast majority of patients with secondary AEF is a reversed, staged procedure consisting of lower extremity revascularization followed after a short interval by infected graft removal and fistula repair.

REFERENCES

1. Bunt TJ. Synthetic vascular graft infections: Secondary graft enteric erosions and graft enteric fistulas. Surgery 94:1-9, 1983.
2. Kuestner LM, Reilly LM, Jicha DL, Ehrenfeld WK, Goldstone J, Stoney RJ. Secondary aortoenteric fistula: Contemporary outcome with use of extraanatomic bypass and infected graft excision. J Vasc Surg 21:184-196, 1995.
3. Reilly LM, Altman H, Lusby RJ, et al. Late results following surgical management of vascular graft infection. J Vasc Surg 1:36-44, 1984.
4. Goldstone J, Moore WS. Infection in vascular prostheses: Clinical manifestation and surgical management. Am J Surg 128:228-233, 1974.
5. Reilly LM, Goldstone J, Ehrenfeld WK, Stoney RJ. Gastrointestinal tract involvement by prosthetic graft infection: The significance of gastrointestinal hemorrhage. Ann Surg 202:342-348, 1985.
6. O'Hara PJ, Hertzer NR, Beven EG, Krajewski LP. Surgical management of infected abdominal aortic grafts: Review of a 25-year experience. J Vasc Surg 3:725-731, 1986.
7. Plate G, Hollier LA, O'Brien P, Pairolero PC, Cherry KJ, Kazmier FJ. Recurrent aneurysms and late vascular complications following repair of abdominal aortic aneurysms. Arch Surg 120:590-594, 1985.
8. Bergeron P, Espinoza H, Rudondy P, et al. Secondary aortoenteric fistulas: Value of initial axillofemoral bypass. Ann Vasc Surg 5:4-7, 1991.

9. Champion MC, Sullivan SN, Coles JC, Goldbach M, Warson WC. Aortoenteric fistula: Incidence, presentation, recognition and management. Ann Surg 195:314-317, 1982.
10. Trout HH III, Kosloff L, Giordano JM. Priority of revascularization in patients with graft enteric fistulas, infected arteries, or infected arterial prostheses. Ann Surg 199:669-683, 1982.
11. Clagett GP, Bowers BL, Lopez-Viego MA, Rossi MB, Valentine RJ, Myers SI, Chervu A. Creation of a neo-aortoiliac system from lower extremity deep and superficial veins. Ann Surg 218:239-249, 1993.

30

The Importance of Age, Sex, and Aortic Size on the Outcome of Aortobifemoral Bypass

R. JAMES VALENTINE, M.D., and G. PATRICK CLAGETT, M.D.

The onset of lower extremity atherosclerosis at an early age has been associated with rapid progression and a high incidence of graft occlusion, amputation, and death.[1-4] Patients with premature atherosclerosis do not enjoy the favorable long-term patency rates usually associated with aortobifemoral bypass (AFB). A high rate of graft failure among young patients has been reported by several authors, with reoperations required in 25% to 34% within 3 to 4 years of the original operation.[2,3,5,6]

Aortic size may also influence patency, and young women with small aortas appear to have a particularly unfavorable prognosis after aortoiliac reconstruction.[1,6] The "hypoplastic aorta syndrome" is more common in women, who tend to present at a younger age with less severe symptoms than do patients with normal aortas.[7-9] The syndrome has also been reported in men, who also tend to have symptoms much earlier than their counterparts with normal-sized aortas. Although aortoiliac reconstruction is technically challenging in patients with hypoplastic aortas, reported cumulative patency rates in some series that include all ages and both sexes are not significantly lower than those in patients with normal-sized aortas. The correlation between small aortic size and young age in both sexes and its influence on outcome have not previously been examined. We hypothesized that this combination of variables has a particularly detrimental effect on patency.[10] To examine this problem we studied the clinical course of patients under the age of 50 years, who were surgically treated for aortoiliac occlusive disease.

We studied 73 patients, aged 49 years and younger, who underwent AFB or aortoiliac thromboendarterectomy (aTEA) for atherosclerotic occlusive disease at our institutions during the past 15 years. There were 36 men (49%) and 37 women (51%) whose respective mean ages at the time of the first operation were 44.0 ± 0.8 years and 43.5 ± 0.7 years.

All patients underwent direct aortoiliac reconstruction as their first procedure. Sixty-five patients (89%) underwent AFB with Dacron grafts, and eight (11%) underwent aTEA with Dacron patch angioplasties. Patency in all cases was documented at discharge by the presence of palpable femoral pulses. The mean follow-up period of the 73 patients was 60 ± 5 months.

Poor results were all too apparent in these young patients. During follow-up, 37 patients (51%) (20 women and 17 men) had at least one documented occlusion of the original vascular repair. Thirty-three patients had thrombosis of a graft limb after AFB, and four patients had iliac artery occlusion after aTEA. Occlusions occurred during a mean time of 27 ± 6 months after the original procedure in the men and 33 ± 10 months in the women. Primary patency rates did not differ between men and women (Fig. 1). The most frequent cause of limb occlusion was distal anastomotic neointimal hyperplasia.

Recurrent distal intimal hyperplasia was a vexing problem leading to reocclusion in the 37 patients with failed reconstructions regardless of sex. Two limb occlusions or iliac artery thromboses ultimately occurred in four women and four men, and three or more failures ultimately occurred in 10 women and 12 men.

The vicious cycle of intimal hyperplasia → limb occlusion → reoperation ultimately led to a major amputation in one fourth of these young patients. Seven women (19%) underwent amputations including one unilateral and two bilateral above-knee amputations and two unilateral and two bilateral hip disarticulations. Ten men (28%) underwent amputations including two unilateral below-knee, four unilateral above-knee, and four bilateral above-knee amputations. Three of the 37 women and 7 of the 36 men died during follow-up. This was a most disappointing outcome in a group of patients whose most common presenting complaint was intermittent claudication.

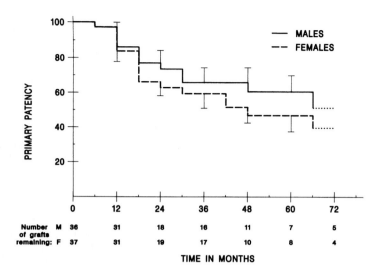

Fig. 1 Cumulative patency rates of men and women following aortoiliac reconstruction; differences are not significant. (From Valentine RJ, Hansen ME, Myers SI, Chervu A, Clagett GP. The influence of sex and aortic size on late patency after aortofemoral revascularization in young adults. J Vasc Surg 21:296-306, 1995.)

Table 1 Comparison of clinical variables between patients with patent vascular repairs and those with occlusions

Variable	Patent (n = 36)	Occluded (n = 37)
Mean age	41.5 ± 1.2	43 ± 1.1
Number of males	19 (53%)	17 (46%)
Smoking	33 (92%)	34 (92%)
Hypertension	15 (42%)	19 (51%)
Hyperlipidemia	12 (33%)	8 (22%)
Diabetes	5 (14%)	9 (24%)
Operative indication		
Claudication	22 (61%)	20 (54%)
Threatened limb	14 (39%)	17 (46%)

Differences between groups were not significant.

To more closely examine this problem, we studied variables associated with loss of patency. When patients with occluded vs. patent grafts were compared, no differences were found in age, sex, symptoms, type or number of atherosclerotic risk factors, operative indications, or operative details (Table 1).

Preoperative arteriograms were reviewed to determine aortic size and to evaluate the patency of runoff vessels. Arterial outflow in the femoral, popliteal, and infragenicular arteries was determined according to standards set by the Society for Vascular Surgery and the International Society for Cardiovascular Surgery.[11] Preoperative arteriograms were available for review in 27 men (75%) and 22 women (59%). Mean runoff scores did not differ between men and women, but mean aortic diameters were smaller among women than among men ($p < .001$). Mean runoff scores did not differ in men or women with occlusions compared to those with patent repairs. However, both men and women who had occlusions had significantly ($p = .002$) smaller aortas than patients who maintained patency.

The small size of the aortas among patients whose treatment failed was particularly striking when compared to age-matched control subjects undergoing angiography for nonatherosclerotic disease (Fig. 2).[9] Among men and women with aortas greater than 1.8 cm in diameter, the 5-year cumulative patency rate was 75%. In comparison, among those with aortic diameters less than 1.8 cm, the 5-year patency rate was 30% ($p = .003$). In subjecting these data to proportional hazards regression analysis, it was found that the relative risk of limb occlusion increased 1.2 times for each 1 mm decrease in aortic diameter. This model predicts a limb occlusion rate higher than 90% for men with an aortic diameter of less than 16 mm and for women with a diameter of less than 13 mm (Fig. 3).

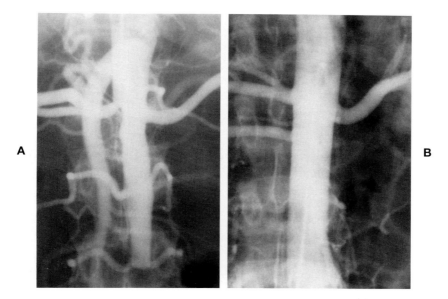

Fig. 2 A, Young male patient with distal aortic occlusion who underwent aortobifemoral bypass and suffered multiple limb occlusions. **B,** Age-matched control subject undergoing aortography for nonatherosclerotic disease.

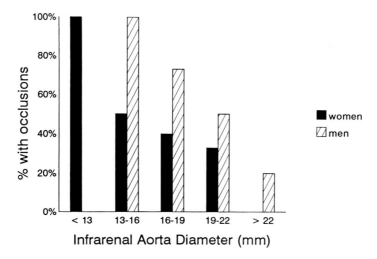

Fig. 3 Prevalence of occlusions among men and women according to aortic size. (From Valentine RJ, Hansen ME, Myers SI, Chervu A, Clagett GP. The influence of sex and aortic size on late patency after aortofemoral revascularization in young adults. J Vasc Surg 21:296-306, 1995.)

CONCLUSION

We conclude that the results of intervention are poor in both young men and young women, particularly those with small aortas. In the absence of limb-threatening ischemia, these patients are best managed conservatively with exercise therapy and risk-factor reduction. Percutaneous balloon angioplasty also appears to be of limited value in these patients and should probably be avoided.[12]

Young adults who undergo aortoiliac reconstruction for limb salvage should be followed closely for graft complications. Young men and young women are equally affected. The present data suggest that graft occlusions will occur within 3 years in most young women with aortic diameters of less than 14 mm and most young men with aortic diameters of less than 18 mm. No proven methods have been found for reducing the risk of occlusion in these young patients. Progression of premature atherosclerosis may be slowed by strict control of atherosclerotic risk factors, especially smoking. Timely intervention to correct graft stenoses can prevent the need for graft replacement, and ultimately amputation can be avoided. Other technical considerations may be important. It has been suggested that aortic thromboendarterectomy is superior to AFB in young patients with small aortas.[13] Bifurcated polytetrafluoroethylene prostheses and routine profundaplasty have been reported to improve patency rates in patients with small aortas.[14] In young patients with small aortas and extremely limited runoff (associated severe superficial femoropopliteal occlusive disease) who have a particularly dismal prognosis, we have a preliminary experience in replacing the aortoiliac system with superficial femoropopliteal vein grafts.[15] Early results are encouraging.

REFERENCES

1. McReady RA, Vincent AE, Schwartz RW, Hyde GL, Mattingly SS, Griffin WO. Atherosclerosis in the young: A virulent disease. Surgery 96:863-868, 1984.
2. Olsen PS, Gustafsen J, Rasmussen L, Lorentzen JE. Long-term results after arterial surgery for arteriosclerosis of the lower limbs in young adults. Eur J Vasc Surg 2:15-18, 1988.
3. Valentine RJ, MacGillivray DC, DeNobile JW, Synder DA, Rich NM. Intermittent claudication caused by atherosclerosis in patients aged forty years and younger. Surgery 107:560-565, 1990.
4. Levy PJ, Hornung CA, Haynes JL, et al. Lower extremity ischemia in adults younger than forty years of age: A community-wide survey of premature atherosclerotic arterial disease. J Vasc Surg 19:873-881, 1994.
5. Najafi H, Ostermiller WE, Ardekani RG, et al. Aortoiliac reconstruction in patients aged 32 to 45 years of age. Arch Surg 101:780-784, 1970.
6. Evans WE, Hayes JP, Vermilion BD. Atherosclerosis in the young patient: Results of surgical management. Am J Surg 154:225-229, 1987.
7. Cronenwett JL, Davis JT, Gooch JB, Garrett HE. Aortoiliac occlusive disease in women. Surgery 88:775-784, 1980.
8. DeLaurentis DA, Friedmann P, Wolferth CC, Wilson A, Naide D. Atherosclerosis and the hypoplastic aortoiliac system. Surgery 83:27-37, 1978.
9. Caes F, Cham B, Van den Brande P, Welch W. Small artery syndrome in women. Surg Gynecol Obstet 161:165-170, 1985.
10. Valentine RJ, Hansen ME, Myers SI, Chervu A, Clagett GP. The influence of sex and aortic size on late patency after aortofemoral revascularization in young adults. J Vasc Surg 21:296-306, 1995.
11. Ad Hoc Committee on Reporting Standards. Suggested standards for reports dealing with lower extremity ischemia. J Vasc Surg 4:80-94, 1986.
12. Levy PJ, Close T, Hornung CA, Haynes JL, Rush DS. Percutaneous transluminal angioplasty in adults less than 45 years of age with premature lower extremity atherosclerosis. Ann Vasc Surg 9:471-479, 1995.
13. van den Akker PJ, van Schilfgaarde R, Brand R, van Bockel JH, Terpstra JL. Long-term results of prosthetic and nonprosthetic reconstruction for obstructive aortoiliac disease. Eur J Vasc Surg 6:53-61, 1992.
14. Burke PM, Herrmann JB, Cutler BS. Optimal grafting methods for the small abdominal aorta. J Cardiovasc Surg (Torino) 28:420-426, 1987.
15. Clagett GP, Bowers BL, Lopez-Viego MA, Rossi MB, Valentine RJ, Myers SI, Chervu A. Creation of a neo-aortoiliac system from lower extremity deep and superficial veins. Ann Surg 218:239-249, 1993.

31

Axillobifemoral Bypass: Current Indications, Techniques, and Results

ROBERT B. RUTHERFORD, M.D.

HISTORICAL PERSPECTIVE

As with any operation, indications influence results and results influence indications. In other words, the patients selected for an operation influence its results, and those results ultimately modify the indications for operation. Nowhere is this continuing interplay between indications and results more evident than with axillobifemoral (AxBF) bypass, but here it would appear that the indications have affected the results more than the results have influenced the indications.

The three decades since its introduction have witnessed changing enthusiasm over the AxBF bypass. The operation was introduced in the early 1960s as an expedient method for dealing with infected grafts or bypassing aortoiliac occlusive disease (AIOD) in prohibitive risk patients, but by the late 1970s progressively liberal application had culminated in the opinion that extra-anatomic bypasses should be used as a matter of "preference rather than compromise."[1] In one series AxBF bypass was offered to "anyone over 65, regardless of risk"[2]; in another series almost 60% of patients receiving AxBF bypass were claudicators.[3] Close to 75% long-term patencies were claimed. At about the same time review of the experience at the San Francisco VA Hospital, from the time of the introduction of the AxBF bypass, reported an 8% mortality and a 33% patency rate.[4] Thus in four reports[2-5] appearing close to each other in the late 1970s, there was a fourfold range in mortality and a twofold range in patency. Ultimately it became apparent that much of this variability between reported results was attributable to differing reporting practices. Specifically, case exclusions could explain the difference in mortality, and primary vs. secondary patency rates accounted for the differences in patency. For example, in one article the reported 76% patency was achieved by reintervention in 43% of the cases,[5] and a difference in patency of 8% to 1.8% in two reports from the same institution[2,5] was the result of excluding urgent or emergent cases in one report. A number of reports followed in which it became apparent that when primary patency rates were considered, the results for AxBF were quite inferior to those for aortobifemoral (AoBF) bypass,[6-8] and vascular surgeons in the 1980s were urged to reserve AxBF bypass for two basic indications—*prohibitive* risk and "hostile" abdominal disease—and to use direct aortic reconstruction in the great majority of aortoiliac reconstructions for occlusive disease. However, in recent years reports of excellent *primary* patencies with AxBF bypass have emerged from two centers in the Northwest: the University of Oregon[9,10] and the Bob Hope Institute in Seattle.[11] The authors have attributed these improved patencies to the use of externally supported grafts (polytetrafluoroethylene and Dacron, respectively), and liberal application of the AxBF bypass is again being advocated. Porter[12] recently stated that "axillobifemoral bypass is about as good as aortobifemoral bypass and should be used more often."

Running parallel to these trends was the use of AxBF bypass in abdominal aortic aneurysms (AAAs). Berguer et al.[13] in Detroit and Karmody et al.[14] in Albany began to use the AxBF bypass, with thrombosis of the bypassed AAA induced by outflow (iliac artery) ligation. Objections to this application soon arose because of (1) the frequent need for enlisting interventional radiologists to occlude residual outflow vessels to finally produce aneurysm thrombosis, (2) the number of secondary procedures needed to maintain AxBF patency, and (3) reports of rupture in spite of successfully induced thrombosis.[15-18] The report of results and complications derived from a national survey by Kim et al.[19] effectively discredited this application of AxBF bypass, although recently Pevec and Blaisdell[20] have pointed out that the results are more acceptable when both inflow and outflow ligation is carried out. However, the exposure required for proximal ligation of an infrarenal aortic aneurysm is such that operative risk is not significantly decreased over a fuller retroperitoneal approach in which either a parallel bypass is performed after oversewing the neck of the aneurysm[21] or a retroperitoneal tube graft repair is feasible when dealing with an aortic aneurysm with no iliac involvement.

However, the third categoric indication for AxBF bypass has remained firm—namely, its use for dealing with infected grafts—and here the main question has to do with sequence of extra-anatomic bypass and graft removal, the current vogue favoring the removal of the infecting graft a few days after AxBF bypass whenever possible.[22] Thus, in looking over the history of the AxBF bypass in relation to its three categoric indications, there are solid indications for its use for infected grafts, rare application for bypass with exclusion of AAAs, and a rekindled debate over its application for AIOD. For this reason, the main focus of this chapter will be on its still controversial use for AIOD.

RESULTS OF AXILLOBIFEMORAL BYPASS

If one studies the reported results of AxBF bypass for AIOD, in trying to explain mortalities ranging from 1.8% to 18% and patencies ranging from 33% to 85%, it is apparent that in addition to the differing reporting practices alluded to previously, there are two other possible explanations: techniques that are changing and improving and differing case selection. In regard to the latter, the dichotomy produced by liberal vs. conservative application of AxBF bypass is impressive and within a given institution greatly affects the comparison of the results of AxBF with those of AoBF bypass. With *liberal application* of AxBF bypass, better risk cases, including claudicators with good runoff, are added to its ledgers, thereby decreasing its mortality rate and improving its patency to the point where they approach those of the AoBF bypass. By contrast, *conservative application*—that is, limiting AxBF bypass mainly to prohibitive risk patients, most of whom have poor runoff and are in a limb salvage situation—produces a much lower primary patency rate and a higher operative mortality and, by taking these patients out of the group on whom AoBF bypass is performed, improves the results of the latter operation and magnifies its apparent advantages. A good example of the impact of conservative application is seen in the Dartmouth experience reported by Schneider et al.[23] Compared with AoBF, those patients with AxBF bypass had approximately three times the history of previous myocardial infarction and five times the history of congestive heart failure; twice as many patients had chronic obstructive pulmonary disease, and only 6% were claudicators (compared with 47% for AoBF). Not surprisingly, the results with AxBF bypass were much worse than with AoBF, with a much higher mortality rate (9% vs. 1%), amputation rate (9% vs. 2%), and hemodynamic failure rate (14% vs. 7%). The subsequent graft limb thrombosis rate was 18% vs. 6%. The same effect has been experienced at the University of Colorado[6,24] where the AxBF bypass has also been applied conservatively, resulting in half the patency rate (47% vs. 86%), twice the hemodynamic failure rate (27% vs. 14%), five times the technical failure rate (10% vs. 2%), and twice the mortality (7% vs. 3%) of AoBF bypass. The striking impact that indication for operation has on results has been nicely demonstrated in a recent report by Schneider and Golan[25] in which 11 well-documented reports of AxBF bypass were ranked in order of patency and analyzed in terms of 15 variables, including operative mortality, survival, primary patency rate, age, and multiple risk factors. It is clear from their analysis that those series with the highest patencies have many fewer patients with limb-threatening ischemia and fewer associated risk factors and, in turn, enjoy lower operative mortality and better patency and long-term survival. As a rough approximation, liberal application produces primary 3-year patency rates of 80% ± 5% with a mortality risk of 3% ± 1%, whereas conservative application results in primary patencies of 55% ± 15% with a mortality of 9% ± 3%.

The group in Oregon[9] have made a case for the use of externally supported prostheses, and this may well have had a positive impact on their results. But it is also apparent from their reports[9,10] that other equally important differences have probably contributed to their observed improved results (compared with historical internal controls)—namely, (1) significantly different anastomotic techniques, (2) improving runoff by concomitant distal bypass, (3) including cases operated on for reasons other than arteriosclerotic occlusive disease (AAA or infected graft), and (4) liberalized indications for this operation. The latter is reflected by the fact that they averaged six cases a year from 1977 to 1982, 12 cases a year from 1983 to 1988,[9] and 16 cases a year from 1983 to 1993,[10] with a zenith of 31 AxBF bypasses in 1991.[12]

In this debate between liberal and conservative application of AxBF bypass, it should be apparent that neither approach has been proved right and that case selection has produced results that in turn are used to justify innate biases regarding the application of this operation. The author pleads guilty to this, having for many years staunchly defended limiting the indications for AxBF bypass to prohibitive risk and hostile abdominal disease and in doing so has produced results that appear to justify this stance.[6]

TECHNICAL CONSIDERATIONS

Technique undoubtedly plays a significant role in determining patency. What is debatable is the degree to which it influences patency (vis-à-vis case selection). There are two controversial aspects that deserve discussion: the best anastomotic configuration[5] and the value of externally supported prostheses. In regard to appropriate anastomotic configuration, a basic underlying consideration is whether AxBF bypass has a better patency than axillounifemoral (AxUF) bypass and, if so, whether this is caused by a higher flow in the axillofemoral stem when it supplies two limbs rather than one. This is important because if it is true, then the graft configuration should try to maximize this flow advantage. Half the articles in the literature have not been able to show a *statistically significant* difference between AxUF and AxBF bypasses, but even in these articles mean patency rates are consistently higher for the AxBF bypass, suggesting a type II error. In the other half of the articles, a statistical significance has been shown.[26] In the author's experience this applied to both primary and secondary patency rates and whether the procedure was performed in the face of good or poor runoff.[6] In the only actual correlation of graft flow with patency, LoGerfo et al.[5] showed that in AxBF bypass graft flow was roughly double that of the flow through an AxUF bypass and in this experience the patency was also twice as good. In view of such hemodynamic considerations, most vascular surgeons believe that the axillofemoral stem should be brought as close to the ipsilateral femoral artery as possible before giving off the crossover femorofemoral graft. This explains the current preference for the so-called h over the inverted y configuration (in which the crossover limb takes off in an antegrade direction higher up). Nevertheless, there are concerns that in the h configuration the double onlay or "piggy back" arrangement at this junction of two grafts produces turbulent retrograde flow that may negate its higher flow advantage. The University of Oregon group have suggested that better results will be achieved by placing these anastomoses in the reverse sequence—that is, instead of applying the femorofemoral graft on top of the axillofemoral graft, they construct the femorofemoral bypass first and then anastomose the axillofemoral stem to the proximal hood of the femorofemoral graft. A number of other solutions have been offered. Blaisdell et al.[27] have recommended anastomosing the femorofemoral graft to the distal end of the divided ipsilateral common femoral artery, thus moving that anastomosis away from the distal axillofemoral anastomosis. For a number of years the author preferred to first perform a crossover axillofemoral bypass to the *opposite* femoral artery and then add a short spur down to the ipsilateral femoral artery, primarily because it simplified the anastomoses. Recently this approach has been further modified along the lines suggested by Blaisdell and associates by anastomosing the distal end of the divided ipsilateral common femoral artery (or the external iliac artery if it is divided higher up) to the side of the single crossover axillofemoral graft. This involves only three instead of four anastomoses, preserves high flow in the axillofemoral graft down to the ipsilateral femoral artery anastomosis, and is configured so that all of the anastomoses are antegrade. All of the above modifications take advantage of the higher flow of the proximal axillofemoral stem and simplify or streamline the crossover graft configuration, thus optimizing patency.

As important as these improved graft configurations are, the current focus in technique is on the use of externally supported prostheses. It is difficult to determine whether the improved patency rates reported by Porter and his associates at the University of Oregon[12] are the result of the use of externally supported prostheses, as claimed, or anastomotic modifications, generic technologic improvements with time, or more liberal application (or a combination of these). Comparisons of externally supported prostheses in other locations have failed to show a patency advantage,[28] and hemodynamic studies of AxBF grafts have *not* shown compromised flow when compressed by the weight of the patient. In fact, the observation that many of these grafts occlude at night may relate more to decreased flow in the sleeping patient (due to reduced cardiac output, blood pressure, and reduced flow demand in the inactive state). Finally, one of the most recently reported experiences with axillofemoral bypass[29] found a *reverse* correlation between externally supported polytetrafluoroethylene prostheses and patency! Therefore in the absence of proof (in the form of randomized prospective comparison) that externally supported prostheses are indeed superior, one must consider the technical difficulties posed by the supporting rings, both in the primary operation and in performing a thrombectomy or "redo" procedure.

A final important technical consideration is the configuration of the axillary anastomosis. The Oregon group have recently called attention to the continuing problem of disruption of the upper anastomosis,[30] noting that the occurrence rate has been 5% in their experience (11 of 200), and that although only 23 cases have been reported in journal articles, there have been 67 cases documented nationwide from 1984 to 1993. The problem has been thought to relate to the angle of anastomosis to the axillary artery and how far out on the axillary artery the anastomosis is made, each potentially producing susceptibility to disruption when the arm is raised over the head. Graft manufacturers have made recommendations regarding the proper angle of this anastomosis (135 degrees), and most authors have realized the importance of placing the anastomosis as far medially as possible. However, Porter[12] recommends that the anastomosis simply be made as acutely angled as possible and the direction of the graft be continued parallel to the native artery for some distance before being gently curved back in a downward direction to follow the usual course of an axillofemoral bypass graft, along the thoracic wall in the midaxillary line. Since adopting this acutely angled anastomosis with generous slack, he has not seen this complication at the University of Oregon in the last 70+ cases.

INDICATIONS FOR AXILLOBIFEMORAL BYPASS IN PATIENTS WITH AORTOILIAC OCCLUSIVE DISEASE

In deciding whether to perform an AxBF or AoBF bypass, the surgeon is basically dealing with a trade-off between mortality and patency. Under the exact same circumstances the AxBF bypass will produce a lower mortality and the AoBF bypass will produce a better patency. It is clear that the AxBF bypass is appropriate in patients with AIOD who really need lower extremity revascularization (i.e., critical ischemia, not claudication) and who have either a prohibitive anesthetic risk or hostile abdominal disease that precludes direct transabdominal reconstruction (e.g., septic graft, abdominal sepsis, radiation, enterostomies, multiple previous operations with adhesions). However, in the author's view the liberalization of the AxBF bypass to include claudicators, or even limb salvage patients *without* significant risk or hostile abdominal disease, does not seem justified in this era of improved perioperative care and monitoring. Furthermore, other alternatives to AxBF bypass must be considered in such settings. For example, by using a small retroperitoneal incision to approach the left side of the aorta (not much larger than one would need for a left-sided sympathectomy), one can fashion an end-to-side or end-to-end anastomosis to the infrarenal aorta and by using a long-stemmed bifurcation graft can bring both limbs of the graft through an extraperitoneal tunnel that emerges in the left groin. Then the left limb of the graft can be anastomosed directly to the left femoral artery while the right limb of the graft is brought across, in a "lazy S" fashion suprapubically, to anastomose to the right femoral artery. In the author's experience this approach has been extremely well tolerated and achieves patency equivalent to the AoBF bypass. Alternatively, a thoracic aortofemoral bypass can be used in patients with good pulmonary function. Finally, although the application of percutaneous balloon angioplasty, with or without stents or adjunctive thrombolysis, has probably been overdone recently, if there ever was an indication for such an approach, it would be in prohibitive risk patients or those with hostile abdominal disease needing aortoiliac reconstruction.

REFERENCES

1. Parsonnet V, Alpert J, Brief DK. Femorofemoral and axillofemoral grafts: Compromise or preference. Surgery 67:26, 1970.
2. Johnson WC, LoGerfo FW, Vollman RW, et al. Is axillo-bilateral femoral graft an effective substitute for aortic-bilateral iliac/femoral graft? An analysis of ten years experience. Ann Surg 186:123-129, 1977.

3. Ray LI, O'Connor JB, Davis CC, et al. Axillofemoral bypass: A critical reappraisal of its role in the management of aortoiliac disease. Surgery 138:117-128, 1979.
4. Eugene J, Goldstone J, Moore WS. Fifteen year experience with subcutaneous bypass grafts for lower extremity ischemia. Ann Surg 186:177-183, 1977.
5. LoGerfo FW, Johnson WC, Corson JD, et al. A comparison of the late patency rates of axillobilateral femoral and axillounilateral femoral grafts. Surgery 81:33-40, 1977.
6. Rutherford RB, Patt A, Pearce WH. Extra-anatomic bypass: A closer view. J Vasc Surg 6:437-446, 1987.
7. Ascer E, Veith FJ, Gupta SK, et al. Comparison of axillounifemoral and axillobifemoral bypass operations. Surgery 97:167-174, 1985.
8. Donaldson MC, Louras JC, Bucknam CA. Axillofemoral bypass: A tool with a limited role. J Vasc Surg 3:757-763, 1986.
9. Harris EJ Jr, Taylor LM Jr, McConnell DB, et al. Clinical results of axillobifemoral bypass using externally supported polytetrafluoroethylene. J Vasc Surg 12:416-421, 1990.
10. Taylor LM Jr, Moneta GL, McConnell D, et al. Axillofemoral grafting with externally supported polytetrafluoroethylene. Arch Surg 129:588-595, 1994.
11. El-Massry S, Saad E, Sauvage LR, et al. Axillofemoral bypass with externally supported, knitted Dacron grafts: A follow-up through twelve years. J Vasc Surg 17:107-115, 1993.
12. Porter JM. When are extraanatomic bypasses preferable to aortofemoral bypass for aortoiliac occlusive disease? Presented at Vascular Diseases 1994: Diagnosis and Treatment. Monterrey, Calif., October 29, 1994.
13. Berguer R, Schneider J, Wilner HI. Induced thrombosis of inoperable abdominal aortic aneurysm. Surgery 84:425-429, 1978.
14. Karmody AM, Leather RP, Goldman M, et al. The current position of nonresective treatment for abdominal aortic aneurysm. Surgery 94:591, 1983.
15. Schwartz RA, Nichols WK, Silver D. Is thrombosis of the infrarenal abdominal aortic aneurysm an acceptable alternative? J Vasc Surg 3:448, 1986.
16. Inahara T, Geary GL, Mukherjee D, et al. The contrary position to the nonresective treatment of abdominal aortic aneurysm. J Vasc Surg 4:42, 1985.
17. Schanzer H, Papa MC, Miller CM. Rupture of surgically thrombosed abdominal aortic aneurysm. J Vasc Surg 2:278-280, 1985.
18. Kwaan JHM, Dahl RK. Fatal rupture after successful surgical thrombosis of an abdominal aortic aneurysm. Surgery 95:235-237, 1984.
19. Kim L, Kohler T, Johansen K. Nonresective therapy for aortic aneurysm: Results of a survey. J Vasc Surg 4:469, 1986.
20. Pevec WC, Holcroft JW, Blaisdell FW. Ligation and extra-anatomic arterial reconstruction for the treatment of aneurysms of the abdominal aorta. J Vasc Surg 20:629-636, 1994.
21. Corson JD, Leather RP, Shah DM, et al. Extraperitoneal aortic bypass with exclusion of the intact infrarenal aortic aneurysm: The in situ management of aortic aneurysms. A preliminary report. J Cardiovasc Surg 28:274-276, 1987.
22. Bandyk DF, Bergamini TM. Infection in prosthetic vascular grafts. In Rutherford RB, ed. Vascular Surgery, 4th ed. Philadelphia: WB Saunders, 1995, pp 588-604.
23. Schneider JR, McDaniel MD, Walsh DB, et al. Axillofemoral bypass: Outcome and hemodynamic results in high-risk patients. J Vasc Surg 15:952-963, 1992.
24. Rutherford RB, Jones DN, Martin S, et al. Serial hemodynamic assessment of aortobifemoral bypass. J Vasc Surg 4:428, 1986.
25. Schneider JR, Golan JF. The role of extraanatomic bypass in the management of bilateral aortoiliac occlusive disease. Semin Vasc Surg 7:35-44, 1994.
26. Rutherford RB, Mitchell MB. Extra-anatomic bypass. In Rutherford RB, ed. Vascular Surgery, 4th ed. Philadelphia: WB Saunders, 1995, pp 815-827.
27. Blaisdell FW, Holcroft JW, Ward RE. Axillofemoral and femorofemoral bypass: History and evolution of technique. In Greenhalgh RM, ed. Extra-anatomic and Secondary Arterial Reconstruction. London: Pitman, 1982.
28. Gupta SK, Veith FJ, Kram HB, Wengerter KR. Prospective randomized comparison of ringed and non-ringed polytetrafluoroethylene femoropopliteal bypass grafts: A preliminary report. J Vasc Surg 13:163-172, 1991.
29. Harrington ME, Harrington EB, Haimov M, et al. Axillofemoral bypass: Compromised bypass for compromised patients. J Vasc Surg 20:195-201, 1994.
30. Taylor LM Jr, Park TC, Edwards JM, et al. Acute disruption of polytetrafluoroethylene grafts adjacent to axillary anastomoses: A complication of axillofemoral grafting. J Vasc Surg 20:520-528, 1994.

32

Reconstruction of the Celiac, Superior Mesenteric, and Left and Right Renal Arteries Using an Extended Left Retroperitoneal Approach: Techniques and Results

R. CLEMENT DARLING III, M.D., DHIRAJ M. SHAH, M.D., BENJAMIN B. CHANG, M.D., PHILIP S.K. PATY, M.D., and ROBERT P. LEATHER, M.D.

The extended left retroperitoneal approach provides excellent exposure of the suprarenal segment of the aorta and its branches.[1,2] However, it is commonly believed that the transperitoneal approach offers greater flexibility for the repair of bilateral renal artery disease and extensive occlusive disease of the superior mesenteric artery (SMA) and celiac axis. Historically, the retroperitoneal approach has been reserved as an option for treatment of proximal "orifice lesions," and many consider this approach a contraindication for right or bilateral renal revascularization. However, since the retroperitoneal approach to the aorta has been suggested for high-risk patients with associated cardiac and respiratory compromise and because this approach offers superb exposure of the suprarenal aorta and its visceral branches, we have expanded its indication to patients who have chronic and acute visceral and renal artery ischemia.[2] This chapter presents our experience with these operative techniques and exposure for the management of these problems.

MATERIALS AND METHODS

From January 1987 through September 1994, 1302 elective aortic procedures were performed through the left retroperitoneal approach. During this time 224 renal artery and 39 visceral artery reconstructions were performed in 220 patients. Hospital charts and office records of all patients undergoing elective renal and visceral artery revascularization using the left retroperitoneal approach were reviewed. Excluded from the study were patients requiring emergent operations and thoracoabdominal aneurysm repairs. During this time 146 patients underwent renal and visceral arterial revascularization using transperitoneal or right retroperitoneal approaches and these were not included. Demographics, indications, operative procedure, complications, and long-term follow-up were obtained. All patients underwent preoperative cardiac evaluation, and arteriography as indicated. Patients with an elevated serum creatinine level received intravenous hydration for 1 day and infusion of mannitol before angiography. Carbon dioxide or magnetic resonance angiography was used for several patients at risk for renal failure.

SURGICAL TECHNIQUE

After placement of a Swan-Ganz catheter and radial artery line, general endotracheal anesthesia is produced. The patient is then positioned in a right lateral decubitus position with the left chest up at an angle of approximately 45 to 60 degrees. The pelvis is maintained at a 30-degree angle to facilitate access to the groins. The patient is held in position by a suction bean bag covered with a heating blanket and a bath blanket extending from the top of the patient's shoulders to just below the buttocks.

A second series of blankets is used to flex the left leg slightly and abduct the hip in order to relax the left iliopsoas muscle and facilitate control of the left iliac artery. The iliac crest is placed at the flexion point on the operating table to generate maximum distance between the costal margin and iliac crest by flexing the table (Fig. 1).

Prior to incision, 25 gm of mannitol is given intravenously to promote vigorous diuresis.

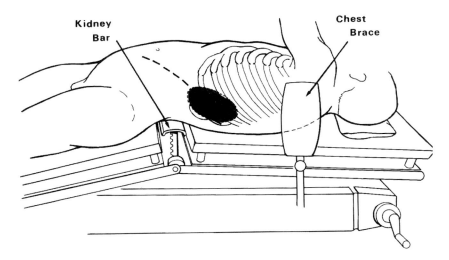

Fig. 1 Diagram showing position of patient on the operating table with flexion using a kidney bar.

The patient then receives 5 gm of mannitol per hour intravenously for 24 hours; 30 U/kg of heparin is given intravenously before aortic cross-clamping. In aneurysm patients distal control is obtained before aortic dissection to avoid distal embolization.

After the patient is prepped and draped from the chest to both groins, an incision is made over the eleventh rib and the tenth interspace is entered. After the musculature is divided, the transversalis fascia is carefully entered laterally in order to avoid entry into the peritoneal cavity. The left kidney and peritoneal contents are mobilized anteriorly, medially, and cephalad to expose the aorta. Stable exposure is facilitated by the use of a Buckwalter retractor.

The lumbar branch of the left renal vein is transected to aid exposure of the left renal artery and infrarenal aorta (Fig. 2). Exposure of the suprarenal aorta and visceral arteries is gained by division of the overlying diaphragmatic crus. The level of aortic clamping is dictated by the proximal extent of the aneurysmal or occlusive disease.

Renal artery reconstructions are performed by means of endarterectomy, bypass, or both. For endarterectomy the aorta is clamped cephalad to the involved artery or arteries. If the aorta does not require replacement, a "trap-door" aortotomy may be performed. Extension of the proximal aortotomy provides intraluminal exposure of the renal and visceral arteries (Fig. 3).

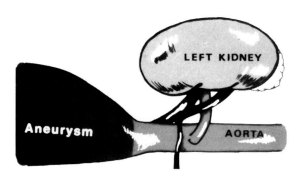

Fig. 2 Operative illustration of aortic root dissection showing a lumbar branch of the left renal vein crossing the aorta just inferior to the left renal artery.

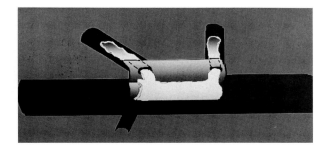

Fig. 3 Diagram of trap door aortotomy for performance of transaortic endarterectomy of orifice lesions of the celiac, superior mesenteric, and renal arteries.

If renal artery bypass is to be performed, the aorta is divided transversely. Anterior and cephalad mobilization of the proximal aorta facilitates right renal artery control (Fig. 4).

Expanded polytetrafluoroethylene (ePTFE) 6 mm grafts for the left and/or right renal arteries are sewn onto the body of the aortic graft beforehand to minimize operating and warm ischemia time. The proximal aortic anastomosis is performed with a parachute technique using a running 48-inch 3/0 polypropylene suture. The right renal artery may then be dissected over a distance of approximately 3 to 4 cm. A curved Cooley clamp is used to obtain stable control of the exposed right renal artery, and an end-to-end anastomosis is usually performed using 6-0 polypropylene continuous suture (Fig. 5). After this is completed, the aortic clamp is moved distally to allow flow to the right renal artery. The left renal artery anastomosis is performed in a similar fashion (Fig. 6).

If visceral artery reconstruction is to be performed, the left kidney can remain in its anatomic position by dissecting anteriorly to Gerota's fascia. The peritoneum is then retracted medially. The origins of the SMA and celiac axis are easily identified after the crus of the left diaphragm is divided along the axis of the aorta. If necessary, each vessel can then be further exposed by dissecting the tissue along the axis of the artery. The SMA can be dissected as it courses between the body and uncinate process of the pancreas and duodenum for approximately 5 to 10 cm (Fig. 7). The vessel branches at this point, but additional exposure may be obtained by incising the peritoneum. The celiac artery can be exposed in a similar manner up to its trifurcation. At this point the left gastric artery courses superiorly and the common hepatic artery courses posteriorly and to the right into the peritoneum. The splenic artery can be followed along its distance by dissecting along the superior border of the body and tail of the pancreas. This provides the additional option of using the splenic artery as an inflow source for left renal artery revascularization. With this technique a sufficient length of SMA and celiac artery may be exposed for the performance of either an endarterectomy or bypass. After completion of these reconstructions, an incision is often made in the peritoneum and the bowel is visually examined. All reconstructed arteries are auscultated by Doppler ultrasound to ascertain the presence of a good flow signal. The perito-

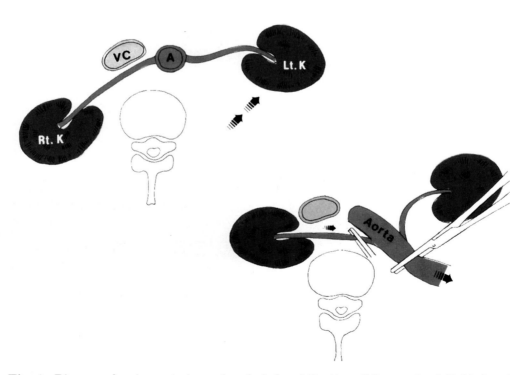

Fig. 4 Diagram showing anterior and cephalad mobilization of the proximal divided aorta for exposure of the right renal artery.

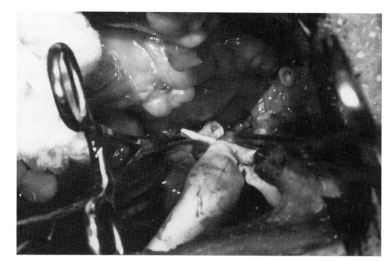

Fig. 5 Photograph showing exposure of the right renal artery and its stabilization by means of a vascular clamp prior to end-to-end anastomosis.

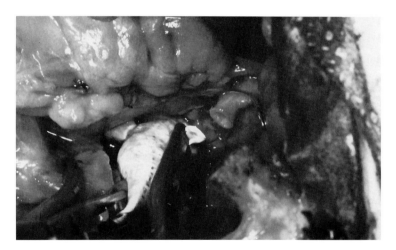

Fig. 6 Same patient as in Fig. 5, after completion of right and left renal artery anastomoses.

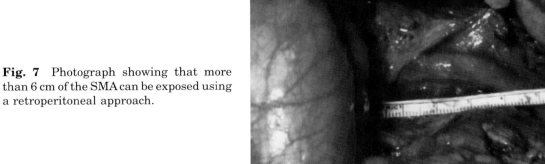

Fig. 7 Photograph showing that more than 6 cm of the SMA can be exposed using a retroperitoneal approach.

neum and the abdominal incisions are closed in layers using nonabsorbable sutures.

RESULTS

Two hundred twenty patients underwent 224 renal and 39 visceral artery procedures through an extended left retroperitoneal approach over a 7-year period. This comprises 17% of the total number of elective aortic operations performed using this approach during the same time period. Demographic information is listed in Table 1. The predominant associated conditions for these procedures were aortic aneurysm (126 patients), aortoiliac occlusive disease (26 patients), renovascular hypertension (39 patients), and mesenteric ischemia (29 patients). One hundred seventy-four reconstructions involved the left renal artery: 142 bypasses, 20 endarterectomies, 11 direct reimplantations into the aortic graft, and one excision of a renal artery aneurysm with primary anastomosis. With the exception of four patients in whom saphenous vein grafts were used, all left renal artery bypasses were completed using 6 mm ePTFE grafts.

The inflow source in 113 of these bypasses was the aortic graft. Other inflow sources included native aorta (21), iliac artery (5), SMA (2), and splenic artery (1). Fifty procedures were performed on the right renal artery using a left retroperitoneal approach. Of these, 36 were bypasses using ePTFE grafts and 14 were endarterectomies. Twenty-nine patients underwent bilateral renal artery revascularization.

Twenty-nine patients presented with symptoms of mesenteric ischemia. Most related a history of chronic abdominal pain and weight loss. Twenty-eight patients underwent SMA reconstructions. Nineteen of these procedures were bypasses. Thirteen of the bypasses were completed with ePTFE grafts; autogenous veins were used in six procedures (5 greater saphenous veins and 1 inferior mesenteric vein). The inflow source was native aorta in eight bypasses, aortic graft in nine, and one each from the left renal artery and left common iliac artery. The remaining procedures were endarterectomies (8) and reimplantation (1). Eleven procedures were performed for celiac artery ischemia. These included seven bypasses (6 ePTFE, 1 vein) and four endarterectomies. The inflow sources for these bypasses were native aorta (9) and aortic graft (2).

The average estimated blood loss for all procedures was 980 ± 714 ml (range, 200 to 4000

Table 1 Patient demographics

Age	68 years (range, 10-92)
Male/female distribution	57%/43%
Diabetis mellitus	10%
Hypertension	83%
Smoking	68%
Creatinine level >1.5 mg/dl	15%

ml). The average length of hospital stay was 9.4 days (range, 4 to 41 days). Patients were followed up for a mean of 15 months (range, 2 to 86 months). During this time all patients underwent a duplex scan, renal flow scan, and/or angiography. There were eight perioperative deaths for an operative mortality of 3.6%. Five deaths were in the group undergoing renal revascularization, and three were in the mesenteric group. Five patients died because of cardiac failure. One patient suffered a massive, fatal stroke the first postoperative day after repair of an abdominal aortic aneurysm (AAA) with bilateral renal artery bypass. One patient died after the development of a necrotic left colon, acute renal failure, and multisystem organ failure following repair of a suprarenal aortic aneurysm with bilateral renal artery bypass. The last patient died of complications from upper gastrointestinal bleeding.

Four of the reconstructions failed during the follow-up period. A 50-year-old woman who underwent a celiac artery and SMA endarterectomy (her fifth operation for mesenteric ischemia and renal hypertension, beginning at age 39) had recurrent chronic symptoms 4 months postoperatively as well as lower extremity ischemia. She underwent an aortobifemoral bypass with SMA bypass through a midline approach.

The second occlusion occurred 8 months after bilateral renal artery bypass with ePTFE grafts for renovascular hypertension. Recurrent hypertension developed in this patient, and she was found to have an atrophic left kidney and a patent right renal artery bypass. She subsequently underwent a left nephrectomy.

The third failure was noted in a 60-year-old man who suffered a left renal infarct 13 months after bypasses for AAA and left renal artery stenosis. A workup indicated a probable thrombosed aortic dissection with false lumen leading to the left renal artery.

The last failure occurred in a patient who required nephrectomy secondary to a necrotic, nonfunctioning kidney.

Eight other complications required returning the patients to the operating room. Two patients required splenectomy for bleeding, most likely secondary to a retractor injury. Two patients required femoral artery embolectomy. One patient needed wound closure after dehiscence of his left flank wound. Necrosis developed in one patient involving the majority of the jejunum and ileum after bilateral renal and SMA endarterectomy and aortoiliac endarterectomy; this occurred despite a functioning reconstruction. The patient ultimately underwent bowel resection and was able to maintain her weight with oral food intake. The last two patients returned to the operating room for a negative "second look" laparotomy after initial presentation for an acute exacerbation of chronic mesenteric ischemia.

Renal failure developed in 10 patients after renal artery bypass; it was temporary in nine patients, with four requiring short-term dialysis (less than 2 weeks). Acute tubular necrosis developed in two of these patients after angiography. One patient who required permanent dialysis had an 8 cm AAA and a history of chronic renal insufficiency with a preoperative creatinine level of 4.8 mg/dl. She required dialysis postoperatively, and a dialysis catheter was placed preoperatively.

Four patients had nonfatal cardiac complications (dysrhythmias and congestive heart failure), and two patients required prolonged mechanical ventilation and eventual tracheostomy. There were four minor wound infections. Paraplegia developed in one patient after aortic aneurysm repair and left renal artery bypass.

DISCUSSION

Vascular exposure for endarterectomy or bypass for intestinal ischemia has most commonly been performed through a transperitoneal route.[3-6] However, we have found that both types of revascularizations can be performed successfully through a posterolateral extended left retroperitoneal approach. Exposure of the visceral and renal arteries through the left retroperitoneum has been previously described.[2] Stoney et al.[5,7] have pioneered visceral reconstructions using medial visceral rotation through a left thoracoabdominal incision. This approach offers excellent exposure of the visceral aorta and has truly facilitated the use of endarterectomy and bypass for this surgical problem.[8] However, it requires entry into both the thoracic and peritoneal cavities to achieve exposure of the retroperitoneal visceral aorta. It would seem only logical that this portion of the aorta can be approached through a totally retroperitoneal exposure. Even those authors who advocate the use of a retroperitoneal aortic exposure generally regard it to be most useful in the treatment of occlusive disease limited to the orifices of the visceral vessels.

Many consider the left retroperitoneal approach to be strictly contraindicated in patients requiring right renal artery revascularization. However, endarterectomy or bypass of this artery may easily be performed through this exposure. Complete transection of the aorta gives access to the right renal artery before or as it dives behind the vena cava. Dissection is not hindered by other structures. Approximately 3 cm of the right renal artery can easily be dissected, and with placement of a curved Cooley clamp, stable exposure is obtained for bypass. The left renal artery is widely visible during the entire dissection and thus bilateral renal artery reconstructions can be performed.

Nypaver et al.[9] demonstrated that pararenal aneurysms can be effectively treated using a retroperitoneal approach and concluded that this approach can facilitate the repair. It should be noted that during our experience with visceral and renal artery revascularization by the extended left retroperitoneal approach, all bypasses and endarterectomies were successfully completed without modifying the approach. If renal artery reconstruction is undertaken during the placement of an aortic graft, the easiest option is to sew 6 mm limbs onto the body of the aortic graft before aortic cross-clamping. These may then be anastomosed to the renal arteries in an end-to-end (our choice) or end-to-side fashion.

Alternatively, the renal artery may be reimplanted directly into the body of the graft. The other major option for revascularization of the renal and visceral arteries is transaortic endarterectomy. Stoney's group[5,7,8,10] has reported extensively on this procedure and demonstrated conclusively that this is a viable reconstructive option requiring no prosthetic material. It does require impeccable surgical technique and access to the midportion of the visceral and renal arteries to be certain that the endarterectomies are terminated satisfactorily. The medial visceral rotation used by Stoney and associates and the extended left retroperitoneal approach used in this report provide virtually identical exposure of the visceral aorta and its branches. The type of aortotomy varies with the extent and type of endarterectomy performed. Usually the aortotomy is made vertically along the posterolateral side of the vessel. Alternatively, a "trapdoor" aortotomy may be made around the arterial orifices to be endarterectomized. If the end point is not satisfactory, an incision into the artery in question may be performed to extend the endarterectomy. Alternatively, a bypass may be performed distal to the endarterectomized artery.

Elective infrarenal aortic surgery has mortality rates ranging from 2% to 5%. The addition of bilateral renal and visceral revascularization in many series has increased mortality and morbidity up to 20%.[11-13] Transperitoneal exposure of the suprarenal aorta is hindered by the left renal vein and pancreas. From a lateral approach, once the lumbar branch of the left renal vein is ligated and the crus of the diaphragm is divided, the left renal vein, pancreas, and visceral structures can be retracted anteriorly, medially, and cephalad, giving superb exposure of the renal and visceral segments of the aorta. Aortic cross-clamping can then proceed at numerous locations above, below, or between the renal and visceral vessels. This minimizes end-organ ischemia. The addition of visceral or bilateral renal artery bypasses does not appear to influence mortality and morbidity substantially when performed by this approach. Operative mortality for our procedures was 3.6% in this series. This does not vary greatly from our reported results with infrarenal aortic reconstructions (2.9%)[14-16] but does differ considerably with the combined aortic and visceral arterial reconstruction results reported by other authors.[10,13] This may be partly attributable to the physiologic benefits reported from the retroperitoneal exposure as opposed to the transperitoneal approach to the aorta. In addition, in our study the average blood loss was 980 ml and the average length of hospital stay was 9.4 days. Although this was not a prospective randomized study, our data showed improved results compared with other recent series.[10-13,17] Also, we find the retroperitoneal exposure clearly superior to that obtained transperitoneally, and this simplifies the technical conduct of the operation. As one becomes more familiar with this approach, the limitations of the exposure become fewer.

Although many surgeons are not comfortable with the extended left retroperitoneal approach, we believe it is a useful adjunct to surgical therapy for bilateral renal and visceral arterial reconstructions. This flank incision causes less respiratory embarrassment and thus is associated with fewer postoperative respiratory complications.[14,17-19] Since the peritoneum and its contents are not exposed, there is less evaporative fluid loss and decreased intraoperative fluid requirements, resulting in small postoperative fluid shifts.[14,15,20] Furthermore, decreased intestinal traction reduces postoperative adynamia, resulting in an earlier return of intestinal function. In patients who had undergone multiple previous intra-abdominal procedures, the retroperitoneal approach gave access to the aorta without the need of enterolysis. Allen et al.[20] recently reported their comparative results in patients undergoing aortic and renal revascularization using the retroperitoneal and transperitoneal approaches. They concluded that the retroperitoneal approach was associated with less intraoperative fluid requirements, earlier resumption of diet, and better long-term survival.

In conclusion, the extended left retroperitoneal approach provides excellent exposure of orificial lesions and distal disease of the visceral and renal arteries. It is hoped that this technique will further increase surgeons' options in treating visceral and bilateral renal artery ischemia.

REFERENCES

1. Ricotta JJ, Williams GM. Endarterectomy of the upper abdominal aorta and visceral arteries through an extraperitoneal approach. Ann Surg 192:633-638, 1980.
2. Saifi J, Shah DM, Chang BB, Kaufman JL, Leather RP. Left retroperitoneal exposure for distal mesenteric artery repair. J Cardiovasc Surg 31:629-633, 1990.
3. Shaw RS, Maynard EP III. Acute and chronic thrombosis of the mesenteric arteries associated with malabsorption: A report of two cases successfully treated by thromboendarterectomy. N Engl J Med 258:874-878, 1958.
4. Crawford ES, Morris GC Jr, Myhre HO, Rochm JOF Jr. Celiac axis, superior mesenteric artery, and inferior mesenteric artery occlusion: Surgical considerations. Surgery 82:856-866, 1977.
5. Stoney RJ, Ehrenfeld WK, Wylie EJ. Revascularization methods in chronic visceral ischemia caused by atherosclerosis. Ann Surg 186:468-476, 1977.
6. Taylor LM Jr, Porter JM. Treatment of chronic intestinal ischemia. Semin Vasc Surg 3:186-199, 1990.
7. Stoney RJ, Skioldebrand CG, Qvarford PG, Reilly LM, Ehrenfeld WK. Juxtarenal aortic atherosclerosis. Ann Surg 200:345-354, 1984.
8. Rapp JH, Reilly LM, Qvarfordt PG, Goldstone J, Ehrenfeld WK, Stoney RJ. Durability of endarterectomy and retrograde grafts in the treatment of chronic visceral ischemia. J Vasc Surg 3:799-806, 1986.

9. Nypaver TJ, Shepard AD, Reddy DJ, Elliott JP Jr, Smith RF, Ernst CB. Repair of pararenal abdominal aortic aneurysms. Arch Surg 128: 803-812, 1993.
10. Stoney RJ, Messina LM, Goldstone J, Reilly LM. Renal endarterectomy through the transected aorta: A new technique for combined aortorenal atherosclerosis—a preliminary report. J Vasc Surg 9:224-233, 1989.
11. Tarazi RY, Hertzer NR, Beven EG, O'Hara PJ, Anton GE, Krajewski LP. Simultaneous aortic reconstruction and renal revascularization: Risk factors and late results in 89 patients. J Vasc Surg 5:707-714, 1987.
12. Dean RH, Keyser JE III, Dupont WD, Nadeau JH, Meacham PW. Aortic and renal vascular disease: Factors affecting the value of combined procedures. Ann Surg 200:336-344, 1984.
13. Atnip RG, Neumeyer MM, Healy DA, Thiele BL. Combined aortic and visceral arterial reconstruction: Risks and results. J Vasc Surg 12:705-715, 1990.
14. Darling RC III, Shah DM, McClellan WR, Chang BB, Leather RP. Decreased morbidity associated with retroperitoneal exclusion treatment for abdominal aortic aneurysm. J Cardiovasc Surg 33:65-69, 1992.
15. Leather RP, Shah DM, Kaufman JL, Fitzgerald KM, Chang BB, Feustel PJ. Comparative analysis of retroperitoneal and transperitoneal aneurysm resection. Surg Gynecol Obstet 168:387-393, 1989.
16. Shah DM, Chang BB, Paty PSK, Kaufman JL, Koslow AR, Leather RP. Treatment of abdominal aortic aneurysm by exclusion and bypass: An analysis of outcome. J Vasc Surg 13:15-22, 1991.
17. Darling RC III, Shah DM, Chang BB, Leather RP. Does concomitant aortic bypass and renal artery revascularization using the retroperitoneal approach increase perioperative risk? Cardiovasc Surg (in press).
18. Judson JC, Wurm WH, O'Donnell TF, et al. Hemodynamics and prostacyclin release in the early phases of aortic surgery: Comparison of transabdominal and retroperitoneal approaches. J Vasc Surg 7:190-198, 1988.
19. Sicard GA, Freeman MB, Van der Woude JC, Anderson CB. Comparison between transabdominal and retroperitoneal approach for reconstruction of infrarenal abdominal aorta. J Vasc Surg 5:19-27, 1987.
20. Allen BT, Rubin BG, Anderson CB, Thompson RW, Sicard GA. Simultaneous surgical management of aortic and renovascular disease. Am J Surg 166:726-733, 1993.

SECTION IV

Advances in the Management of Lower Extremity Ischemia

This section describes important advances in the management of lower extremity ischemia including a prospective comparison of epidural and general anesthesia, optimal treatment of vein and anastomotic lesions, use of the superficial vein as a bypass graft, and use of free flaps in association with distal bypasses. Conflicting views on the value of angioscopy are offered, and an important chapter discussing the optimal treatment of intermittent claudication is presented.

33

Randomized Prospective Comparison of Epidural and General Anesthesia for Infrainguinal Bypass Surgery

BRUCE A. PERLER, M.D.

Exclusive of carotid endarterectomy, infrainguinal bypass grafts are the most frequently performed peripheral vascular operations in this country, and long-term patency is excellent. Nevertheless, even in the most favorable reports, 20% to 30% of grafts have failed during follow-up.[1,2] Most graft occlusions occur early, including some within the immediate postoperative period. Technical or judgment errors on the part of the surgeon have been the most frequently cited causes of acute postoperative graft thrombosis. More recently, an increasing number of acute graft occlusions have been attributed to underlying hypercoagulability that in many cases was not recognized preoperatively. However, little attention has been paid to the impact of other perioperative physiologic processes and the factors that influence them, such as method of anesthesia, on early graft patency. Although the current study was undertaken to investigate the influence of the method of anesthesia on perioperative cardiac morbidity, it provided an intriguing insight into the potential impact of the anesthesia method on early graft patency.[3,4]

BACKGROUND
Theoretical Issues

It is well recognized that the successful infrainguinal bypass graft is associated with a pronounced distal hyperemia that is maximal within the first 24 hours postoperatively, generally does not normalize until 72 to 96 hours postoperatively, and predominantly reflects a reduction in peripheral vascular resistance.[5,6] On the other hand, increased outflow resistance can result in a predisposition to early graft occlusion.[7,8] It is logical to assume, therefore, that any intervention mediating a reduction in peripheral vascular resistance might promote early graft patency. Epidural anesthesia produces a transient sympathetic blockade that has been shown to result in increased arterial flow, venous emptying, and venous capacitance when compared to the effects experienced by patients who receive general anesthesia.[9,10] Increased blood flow to the skin is manifested by increased skin temperature in patients who receive regional anesthesia.[9] In addition to avoiding the potential reduction in cardiac output associated with general anesthesia and its deleterious impact on peripheral perfusion in the older patient population with significant arteriosclerotic cardiovascular disease, regional anesthesia may promote graft patency via its peripheral sympatholytic effect.[11] This benefit may continue in the postoperative period in patients who continue to receive epidural analgesia.

In fact, the physiologic effects of both types of anesthesia are quite complex, and the potential influence of the method of anesthesia on graft patency may be multifactorial. It is perhaps most important to consider the normal surgical stress response. The trauma of surgical intervention is associated with a variety of acute biochemical and hematologic changes. Specifically, surgical stress has been associated with a rise in the levels of circulating catecholamines, renin, angiotensin, and aldosterone. Elevated levels of catecholamines and other vasoconstricting agents may increase peripheral vascular resistance and thus have a deleterious impact on graft flow and early patency. Numerous studies have demonstrated that epidural anesthesia and analgesia effectively modulate the normal physiologic response to surgical stress by blocking afferent and efferent neural pathways.[12-21]

The surgical stress response is also characterized by a number of alterations in the coagulation and fibrinolytic systems, and these observations may be particularly relevant in patients with severe peripheral arterial occlusive disease. Several studies have confirmed increased concentrations of factor VIII, von Willebrand factor, fibrinogen, decreased concentrations of coagulation inhibitors, and inhibition of fibrinolysis in the postoperative state.[21-24] Increased levels of catecholamines and angiotensin as part of the surgical stress response can increase platelet aggregation.[25,26] Specifically, increased platelet reactivity, increased levels of factor VIII–related antigen, and decreased levels of antithrombin III have been identified postoperatively among patients undergoing peripheral arterial surgery and have been associated with early bypass graft occlusions.[12,27,28] However, there is growing evidence that epidural anesthesia and postoperative analgesia may modulate this hypercoagulability tendency, at least in part, by attenuating the surgical stress response resulting in higher levels of antithrombin III, lower levels of fibrinogen, and reduced platelet reactivity postoperatively.[14,29-31]

Clinical Experience

Several investigators have studied the influence of regional anesthesia on the incidence of deep venous thrombosis among patients undergoing major orthopedic surgery, and the preponderance of evidence supports the theoretical potential of regional anesthesia to ameliorate postoperative hypercoagulability.[32] A significantly reduced incidence of calf and more proximal deep venous thrombosis was reported among patients undergoing total hip replacement under epidural anesthesia as compared to general anesthesia in two recent studies.[17,33] In another study of patients undergoing total hip replacement, the use of epidural anesthesia was associated with a significant reduction only in the incidence of calf vein thrombosis.[34] Others have reported a significantly lower incidence of both calf and more proximal deep venous thrombosis among patients undergoing total hip replacement under spinal anesthesia as compared with those receiving general anesthesia.[35] Epidural anesthesia and postoperative analgesia have also been associated with a reduced incidence of deep venous thrombosis among patients undergoing total knee replacement surgery.[36]

On the other hand, although there has been considerable interest in the relationship between the method of anesthesia and perioperative cardiac morbidity, little attention has been paid to the influence of the method of anesthesia on arterial bypass graft patency. For example, in a prospective study of 213 patients undergoing infrainguinal bypass surgery, and in which regional and general anesthesia was associated with equivalent cardiac risk, early graft patency was not reported.[37] In a randomized prospective trial, 80 patients undergoing arterial bypass surgery under general anesthesia received either on-demand narcotic analgesics or continuous epidural analgesics postoperatively. Early postoperative graft occlusion occurred in only two (5%) patients who received epidural analgesia compared to eight (20%) who did not ($p = .007$). Unfortunately, the specific grafts performed and other important surgical variables known to influence graft patency were not provided.[12] The current study was therefore undertaken to critically examine the potential influence of method of anesthesia on early infrainguinal bypass graft patency.

CLINICAL TRIAL
Protocol

One hundred patients scheduled to undergo elective peripheral vascular reconstruction were randomized to receive either general anesthesia and postoperative intravenous patient-controlled analgesia (GEN) or epidural anesthesia and postoperative epidural analgesia (EPI).[3,4] In view of the heterogeneous mix of arterial reconstructions performed, a subset of 78 patients, including 41 GEN and 37 EPI, who underwent only femoropopliteal or femorotibial grafts for chronic occlusive disease were selected for this analysis to more specifically study the influence of the method of anesthesia on early graft patency. General anesthesia was induced with intravenous thiamylal and fentanyl and was maintained with nitrous oxide in oxygen, 0.3% enflurane, and pancuronium after endotracheal intubation. Epidural anesthesia was achieved with 0.75% bupivacaine. The respective postoperative analgesic regimens were continued until the patients were transferred from the ICU to the regular nursing floor where morphine was administered intramuscularly as needed.

All patients underwent anticoagulation therapy with heparin before arterial clamping, and the heparin effect was not reversed at the completion of the procedure. With rare exceptions, completion angiography was performed and peripheral arterial flow was assessed by Doppler ultrasound in all cases before leaving the operating room. An infusion of low-molecular-weight dextran (Dextran-40) was begun in the operating room and continued for 48 hours postoperatively unless the surgeon elected to use anticoagulation therapy with heparin.

Patients were monitored in the ICU for 18 to 24 hours postoperatively unless peripheral vascular, cardiac, pulmonary, or other morbidity warranted a more prolonged stay. Graft occlusion was detected by a deterioration in clinical status and Doppler flow and in all cases was confirmed at surgical exploration, either for attempted thrombectomy or limb amputation. In addition to routine postoperative hematologic and blood chemistry analyses, levels of circulating plasminogen activator inhibitor-1 (PAI-1) were measured in all patients before the induction of anesthesia and at 24 and 72 hours postoperatively.

One patient in each group died of cardiac complications, yielding an operative mortality of 2.6% and leaving 76 patients available for graft patency analysis. The GEN patients ranged in age from 44 to 91 years (mean, 66 years) and the EPI patients from 37 to 94 years (mean, 65 years). Fifty-five percent of the GEN and 58% of the EPI patients were men. There were no significant differences in the prevalence of hypertension (72% vs. 58%), diabetes mellitus (45% vs. 33%), or history of smoking (80% vs. 92%) between the GEN and EPI groups, respectively. The indications for operation were limb-threatening ischemia in 83% of the GEN and 86% of the EPI patients. The ankle/arm index ranged from 0.00 to 0.64 (mean, 0.34) in the GEN and from 0.00 to 0.63 (mean, 0.33) in the EPI patients. The infrainguinal graft was constructed to the tibial level in 43% of the GEN and 39% of the EPI patients. The grafts were constructed of saphenous vein in 83% of the GEN and 83% of the EPI patients. Multiple vein segments were required in 9% of the GEN and 10% of the EPI patients. The bypass operation was a reoperative procedure in 28% of the GEN and 25% of the EPI patients. None of these differences was statistically significant (Table 1). Poor runoff (fewer than two vessels) was noted in 57% of the GEN and 30% of the EPI patients with femoropopliteal grafts. In addition, heparin was administered postoperatively to 30% of the GEN and 14% of the EPI patients. Although these differences did not achieve statistical significance, they suggested a trend toward more severe disease in the GEN group (see Table 1).

RESULTS

Acute postoperative graft thrombosis occurred in 11 (14%) patients from 1 to 7 days postoperatively. Graft occlusion occurred in nine (22%)

Table 1 Patient and vascular characteristics

	GEN (n = 40)	EPI n = 36)
Age (yr)	44-91	37-94
	($\bar{x}$ = 66 ± 2)	($\bar{x}$ = 65 ± 2)
Males (%)	55	58
Risk factors		
Hypertension (%)	73	58
Diabetes (%)	45	33
Smoking (%)	80	92
Limb salvage (%)	82	86
Ankle/arm index	0.00-0.64	0.00-0.63
	($\bar{x}$ = 0.34 ± 0.004)	($\bar{x}$ = 0.33 ± 0.04)
Grafts		
FP (%)	57	61
FT (%)	43	39
Greater/lesser saphenous vein (%)	83	83
Multiple vein segments (%)	28	25
Reoperative procedure (%)	28	25
Poor FP runoff (%)	57	30
Postoperative heparin (%)	30	14

GEN = general anesthesia; EPI = epidural anesthesia; FP = femoropopliteal; FT = femorotibial.

GEN and two (6%) EPI patients ($p < .05$). There were two (4%) femoropopliteal occlusions, both of which occurred in GEN (9%) patients. Nine (29%) femorotibial grafts acutely occluded, including seven (41%) in GEN and two (14%) in EPI patients. Graft occlusion occurred in 11 (17%) of the procedures performed for limb salvage, including nine (27%) of the GEN and two (6%) of the EPI patients ($p < .05$). None of the grafts performed for intermittent claudication failed. Seven (13%) of 55 grafts constructed with greater saphenous vein failed in the early postoperative period, including six (22%) in GEN and one (4%) in EPI patients ($p < .05$). According to univariate analysis, only femorotibial grafts ($p < .01$) and general anesthesia ($p < .05$) were predictive of early graft failure (Table 2). By multivariate analysis, femorotibial grafts, general anesthesia, and preoperative PAI-1 levels were predictive of early graft thrombosis ($p < .05$).

The mean PAI-1 level 24 hours postoperatively among patients who experienced graft thrombosis (31 ± 8 activity units [AU]/ml) was significantly higher than the preoperative level (17.5 ± 5 AU/ml) ($p < .05$) and was significantly higher than the mean PAI-1 level at 24 hours

Table 2 Graft occlusion: Univariate analysis

	Patent (n = 65)	Occluded (n = 11)	p Value
FT	34%	82%	<.01
GEN	48%	82%	<.05
Reoperative	23%	45%	NS
Limb salvage	82%	100%	NS
Poor runoff	62%	82%	NS
Greater saphenous vein	74%	64%	NS
Greater and lesser saphenous veins	82%	91%	NS
Active smokers	37%	27%	NS
Diabetes	38%	45%	NS
Preoperative PAI-1 (AU/ml)	14.7 ± 2	17.5 ± 5	NS

FT = femorotibial; GEN = general anesthesia; PAI-1 = plasminogen activator inhibitor-1; NS = not significant.

(16 ± 1.7 AU/ml) among the patients who did not experience graft thrombosis ($p < .05$). In addition, the mean PAI-1 level among the GEN group increased from 16.3 ± 2.8 AU/ml) preoperatively to 22.4 ± 3.2 AU/ml 24 hours postoperatively ($p < .05$) and decreased to 14 ± 2.3 AU/ml 72 hours postoperatively. A similar increase was not observed in the EPI group as a whole.

Secondary Procedures

Two of the GEN patients who experienced graft occlusion were thought to have end-stage disease and underwent below-knee amputation, whereas graft salvage was attempted in the other seven patients. Three patients underwent thrombectomy without revision, and two grafts reoccluded, resulting in the need for below-knee amputation. The other four patients underwent graft thrombectomy and revision; three of these grafts were salvaged, but the fourth graft rethrombosed, resulting in below-knee amputation. In summary, four (44%) of the nine grafts were ultimately salvaged, yielding a 30-day secondary patency rate of 88% and a limb salvage rate of 90%. Both patients in the EPI group who experienced acute postoperative graft thrombosis were thought to have end-stage disease and underwent below-knee amputation without further attempts at revascularization. Therefore the 30-day secondary patency and limb salvage rate among the EPI patients was 94%, which was not significantly different from the 30-day result in the GEN group.

CONCLUSION

This trial represents the first investigation in which the influence of the method of anesthesia and postoperative analgesia specifically on early infrainguinal bypass graft patency was critically assessed. Although the apparent benefit of regional anesthesia and postoperative analgesia is intriguing and consistent with its known physiologic and hematologic effects, as well as with its documented potential to reduce the incidence of postoperative deep venous thrombosis among patients undergoing orthopedic surgery, the enhanced early graft patency seen in patients who received epidural anesthesia and postoperative analgesia must be viewed with some caution. First, poor runoff was noted much more often among the GEN patients (see Table 1). Although this difference did not achieve statistical significance, it nevertheless suggests a greater tendency for early graft thrombosis among the GEN group as a result of disadvantaged outflow. Second, formal anticoagulation with heparin was administered roughly twice as often in the GEN group (see Table 1). One may infer from this that the responsible surgeons in these cases were concerned about the risk of early graft failure because of the disadvantaged outflow, as noted previously, or other factors. Third, since secondary patency rates in the GEN and EPI groups were comparable, one might speculate that technical or judgmental errors contributed to at least some of the initial graft thromboses in the GEN group, although in view of the successful randomization of patients and surgeons, this is not likely. Finally, it is impossible from the design of this study to differentiate the effects of the anesthetic regimen from the method of postoperative analgesia. It is hoped that this work will stimulate others to continue to investigate this important clinical problem. Nevertheless, at present, unless the patient scheduled to undergo infrainguinal bypass surgery has a specific contraindication to regional anesthesia, there is growing evidence to support performing that operation under epidural anesthesia.

REFERENCES

1. Mannick JA, Whittemore AD, Donaldson MC. Autologous vein grafts in infrainguinal arterial reconstruction: A 10-year experience. In Veith FJ, ed. Current Critical Problems in Vascular Surgery, vol 3. St. Louis: Quality Medical Publishing, 1991, pp 71-72.
2. Taylor LM Jr, Phinney ES, Porter JM. Present status of reversed vein bypass grafting: Five-year results of a modern series. J Vasc Surg 11:193-206, 1990.
3. Christopherson R, Beattie C, Frank S, et al. Perioperative morbidity in patients randomized to epidural or general anesthesia for lower extremity vascular surgery. Anesthesiology 79:422-434, 1993.
4. Rosenfeld BA, Beattie C, Christopherson R, et al. The effects of different anesthetic regimens on fibrinolysis and the development of postoperative arterial thrombosis. Anesthesiology 79:435-447, 1993.
5. Renwick S, Gabe IT, Shillingford JP, Martin P. Blood flow after reconstructive arterial surgery measured by implanted electromagnetic flow probes. Surgery 64:544-553, 1968.
6. Wellington JL, Olszewski V, Martin P. Hyperaemia of the calf after arterial reconstruction for atherosclerotic occlusion. Br J Surg 53:180-184, 1966.
7. Ascer E, Veith FJ, Morin L, et al. Components of outflow resistance and their correlation with graft patency in lower extremity arterial reconstructions. J Vasc Surg 1:817-828, 1984.
8. Bandyk DF, Cato RF, Towne JB. A low flow velocity predicts failure of femoropopliteal and femorotibial bypass grafts. Surgery 98:799-809, 1985.
9. Cousins MJ, Wright CJ. Graft, muscle, skin blood flow after epidural block in vascular surgical procedures. Surg Gynecol Obstet 133:59-64, 1971.
10. Modig J, Malmberg P, Karlstrom G. Effect of epidural versus general anesthesia on calf blood flow. Acta Anaesthesiol Scand 24:305-309, 1980.
11. Halijame H, Frid I, Holm J, Akerstrom G. Epidural versus general anesthesia and leg blood flow in patients with occlusive atherosclerotic disease. Eur J Vasc Surg 2:395-400, 1988.
12. Tuman KJ, McCarthy RJ, March RJ, DeLaria GA, Patel RV, Ivankovich AD. Effects of epidural anesthesia and analgesia on coagulation and outcome after major vascular surgery. Anesth Analg 73:696-704, 1991.
13. Carli F, Webster P, Nandi I, MacDonald A, Pearson J, Mehta R. Thermogenesis after surgery: Effect of perioperative heat conservation and epidural anesthesia. Endocrinol Metab 26:E441-E447, 1992.
14. Christensen P, Brandt M, Rem J, Keblet H. Influence of extradural morphine on the adrenocortical and hyperglycemic response to surgery. Br J Anaesth 43:23-27, 1982.
15. Brandt MR, Olguard K, Keblet H. The blocking effects of epidural analgesia on the adrenocortical and hyperglycemic responses to surgery. Acta Anaesthesiol Scand 21:330-335, 1977.
16. Engquist A, Fog-Moller F, Christensen C, Thode J, Anderson T, Nestrop-Madsen S. Influence of epidural analgesia on the catecholamine and cyclic AMP response to surgery. Acta Anaesthesiol Scand 24:17-21, 1980.
17. Modig J, Borg T, Bagge L, Saldeen T. Role of extradural and of general anesthesia in fibrinolysis and coagulation after total hip replacement. Br J Anaesth 55:625-628, 1983.
18. Borg T, Modig J. Potential antithrombotic effects of local anesthetics due to their inhibition of platelet aggregation. Acta Anaesthesiol Scand 29:739-742, 1985.
19. Nielsen TH, Nielson HK, Husted SE, Hansen SL, Olson KH, Fjeldborg N. Stress response and platelet function in minor surgery during epidural bupivicane and general anesthesia: Effect of epidural morphine addiction. Eur J Anaesthesiol 6:409-417, 1989.
20. Rutberg H, Hakanson E, Anderberg B, Jorfeldt L, Martensson J, Schildt B. Effects of the epidural administration of morphine, or bupivicane, on the adrenocortical response to upper abdominal surgery. Br J Anaesth 56:233-238, 1984.
21. Kehlet H, Brandt MR, Prange-Hansen A, Alberti KFMM. Effects of epidural analgesia on metabolic profiles during and after surgery. Br J Surg 66:543-546, 1979.
22. Bredbacka S, Blomback M, Hagnerik K, Irestedt L, Raabe N. Pre-and postoperative changes in coagulation and fibrinolytic variables during abdominal hysterectomy under epidural or general anesthesia. Acta Anaesthesiol Scand 30:204-210, 1986.
23. Kuitunen A, Hynynem M, Salmenpera M, et al. Anesthesia affects plasma concentrations of vasopressin, von Willebrand factor and coagulation factor VIII in cardiac surgical patients. Br J Anaesth 70:173-180, 1993.
24. Anderson TR, Berner NS, Larsen ML, Odegaard OR, Abildgaard U. Plasma heparin cofactor II, protein C and antithrombin in elective surgery. Acta Chir Scand 153:291-296, 1987.
25. Ardlie NG, Cameron HA, Garrett J. Platelet activation by circulating levels of hormones: A possible link in coronary heart disease. Thromb Res 36:315-322, 1984.
26. Uza G, Crisnic I. Effects of angiotensin II upon platelet adhesiveness and the thrombelastogram in patients with essential arterial hypertension. Pathol Eur 10:327-332, 1975.
27. McDaniel MD, Pearce WH, Yao JST, et al. Sequential changes in coagulation and platelet function following femorotibial bypass. J Vasc Surg 1:261-268, 1984.
28. Flinn WR, McDaniel MS, Yao JST, Fahey VA, Green D. Antithrombin III deficiency as a reflection of dynamic protein metabolism in patients undergoing vascular reconstruction. J Vasc Surg 1:888-895, 1984.
29. Simpson PJ, Radford SG, Lockyear JA. The influence of anaesthesia on the acute phase protein response to surgery. Anaesthesia 42:690-696, 1987.
30. Brandt R, Fernandes A, Mordhorst R, Keblet H. Epidural analgesia improves postoperative nitrogen balance. Br Med J 1:1106-1108, 1978.
31. Prins MH, Hirsh J. A comparison of general anesthesia and regional anesthesia as a risk factor for deep vein thrombosis following hip surgery: A critical review. Thromb Haemost 64:497-500, 1990.
32. Modig J, Borg T, Karlstoem G, Maripuu E, Sahlstedt B. Thromboembolism after total hip replacement: Role of epidural and general anaesthesia. Anaesth Analg 62:174-180, 1983.

33. Thoburn J, Louden JR, Vallarie R. Spinal and general anaesthesia in total hip replacement: Frequency of deep venous thrombosis. Br J Anaesth 52:1117-1121, 1980.
34. Modig J, Hjelmstedt A, Sablstedt B, Maipuu E. Comparative influences of epidural and general anaesthesia on deep vein thrombosis and pulmonary embolism after total hip replacement. Acta Chir Scand 142:125-130, 1981.
35. Sharrock NE, Haas SB, Hargett JM, Urguhart B, Insall JN, Scuderi G. Effects of epidural anesthesia on the incidence of deep-vein thrombosis after total knee arthroplasty. J Bone Joint Surg (Am) 73:502-506, 1991.
36. Jorgensen LN, Rasmussen LS, Nielsen PT, Leffers A, Albrecht-Beste E. Antithrombotic efficacy of continuous extradural analgesia after knee replacement. Br J Anaesth 66:8-12, 1991.
37. Rivers SP, Scher LA, Sheehan E, Veith FJ. Epidural versus general anesthesia for infrainguinal arterial reconstruction. J Vasc Surg 14:764-770, 1991.

34

Optimal Treatment of Vein and Anastomotic Lesions Responsible for Failing Vein Grafts: When Is PTA Appropriate?

LUIS A. SANCHEZ, M.D., WILLIAM D. SUGGS, M.D., MICHAEL L. MARIN, M.D., KURT R. WENGERTER, M.D., and FRANK J. VEITH, M.D.

Advances in vascular surgery and interventional radiology have resulted in improved primary and secondary patency rates for lower extremity bypass grafts with improved limb salvage rates.[1] However, vein grafts have a steady rate of attrition because of thrombosis secondary to the development of graft stenoses. These lesions develop in 11% to 33% of all vein grafts, and it is widely agreed that they should ideally be detected and treated in the "failing state" before they cause graft thrombosis. However, there has been considerable disagreement regarding the best treatment for these lesions.[2-16]

Percutaneous transluminal balloon angioplasty (PTA) is a well-established treatment for stenotic lesions of native arteries. Early successes using PTA in the treatment of certain vein graft stenotic lesions prompted some investigators to use this modality more extensively.[2,3] However, some groups have found angioplasty of vein graft stenoses to be of less value than surgical repair in maintaining the patency of failing vein grafts.[10,11]

Over a 14-year period (January 1, 1980, to December 31, 1993), 87 patients at our institution were found to have patent vein grafts associated with hemodynamically significant graft lesions (intragraft and anastomotic). The treatment modality used (PTA or surgery) was decided by the attending surgeon in consultation with the attending interventional radiologist. PTA was generally used for intragraft and anastomotic lesions less than 5 cm in length, although this criterion was not absolute. Anastomotic lesions were defined as vein graft lesions that occurred within the proximal or distal 2 cm of the graft. Any other lesions were considered to be within the body of the graft. Over the last 4 years of our review, surgery was increasingly used because of the limited success of long-lesion PTA in our own patients and the reported limitations of PTA in the treatment of vein graft lesions.

There were 37 men and 50 women in the study and their ages ranged from 45 to 85 years (mean, 67 years). In all cases critical limb-threatening ischemia was the indication for the initial bypass procedure. A total of 125 lesions within 87 vein grafts were treated over the period reviewed. Ninety-five lesions were treated with PTA and 30 with simple surgical interventions. The patients were monitored for 1 to 82 months after their initial operation, with a mean follow-up of 22 months.

Sixty-four vein grafts in 62 patients (31 men and 31 women) were identified to be in the failing state (20 femoropopliteal, 30 femorodistal, and 14 popliteal-distal). A total of 95 graft lesions were identified and treated: 25 (26%) at the proximal anastomosis, 58 (61%) within the body of the graft, and 12 (13%) at the distal anastomosis. Twelve of the 95 lesions treated had recurred after an initial PTA. Seventy-eight lesions were within reversed saphenous vein grafts, 12 within in situ vein grafts, three within cephalic vein grafts, one within a nonreversed, translocated greater saphenous vein graft, and one within a composite graft of greater and lesser saphenous veins. Sixty-five of the lesions (68%) were first seen within 12 months of the original operation, 73 (77%) within 18 months, 81 (85%) within 2 years, and 14 (15%) more than 2 years after the initial operation.

Lesion and graft characteristics that could

Supported in part by the James Hilton Manning and Emma Austin Manning Foundation, The Anna S. Brown Trust, and the New York Institute for Vascular Studies.

Table 1 Individual life-table comparisons of lesions treated with PTA distributed by individual treatment variables

Variable evaluated	Comparison	Results
Lesion length	<15 mm vs. ≥15 mm	60% vs. 38% patency (12 mo)*
Lesion location	Proximal anastomosis vs. midgraft vs. distal anastomosis	No difference betwen groups when compared separately
Lesion type	Single vs. multiple	59% vs. 29% patency (12 mo)†
	Nonrecurrent vs. recurrent	67% vs. 40% patency (6 mo)*
Minimum vein graft diameter	≥3 mm vs. <3 mm	63% vs. 14% patency (12 mo)†
Combination of variables	Simple vs. complex	66% vs. 17% patency (24 mo)‡

*Nonsignificant trend.
†$p < .05$.
‡$p = .001$.

potentially influence the patency of vein graft lesions after PTA were evaluated (Table 1). These included lesion length (<15 mm vs. ≥15 mm), minimal graft diameter (<3 mm vs. ≥3 mm), lesion location (proximal anastomosis, mid-graft, distal anastomosis), and lesion type (single vs. multiple, recurrent vs. nonrecurrent). In addition, the lesions were divided into two groups: simple and complex. Simple lesions were defined as single, nonrecurrent, less than 15 mm in length, and within vein grafts that were greater than or equal to 3 mm in minimal diameter, whereas complex lesions were multiple, recurrent, greater than or equal to 15 mm in length, or within grafts less than 3 mm in minimal diameter. The initial technical success rate for all PTAs was 95%. There were no deaths associated with PTA but there were three major (two ruptured grafts and one graft occlusion) and four minor complications (localized hematomas).

The 24-month extended patency rate for all lesions treated with PTA was 42%. PTA-treated single vein graft lesions had significantly better ($p < .05$) extended patency rates at 12 months (59%) than PTA-treated multiple lesions (29%). When PTA-treated lesions were compared according to the size of the grafts in which they were present, a significant difference ($p < .05$) was found at 12 months between lesions within grafts that were greater than or equal to 3 mm in minimal diameter (63%) and lesions within grafts less than 3 mm in diameter (14%). Trends that did not reach statistical significance were noted at 12 months when comparing lesions less than 15 mm in length (60%) with lesions greater than or equal to 15 mm in length (38%) and at 6 months when comparing recurrent (40%) and nonrecurrent (67%) lesions. The extended patency rates of proximal anastomotic lesions, midgraft lesions, and distal anastomotic lesions were compared separately. There was no difference at 6 months following PTA. In addition, simple lesions had a significantly better extended patency rate at 24 months (66%) when compared with complex lesions (17%) ($p = .001$) (Fig. 1).

Twenty-five other grafts in 25 patients (19 women and six men) were identified to be in the failing state (seven femoropopliteal, 15 femorodistal, and three popliteal-distal). A total of 30 lesions were identified and surgically treated with extensions or interposition grafts (24 within reversed saphenous vein grafts, three within in situ grafts, two within nonreversed, translocated greater saphenous vein grafts, and one within a composite of two segments of saphenous vein). Eighty percent of the lesions treated were first seen within 18 months of the original operation. There were no deaths associated with the surgical therapy and only one minor complication (wound infection) was noted.

The 21-month extended patency rate of lesions treated surgically (86%) was significantly better than the patency rate for all lesions treated with PTA (42%) ($p < .01$) (Fig. 1). In contrast, there was no significant difference when the 21-month extended patency rates of surgically treated lesions (86%) and simple lesions treated with PTA (66%) were compared ($p = .25$).

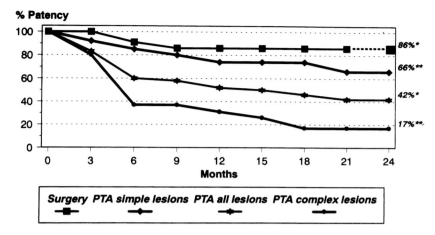

Fig. 1 Cumulative extended patency rates for failing graft lesions treated with surgery. There was a significant difference ($p < .01$) at 21 months between the surgically treated lesions (■, 86%) and all lesions treated with PTA (*, 42%). In addition, a significant difference ($p = .001$) was noted at 24 months when comparing the extended patency rates of simple lesions treated with PTA (♦, 66%) and complex lesions (•, 17%). No significant difference ($p = .25$) was noted between the surgically treated lesions (■, 86%) and the simple lesions (♦, 66%) treated with PTA. (From Sanchez LA, Suggs WD, Marin ML, Panetta TF, Wengerter KR, Veith FJ. Is percutaneous balloon angioplasty appropriate in the treatment of graft and anastomotic lesions responsible for failing vein bypasses. Am J Surg 168:97-101, 1994.)

COMMENTS

Recent studies have suggested that PTA is initially effective in more than 90% of vein graft stenoses.[2-4,10,11] However, lesions treated in this manner appear to have a high recurrence rate and associated poor long-term patency.[10,11] In contrast, studies by Berkowitz et al.[2] and Taylor et al.[3] suggested high initial success rates, lower recurrence rates (25% to 35%), and patency rates greater than 60% at 2 years following PTA. In view of these reports, as well as our earlier large experience with vein graft PTA,[9,14] we evaluated a variety of lesion and graft characteristics that could influence the success of PTA and long-term patency. Lesion length has been considered an important characteristic in the successful PTA of arterial and vein graft lesions.[3,9] A trend suggesting improved patency was noted when lesions less than 15 mm in length (60%) were compared with lesions greater than or equal to 15 mm in length (38%). This trend did not reach statistical significance at 6 months. This fact correlates well with the report by Taylor et al.[3] who suggested that PTA of vein graft lesions less than 1 cm in length results in better late patency rates than those of longer lesions.[3] Single vein graft lesions in our patients had significantly better patency rates at 12 months (59%) compared with multiple lesions (29%). Vein grafts with multiple lesions may be diffusely abnormal and lesion treatment may be followed by early progression of abnormalities elsewhere in the graft leading to failure. In addition, the treatment of sequential lesions is more likely to lead to complications or graft failure because of the additive failure potential of each lesion. Several lesions (<10%) that recurred following a technically successful initial PTA were treated with PTA. A trend that did not reach statistical significance was noted at 6 months with regard to the superiority of patency rates after PTA of primary lesions (67%) as compared with those after PTA of recurrent lesions (40%). Although Whittemore et al.[11] reported poor results with PTA of vein graft lesions, their data suggested favorable results in selected patients with lesions that required a single dilatation. This is consistent with our improved results with single and primary lesions.

We also evaluated the treatment of lesions within small vein grafts. At 12 months there was a significant difference in patency between vein graft lesions treated by PTA within grafts greater than or equal to 3 mm in minimal distended diameter (63%) and those within grafts less than 3 mm in minimal distended diameter (14%) at the time of arteriography for a failing graft. We previously reported that small vein grafts (<3 mm in distended diameter at operation) have a decreased patency rate compared with larger diameter veins.[17] Thus small vein grafts seem to fare poorly with or without any intervention. Berkowitz et al.[2] noted the importance of lesion location when they reported that lesions within reversed saphenous vein grafts were more common in the proximal 4 cm of the graft, including the proximal anastomosis. In addition, they noted that these lesions had better patency after PTA compared with lesions in the body of the graft or at the distal anastomosis. These investigators did not discuss any other factors that might influence the success of PTA. In our series, individual comparisons of lesions were made based on their location (proximal anastomosis, mid-graft, distal anastomosis). If this is the only factor analyzed, there was no difference in patency rates at 6 months following PTA. Finally, multiple factors that could influence vein graft patency were considered together and the lesions treated by PTA were divided into simple and complex groups. Simple lesions (single, nonrecurrent, <15 mm in length, and within vein grafts that were ≥3 mm in minimal diameter) treated with PTA had significantly better patency rates at 24 months (66%) compared with complex lesions (17%).

Surgical revision has been advocated as the treatment of choice for hemodynamically significant vein graft lesions.[4-11,13-16] Over the past 7 years we have treated 30 vein graft lesions with surgical interventions. The 21-month patency rate for the surgically treated lesions (86%) was significantly better than the patency rate for all lesions treated with PTA (42%). This difference is particularly noteworthy in view of the fact that in our series the more difficult lesions were treated surgically. We suspect that comparison of similar lesions subjected to surgery or PTA would reveal an even greater superiority for the surgically treated group. In addition, the morbidity (3.3%) and mortality (0%) rates associated with these surgical interventions were very low. Finally, there was no significant difference at 21 months between the patency rates of lesions treated surgically (86%) and simple lesions treated with PTA (66%). All of these data clearly support the use of surgical interventions to treat vein graft lesions. However, they appear to define a small group of patients that can potentially be treated by PTA with reasonable success, particularly if operative repair is difficult or contraindicated.

The importance of vein graft salvage before thrombosis cannot be overemphasized, especially in patients requiring an arterial reconstruction for limb salvage. Once thrombosis has occurred, complex surgical procedures are required with increased operative morbidity, mortality, and decreased patency.[15,18-20] Efforts to treat thrombosed vein grafts by initial thrombolytic therapy with or without secondary reconstructions of the underlying causative lesions have also been discouraging.[21,22] Early recognition of failing vein grafts requires a protocol of close postoperative surveillance using clinical evaluation and noninvasive testing. Graft-threatening lesions usually are seen within the first 18 months after surgery.[2-11,16] In our series 77% of the lesions were noted within 18 months, 85% within 2 years, and 15% more than 2 years afterward. These observations confirm the importance of noninvasive surveillance during the first 18 to 24 months after the surgical procedure. However, it is also necessary to continue the surveillance after 2 years, since 15% of the lesions will occur after that time and progression of distal or proximal disease becomes an increasingly common cause of vein graft failure.[9]

CONCLUSION

Hemodynamically significant vein graft lesions will lead to vein graft failure. Until further medical advances permit prevention of these lesions, current therapy will continue to be directed toward treatment of the established lesion. Vein graft lesions detected by noninvasive evaluation or by changes in the clinical evaluation should be localized by arteriography and treated with simple surgical interventions using autogenous vein when medically safe and technically feasible. PTA can be used to maintain graft patency until an operation can be safely performed and to treat simple lesions that are difficult to access surgically or in patients with medical contraindications to surgical treatment.

REFERENCES

1. Veith FJ, Gupta SK, Wengerter KR, et al. Changing arteriosclerotic disease patterns and management strategies in lower limb threatening ischemia. Ann Surg 212:402-414, 1990.
2. Berkowitz HD, Fox AD, Deaton DH. Reversed vein graft stenosis: Early diagnosis and management. J Vasc Surg 15:130-142, 1992.
3. Taylor PR, Gould D, Harris P, Al-Kutoubi A, Wolfe JH. Balloon dilation of graft stenoses —reasons for failure. Br J Surg 78:371, 1991.
4. Bandyk DF, Schmitt DD, Seabrook GR, Adams MB, Towne JB. Monitoring functional patency of in situ saphenous vein bypasses: The impact of a surveillance protocol and elective revision. J Vasc Surg 9:286-296, 1989.
5. Taylor PR, Wolfe JHN, Tyrrell MR, Mansfield AO, Nicolaides AN, Houston RE. Graft stenosis: Justification for 1 year surveillance. Br J Surg 77:1125-1128, 1990.
6. Sladen JG, Reid JDS, Cooperberg PL, et al. Color flow duplex screening of infrainguinal grafts combining low- and high-velocity criteria. Am J Surg 158:07-112, 1989.
7. Donaldson MC, Mannick JA, Whittemore AD. Causes of primary graft failure after in situ saphenous vein bypass grafting. J Vasc Surg 15:113-120, 1992.
8. Mills JL, Fujitani RM, Taylor SM. The characteristics and anatomic distribution of lesions that cause reversed vein graft failure: A five year prospective study. J Vasc Surg 17:195-206, 1993.
9. Sanchez LA, Gupta SK, Veith FJ, et al. A ten-year experience with one hundred fifty failing or threatened vein and polytetrafluoroethylene arterial bypass grafts. J Vasc Surg 14:729-738, 1991.
10. Perler BA, Osterman FA, Mitchell SE, Burdick JF, Williams GM. Balloon dilatation versus surgical revision of infrainguinal autogenous vein graft stenoses: Long-term follow-up. J Cardiovasc Surg 31:656-661, 1990.
11. Whittemore AD, Donaldson MC, Polak JF, Mannick JA. Limitations of balloon angioplasty for vein graft stenosis. J Vasc Surg 14:340-345, 1991.
12. O'Mara CS, Flynn WR, Johnson ND, et al. Recognition and surgical management of patent but hemodynamically failed arterial grafts. Ann Surg 193:467-476, 1981.
13. Smith CR, Green RM, DeWeese JA. Pseudoocclusion of femoropopliteal bypass grafts. Circulation 68(Suppl II):88-93, 1983.
14. Veith FJ, Weiser RK, Gupta SK, et al. Diagnosis and management of failing lower extremity arterial reconstructions prior to graft occlusion. J Cardiovasc Surg 25:381-384, 1984.
15. Cohen JR, Mannick JA, Couch NP, Whittemore AD. Recognition and management of impending vein-graft failure. Arch Surg 121:758-759, 1986.
16. Berkowitz HD, Greenstein SM. Improved patency in reversed femoral-infrapopliteal autogenous vein grafts by early detection and treatment of the failing graft. J Vasc Surg 5:755-761, 1987.
17. Wengerter KR, Veith FJ, Gupta SK, et al. Prospective randomized multicenter comparison of in situ and reversed vein infrapopliteal bypasses. J Vasc Surg 13:189-199, 1991.
18. Veith FJ, Gupta SK, Ascer E, et al. Improved strategies for secondary operations on infrainguinal arteries. Ann Vasc Surg 3:85-93, 1990.
19. Bartlett ST, Olinde AJ, Flinn WR, et al. The reoperative potential of infrainguinal bypass: Long-term limb and patient survival. J Vasc Surg 5:170-179, 1987.
20. Whittemore AD, Clowes AW, Couch NP, Mannick JA. Secondary femoropopliteal reconstruction. Ann Surg 193:35-42, 1981.
21. Gardiner GA, Harrington DP, Koltun W, et al. Salvage of occluded arterial bypass grafts by means of thrombolysis. J Vasc Surg 9:426-431, 1989.
22. Belkin M, Donaldson MC, Whittemore AD, Polak VF, Grassi CJ, Harrington DP, Mannick JA. Observations on the use of thrombolytic agents for thrombotic occlusion of infrainguinal vein grafts. J Vasc Surg 11:289-296, 1990.

35

The Superficial Femoral Vein as a Bypass Graft: Indications, Techniques, Results, Morbidity, and "Spinoffs"

MARTIN L. SCHULMAN, M.D., and LEE G. SCHULMAN, M.D.

Use of deep veins of the thigh and knee (DLVs) as arterial grafts in the lower extremity is not a new concept. We are aware of their placement in 21 limbs prior to our first use of these grafts in 1974. Goyanes[1] used the popliteal vein to replace a popliteal aneurysm in 1906. Fontaine and Hubinont[2] used 10 DLVs as femoropopliteal (FPB) grafts in 1950. In Kunlin's[3] report of 17 FPB grafts in 1951, a segment of superficial femoral vein (SFV) was used to lengthen a saphenous vein graft. Two obstructed superficial femoral arteries were replaced with SFVs by Julian et al.[4] in 1952. Concerns about weakness of the vein wall, which have proved to be unfounded in our experience, prompted Palma[5] to wrap two SFVs in the adventitia of the native arteries in 1960. Ejrup et al.,[6] in 1961, reported early atherosclerotic changes in a SFV recovered at autopsy 39 months after insertion. In 1970 Awe and Krippaehne,[7] in a report that inspired our use of DLVs, described the use of four SFV segments as FPB grafts. Although follow-up was limited in most reports, no significant lower extremity sequelae were noted in the five extremities followed for more than 2 years.

This report is based on the use of 152 DLVs as FPB grafts over a 20-year period. It will focus on five areas: indications, techniques, results, morbidity, and derivative information or "spinoffs."

INDICATIONS

We have been committed to the use of autogenous veins for infrainguinal reconstruction since 1964. During that time, 1003 infrainguinal bypasses were performed, with prosthetic materials used in only 7% of cases.

Indications for the use of DLVs have gradually expanded over the past 20 years. From 1974 to 1979, six DLVs were used after both the greater saphenous vein and the veins of one arm were found to be unavailable. Use of arm veins was abandoned in 1979, and over the next 2 years 14 additional DLVs were used when both saphenous veins were rejected. A series comparing greater saphenous and DLVs was carried out from 1981 to 1985, and during that period 65 grafts were used.[8] Since 1985, during a period of selective preferential DLV use with saphenous preservation, 67 grafts were employed.[9]

During most of this experience, graft use was restricted to limbs with critical ischemia. Ten grafts were recently placed in claudicants.

For those acquiring initial experience with DLVs, a small patient with unavailable saphenous veins requiring a primary FPB for limb salvage is ideal.

Contraindications

DLVs should not be used in secondary bypasses, because the veins become adherent to prior anastomotic sites and the reoperative experience is both difficult and traumatic. The common femoral vein should never be resected and tibial veins should not be used as bypass grafts. All of our infrainguinal reconstructions using DLVs have been FPBs and most have included the popliteal vein; concerns about disparity in vessel diameter have made us reluctant to use these large grafts for tibial reconstruction.

TECHNIQUES

Resection of the major thigh, knee, and upper calf veins is an essentially straightforward dissection, and relatively few changes have been made since our first operation in 1974.[9] Two principles essential to successful graft use have remained constant: the shortest possible bypass is performed (superficial femoral or deep femoral origins were used in three fourths of patients) and the deep femoral vein is always preserved. A third tenet, adopted in 1985, is the construction of moderately tapered 3 cm proximal and distal anastomoses[10]; this will be discussed under "Spinoffs."

Either one long medial incision or two incisions with a short intervening skin bridge are used. As a result of the additional time spent for DLV resection and construction of long anastomoses, operating time is increased by approximately 45 minutes in comparison to that needed for saphenous veins. To facilitate popliteal vein exposure during harvest, the adductor magnus and medial tendons at the knee are usually transected. Although no repair is carried out, limb function is unimpaired.

Grafts may be placed in the nonreversed position following valve ablation, or, as was done in most cases, reversed. On four occasions additional graft length was obtained without incident by including the tibioperoneal trunk[11]; in those situations valves were ablated and grafts placed in the nonreversed position to avoid the size disparity that would have occurred if the most proximal SFV were anastomosed to the smaller popliteal artery.

Unlike the in situ saphenous operation, no special instruments or techniques are necessary for DLV bypass. An obvious exception is the valve ablation required when nonreversed graft placement is chosen.

Because the SFV originates 8 cm distal to the superficial femoral artery, even a graft that includes the superficial femoral, popliteal, and tibioperoneal veins will not be long enough for a bypass from the common femoral to the most distal popliteal artery. Fortunately, only one patient has been encountered in whom it was not possible to either use a distal graft origin or anastomose the graft to a more proximal portion of the popliteal artery. In that unique situation an endarterectomy and patch graft of the origin of the profunda femoris artery allowed a bypass from the profunda femoris distal to the patch to the farthest popliteal artery.

In our early experience an average size for each DLV was calculated by filling each graft with heparin-saline solution, measuring its length, and calculating the fluid capacity per centimeter.[12] We now believe that reduced graft ischemic time is desirable. To that end, arterial exposures are performed before vein resection and, after harvest, the graft is used immediately without placing it in storage solution or taking measurements.

In patients in whom DLVs are used preferentially,[9] several additional technical points are pertinent. When a distal graft origin is planned, as is usually the case, dissection of the groin lymphatic vessels is avoided by starting the proximal incision 5 to 8 cm below the inguinal ligament, at the level of origin of the SFV. No attempt is made to explore the saphenous vein but when it is encountered, great care is taken to avoid injury and preserve it for future use.

One group has used SFVs in situ for FPB. We would caution against that approach, since the vein has many deep branches and a late arteriovenous fistula deep in the thigh would present significant problems and negate any potential benefit from in situ use. As a practical matter, carefully reviewing reports of DLV use will facilitate early experience and enhance late results.[8-12]

RESULTS

How can the intrinsic value of any graft or technique for femoropopliteal bypass be determined? The four parameters by which a comprehensive evaluation may be made are: (1) statistical data (cumulative life-table method patency rates), (2) examination of late graft structural changes (aneurysmal degeneration), (3) randomized comparison with reversed saphenous vein grafts, and (4) analysis of graft failures. Other factors that might influence the selection of one graft over another but are not measures of intrinsic graft function are late limb morbidity, ease of insertion, prior experience of the operator, resistance to infection, expense, ease of revision, and availability.

Statistical Data

Life-table patency rates for the most recent 97 primary FPBs using DLVs are shown in Fig. 1 and Table 1. Although the 97 bypasses include several potentially avoidable failures caused by distal anastomotic hyperplasia (DAH) when short anastomoses were constructed,[10] the primary and secondary patency rates of 82% and 90%, respectively, at 5 years, with 35 grafts followed for that length of time, compare favorably with reported saphenous vein results.

Table 1 Patency rates for FPB using DLVs

Interval (mo)	At risk	Failed	Duration	Lost	Death	Interval patency	Cumulative patency	Standard error (%)*
Primary patency of 97 DLVs used as FPB grafts								
0-1	97	3	0	0	2	.9688	.9688	1.7
2-12	92	10	8	0	6	.8824	.8549	3.5
13-24	68	0	0	2	6	1.000	.8549	4.1
25-36	60	2	0	0	6	.9649	.8249	4.5
37-48	52	0	0	2	8	1.000	.8249	4.9
49-60	42	0	3	2	2	1.000	.8249	5.3
Secondary patency of 97 DLVs used as FPB grafts								
0-1	97	2	0	0	2	.9792	.9792	1.5
2-12	93	4	10	0	7	.9527	.9329	2.5
13-24	72	0	0	2	6	1.000	.9329	2.8
25-36	64	2	1	0	7	.9667	.9018	3.5
37-48	54	0	0	2	8	1.000	.9018	3.8
49-60	44	0	3	2	2	1.000	.9018	4.3

*Calculated in accordance with Rutherford RB, Flanigan DP, Gupta SK, et al. Suggested standards for reports dealing with lower extremity ischemia. J Vasc Surg 4:80-94, 1986.

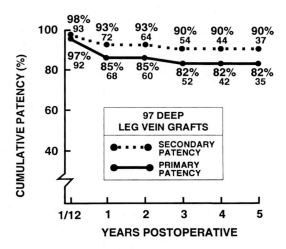

Fig. 1 Primary and secondary patency rates of 97 primary FPBs using DLVs. Each time interval shows the number and percentage of grafts observed to be patent for that length of time.

Late Structural Changes

As might be expected with autogenous tissue, there were no anastomotic aneurysms. The only instance of aneurysmal change was detected on routine postoperative angiography in an asymptomatic patient in the eighth postoperative year; it was not treated and the graft was patent when the patient died 2 years later.

Comparative Series

A prospective, randomized series comparing reversed saphenous vein bypass with another graft or technique is probably the best single indicator of the value of that graft or technique. Unfortunately the randomized comparative series of DLVs and reversed saphenous veins reported in 1987 was fundamentally flawed.[8] It was started too early in our DLV experience; significant changes in graft use were made during the course of the study. Although there was no difference in patency rates of DLVs and reversed saphenous veins at 3 years, the value of DLVs vis-à-vis saphenous veins still awaits a randomized comparative study by investigators skilled in both techniques.

Analysis of Graft Failures

As part of a program of periodic postoperative angiographic follow-up of grafts, 537 conventional femoral arteriograms were performed on 125 DLVs. This enabled us to observe late graft changes and, in most instances, draw highly informed conclusions regarding the cause of failure. In some cases, however, either because appropriately timed arteriograms were not available or because several processes were occurring simultaneously, the mechanism was less certain and the conclusions drawn less firm. Primary failure occurred in 15 of the 97 grafts.

Two of the three failures within the first

month were the result of errors in judgment. One patient was, in retrospect, clearly inoperable. Another graft, brought to a proximal portion of the popliteal artery, occluded postoperatively but was salvaged with a distal graft extension. The third early failure was presumed to be technical in origin.

There were 10 primary failures between 1 month and 1 year. Seven were caused by DAH, which was detected more often on follow-up angiography than by noninvasive testing. In two additional grafts failure was attributed to progression of distal disease during the first year. The remaining failure was believed to be embolic in origin; the patient had atrial fibrillation and, subsequent to the occlusion, pedal pulses returned suggesting that recanalization had occurred.

The two failures in the third year were due to progression of distal disease. One was in a graft to an above-knee isolated popliteal segment, and the other was in a small female patient with hypoplastic vessels.

It is important to examine the incidence of *intrinsic* graft failure in this series, that is, failures caused by changes within the graft itself. None of the perioperative failures were intrinsic, but 7 of the 10 failures between 1 month and 1 year were—that is, they were caused by DAH. Both of the third year failures were *extrinsic*, occurring after popliteal occlusion.

It has been shown, primarily in saphenous aortocoronary bypass grafts, that graft atherosclerosis is a significant cause of late saphenous occlusion.[13] The development of atherosclerosis was also detected angiographically in DLVs, but at a rate that may be slower than that in saphenous grafts. Testimony to this delayed progression of atherosclerosis is the fact that in this group of 97 grafts, none of the occlusions during the first 5 years were due to graft atherosclerosis. We have, however, seen atherosclerosis as a cause of intrinsic failure in grafts followed more than 5 years.

MORBIDITY

The evaluation of morbidity after resection of major knee and thigh veins may be approached from three perspectives: first and foremost is clinical evaluation of the limbs; second, results of laboratory tests may be examined; and third, one may review the literature relating to late sequelae in limbs in which major deep veins have

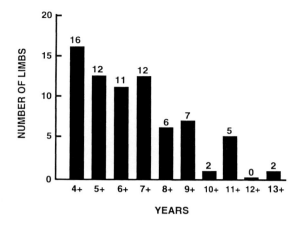

Fig. 2 Periods of observation of 73 limbs with DLV resection.

been ligated after isolated venous trauma or in the treatment or prophylaxis of pulmonary embolism.

Clinical Evaluation

A major concern during our early cautious use of DLVs was the possibility of significant late morbidity after resection of the principal venous trunks at the knee and thigh. That concern, coupled with the absence of data regarding late graft changes and patency, tempered our initial enthusiasm. Careful observation of these patients over a 20-year period, with 73 limbs followed for more than 4 and as long as 13 years (Fig. 2), leads to the conclusion that significant late morbidity as a result of DLV resection does not occur. If late morbidity were to occur, it would take the form of swelling, ulceration, or stasis changes.

Swelling. Since 1981, ankle circumference measurements of operated and unoperated control limbs have been taken at each follow-up visit in all patients. As shown in Fig. 3, the increase in the ankle circumference of operated vs. nonoperated limbs was greater with DLVs compared to saphenous veins at all time points. With both grafts, however, edema gradually receded and that improvement has been maintained in patients followed for as long as 13 years. Mild-to-moderate late lymphedema was seen in an occasional DLV limb (and rarely in a saphenous vein limb) but has not been a clinical problem. Although salt restriction was advised, no active

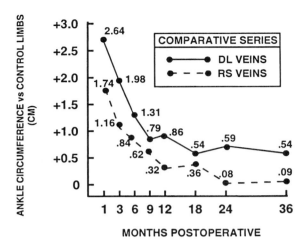

Fig. 3 Ankle circumferences in reversed saphenous vein and DLV limbs vs. contralateral unoperated control limbs (data taken from comparative series[8]). Numbers indicate the average increase in ankle circumference at each time interval.

therapy with diuretics or elastic support was employed. More significantly, in response to specific questioning, none of the patients complained of any disability caused by late leg swelling, and in the few limbs with late edema no stasis changes or ulceration were present.

Ulceration. In one patient an intractable and painful ankle ulcer caused by combined arterial and venous insufficiency was the indication for bypass. Although ulcer healing was prolonged, pain was relieved immediately. The only instance of new stasis ulceration was in the seventh postoperative year in a patient who had stasis changes preoperatively. It healed rapidly with compression bandaging.

Stasis Changes. Stasis changes in the form of ankle induration and discoloration were present in several patients preoperatively. With the exception of the patient mentioned in the preceding paragraph, no worsening of these changes occurred. New stasis changes were seen in one patient whose popliteal vein was thickened at surgery and in whom extensive calf vein phlebitis was demonstrated at venography 6 months postoperatively. No patient developed a thickened, indurated, and discolored lower extremity, bolstering our belief that postphlebitic changes are caused by venous reflux rather than the absence of major venous conduits.

Laboratory Testing

Schanzer et al.[14] investigated functional changes in 25 limbs following DLV resection and compared them with changes in a control group of 22 extremities in which saphenous vein or polytetrafluoroethylene (PTFE) was used for FPB. The groups were comparable in terms of age, sex, and time from surgery to the venous testing. There was no significant increase in early or late swelling in the DLV group. Plethysmographic examination showed a pattern consistent with venous outflow obstruction in 21 (84%) of 25 DLV extremities and in 11 (50%) of 22 control limbs. Thus, although an obstructive pattern was more frequent in DLV limbs, there were no significant clinical differences between the two groups.

Review of the Literature

The fact that late sequelae occur so infrequently is not surprising.[15] All evidence purporting to show the dangers of resecting or ligating these veins is flawed in one of three areas.

Early vs. Late Results. In 1976 Rich et al.[16] reported edema in 51% of ligations and 13% of repairs of 110 isolated popliteal vein injuries. No time frame for these observations was given; only 28 patients were seen in the "late follow-up period." The 51% and 13% figures were repeated in 10 different reports with no deviation from the original data.[15] It appears that Rich et al.[16] were reporting their early observations; in addition to the absence of specific follow-up data, it is not possible to follow 110 patients with any dynamic vascular problem and find no change in results over 10 years. Most other reports of lower extremity venous trauma also present only early results; their analysis is further complicated by the failure to separate isolated venous injuries from more complex injuries, and the tendency to group common femoral, superficial femoral, and other venous injuries of the lower extremity together. In those reports presenting late data, morbidity after isolated superficial femoral and popliteal vein ligation was minimal or absent.[15,17]

Superficial Femoral or Popliteal vs. More Proximal Venous Ligations. In the late 1940s, common femoral or SFV ligation was performed frequently for venous thrombosis or prophylacticly to prevent pulmonary embolism.[18-21] In patients with established deep phlebitis, SFV ligation resulted in fewer sequelae than common femoral or vena cava ligation.[18,19] There was no morbidity from prophylactic SFV ligation.[21] The venographic studies of Szilagyi and Alsop[20] showed that, following SFV ligation, thrombosis of the SFV occurred in 57% and thrombosis of the popliteal vein occurred in 32% of limbs. Authors correlating postligation edema with length of follow-up noted progressive limb improvement,[20,21] paralleling our observations after DLV resection. Confirmation of these earlier studies has been provided by Masuda et al.[22] who reported minimal morbidity in 35 limbs followed for an average of 13.5 years after SFV ligation for acute or chronic venous disease.

"Postphlebitic" vs. Otherwise Normal Limbs. Results of attempts to relieve symptoms in postphlebitic limbs by resecting deep veins and observations derived from patients with established chronic venous insufficiency cannot be used to predict late sequelae in limbs from which normal veins have been removed.[23,24] The misnamed "postphlebitic syndrome" has a variety of causes, and ligation or resection of normal superficial femoral and popliteal veins has never been shown to be one of them.

DERIVATIVE INFORMATION OR "SPINOFFS"

Although our advocacy of DLVs as FPB grafts has not been widely accepted, this work has yielded considerable derivative information and has inspired others to use DLVs in brilliantly innovative ways. These areas will be described briefly.

Distal Anastomotic Hyperplasia

Early in our experience, when blunt 2 cm ("cobra head") anastomoses were constructed, DAH was noted on routine follow-up angiography in 31% of limbs. With 3 cm moderately tapered ("fish mouth") anastomoses, the incidence of DAH was reduced to 8%.[10] Despite voluminous literature, the cause of DAH is unknown. We have, however, demonstrated in patients that by diluting whatever the etiologic factors are (i.e., by anastomotic lengthening), the incidence of DAH can be significantly reduced. Another fascinating observation was that with long anastomoses the only patients who developed DAH were diabetic females.

It is also important to point out that intimal hyperplasia of the graft body, the most common cause of saphenous graft failure, is not seen in DLVs. Conversely, the hyperplastic lesions found at DLV distal anastomoses are rarely seen in saphenous grafts.[10] Although reasons for the difference are unknown, it is clear that saphenous veins and DLVs develop different hyperplastic lesions when placed in the arterial system.

Anatomy and "Unusual" Grafts

Although undescribed in anatomy texts, in 7% of limbs the popliteal vein drains into the profunda femoris vein, and the SFV is a smaller vein originating in the distal thigh (Fig. 4).[11] This anomaly was responsible for 11 grafts in this series; one nondominant SFV, used as a short graft, and 10 profunda femoris–popliteal veins used as FPB grafts. Other "unusual" DLVs employed were two nondominant profunda femoris veins, two contralateral SFVs, and four tibioperoneal trunks. Results achieved with these grafts did not differ from those with superficial femoropopliteal veins.

Two "unusual" grafts were unacceptable: early postoperative hemorrhage necessitated removal of a posterior tibial vein, and common femoral vein resection was associated with excessive edema, wound slough, and eventual graft hemorrhage. Based on these two misadventures, we suggest these veins not be used as grafts.

Saphenous Hypertrophy

In seven cases in which DLVs were used preferentially, preserved saphenous veins (saphenous "spare tires") were later harvested as arterial grafts. All were superb—thin-walled and at least 5 mm in diameter—indicating that saphenous hypertrophy occurs after DLV resection. Additional evidence suggesting saphenous enlargement after DLV resection was provided by two patients in whom "spare tires" were removed from one limb and normal saphenous veins from the other. In contrast to the superb quality of the "spare tires," one normal saphenous vein was too small to use and the other was a thickened but usable 4 mm vein. Patency has been maintained in all of these grafts, with an average follow-up of 5.4 years.

Morbidity

The finding that, with the exception of occasional mild-to-moderate edema, there is no significant late limb morbidity after DLV resection and the observation that swelling, when present,

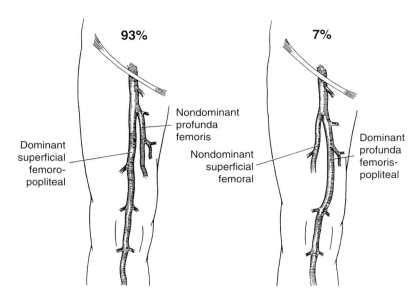

Fig. 4 Anatomy of major thigh and knee veins. The profunda femoris–popliteal vein, present in 7% of limbs, follows a variable deep intermuscular course but is always accessible through a long medial incision.

recedes rather than increases with time, strongly support two concepts that are rapidly gaining acceptance: (1) stasis changes are caused primarily by venous reflux and not by the absence or complete obstruction of major venous channels,[25] and (2) edema after lower extremity arterial reconstruction is lymphatic not venous in origin.[26] (When harvesting DLVs, it is impossible to avoid trauma to the superficial lymphatic vessels of the thigh, which course in the medial subcutaneous tissues, and to the deep lymphatics, which accompany the superficial femoral and popliteal vessels.[27])

We have stressed the importance of preserving the deep femoral vein. One exception has been made, however, and that exception serves to illustrate the remarkable resiliency of the lower extremity venous system.[28]

Case Report

A 67-year-old man with diabetes underwent a right femorotibial bypass using the right greater saphenous vein. Three months later a stenosis in the right saphenous graft was bypassed using the left deep femoral vein (the left greater saphenous vein had been used for coronary bypass). Two months later the left superficial femoropopliteal-tibioperoneal vein was used as a left FPB graft. No unusual swelling of the left leg was noted postoperatively. The patient died 13 months after the last operation. Just prior to death, both legs were healed and pain free, but mild ankle edema was present bilaterally (left ankle circumference 1.4 cm greater than right).

There are several possible explanations for the absence of late morbidity in a limb from which every major vein below the common femoral has been removed. They are as follows: (1) there was insufficient time postoperatively for postphlebitic changes to occur; (2) limited distal runoff resulted in reduced flow rates that could be accommodated by the available venous collaterals; or (3) the venous resections were staged, without which early morbidity might have been prohibitive. Although all of the previous explanations may have been operative to some extent, we believe the benign course observed in the donor limb is best explained by a more fundamental concept—that is, the reserve and regenerative capacity of the normal (i.e., nonrefluxive) venous system is much greater than is generally appreciated, and that inherent capacity was the single most important factor in the ability of the limb to tolerate these extensive venous resections.

Autogenous Strategy

Extensive use of these grafts has been an integral part of an overall autogenous strategy. The increasing use of DLVs without reservation has led to a marked reduction in the use of prostheses. In 114 of 115 recent infrainguinal reconstructions, it was possible to use autogenous lower extremity veins exclusively (superficial femoral, superficial femoral-popliteal, profunda femoris–popliteal, profunda femoris, and greater and lesser saphenous).

Alternative Graft Uses

Others have used DLVs as arterial and venous grafts in a variety of innovative ways.

Arterial Grafts. Clagett et al.[29] reported the extraordinary performance of DLVs used to replace infected abdominal aortic grafts. Clagett created neoaortoiliac systems in 20 patients using DLVs, greater saphenous veins, or both. With a mean follow-up of 22.5 months, patency of greater saphenous veins and DLVs was 34% and 100%, respectively. Failure of saphenous veins was caused by diffuse neointimal hyperplasia; consonant with what was stated earlier in this report, neointimal hyperplasia of the graft body was not seen in DLVs. In patients whose DLVs were harvested, limb edema and other signs of venous hypertension were minimal. Nevelsteen et al.[30] reported four patients treated with a similar operation; after a mean follow-up of 6 months, all grafts were patent and there were no signs or symptoms of chronic venous stasis.

SFVs have also been used as the distal component of composites for tibial bypass, as replacements for infected femorofemoral grafts, in vascular access procedures, as popliteal aneurysm replacements, for iliofemoral and femorofemoral bypass, and as replacements for prostheses in the repair of false aneurysms.

Venous Grafts. DLVs have the potential to be ideal replacements in the venous system. Their large caliber, adequate length, and autogenous nature offer distinct advantages when compared with spiral saphenous grafts and prosthetic materials.

Gladstone et al.[31] used SFVs to bypass obstructed superior venae cavae in five patients. With follow-up periods of less than 1 year, all grafts were patent and postoperative edema was not a problem. Successful use of the SFV to replace the internal jugular, inferior vena cava, and portal vein was reported by Schanzer et al.[14]

CONCLUSION

Deep veins of the thigh and knee should be viewed as potential spare parts. Their use as FPB grafts has markedly reduced the need for prostheses, without incurring significant late morbidity. Primary and secondary patency rates were 82% and 90%, respectively, at 5 years. In addition, this work demonstrates that DAH can be reduced by constructing long anastomoses, provides evidence of the remarkable reserve and regenerative capacity of the lower extremity venous system, and helps confirm the lymphatic origin of postreconstruction edema. It has also inspired others to use DLVs successfully to replace infected abdominal aortic grafts and as grafts in the venous system.

REFERENCES

1. Goyanes J. El Siglo Med 53:561, 1906.
2. Fontaine R, Hubinont J. Le traitement des obliterations arterielles par autogreffes fraiches et segmentaires de veines. Acta Chir Bel 4:397-427, 1950.
3. Kunlin J. Le traitement de l'ischemie arteritique par la greffe veineuse longue. Rev Chir 70:206-235, 1951.
4. Julian OC, Dye WS, Olwin JH, et al. Direct surgery of arteriosclerosis. Ann Surg 136:459-474, 1952.
5. Palma EC. Treatment of arteritis of the lower limbs by autogenous vein grafts. Minerva Cardioangiol Eur 8:36-49, 1960.
6. Ejrup B, Hiertonn T, Moberg A. Atheromatous changes in autogenous venous grafts. Acta Chir Scand 121:211-218, 1961.
7. Awe WC, Krippaehne WW. Use of the superficial femoral vein for femoropopliteal bypass. Am J Surg 120:149-152, 1970.
8. Schulman ML, Badhey MR, Yatco R. Superficial femoral-popliteal veins and reversed saphenous veins as primary femoropopliteal bypass grafts: A randomized comparative study. J Vasc Surg 6:1-10, 1987.
9. Schulman ML, Badhey MR, Yatco R, Pillari G. A saphenous alternative: Preferential use of superficial femoral and popliteal veins as femoropopliteal bypass grafts. Am J Surg 152:231-236, 1986.
10. Schulman ML, Badhey MR, Schulman LG, Lledo-Perez AM. Distal anastomotic hyperplasia in superficial femoral-popliteal vein femoropopliteal bypass grafts. Vasc Surg 25:618-627, 1991.
11. Schulman ML, Schulman LG, Lledo-Perez AM. Unusual autogenous vein grafts. Vasc Surg 26:257-264, 1992.
12. Schulman ML, Badhey MR, Yatco R, Pillari G. An 11-year experience with deep leg veins as femoropopliteal bypass grafts. Arch Surg 121:1010-1015, 1986.
13. Campeau L, Enjalbert M, Lesperance J, et al. Atherosclerosis and late closure of aortocoronary saphenous vein grafts: Sequential angiographic studies at 2 weeks, 1 year, 5 to 7 years, and 10 to 12 years after surgery. Circulation 68(Suppl II):11-1–II-7, 1983.
14. Schanzer H, Chiang K, Mabrouk M, Peirce EC III. Use of lower extremity deep veins as arterial substitutes: Functional status of the donor leg. J Vasc Surg 14:624-627, 1991.
15. Schulman ML, Schulman LG. Deep leg veins as femoropopliteal bypass grafts. World J Surg 14:843-846, 1990.

16. Rich NM, Hobson RW, Collins GJ, Andersen CA. The effect of acute popliteal venous interruption. Ann Surg 183:365-368, 1976.
17. Timberlake GA, O'Connell RC, Kerstein MD. Venous injury: To repair or ligate, the dilemma. J Vasc Surg 4:553-558, 1986.
18. Robinson JR, Moyer CA. Comparison of late sequelae of common and superficial femoral vein ligations. Surgery 35:690-694, 1954.
19. Nabatoff RA, Blum L, Touroff ASW. Long-term sequelae of common femoral vein ligation in the treatment of thromboembolic disease. Surgery 67:272, 1970.
20. Szilagyi DE, Alsop JF. Early and late sequelae of therapeutic vein ligation for thrombosis of veins of lower limbs. Arch Surg 59:633-666, 1949.
21. Allen AW. The present evaluation of the prophylaxis and treatment of venous thrombosis and pulmonary embolism. Surgery 26:1-7, 1949.
22. Masuda EM, Kistner RL, Ferris EB III. Long-term effects of superficial femoral vein ligation: Thirteen-year follow-up. J Vasc Surg 16:741-749, 1992.
23. Bauer G. The etiology of leg ulcers and their treatment by resection of the popliteal vein. J Int Chir 8:937-967, 1948.
24. Linton RR, Hardy IB Jr. Postthrombotic sequelae of the lower extremity. Treatment by superficial femoral vein interruption and stripping of the saphenous vein. Surg Clin North Am 27:1171-1177, 1947.
25. Labropoulos N, Leon M, Nicolaides AN, et al. Venous reflux in patients with previous deep venous thrombosis: Correlation with ulceration and other symptoms. J Vasc Surg 20:20-26, 1994.
26. AbuRahma AF, Woodruff BA, Lucente FC. Edema after femoropopliteal bypass surgery: Lymphatic and venous theories of causation. J Vasc Surg 11:461-467, 1990.
27. Pflug JJ, Calnan JS. The normal anatomy of the lymphatic system in the human leg. Br J Surg 58:925-930, 1971.
28. Schulman ML, Schulman LG. Extended vein graft donation from a single lower extremity. J Vasc Surg 12:631-632, 1990.
29. Clagett GP, Bowers BL, Lopez-Viego MA, et al. Creation of a neo-aortoiliac system from lower extremity deep and superficial veins. Ann Surg 218:239-249, 1993.
30. Nevelsteen A, Lacroix H, Suy R. The superficial femoral vein as autogenous conduit in the treatment of prosthetic arterial infection. Ann Vasc Surg 7:556-560, 1993.
31. Gladstone DJ, Pillai R, Paneth M, Lincoln JCR. Relief of superior vena caval syndrome with autologous femoral vein used as a bypass graft. J Thorac Cardiovasc Surg 89:750-752, 1985.

36

Free Flaps in Association With Distal Bypasses to Extend Limb Salvage

RICHARD M. GREEN, M.D., and JOSEPH M. SERLETTI, M.D.

Arterial bypass alone is insufficient for complete lower extremity reconstruction in patients with exposed tendon or bone proximal to the metatarsal-phalangeal joints. Amputation is required for these severely ischemic wounds of the distal leg, ankle, and proximal foot. During the past 44 months, 30 patients at the University of Rochester Medical Center in whom primary amputation would have potentially compromised either independent activity or ambulation were chosen for vascular reconstruction with free tissue transfer. The patients were selected by an interdisciplinary team of plastic surgeons, vascular surgeons, and orthopedic surgeons. All 30 patients ambulated independently prior to the development of their soft tissue defects. Combined vascular reconstruction with free tissue transfer for coverage of these wounds permits extended limb salvage in this population as well as others reported in the literature.[1-6]

PATIENT SELECTION

Twenty-one patients were diabetic and had evidence of significant bilateral occlusive disease. Five of these patients had a prior contralateral amputation. The remaining nine patients had atherosclerosis alone and were stratified into two subgroups based on the severity of their medical illnesses using criteria established by the American Society of Anesthesiologists (ASA classification).[7] There were four patients in ASA classes I to III who refused amputation and five in ASA class IV or V who were believed to be unlikely to function independently with a major amputation. One of these patients had a prior amputation.

All 30 patients had ischemic wounds of the lower extremity with significant bone, tendon, and/or joint exposure and arterial reconstruction, and minor amputation or split-thickness skin grafting would not have resulted in a functional and stable lower extremity. Thirteen patients had a concomitant diagnosis of osteomyelitis confirmed by bone biopsy. Preference was given whenever possible to simultaneous vascular and free soft tissue reconstruction.

VASCULAR PROCEDURES

Arterial reconstructions were performed to revascularize the lower extremity with a direct connection into a vessel perfusing the foot. The distal anastomosis was placed at a site that could also be used for attachment to the free flap whenever possible. Autogenous venous bypasses were performed to the popliteal artery in six patients and the infrapopliteal arteries in 18. Grafts were reversed or left in situ based on the characteristics of the vein and the preference of the operating surgeon. Five patients lacked an adequate outflow vessel and the distal anastomosis of the vein graft was placed directly into the free flap artery. One patient underwent an aortobifemoral reconstruction for iliac occlusive disease. Patients were followed by monitoring independent Doppler signals for both the bypass graft and the free flap. Aspirin (325 mg) was given to all patients 1 day before the operation and was continued throughout the follow-up period. The 18 patients who underwent infrapopliteal bypasses were treated with heparin during the operation and for 5 days postoperatively.

FREE FLAPS

Specific flaps were selected for the quality of the donor vessels and the length of reliable soft tissue and to minimize contour deformity. Wounds of the foot required thick durable skin, whereas calf wounds often required muscle bulk. The free flap donor tissues included the rectus abdominis muscle, the latissimus dorsi muscle, the radial forearm flap, the scapular flap, and the omentum. Inflow to the flap was directly from the bypass graft in 15 of the 18 patients who underwent infrapopliteal vascular reconstruction. Five patients with nonreconstructible distal vascular disease had an end-to-end microarterial anastomosis to a proximal vein graft. In the remaining 10 patients the reperfused anterior or posterior tibial artery closest to the wound was used. Outflow (venous anastomosis) for the flap was from the tibial vein closest to the soft-tissue defect.

RESULTS

There were no in-hospital deaths. The major morbidity was congestive heart failure in six patients. Hospitalization for all patients from the day of admission to the day of discharge averaged 50 days (range, 9 to 119 days). Hospitalization after free flap reconstruction was 33 days (range, 4 to 102 days). Patients in ASA classes I to III had a mean stay of 18 days; patients in ASA class IV or V were hospitalized for an average of 60 days. Diabetic patients were hospitalized for a mean of 53 days and patients with a prior contralateral below-knee amputation required 77 days of hospitalization.

The combined procedures were initially successful in 27 of these 30 patients. The three immediate failures resulted in below-knee amputations. Each failure occurred because of inadequate outflow for the arterial reconstruction. Twenty-two of the 27 patients with successful operations walked independently over the mean follow-up period of 22 months (range, 5 to 44 months). Twelve of the 22 independently ambulating patients required the following minor secondary procedures: drainage of recipient site hematomas in three, donor site hematomas in two, redebridement of an osteomyelitis in two, limited repeat skin grafts in three, delayed toe amputation in two, and flap debulking in one. Five of these 22 ambulating patients developed contralateral lower extremity ischemic disease requiring intervention. Four of these five patients underwent contralateral lower extremity revascularization and two of these four had a subsequent contralateral below-knee amputation. Each continued to ambulate independently with the reconstructed lower extremity and a contralateral prosthesis. One patient had a contralateral transmetatarsal amputation and continued to ambulate independently.

Five patients with successful reconstructions had ongoing infection and ischemia in the adjacent (nonflap) soft tissues. Each of these patients had the vein graft anastomosed directed only into the free flap artery. Although the arterial reconstruction remained patent in each instance, these patients all required a delayed below-knee amputation and none regained the ability to ambulate.

FLAP TYPES

Free flap tissues included the rectus abdominis muscle in 13, the latissimus dorsi muscle in seven, the radial forearm fasciocutaneous flap in five, the scapular fasciocutaneous flap in three, and the omentum in two. The flap choice in each case was dependent on contour, skin thickness, and flap length. The fanning shape of the distal latissimus dorsi has been particularly useful for large surface area defects. Unfortunately, necrosis of the distal 2 cm of the latissimus dorsi in most of our patients prompted our switch to the rectus abdominis when a muscle flap is required. Another advantage of the rectus flap was the ability to position the patient in a supine position, thereby allowing two teams to work simultaneously. The radial forearm flap was the flap of choice when contour problems arose in covering wounds on the dorsum of the foot. Muscle flaps around the foot and ankle remained bulky for many months following the operation and should be avoided in this area. The scapular fasciocutaneous flap was the flap of choice for large defects on the weight-bearing plantar surface because of its thickness and durability. The most effective means of limiting the length of free flap required was to place the bypass graft as close to the soft tissue defect as possible. This is not always possible because adequate lengths of saphenous vein were not always available. The omentum was the flap of choice[8] when the bypass graft could not be placed near the soft tissue defect.

WOUND TYPES

Ten patients had dorsal foot wounds, which typically resulted in exposure of the midfoot skeleton and anterior compartment tendons (Fig. 1). These wounds were best covered with a radial forearm flap and since the weight-bearing surface was not involved produced the best functional results. Ten patients had plantar wound (Fig. 2). Nine of these patients had diabetes as well as sensory neuropathy. These wounds were best covered with a scapular flap. The remaining patients had an assortment of wounds around the malleoli and distal tibia, which required muscle for bulk and were best covered with rectus flaps (Fig. 3).

JUSTIFICATION

These patients with bone, tendon, and joint exposure cannot be compared with those re-

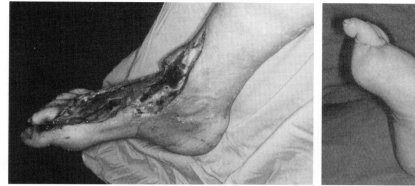
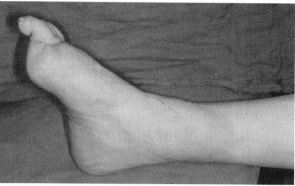

Fig. 1 **A,** Soft tissue defect after diabetic foot infection with exposure of dorsal skeleton and anterior compartment tendons. **B,** Postoperative result at 1 year after femoral-to-dorsalis pedis bypass and free rectus abdominis transfer with skin graft. This flap does produce increased bulk and the current preference in this area is the radial forearm flap.

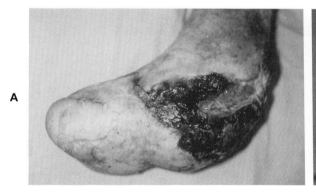
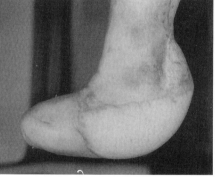

Fig. 2 **A,** Severe necrosis of the plantar surface of the heel with osteomyelitis of the calcaneus in a diabetic patient who had already undergone a transmetatarsal amputation. **B,** Healed postoperative result at 2 years after femoral-to-popliteal bypass and free scapular fasciocutaneous flap to weight-bearing surface of foot.

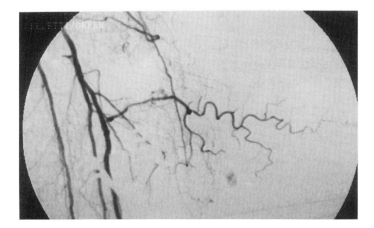

Fig. 3 Arteriogram at 1 year following a rectus flap to cover an exposed knee prosthesis. The free flap artery (inferior epigastric) can be seen coming off the femoral-to-posterior tibial venous bypass graft.

ported in studies comparing amputation with vascular reconstruction alone. Vascular reconstruction has been shown to be comparable to amputation in terms of overall success and total costs when the costs of the prosthesis and rehabilitation were considered.[9] Furthermore, the likelihood of ambulation with a below-knee prosthesis in this patient population was only 45%.[10,11] The ambulation rate of 73% in our patients was comparable to that of any amputation series.

REFERENCES

1. Chowdary RP, Celani VJ, Goodreau JJ, McCullough JL, McDonald KM, Nicholas GG. Free-tissue transfers for limb salvage utilizing in situ saphenous vein bypass conduit as the inflow. Plast Reconstr Surg 87:529, 1991.
2. Cronenwett JL, McDaniel MD, Zwolak RM, et al. Limb salvage despite extensive tissue loss: Free tissue transfer combined with distal revascularization. Arch Surg 124:609, 1989.
3. Greenwald LL, Comerota AJ, Mitra A, Grosh JD, White JV. Free vascularized tissue transfer for limb salvage in peripheral vascular disease. Ann Vasc Surg 4:244, 1990.
4. Serletti JM, Hurwitz SR, Jones JA, Herrera HR, Reading GP, Ouriel K, Green RM. Extension of limb salvage by combined vascular reconstruction and adjunctive free-tissue transfer. J Vasc Surg 18:972, 1993.
5. Shenaq SM, Dinh TA. Foot salvage in arteriolosclerotic and diabetic patients by free flaps after vascular bypass: Report of two cases. Microsurgery 10:310, 1989.
6. Shestak KC, Fitz DG, Newton ED, Swartz WM. Expanding the horizons in treatment of severe peripheral vascular disease using microsurgical techniques. Plast Reconstr Surg 85:406, 1990.
7. Dripps RD, Lamont A, Eckenhoff JE. The role of anesthesia in surgical mortality. JAMA 178:261, 1961.
8. Herrera HR, Geary J, Whitehead P, Evangelisti S. Revascularization of the lower extremity with omentum. Clin Plast Surg 18:491, 1991.
9. Mackey WC, McCullough JL, Conlon TP, et al. The costs of surgery for limb-threatening ischemia. Surgery 99:26, 1986.
10. High RM, McDowell DE, Savrin RA. A critical review of amputation in vascular patients. J Vasc Surg 1:653, 1984.
11. Harris KA, van Schie L, Carroll SE, et al. Rehabilitation potential of elderly patients with major amputations. J Cardiovasc Surg 32:463, 1991.

37

Tibiotibial Bypass for Limb Salvage

ROSS T. LYON, M.D., and FRANK J. VEITH, M.D.

Although lower extremity arterial bypass procedures have more than a 30-year history of clinical application, the technical aspects of these procedures have continued to evolve (Fig. 1).[1] Refinements have improved patency and further extended the limits of limb salvage. Femoropopliteal and subsequently femorotibial bypasses have allowed successively more distal infrainguinal arterial occlusive lesions to be treated. Femoropedal arterial bypasses exemplify the use of very long bypasses for the treatment of very distal diseases.[2] Despite the success of these procedures, the ability to obtain sufficient suitable autologous vein for such long bypasses is a significant limitation. In the absence of an adequate length of vein, a prosthetic conduit is often used for bypasses above the knee or proximal to the tibial arteries. Yet when bypass to the infrapopliteal arteries is needed, prosthetic conduits are of limited value and often require long-term anticoagulation therapy to allow even short-term patency.

Although the common femoral artery has been the preferred site of origin for lower extremity bypasses, use of more distal arteries for inflow has allowed revascularization of the foot with autologous vein in patients that otherwise would not have had sufficient vein for distal bypass procedures.[3,4]

Tibiotibial bypass allows very distal revascularization with a limited length of autologous vein (Fig. 2). We currently use this bypass in patients with nonhealing foot lesions and occlusive lesions limited to the distal infrapopliteal arteries who also have a saphenous or upper extremity vein that is inadequate for a more proximal bypass origin.

Circumstances where tibiotibial bypass should be considered are relatively infrequent. In a consecutive series of 2473 lower extremity revascularization procedures done at Montefiore Medical Center in New York over an 11-year period, only 42 (1.7%) were tibiotibial bypasses. Nevertheless, in selected patients it is a valuable option when a more standard bypass is not possible because of limited autologous vein.

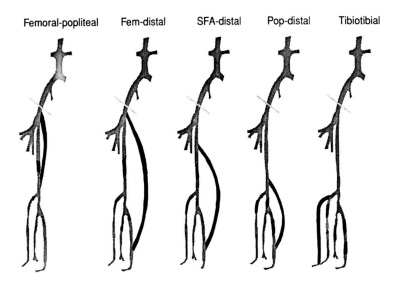

Fig. 1 The evolution of the different types of lower extremity arterial bypass procedures, progressing to more distal anastomotic sites for runoff and the subsequent utilization of more distal inflow sites.

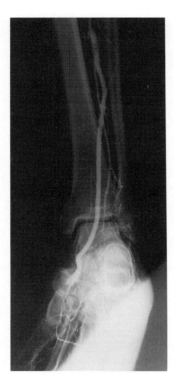

Fig. 2 Intraoperative angiogram of a proximal to distal anterior tibial artery bypass in a patient with partial forefoot necrosis and an absent pedal arch. This bypass has remained patent for more than 4 years.

INFLOW SITES FOR LOWER EXTREMITY BYPASS

Although atherosclerosis is a systemic disease process potentially involving all of the large and medium-sized arteries, plaque deposition is not uniform. Some patients develop lesions localized to the aorta and iliac arteries yet have minimal involvement of the femoral or tibial arteries. Others have predominantly infrapopliteal disease or isolated superficial femoral artery occlusions. The absence of occlusive lesions of the aortoiliac and femoral arteries allows bypasses for distal lesions to be originated below these sites without compromising inflow to the graft.

In the absence of significant proximal occlusive lesions, the superficial femoral, popliteal, tibial, and peroneal arteries have been used successfully as sites for originating distal arterial bypasses. A short bypass is attractive not only because it requires less vein but also because the extent of surgical dissection that is required is limited, reducing the operative time and the likelihood of postoperative wound complications. Additionally, short vein bypasses may be inherently less prone to thrombosis because of the decreased likelihood of intrinsic vein graft lesions.[5]

INFLUENCE OF BYPASS CONDUIT ON PATENCY

Despite the importance of suitable inflow and quality of the runoff vessels to the clinical success of a bypass, the most important determinant of bypass patency is the quality of the bypass conduit.[6] In the absence of intrinsic lesions, autologous saphenous vein is the conduit that has resulted in the highest long-term patency rates for lower extremity bypasses. Lesser saphenous and upper extremity cephalic vein are alternative sources, although they are not as reliable as the greater saphenous vein because of a higher incidence of intrinsic defects and increased likelihood of the development of hyperplastic lesions in arm veins. Prosthetic arterial conduits have high patency rates when used for aortic reconstructive procedures but only moderate patency for infrainguinal revascularization below the knee.[7] Long-term oral anticoagulation has decreased the spontaneous thrombosis rate of distal prosthetic grafts, but the patency of these bypasses remains substantially inferior to that for autologous vein. Patency of cryopreserved allograft vein bypasses at 1 year is below that for prosthetic conduit bypasses. Tibiotibial bypass allows use of even very short segments of autologous vein for distal revascularization procedures and therefore avoids the use of more thrombogenic alternative conduits in patients with a limited length of suitable vein.

LENGTH OF BYPASS

Although bypasses from the common femoral artery to the inframalleolar vessels using autologous vein have been shown to allow prolonged patency, the likelihood of a preexisting intrinsic defect of the development of a secondary lesion increases with the length of required vein. Unfortunately, a vein graft is only as good as its worst portion, and inadequate diameter or length, sclerotic segments, and varicose changes are all more likely to occur in longer segments of vein in instances in which the entire length must be used. Tibiotibial bypass has the advantage of requiring only a very short length of vein even for very distal revascularization procedures. It therefore increases the use of other inadequate lengths of autologous vein segments and decreases the likelihood of intrinsic vein defects.

PREEXISTING PROXIMAL OCCLUSIVE DISEASE

Most patients with severe lower extremity arterial insufficiency have multilevel arterial occlusive disease that is not limited to the mid- or distal tibial and peroneal vessels. In these instances, if there is only enough available autologous vein for bypass of one level of disease, yet the clinical situation requires multilevel revascularization, we would prefer to do balloon angioplasty or proximal reconstruction (e.g., aortofemoral or femoropopliteal bypass) with a prosthetic graft and a separate popliteal-distal or tibiotibial bypass, with the available autologous vein, for the more distal lesions. Proximal stenoses of the inflow vessels that produce less than a 30% luminal narrowing and do not result in a drop in resting pressure measured intraoperatively are left untreated.

NONINVASIVE TESTING

Because of the absence of significant occlusive disease proximal to the tibial arteries in these patients, segmental cuff occlusion pressures should be normal at the below-knee level and are usually only moderately reduced at the ankle. Ankle pressures or pulse volume recordings (PVRs) are not sufficient to determine the potential for healing of open foot lesions and the need for a bypass. Forefoot and toe tracings provide the most useful indicators of the adequacy of arterial supply for healing of an open foot wound in these patients. A forefoot PVR amplitude of more than 10 mm is usually sufficient to allow spontaneous healing, whereas an amplitude of less than 5 mm is not.

PROGRESSION OF PROXIMAL DISEASE

Because atherosclerosis is a chronic and progressive disease, the most distal a bypass is originated, the more likely it is to be vulnerable to progression of proximal occlusive lesions. Additionally, because the infrapopliteal vessels are smaller, lesion progression can seem to occur at a faster rate (of diameter stenosis) than in larger, more proximal arteries. We therefore do not recommend the use of the tibiotibial bypass technique when an adequate length of suitable autologous vein exists for a more proximal origin bypass, such as a popliteal-distal bypass.

TECHNIQUES

Vein harvest, surgical exposure, proximal and distal vascular control, and routing of the bypass are all simplified during a tibiotibial bypass compared with longer conventional bypasses, primarily because of the shorter distance between the proximal and distal anastomotic sites. When performing a bypass to the dorsalis pedis artery, use of the proximal anterior tibial artery for inflow obviates the need for tunneling through the interosseous fascia or over the bony prominence. Clamping and circumferential dissection of the inflow and outflow vessel are avoided by using a pneumatic arterial tourniquet at the above-knee level. The entire tibiotibial bypass can then be done in a bloodless field that is unencumbered by clamps and vessel loops.

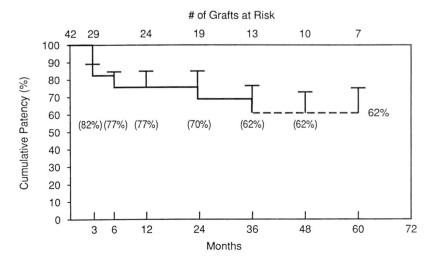

Fig. 3 Primary bypass patency in 42 consecutive tibiotibial bypass procedures.

RESULTS

In a consecutive series of 42 tibiotibial bypasses performed over an 11-year period at Montefiore Medical Center, 77% of the bypasses were patent at 1 year and 62% after 5 years (Fig. 3). Limb salvage rates were 81% and 74%, respectively.

CONCLUSION

Tibiotibial bypass is an effective and durable limb salvage procedure in patients with occlusive lesions that are limited to the mid- or distal tibial arteries and limited autologous saphenous vein. It allows distal lower extremity revascularization with autologous vein in circumstances where more standard bypass procedures are not possible.

REFERENCES

1. Veith FJ, Gupta SK, Wengerter KR, et al. Changing arteriosclerotic disease patterns and management strategies in lower-limb-threatening ischemia. Ann Surg 212:402-414, 1990.
2. Andros G, Harris RW, Salles-Cunha SX, et al. Bypass grafts to the ankle and foot. J Vasc Surg 7:785-794, 1988.
3. Veith FJ, Gupta SK, Samson RH, et al. Superficial femoral and popliteal arteries as inflow sites for distal bypasses. Surgery 90:980-990, 1981.
4. Veith FJ, Ascer E, Gupta SK, et al. Tibiotibial vein bypass grafts: A new operation for limb salvage. J Vasc Surg 2:552-557, 1985.
5. Panetta TF, Marin ML, Veith FJ, et al. Unsuspected preexisting saphenous vein disease: An unrecognized cause of vein bypass failure. J Vasc Surg 15:103-110, 1992.
6. Donaldson MC, Mannick JA, Whitemore AD. Causes of primary graft failure after in situ saphenous vein bypass grafting. J Vasc Surg 15:113-120, 1992.
7. Londrey GL, Ramsey DE, Hodgson KJ, et al. Infrapopliteal bypass for severe ischemia: Comparison of autogenous vein, composite and prosthetic grafts. J Vasc Surg 13:631-632, 1991.

38

Is Routine Vein Graft Angioscopy Worthwhile in Infrainguinal Bypass Surgery?

DANIEL G. CLAIR, M.D., MICHAEL A. GOLDEN, M.D., JOHN A. MANNICK, M.D., ANTHONY D. WHITTEMORE, M.D., and MAGRUDER C. DONALDSON, M.D.

Angioscopy has been used in vein preparation and evaluation of anastomoses during infrainguinal bypass grafting.[1-8] Incomplete valve lysis, unligated venous branches, and wound healing problems can contribute to operative morbidity in infrainguinal vein grafting, and angioscopy has been recommended as an aid to improve surgical outcomes by ensuring complete valve lysis, identifying significant venous tributaries, and detecting venous abnormalities that require intraoperative correction. However, concerns have been raised about angioscopy, including the potential for infusion of unacceptably large volumes of fluid and endothelial injury from either prolonged distention with nonphysiologic fluid or from the angioscope itself. We therefore undertook a prospective evaluation of angioscopy in in situ vein grafting to determine whether its use decreased wound morbidity and limited early failures from technical problems associated with vein preparation.[9] We also hoped to document the significance of any of the proposed shortcomings of angioscopically assisted surgery.

METHODS

During a 48-month period ending in August 1993, 59 patients requiring primary infrainguinal in situ vein reconstruction to the distal popliteal artery or to a tibial vessel were randomized to one of two groups before surgery. Exclusion criteria included a need for secondary revision procedures, a history of prior inflow grafting, evidence of aneurysmal disease, or a need for composite vein grafting. Patients in the first group (angioscopy) underwent in situ saphenous vein grafting with angioscopic assistance for valve lysis and vein branch identification. The patients in this group had the femoral artery and proximal saphenous vein exposed in the groin. Sufficient distal vein and the outflow target vessel were then exposed through a separate incision in the lower leg. In three instances the external diameter of the distal vein was less than 3 mm after gentle distention with heparinized crystalloid solution and these patients were switched to the no-angioscopy arm of the study to undergo conventional in situ vein bypass.

After intravenous heparinization the saphenofemoral junction was clamped and a 2.2 mm steerable angioscope (Olympus Corporation, Lake Success, N.Y.) was introduced through a sheath secured into a branch of the saphenous vein at the bulb. Heparinized crystalloid solution was introduced for flushing via the side port of the sheath; a pump operated by a foot pedal switch allowed low-flow (50 ml/min) and high-flow (200 ml/min) irrigation. After inserting the angioscope, a deflated 3 Fr Fogarty balloon catheter was advanced from the distal end of the vein to confirm the course of the vein and the absence of gross obstructions before passing the valvulotome. The Fogarty catheter was then removed, and a modified Mill's valvulotome with a long flexible shaft (Olympus Corporation) was advanced from the distal end of the vein. During the last half of the study a distal side branch of the vein was intermittently perfused with a 20-gauge plastic cannula connected to the flush pump by means of a Y connector, facilitating advancement of the valvulotome and reducing flush volumes necessary for visualization. While advancing the angioscope, valves were lysed under direct vision and branches of the vein were marked with skin pencil or staples guided by transillumination from the light on the tip of the angioscope. On completion of valve lysis the distal vein was clamped and the side branches were ligated by small skin incisions. The proximal saphenous vein was then detached from the femoral vein, and the proximal and distal anastomoses were performed in standard fashion. Completion angiograms were taken to evaluate the graft and the anastomoses, and a sterile Doppler probe was used to check for residual arteriovenous fistulas.

Patients in the second group (no angioscopy) underwent in situ vein grafting by the conventional technique. The entire saphenous vein, the femoral artery, and outflow vessels were exposed through a single incision. When encountered, branches of the vein were either ligated or retained for use as valvulotome insertion sites. After heparinization the proximal saphenous vein was separated from the femoral vein, which was oversewn with 5-0 polypropylene sutures. The proximal anastomosis was then created, followed by valve lysis with the Mill's valvulotome introduced through multiple side branches. After completion of the distal anastomosis, angiography was performed as before to confirm the quality of vein preparation, the technical adequacy of the anastomoses, and the presence of any residual fistulas. Ultrasound was again used to check for unidentified fistulas.

From the first postoperative day patients from both groups ambulated. Wounds were carefully evaluated for infection, necrosis, phlebitis, or hematoma. Postoperative graft monitoring included assessment of symptoms and examination of pulses and segmental limb pressures. Color-flow duplex scanning was also used to detect localized graft lesions. Graft patency was then determined from actuarial life-table analysis. An evaluation of primary patency applied to all grafts requiring no revision after leaving the operating room. Primary assisted patency comprised grafts needing no revision plus grafts requiring revision while still patent. Tests of statistical significance were done with the chi-square method and analysis of variance, and life-table estimates were compared using the Mantel-Cox (log-rank) test.

RESULTS

Initially 35 patients were randomized to the angioscopy group; three patients required transfer to the no-angioscopy group because of small infrageniculate veins, which resulted in 32 patients in the angioscopy group and 27 patients in the no-angioscopy group. Preoperative characteristics for the two groups were similar (Table 1); most patients in both groups required surgery for limb salvage. There were slightly greater percentages of patients with diabetes and patients with threatened limbs in the no-angioscopy group, but neither of these differences were significant. The incidence of claudication as an indication for surgery was considerably higher in the angioscopy group; this difference approached, but did not reach, statistical significance ($p = .07$). There were more patients with tissue necrosis of some form in the no-angioscopy group ($p < .003$). Nearly half the patients had some form of tissue loss related to ischemia.

Table 2 summarizes the operative results for the two groups of patients. There was a slightly increased mean operating time for patients in the angioscopy group, and despite the volume required for angioscopy (1131 ml) there was no significant difference in the overall intraoperative fluid load given to the two groups. A small percentage of patients in each group required attention for an ischemic foot ulceration or localized gangrene at the time of initial bypass grafting. Most grafts in both groups were infrapopliteal, with no differences in target vessels or runoff between the groups.

Analysis of postoperative outcome in these patients (Table 3) shows a similar incidence of postoperative myocardial events and overall major morbidity. In the entire group there was one death, a result of multisystem organ failure following cardiac failure; this occurred in the no-angioscopy group. The total length of stay and postoperative length of stay were similar for the two groups, with wide ranges in each group. The incidence of wound problems in both groups was remarkably similar, and each group had two early graft occlusions.

The mean postoperative follow-up for the entire group was 13.6 months, and 12% of the grafts had not been assessed within 6 months of the last follow-up visit. Graft revisions for stenosis were required in seven patients (11.9%) during the follow-up: three of the 32 angioscopy grafts and four of the 27 no-angioscopy grafts. Four grafts were revised by vein patch angioplasty, two were repaired by percutaneous angioplasty, and one graft was treated with percutaneous atherectomy of a stenotic segment. Eight grafts occluded during the course of follow-up: five of the angioscopy grafts and three of the no-angioscopy grafts. Five of the occluded grafts were treated by thrombectomy and graft revision, and the other three required a new vein graft.

Life-table analysis of patency rates for these

Table 1 Preoperative characteristics of 59 patients randomized into study of angioscopically assisted in situ bypass

	Angioscopy (n = 32)	No angioscopy (n = 27)	Overall
Mean age (yr)	71.0	71.2	71.1
Risk factors			
Diabetes	11 (34.4%)	12 (44.4%)	23 (39.0%)
Smoking	12 (37.5%)	12 (44.4%)	24 (40.7%)
Hypertension	19 (59.4%)	18 (66.7%)	37 (67.2%)
Coronary artery disease	14 (43.8%)	13 (48.2%)	27 (45.8%)
Indication			
Claudication	11 (34.4%)	5 (18.5%)	16 (27.1%)
Limb salvage	21 (65.6%)	2 (81.5%)	43 (72.9%)
Rest pain	11 (34.4%)	5 (18.5%)	16 (27.1%)
Ulcer	10 (31.2%)	11 (40.7%)*	21 (35.6%)
Gangrene		6 (22.2%)	6 (10.2%)

*$p < .003$ tissue necrosis (ulcer/gangrene) for angioscopy vs. no-angioscopy groups.

Table 2 Intraoperative characteristics of 59 patients in study of angioscopically assisted in situ bypass

	Angioscopy (n = 32)	No angioscopy (n = 27)	Overall
Mean operating room time (min)	239	206*	224
Vein graft size (mm)	3.6	3.3	3.5
Mean operating room fluid (ml)	2640	2238	2436
Distal anastomosis			
Distal popliteal	15 (46.9%)	10 (37.0%)	25 (42.4%)
Anterior tibial	6 (18.8%)	3 (11.1%)	9 (15.5%)
Posterior tibial	6 (18.8%)	5 (18.5%)	11 (18.6%)
Peroneal	3 (9.3%)	7 (25.9%)	10 (16.9%)
Dorsalis pedis	2 (6.2%)	2 (7.4%)	4 (6.8%)
Secondary procedure at bypass			
Toe amputation	2 (6.3%)	2 (7.4%)	4 (6.8%)
Debridement	1 (3.1%)	2 (7.4%)	3 (5.1%)

*$p < .05$ mean operating room time for angioscopy vs. no-angioscopy groups.

Table 3 Postoperative morbidity and mortality after 59 in situ bypass grafts with randomized angioscopy*

	Angioscopy (n = 32)	No angioscopy (n = 27)	Overall
Complications			
Local			
Wound infection	1 (3.1%)	1 (3.7%)	2 (3.4%)
Hematoma	2 (6.1%)	0 0	2 (3.4%)
Early occlusion	2 (6.2%)	2 (7.4%)	4 (6.8%)
Systemic			
Myocardial infarction	1 (3.1%)	1 (3.7%)	2 (3.4%)
Dysrhythmia	0 0	1 (3.7%)	1 (1.7%)
Stroke	1 (3.7%)	1 (1.7%)	0 0
Pneumonia	0 0	1 (3.7%)	1 (1.7%)
Mean length of stay (range)			
Total (days)	10.5 (4-27)	10.7 (4-23)	10.6 (4-27)
Postoperative (days)	8.0 (2-25)	8.6 (2-21)	8.2 (2-25)
Mortality rate	0 0	1 (3.7%)	1 (1.7%)

*No statistically significant difference in early postoperative outcomes between the angioscopy and no-angioscopy groups.

Table 4 Cumulative primary revised patency rates comparing angioscopy and no-angioscopy groups

Interval	No. of grafts at risk	No. of grafts failing	No. of grafts withdrawn	Interval patency (%)	Cumulative patency (%)	SE
0-3 mo						
Overall	59	6	8	89.2	89.2	4.3
Angioscopy	32	3	4	90.3	90.3	5.3
No angioscopy	27	3	4	88.0	88.0	6.6
3-6 mo						
Overall	45	1	6	97.6	87.0	4.6
Angioscopy	25	1	2	95.8	86.5	6.3
No angioscopy	20	0	4	100.0	88.0	6.6
6-12 mo						
Overall	38	0	9	100.0	87.0	4.6
Angioscopy	22	0	5	100.0	86.5	6.3
No angioscopy	16	0	4	100.0	88.0	6.6
12-24 mo						
Overall	29	1	13	95.6	83.2	5.6
Angioscopy	17	1	7	92.6	80.1	8.5
No angioscopy	12	0	6	100.0	88.0	6.6
24-36 mo						
Overall	15	0	9	100.0	83.2	5.6
Angioscopy	9	0	5	100.0	80.1	8.5
No angioscopy	6	0	4	100.0	88.0	6.6
36-48 mo						
Overall	6	0	6	100.0	83.2	5.6
Angioscopy	4	0	4	100.0	80.1	8.5
No angioscopy	2	0	2	100.0	88.0	6.6

grafts yielded an overall 48-month primary patency rate of 61.6%: 63.2% for the angioscopy group and 60.0% for the no-angioscopy group. With careful graft surveillance and appropriate therapy for stenotic lesions, an overall primary revised patency rate of 83.2% was achieved. The primary revised patency was 80.1% for the angioscopy group and 88.0% for the no-angioscopy group (Table 4). Major amputations were performed in two limbs during the entire follow-up period.

DISCUSSION

The use of the angioscope in infrainguinal reconstructions has been advocated by several groups.[1-8] Although proponents have claimed increased intraoperative sensitivity, excellent short-term patency, and a trend toward reduced morbidity, the improved safety and efficacy of angioscopically assisted venous bypass over conventional techniques remains to be proved. Concern regarding the use of the angioscope is related to its possible detrimental effects on the venous endothelium (with reduction in long-term patency) and volume load given to elderly patients with cardiac disease during the course of the angioscopy.

Maini et al.[8] performed a study of angioscopically assisted in situ bypasses similar to that in this report. These authors noted a significant reduction in postoperative length of stay and wound complication rates and no differences in 12-month patency rates. The present study confirms the absence of impact of angioscopy on patency rates but does not show a reduction in length of stay or wound complication rates. These findings were recorded despite several potential biases in the present study favoring the angioscopy group. Patients with external vein diameters believed to be too small for angioscopy (less than 3 mm) were crossed over to the conventional group. A larger number of patients in the angioscopy group had claudication as an indication for surgery, although this was not statistically significant. Finally, a significantly higher percentage of patients in the no-angioscopy group had tissue necrosis as a presenting complaint.

The preoperative characteristics of patients and the indications for surgery in this study are similar to several larger series of in situ vein grafts previously reported.[10-12] The distribution of sites of distal anastomoses and the operative time are also consistent with earlier studies. A longer operative time in the angioscopy group very likely represents extra time required to set up the equipment and perform the angioscopy. However, the total mean intraoperative fluid volume in the angioscopy group was kept to the same amount as that administered to the no-angioscopy group despite the volume used for flushing (1131 ml) during performance of the angioscopy. Fluid volume administered to patients during angioscopy can be limited by several techniques, including the use of a distal flush cannula as in this study and the use of preoperative vein mapping to allow ligation of branches before the angioscopy is performed. Maini et al.,[8] for example, used the preoperative vein mapping technique and reduced mean flush volume to 400 ml.

This study clearly demonstrates the safety of both conventional and angioscopically assisted vein grafting methods, with limited major morbidity in both groups. This study also reemphasizes the low incidence of postoperative wound problems in patients undergoing conventional in situ bypass grafting. We had hypothesized that wound morbidity would be reduced in the angioscopy group. Longitudinal skin incisions for vein branch ligations and attempts to ligate more than one branch by a single incision may lead to delayed healing. The liberal use of transverse skin incisions for vein branch ligation may be preferable. Although in the present study the angioscope could not be shown to reduce early or late graft stenosis or occlusion, this small series also shows no clear detrimental effect on graft patency from the use of the angioscope. The acceptable 36- and 48-month patency rates reduce concern regarding long-term patency problems caused by endothelial injury from the angioscope.

This evaluation of the angioscope involves a small number of patients, and small but significant differences would be impossible to prove. For this reason, further prospective trials with larger numbers of patients might help to identify subgroups of patients who could benefit from the use of the angioscope. In this study the angioscope was not assessed as a method of evaluating the quality of graft preparation or anastomoses.

REFERENCES

1. White GH, White RA, eds. Angioscopy: Vascular and Coronary Applications. Chicago: Year Book, 1989.
2. Miller A, Stonebridge PA, Tsoukas AI, et al. Angioscopically directed valvulotomy: A new valvulotome and technique. J Vasc Surg 13:813-821, 1991.
3. Lamuraglia GM, Cambria RP, Brewster DC, et al. Angioscopy-guided semiclosed technique for in situ bypass. J Vasc Surg 12:601-604, 1990.
4. Stierli P, Aeberhard P. Angioscopy-guided semiclosed technique for in situ bypass with a novel flushing valvulotome: Early results. J Vasc Surg 15:564-568, 1992.
5. Baxter TB, Rizzo RJ, Flinn WR, et al. A comparative study of intraoperative angioscopy and completion arteriography following femorodistal bypass. Arch Surg 125:997-1002, 1990.
6. Gilbertson JJ, Walsh DB, Zwolak RW, et al. A blinded comparison of angiography, angioscopy, and duplex scanning in the intraoperative evaluation of in situ saphenous vein bypass grafts. J Vasc Surg 15:121-129, 1992.
7. Miller A, Marcaccio EJ, Tannenbaum GA, et al. Comparison of angioscopy and angiography for monitoring infrainguinal bypass vein grafts: Results of a prospective randomized trial. J Vasc Surg 17:382-398, 1993.
8. Maini BS, Andrews L, Salimi T, et al. A modified, angioscopically assisted technique for in situ saphenous vein bypass: Impact on patency, complications, and length of stay. J Vasc Surg 17:1041-1049, 1993.
9. Clair DG, Golden MA, Mannick JA, Whittemore AD, Donaldson MC. Randomized prospective study of angioscopically assisted in situ saphenous vein grafting. J Vasc Surg 19:992-1000, 1994.
10. Leather RP, Shah DM, Chang BB, Kaufman JL. Resurrection of the in situ saphenous vein bypass: 1000 cases later. Ann Surg 208:435-442, 1988.
11. Bergamini TM, Towne JB, Bandyk DF, et al. Experience with in situ saphenous vein bypasses during 1981 to 1989: Determinant factors of long-term patency. J Vasc Surg 13:137-149, 1991.
12. Donaldson MC, Mannick JA, Whittemore AD. Femoraldistal bypass with in situ greater saphenous vein: Long-term results using the Mills valvulotome. Ann Surg 213:457-465, 1991.

39

Why Angioscopy Is Worthwhile in Infrainguinal Bypass Surgery: How to Make It Work

ARNOLD MILLER, M.B., Ch.B., and JUHA P. SALENIUS, M.D., Ph.D.

Angioscopy is the only method of endoluminal examination that allows direct in vivo visualization of the interior of the blood vessels in real-life colors. Subtle variations of the different endoluminal states, both normal and pathologic, can be appreciated. Evaluation of angioscopy as a new technology with regard to its efficacy has traditionally been narrowly defined, comparing only early and late graft patency with or without intraoperative angioscopy. The superiority of one monitoring modality over another, defined only as the "patency" of a graft or artery, is a goal that may be deceptively difficult to achieve; determinants of the patency of a graft are multiple and variable and include surgical skill, extent of the disease, and biologic factors for a particular patient.

This narrow definition also ignores other benefits derived from direct intraluminal observation in normal and diseased states. It does not take into consideration the impact of the recognition of new or previously unappreciated intraluminal pathologies, nor the affect on the surgical decision-making process, where unsuspected angioscopic information on the endoluminal state remote from the operation site is available. Such information may minimize, alter, or even result in abandonment of the proposed surgical procedure. Such decisions resulting from more precise knowledge of the endoluminal state are difficult to account for when patency of a particular surgical bypass graft is the only parameter of success to justify use of the technology. How can the benefits of the technology as a method of teaching surgical technique be factored into the equation when efficacy is defined only as patency? Similar to the initial underestimation by some vascular surgeons of the value of enhanced lighting and loupe magnification, the benefits derived from direct endoluminal observation with minimization of the "judgment" factor and mystique of "experience" may not be fully appreciated. Just as with the introduction of enhanced lighting and loupe magnification, which initially met with resistance by some vascular surgeons, benefits from direct endoluminal observation, with minimization of the judgment factor and experience and mystique from the practice of vascular surgery may be underestimated. Finally, it should be appreciated that endoscopic vascular surgery is in its infancy, both in the evolution of instrumentation and in techniques, and remains one of the exciting and challenging areas of exploration in vascular surgery.

In this chapter we will review our experience, discuss how to make angioscopy work, and show how routine application of angioscopy during infrainguinal bypass grafting improves the surgical results and makes it worthwhile.

INDICATIONS

Our current indications for angioscopy are summarized below.

Diagnostic

Monitoring of surgical-interventional procedures
- Bypass, endarterectomy, thrombectomy, embolectomy, vascular access, preparation of renal transplants, and valvuloplasty for venous insufficiency
- Angioplasty, atherectomy, stenting, and endoluminal grafting

Clinicopathologic correlation
- Lesions responsible for anginal syndromes
- Endoscopic findings and graft failure

Therapeutic

Surgical
- Endoluminal vein graft preparation (valvulotomy and tributary occlusion)

- Catheter-directed thrombectomy or embolectomy

Percutaneous
- Thrombolysis
- Assisted interventions (angioplasty, atherectomy, stenting, and endoluminal grafting)

The usefulness and varied applications of angioscopy depend on the ingenuity and creativity of the individual surgeon. We conceptualize and use the angioscope as an adjunctive tool to see inside vessels, so that rational and informed clinical and surgical decisions can be made with objective findings. We do not rely simply on experience.

Initially we used angioscopy as a simple alternative or adjunct to the operative angiogram, as a means to avoid or correct technical errors. However, we soon appreciated that the rich and detailed endoluminal information not only provides a sensitive and accurate method for the detection of technical errors but allows continual assessment of technical proficiency. It has become an excellent teaching tool, improving and refining the surgical technique of the surgeons and residents. Angioscopy has also identified new or previously unappreciated endovascular pathologies which have enhanced our understanding of the pathogenesis of graft failure[1] and fostered the development and design of new instrumentation for intraluminal manipulations such as valve cutters, tributary occluders, and various grabbing and cutting intraluminal instruments.[2-5]

TECHNICAL ASPECTS

Angioscopy, like endoscopy in all other systems, requires practice. There is a significant learning curve to achieve proficiency with the technique. Routine and frequent usage reduces the frustration generated by poor-quality or unsuccessful procedures and ensures reliable high-quality studies.

Our techniques and details of the equipment for angioscopy in infrainguinal bypass surgery have been previously described in detail.[6,7] Understanding the mechanics and physical constraints of irrigation to clear the visual field for successful angioscopy is essential.[8] The principles of irrigation with saline solution are outlined as follows.*

---

*From Miller A, Lipson W, Isaacsohn J, et al. Intraoperative angioscopy: Principles of irrigation and description of a new dedicated irrigation pump. Am Heart J 118:391-399, 1989.

Aim
- To establish and maintain a *column of clear fluid* within the vessel

Requirements
- No antegrade flow in the main vessel or collateral vessels
- Initial fluid bolus of large volume and high flow rate to establish column of clear fluid
- Subsequent small volume and low flow rate, with pressure in excess of backflow pressure, to maintain clear fluid column

The safety of irrigation with saline solution in a group of patients undergoing bypass surgery has been prospectively and systematically studied.[9] The average fluid volume required for optimal studies has consistently been less than 500 ml and is well tolerated. Carefully and skillfully performed angioscopy does not require unmanageable volumes of irrigation fluid. With time and increasing experience, the volume of saline irrigation we use for completion monitoring angioscopy has diminished.

To concentrate the initial experience and improve familiarity with the technique and instrumentation, we established a separate angioscopy service in our institution. Every angioscopic procedure was performed by the operating surgeon in association with a separate angioscopy team. The "team" tended to all the needs of each angioscopic procedure. This included setting up the instrumentation, participating in the procedure as well as recording, reviewing, and reporting its outcome, and finally, cleaning and packaging of the used angioscopes for resterilization. In a short time, a large experience accrued. This information was easily taught to new personnel with little loss of efficiency. Most important, the high volume of cases allowed systematic data collection in a large variety of vascular procedures. Associated with this accumulated experience was a dramatic reduction in breakage of the delicate angioscopes. The improved durability of the angioscopes was critical in making the procedure cost effective.

Although the "separate" team setup works well in a large institution with a high volume of cases, with the new user friendly angioscopy systems available today, routine high-quality angioscopy can be achieved by any educated surgeon who surmounts the learning curve and makes the appropriate arrangements with the operating room support staff. Frustration and poor results will soon cause the casual angioscopist to reject the technology.

CLINICAL EXPERIENCE

Our clinical studies have been directed to systematically evaluating this new technology and its place in the modern practice of vascular surgery. Introducing a new technology into surgery raises several questions: Is it feasible in a busy clinical setting or is it really only a research tool? Is it safe? Does it facilitate the particular surgical procedure? Does it provide new information unavailable by standard or other technology? If so, is this information useful? Does it influence and alter clinical and operative surgical decisions? And finally, how do these new findings affect the results of the surgery as measured by clinical outcome or graft patency, both in the short and long term?

From our first clinical angioscopy on May 1, 1987, to November 1993, we performed intraoperative angioscopy during more than 1400 revascularization procedures (Table 1), including infrainguinal bypass grafting, reoperative surgery, vascular access surgery, carotid endarterectomy, and coronary artery bypass grafting.

Our largest experience with angioscopy has accumulated with infrainguinal bypass grafting.[1,7,10-12] Others have studied the role of angioscopy during carotid endarterectomy,[13,14] thrombectomy, and embolectomy,[15-17] coronary artery bypass grafting,[18,19] venous valvular repair,[20] and vascular access surgery.[21,22]

In infrainguinal bypass grafting, angioscopy has proved most valuable and clinically useful in monitoring the surgical success of the technical aspects of the procedure, vein conduit preparation, and in reoperation for the failing or failed bypass graft.

Monitoring Infrainguinal Bypass Grafts

Our early studies showed that routine angioscopy for monitoring infrainguinal bypass grafting is feasible, safe, and a clear-cut alternative to routine intraoperative completion angiography, except in cases in which the runoff status is not delineated on the preoperative angiogram. In this situation we often perform an adjunctive intraoperative angiogram confined to the distal graft and runoff vasculature. Analysis of the first 355 angioscopies during infrainguinal bypass grafting consolidated our technique of intraoperative angioscopy.[6,10,11,23] It also delineated the most useful size of angioscope for a given procedure and the volume of irrigation fluid required for consistent high-quality studies (Table 2). Most important is that these studies also showed that the angioscopic findings significantly modified the process of intraoperative surgical decision making (Table 3).

Table 1 Types of procedures in 1466 intraoperative angioscopies

Operation	No.
Infrainguinal bypass	1288
Femoropopliteal	263
Femoro/popliteodistal	942
Reoperative surgery	83
Vascular access surgery	86
Carotid endarterectomy	36
Coronary artery bypass surgery	10
Miscellaneous	26
TOTAL	1446

Table 2 Size of angioscope and mean volume of irrigation fluid used in 355 infrainguinal bypass operations

Outer diameter (mm)	No.	0.8	1.4	2.2	2.8	3.0	Mean fluid volume (range in ml)
Femoral-AKP	28	—	16	11	1	—	458 (64-1412)
Femoral-BKP	53	2	29	20	1	1	410 (51-904)
Femoral-tibial	163	10	130	20	1	2	419 (50-1098)
Femoral-pedal	57	8	41	8	—	—	433 (77-1160)
Popliteal-distal	54	7	45	2	—	—	218 (37-625)
TOTAL	355	27	261	61	3	3	397 (37-1412)

From Miller A, Stonebridge P, Kwolek C. The role of routine angioscopy for infrainguinal bypass procedures. In Ahn S, Moore W, eds. Endovascular Surgery, 2nd ed. Philadelphia: WB Saunders, 1992, pp 58-69.
AKP = above-knee popliteal; BKP = below-knee popliteal.

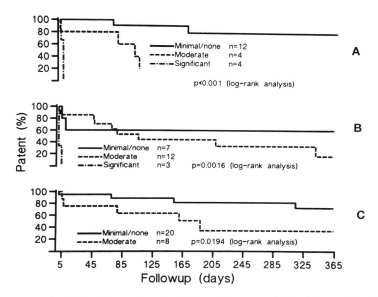

Fig. 4 Graft patency by life-table analysis within subgroups defined by residual thrombus within the graft. **A**, Early graft failure ($p < .001$, log rank analysis). **B**, Late failed grafts ($p = .0016$, log rank analysis). **C**, late failing grafts ($p = .0194$, log rank analysis). (From Hölzenbein T, Miller A, Tannenbaum A, et al. Role of angioscopy in reoperation for the failing or failed infrainguinal vein bypass graft. Ann Vasc Surg 8:74-91, 1994.)

identifies the cause of the graft failure, but also localizes the problem and its extent, thereby minimizing the surgical exposure necessary for the revision surgery. In a retrospective study of 76 reoperations for failing or failed infrainguinal bypass grafts, in 34 (44%) of the bypass operations additional interventions were performed after angioscopic examination.[43] These included removal of unsuspected thrombus, detection, localization, and correction of unsuspected pathologic conditions, and demonstration of usable graft despite the fact that this could not be visualized on the preoperative angiogram.

The more residual thrombus at the end of the reoperation within the graft conduit, anastomosis, and runoff artery, the poorer the early patency ($p < .001$) and long-term patency for each of the three groups (Fig. 4). This may explain the consistent finding that despite an initial high "success" rate, 48% to 86% for thrombolysis, and even with correction of underlying lesion, the long-term patency of failed grafts is disappointing, only 20% to 77% at 1 year[44,45]—so much so that some recommend abandonment of the old graft and establishment of a new graft if sufficient autogenous vein is available.[46] The fate of graft endothelium and intimal surfaces following thrombosis is unknown, but it has been suggested that ischemic or inflammatory changes occur during the time of thrombosis until resumption of arterial blood flow can be achieved, revitalizing the endothelium.[47] Others have suggested intimal injury, attributed to balloon thrombectomy or some unknown direct action of the thrombolytic agents to the endothelium, may be the critical factors in graft durability. The angioscopic appearance of the graft luminal surface following thrombolysis and thrombectomy may provide a clue to the "health" of the vascular endothelium. Grafts that cannot be adequately cleared of adherent thrombus may contain large areas of dead or dysfunctional endothelium while grafts with intact cellular linings can resist the adherence of thrombus through the action of their surface anticoagulant glycoproteins or other unknown mediators.

In these complicated and challenging procedures, angioscopy not only provides additional and useful information to the preoperative angiogram but may provide insights into the pathogenesis of graft failure.

CONCLUSION

Review of the literature reveals a progressive improvement in the patency rates for infrainguinal bypass grafts despite operating in the most severely threatened limbs and ill and elderly patients and extending the grafts more distally in the leg and foot. It appears that if the vein conduit is of good quality and the surgeon proficient in the surgical techniques, good and durable results are possible. In those bypasses in which the vein conduit is of good quality, the runoff vasculature adequate, and the surgeon proficient in the technique, monitoring the bypass surgery for technical or correctable errors by any means does not appear to significantly alter the early graft patency. However, with a conduit of less than optimal quality or a borderline runoff, the role of monitoring of the bypass surgery assumes a new significance.

These studies clearly show that routine intraoperative angioscopy during infrainguinal bypass grafting is worthwhile. It provides the surgeon with additional information of the endoluminal state of the conduit and native vessels that may not only influence the conduct of the bypass surgery and improve the results, but may also enhance our understanding of the factors influencing the durability of infrainguinal bypass grafts. Finally, with the development of new instrumentation and new endovascular techniques, the endoluminal preparation of the vein conduit will become routine, minimizing the extent of the surgery with a concomitant reduction in patient morbidity, hospitalization, and overall medical costs.

REFERENCES

1. Miller A, Jepsen S, Stonebridge P, et al. New angioscopic findings in graft failure after infra-inguinal bypass grafting. Arch Surg 125:749-755, 1990.
2. Mehigan J. Angioscopic preparation of the in situ saphenous vein for arterial bypass: Technical considerations. In White G, White R, eds. Angioscopy: Vascular and Coronary Applications. Chicago: Year Book Medical Publishers, 1989, pp 72-75.
3. White G, White R, Kopock G, et al. Endoscopic intravascular surgery removes intraluminal flaps, dissections, and thrombus. J Vasc Surg 11:280-288, 1990.
4. Miller A, Stonebridge P, Tsoukas A, et al. Angioscopically directed valvulotomy: A new valvulotome and technique. J Vasc Surg 13:813-821, 1991.
5. Stierli P, Aeberhard P. Angioscopy-guided semiclosed technique for in situ bypass with a novel flushing valvulotome: Early results. J Vasc Surg 15:546-548, 1992.
6. Miller A, Jepsen S. Angioscopy in arterial surgery. In Bergan J, Yao JST, eds. Techniques in Arterial Surgery. Philadelphia: WB Saunders, 1990, pp 409-416.
7. Miller A, Hölzenbein T. Angioscopy in peripheral vascular surgery. In White R, Hollier L, eds. Vascular Surgery: Basic Science and Clinical Correlations. Philadelphia: JB Lippincott, 1994, pp 513-530.
8. Miller A, Lipson W, Isaacsohn J, et al. Intraoperative angioscopy: Principles of irrigation and description of a new dedicated irrigation pump. Am Heart J 118:391-399, 1989.
9. Kwolek C, Miller A, Stonebridge P, et al. Safety of saline irrigation for angioscopy: Results of a prospective randomized trial. Ann Vasc Surg 6:62-68, 1992.
10. Miller A, Campbell D, Gibbons G, et al. Routine intraoperative angioscopy in lower extremity revascularization. Arch Surg 124:604-608, 1989.
11. Miller A, Stonebridge P, Jepsen S, et al. Continued experience with intraoperative angioscopy for monitoring infrainguinal bypass grafting. Surgery 109:286-293, 1991.
12. Miller A, Marcaccio E, Tannenbaum G, et al. Comparison of angioscopy and angiography for monitoring infrainguinal bypass grafts: Results of a prospective randomized trial. J Vasc Surg 17:382-398, 1992.
13. Towne J, Bernhard V. Vascular endoscopy: An adjunct to carotid surgery. Stroke 8:569-571, 1977.
14. Mehigan J, DeCampli W. Angioscopic control of carotid endarterectomy. In Ahn S, Moore W, eds. Endovascular Surgery, 2nd ed. Philadelphia: WB Saunders, 1992, pp 102-105.
15. White G, White R, Kopchok B, et al. Angioscopic thrombectomy: Preliminary observations in a recent technique. J Vasc Surg 7:318-325, 1988.
16. White G, Kopchok G, White R. Current role of intraoperative angioscopy for monitoring peripheral vascular surgery. Semin Vasc Surg 2:60-67, 1989.
17. Segalowitz J, Grundfest W, Treiman R, et al. Angioscopy for intraoperative management of thromboembolectomy. Arch Surg 125:1357-1362, 1990.
18. Grundfest W, Litvack F, Glick D, et al. Intraoperative decisions based on angioscopy in peripheral vascular surgery. Circulation 78(Suppl I):I-13–I-17, 1988.
19. Forrester J, Litvack F, Grundfest W, et al. A perspective of coronary disease seen through the arteries of living man. Circulation 75:505-513, 1987.
20. Welch H, McLaughlin R, O'Donnell T. Femoral vein valvuloplasty: Intraoperative angioscopic evaluation and hemodynamic improvements. J Vasc Surg 16:694-700, 1992.
21. Miller A, Marcaccio E, Goodman W, et al. The role of angioscopy in vascular access surgery. In Henry M, Ferguson R, eds. Vascular Access for Hemodialysis - III. W.L. Gore, 1993, pp 210-218.
22. Hölzenbein T, Miller A, Gottlieb M, et al. The role of angioscopy in vascular access surgery. J Endovasc Surg 2:210-225, 1994.
23. Miller A, Stonebridge P, Kwolek C. The role of routine angioscopy for infrainguinal bypass procedures. In Ahn S, Moore W, eds. Endovascular Surgery, 2nd ed. Philadelphia: WB Saunders, 1992, pp 58-69.
24. Williams L, Flanigan D, Schuler J, et al. Intraoperative assessment of limb revascularization by Doppler-derived segmental blood pressure measurements. Am J Surg 144:578-579, 1982.
25. Stonebridge P, Miller A, Tsoukas A, et al. Angioscopy of arm vein infrainguinal bypass grafts. Ann Vasc Surg 5:170-175, 1991.

26. Baxter B, Rizzo R, Flinn W, et al. A comparative study of intraoperative angioscopy and completion arteriography following femorodistal bypass. Arch Surg 125:997-1002, 1990.
27. Gilbertson J, Walsh D, Zwolak R, et al. A blinded comparison of arteriography, angioscopy, and duplex scanning in the intraoperative evaluation of in situ saphenous vein bypass grafts. J Vasc Surg 15:121-129, 1992.
28. Marcaccio E, Miller A, Tannenbaum G, et al. Angioscopically directed interventions improve arm vein bypass grafts. J Vasc Surg 17:994-1004, 1993.
29. Hölzenbein T, Pomposelli F, Miller A, et al. Arm veins for infrainguinal bypass: The first alternative to ipsilateral saphenous vein grafts? [abst]. Presented at the twenty-first annual meeting of the New England Society of Vascular Surgeons. Newport, R.I.: September 29-30, 1994, p 18.
30. Chalmers R, Hoballah J, Kresowik T, et al. The impact of color duplex surveillance on the outcome of lower limb bypass with segments of arm veins. J Vasc Surg 19:279-288, 1994.
31. Veith F, Moss C, Daly V, et al. New approaches in limb salvage by extended extraanatomic bypasses and prosthetic reconstructions to foot arteries. Surgery 84:764-774, 1978.
32. Leather R, Shah D, Chang B, et al. Resurrection of the in situ vein bypass: 1000 cases later. Ann Surg 208:435-442, 1988.
33. Taylor L, Edwards J, Porter J. Present status of reversed vein bypass: Five-year results of a modern series. J Vasc Surg 11:207-215, 1990.
34. Logerfo W, Gibbons G, Pomposelli F, et al. Evolving trends in the management of the diabetic foot. Arch Surg 127:617-621, 1992.
35. Donaldson M, Mannick J, Whittemore A. Causes of primary graft failure after in situ saphenous vein bypass grafting. J Vasc Surg 15:113-120, 1992.
36. Corson J, Karmody A, Shah D, et al. Retrograde valve incision for in situ vein-arterial bypass utilising a valvulotome. Ann R Coll Surg Engl 66:173-174, 1984.
37. Fleisher HI, Thompson B, McCowan T, et al. Angioscopically monitored saphenous vein valvulotomy. J Vasc Surg 4:360-364, 1986.
38. Matsumoto T, Yang Y, Hashizume M. Direct vision valvulotomy for nonreversed vein graft. Surg Gynecol Obstet 165:181-183, 1987.
39. Chin A, Fogarty T. Specialized techniques of angioscopic valvulotomy for in situ vein bypass. In White G, White R, eds. Angioscopy: Vascular and Coronary Applications. Chicago: Year Book, 1989, pp 76-83.
40. La Muraglia G, Cambria R, Brewster D, et al. Angioscopy facilitates a closed technique for in-situ vein bypass. J Vasc Surg 12:601-604, 1990.
41. Maini B, Andrews L, Salimi T, et al. A modified, angioscopically assisted technique for in situ saphenous vein bypass: Impact on patency, complications, and length of stay. J Vasc Surg 17:1041-1049, 1993.
42. Rosenthal D, Herring M, O'Conovan T, et al. Endoluminal in situ femoropopliteal bypass: Will this replace a classical procedure. International Congress V. Angiology 43(Suppl):274-275, 1992.
43. Hölzenbein T, Miller A, Tannenbaum A, et al. Role of angioscopy in reoperation for the failing or failed infrainguinal vein bypass graft. Ann Vasc Surg 8:74-91, 1994.
44. van Breda A, Robison J, Feldman M, et al. Local thrombolysis in the treatment of arterial graft occlusions. J Vasc Surg 1:103-112, 1984.
45. Gardiner G, Harrington D, Koltun W, et al. Salvage of occluded arterial bypass grafts by means of thrombolysis. J Vasc Surg 9:426-431, 1989.
46. Edwards JE, Taylor LM Jr, Porter JM. Treatment of failed lower extremity bypass grafts with new autogenous vein bypass grafting. J Vasc Surg 11:136-145, 1990.
47. Cox J, Chiasson D, Gottlieb A. Stranger in a strange land: The pathogenesis of saphenous vein graft stenosis with emphasis on structural and functional differences between veins and arteries. Prog Cardiovasc Dis 34:45-68, 1991.

40

Diagnosis and Treatment of Paradoxical Arterial Emboli: An Unrecognized Entity

ALI F. ABURAHMA, M.D.

Paradoxical embolism was first described by Cohnheim[1] in 1877. Although there are fewer than 40 reported cases of paradoxical emboli diagnosed during life, it is probably much more common. Chaikof et al.[2] reported six cases occurring over a 5-year period and Meister et al.[3] reported five cases occurring over a 2-year period, presenting a variety of clinical manifestations and diagnosed prior to death.

The diagnosis may be difficult because of the variable nature of the systemic embolization. The presenting manifestation may be acute myocardial infarction, acute mesenteric ischemia, a cerebrovascular accident, or a peripheral vascular deficit. According to Johnson,[4] paradoxical embolism may be considered to be proved when a venous thrombus is found lodged within an intracardiac septal defect at autopsy. A presumptive diagnosis may be based on the presence of (1) venous thrombosis with or without pulmonary embolism, (2) an intracardiac defect showing a right-to-left shunt, or (3) an arterial embolism without a corresponding source in the left heart or the proximal arterial tree. A favorable pressure gradient must exist at some time in the cardiac cycle to promote right-to-left shunting.

Recently a subset of patients who presented with arterial embolism has been identified in whom no clearly definable cardiac or arterial source for the embolism is apparent. It is in this group of patients that paradoxical embolism must be considered and among whom the prevalence of the disease is likely to be much greater than was previously considered. With the advances in echocardiography, in particular the development of noninvasive maneuvers during imaging that define patent foramen ovale,[5-9] the accurate diagnosis of presumptive paradoxical embolism has been facilitated in patients with arterial embolism.

ETIOLOGY AND PATHOPHYSIOLOGY

Paradoxical embolism is commonly defined as the passage into the systemic arterial tree of any material from the venous circulation through an abnormal communication accompanied by a right-to-left shunt. This displacement of material is only possible in the face of increased right intracardiac pressures. Various mechanisms have been proposed to explain this inversion of atrial pressure ratios and the paradoxical passage of an embolus.[10,11] In one instance, however, paradoxical embolism has been reported through a left-to-right shunt.[12] Although paradoxical embolism is most often a venous thrombus, it can consist of air,[13] foreign bodies,[14] or septic material.[15]

The three prerequisites for the occurrence of paradoxical embolism are as follows:
1. A venous thrombus is usually formed.
2. A right-to-left shunt must be present.
3. The thrombus must embolize to the arterial circulation.

Patients may have a ventricular septal defect, an atrial septal defect, a patent ductus arteriosus, or a pulmonary arteriovenous malformation. The most common cardiac defect associated with paradoxical embolism is a patent foramen ovale. Thompson and Evans[16] examined a random series of 1000 autopsies and found a pencil-patent foramen ovale (0.6 to 1.0 cm in diameter) in 6% of cases, whereas a probe-patent foramen ovale (0.2 to 0.5 cm in diameter) was noted in 29%. Recently Cheng[7] described a catheter-patent foramen ovale in 10% of patients.

For a venous thrombus to cross a foramen ovale, a right-to-left pressure gradient must exist. Elevation of the right atrial pressure may be secondary to a chronic condition, as in obstructive lung disease with cor pulmonale, mitral stenosis, tricuspid valve disease, or pulmonary hypertension. More commonly the pressure gradient is caused by an acute process. Substantial pulmonary embolism with acute right ventricular and atrial hypertension is the most common cause of fixed pulmonary right-sided pressure elevations.

Right-to-left shunting might not be demonstrated in many of these patients with foramen ovale without provocative measures to transiently increase right atrial pressure. Valsalva's maneuver and cough are two means by which transient increases in right-sided pressures may be produced.

Seward et al.[17] and Valdes-Cruz et al.[18] have demonstrated the usefulness of contrast echocardiography for the detection of intracardiac right-to-left shunts. Various contrast agents including normal saline solution, the patient's own blood, dextrose water, and indocyanine green can be used since the contrast effect is most likely secondary to microcavitation of bubbles produced in the patient's blood during rapid injection of the contrast medium.[19] These microcavitation bubbles reflect sound waves, thus producing a contrast effect as viewed with two-dimensional and/or M-mode echocardiography. Valsalva's maneuver has been used to detect small defects in the atrial system.[20] Release of Valsalva's maneuver poses transient reversal of the normal resting intra-arterial pressure gradient, and the pressure in the right atrium will exceed that in the left atrium.

Contrast echocardiograms are usually obtained using an apical four-chamber approach and rapid injection of 10 ml of agitated sterile normal saline solution through a peripheral intravenous cannula. At least four saline injections are given and recorded for each patient. All injections are administered during normal quiet respiration and following Valsalva's maneuver. A contrast echocardiogram is considered abnormal if microbubbles appear either in the left atrium or the left ventricle no later than two to three cardiac cycles after their initial appearance in the right atrium.

The incidence of paradoxical embolism in the hospitalized adult population is difficult to assess primarily because of the diagnostic difficulties of defining temporary interatrial shunts and because many of these arterial emboli are clinically silent.[21] Paradoxical embolism may have a significant clinical impact on patients with embolic stroke. Biller et al.[22] reported that among 132 patients aged 15 to 45 years with acute non-hemispheric cerebral infarction, five cases of paradoxical embolism were detected. They concluded that in young patients with cerebral embolism of unknown etiology, if routine M-mode and two-dimensional echocardiograms are normal, contrast echocardiography should be performed to rule out intracardiac shunts and the possibility of paradoxical cerebral embolism. In another study by Biller et al.,[23] which included eight patients with possible or probable paradoxical cerebral embolism, ischemic symptoms occurred following Valsalva's maneuver in three cases and others were linked to placement of a Swan-Ganz catheter, deep venous thrombosis, pulmonary embolism, right atrial myxoma, and use of oral contraceptives. In six of these patients contrast echocardiography showed right-to-left shunting. Cardiac catheterization showed a patent foramen ovale in three patients and one had an atrial septal defect. They concluded that with the use of contrast echocardiography, pulsed Doppler echocardiography, and cardiac CT and MRI scanning, otherwise unsuspected cardiac abnormalities that predispose patients to paradoxical cerebral embolism can be diagnosed. Caplan et al.[24] have shown that 36% of 127 patients meeting strict criteria for embolic stroke had no identifiable intracardiac or arterial source. Although studies in some of these patients were incomplete, the number of patients with this very common clinical disorder suggests that as yet poorly characterized pathophysiologic phenomena may be important contributing factors.

Paradoxical embolism through a patent foramen ovale from deep venous thrombosis in elderly, sedentary patients during coughing or defecation may be one such mechanism for stroke in this population. Lechat et al.,[25] in a study of the prevalence of a patent foramen ovale in patients with stroke, reported that the cause of ischemic stroke in younger adults is undefined in as many as 35%. The prevalence of a patent foramen ovale was significantly higher in patients with stroke (40%) compared to a control group (10%). Among patients with stroke, the prevalence of a patent foramen ovale was 21% in 19 patients with an identifiable cause of stroke, 40% in 15 patients with no identifiable cause but a risk factor for stroke such as mitral valve prolapse, migraine, or use of contraceptive agents, and 50% in 20 patients with no identifiable cause. These data suggest that because of the high prevalence of clinically latent venous thrombosis, paradoxical embolism through a patent foramen ovale may be responsible for stroke more often than is usually suspected.

DIAGNOSIS

Clinically the diagnosis of paradoxical embolism is presumptive, relying on circumstantial evidence. A high index of suspicion should be maintained in all patients with arterial embolism without clinical evidence of the source of emboli from the left heart or the proximal arterial tree, especially if either concomitant deep venous thrombosis or pulmonary embolism is present.

The prognosis of paradoxical embolism varies with the severity of pulmonary embolism and the presence or absence of cerebral embolism. Processes that cause only a transient elevation in right atrial pressure can confound the diagnosis of paradoxical embolus unless the physician's index of suspicion is high. Because systemic embolization may involve any artery, the diagnosis of paradoxical embolism should be considered in patients who present with neurologic manifestations after deep venous thrombosis or pulmonary embolism, myocardial infarction after deep venous thrombosis or pulmonary embolism, or postoperative arterial emboli.

The diagnosis of paradoxical emboli should also be considered in any postoperative patient who has an unexpected arterial embolism or arterial embolism of undetermined etiology. Although simultaneous pulmonary embolism is indicative of paradoxical embolism, it is not a prerequisite. In some of these patients pulmonary embolism may go undiagnosed. Demonstration of the right-to-left shunt is often difficult. If the patient is studied after the event, the pulmonary embolus may have dissolved, with a return of the right atrial pressure to normal. Cardiac catheterization, which is one method of demonstrating such a cardiac defect, may be unrevealing.

The safety and accuracy of defining intracardiac shunting through the foramen ovale has been greatly improved by the use of contrast echocardiography with provocative maneuvers. Using Valsalva's maneuver and contrast echocardiography, Lynch et al.[26] demonstrated a right-to-left shunt in 18% of normal volunteers and 5% had shunting at rest without Valsalva's maneuver. Therefore a mild degree of right-to-left shunting may occur in normal persons.

Until the introduction of contrast echocardiography and/or transesophageal cardiography, cardiac catheterization was the only premorbid method available to define transient intracardiac shunting.

Contrast or transesophageal echocardiography should also be performed in all young patients with arterial emboli, even if all other cardiac findings and studies are normal. Several studies used transesophageal echocardiograms in the diagnosis of several cases of paradoxical embolism.[8,27,28] Nellessen et al.[8] reported a case of impending paradoxical embolism from an arterial thrombus, which was correctly diagnosed by transesophageal echocardiography and prevented by surgery. It was reported as the first case in which an embolus already overriding the interatrial septum could unequivocally be visualized by transesophageal echocardiography allowing successful surgical removal.

Therefore the differential diagnosis of arterial embolism in patients with associated deep venous thrombosis or pulmonary embolism should include (1) paradoxical embolism, (2) acute myocardial infarction with mural thrombi in the left ventricle, occurring concurrently with pulmonary emboli from deep venous thrombosis, (3) emboli arising from infective endocarditis involving both left- and right-sided heart valves, (4) primary cardiomyopathy with mural thrombi in both chambers of the heart, and (5) emboli from myxomas of both the right and left atria.

In patients with cyanotic congenital heart disease and arterial embolism, the diagnosis of paradoxical embolism is extremely likely. In view of the more recent diagnostic advances, a reasonable diagnostic approach for patients with suspected paradoxical embolism is outlined in Fig. 1.

TREATMENT

Various treatment modalities have been used in the management of patients with paradoxical embolism. Most authorities throughout the 1970s recommended surgical interruption of the inferior vena cava as the treatment of choice for paradoxical emboli. In a 1981 review, however, Leonard et al.[5] suggested immediate anticoagulation with heparin. They believed that interruption of the inferior vena cava should be undertaken only in patients with permanent right-to-left shunts. If the site of the paradoxical emboli is not in the brain, thrombolytic therapy should be considered.

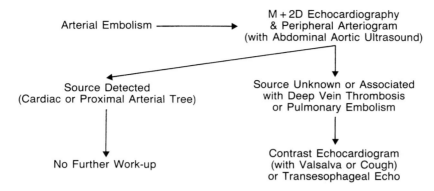

Fig. 1 Diagnostic workup in patients with suspected paradoxical embolism.

Although no single approach can be endorsed for all patients, a multifaceted approach for treatment should be considered. If there are no contraindications to anticoagulation, 7 to 10 days of intravenous heparin followed by 3 to 6 months of warfarin is recommended. If significant acute cor pulmonale develops as a result of acute pulmonary embolism, or if peripheral arterial emboli jeopardize limb viability, thrombolytic therapy should be considered, provided that there are no contraindications for its use. If anticoagulation or thrombolytic therapy is contraindicated, inferior vena cava interruption is recommended and peripheral and/or pulmonary embolectomy should be attempted as hemodynamic compromise dictates. In the rare instances in which an impending paradoxical embolism is noted on echocardiography, intracardiac embolectomy may be attempted and closure of large intracardiac defects undertaken in conjunction with inferior vena cava interruption. Chaikof et al.[2] recommended closure of the foramen ovale after a significant or recurrent paradoxical embolus.

OUR CLINICAL EXPERIENCE

Between December 1986 and December 1993, we encountered five cases of paradoxical embolism and seven others that were diagnosed as possible paradoxical embolism. The five cases of paradoxical emboli had the classic triad of venous thrombus (with or without pulmonary embolism), an intracardiac defect with a right-to-left shunt, and peripheral arterial embolization. The seven cases of possible paradoxical emboli included patients who had unexpected peripheral arterial emboli following venous thrombosis of undetermined etiology, that is no definite cardiac or proximal arterial pathology to explain the source of the arterial emboli.

In a previously published study,[29] nine (22%) of 41 patients who were admitted with a diagnosis of acute arterial embolism were less than 50 years of age, and in this group five (56%) had probable (two cases) or possible (three cases) paradoxical embolism. In this subset of patients paradoxical emboli must be looked at very carefully. The following case reports are three examples of a diagnosis of paradoxical embolism that was confirmed.

Case 1

A 29-year-old man was transferred from a nearby hospital after being hospitalized for treatment of diabetes mellitus. Twelve hours prior to his transfer to our medical center, the patient developed a cold, painful right leg and foot. He had a history of pain and tenderness of the left calf and was said to have deep venous thrombosis. The clinical examination was unremarkable except for a pulseless, cold, pale right leg from the midthigh down to the foot. Chest x-ray film and ECG were unremarkable. M-mode and two-dimensional echocardiograms were normal. Noninvasive vascular testing showed probable occlusion of the right femoral artery by segmental Doppler pressures and impedance plethysmography demonstrated deep venous obstruction of the left leg. An arteriogram showed acute embolization to the right femoropopliteal arteries with a normal proximal arterial tree. A venogram confirmed deep venous thrombosis of the left femoral popliteal veins. A ventilation-perfusion lung scan was inconclusive. The patient was treated with intra-arterial urokinase thrombolysis with a successful outcome as con-

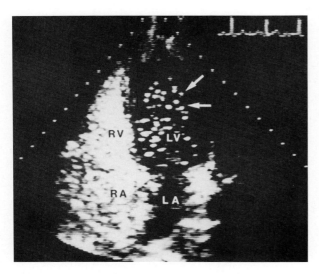

Fig. 2 Contrast saline echocardiography showing patent foramen ovale with right-to-left shunt on coughing. Note white contrast medium in the right and left heart chambers.

firmed by arteriogram. The postoperative Doppler ankle/arm index was 1.0 (in comparison to a preoperative index of 0.48). Contrast saline echocardiography showed a patent foramen ovale with right-to-left shunt on coughing (Fig. 2). The patient was discharged on Coumadin and did not return for definitive treatment of the cardiac defect.

Case 2

A 34-year-old woman was admitted because of sudden onset of a painful, cold, numb right arm of 6 hours' duration. Medical and surgical history was unremarkable, except that 2 weeks prior to this admission she had experienced pain, tenderness, and mild swelling of the right lower leg for 2 days. She had had no shortness of breath or chest pain. General examination was unremarkable. Vascular examination showed mild right calf and thigh tenderness with an equivocal Homan's sign. Pulses in the lower extremities were normal. Right brachial, radial, and ulnar pulses were absent. The arm was cold from the elbow down. Chest x-ray film and ECG were normal. Noninvasive vascular testing by means of impedance plethysmography showed an abnormality of the right leg. M-mode and two-dimensional echocardiograms were normal. A ventilation-perfusion lung scan was positive for right pulmonary emboli. An arteriogram showed acute embolization of the right brachial artery and its bifurcation. The source of arterial emboli was not seen on the peripheral arteriogram. The patient underwent right brachial thromboembolectomy and was maintained on Coumadin postoperatively. Paradoxical embolism was considered in this case; however, the patient refused a cardiac workup at that time. One month later the patient underwent cardiac catheterization, which showed a patent foramen ovale with right-to-left shunt on sustained Valsalva's maneuver.

Case 3

A 41-year-old woman was admitted because of a painful, cold, left lower extremity of 4 hours' duration. Medical and surgical history was unremarkable except for a history of right calf and thigh pain, tenderness, and swelling 1 month prior to this admission. She did not complain of any chest pain. Physical examination was unremarkable except for absent pulses of the left lower extremity, a cold left lower leg with decreased sensation, right calf tenderness, and a positive Homan's sign. Chest x-ray film, ECG, and M-mode and two-dimensional echocardiograms were normal. An arteriogram showed acute embolization to the left femoral, popliteal, and tibial arteries, and the patient therefore underwent embolectomy. Venous plethysmography demonstrated deep venous obstruction of the right leg, which was confirmed by venography. The patient's postoperative course was uneventful and she was discharged on Coumadin. A transesophageal echocardiogram at late 6-month follow-up confirmed the presence of a patent foramen ovale.

CONCLUSION

Paradoxical embolization should be considered whenever unexplained arterial occlusion occurs, particularly in younger patients. A complete diagnostic workup should include a lung scan to determine the presence of pulmonary emboli, venous duplex imaging, and/or peripheral venography to determine the site of venous thrombosis, and a complete cardiac workup. If M-mode and/or two-dimensional echocardiograms and peripheral arteriogram or abdominal aortic sonogram do not show the source of emboli, contrast saline echocardiography with Valsalva's maneuver or transesophageal echocardiography should be performed to rule out a cardiac defect.

REFERENCES

1. Cohnheim J. Thrombose und Embolie. In Vorlesungen uber Allgemeine Pathologie, vol 1. Berlin: Hirschwald, 1877, p 134.
2. Chaikof EL, Campbell BE, Smith RB III. Paradoxical embolism and acute arterial occlusion: Rare or unsuspected? J Vasc Surg 20:377, 1994.
3. Meister SG, Grossman W, Dexter L, Dalen JE. Paradoxical embolism—diagnosis during life. Am J Med 53:292, 1972.
4. Johnson BJ. Paradoxical embolism. J Clin Pathol 4:316, 1951.
5. Leonard RCF, Neville E, Hall RJC. Paradoxical embolism associated with a patent foramen ovale. Postgrad Med J 57:717, 1981.
6. Higgins JR, Strunk BL, Schiller NB. Diagnosis of paradoxical embolism with contrast echocardiography. Am Heart J 107:375, 1984.
7. Cheng TO. Echocardiogram and paradoxical embolism. Ann Intern Med 95:515, 1981.
8. Nellessen U, Daniel WG, Matheis G, Oelert H, Depping K, Lichtlen PR. Impending paradoxical embolism from atrial thrombus— correct diagnosis by transesophageal echocardiography and prevention by surgery. J Am Coll Cardiol 5:1002, 1985.
9. Rodgers DM, Singh S, Meister SG. Contrast echocardiographic documentation of paradoxical embolism. Am Heart J 107:1270, 1984.
10. Elliott GB, Beamish RE. Embolic occlusion of patent foramen ovale. A syndrome occurring in pulmonary embolism. Circulation 8:394, 1953.
11. Blanck C, Olanders S. Paradoxical coronary embolism. J Pathol Bact 86:527, 1963.
12. Katz D, Cooper JA, Frieden J. Bacterial endocarditis presenting as complete heart block with paradoxical (left-to-right) pulmonary emboli. Am Heart J 85:108, 1973.
13. Merkel H. Uber die Bedeutung der sog. Paradoxen oder gekreuzten embolie fur die gerichtliche Medizin. Dtsch Ztsch Ges Gerichtlich Med 23:338, 1934.
14. Nash G, Moylan JS. Paradoxical catheter embolism. Arch Surg 102:213, 1971.
15. Corrin B. Paradoxical embolism. Br Heart J 26:549, 1964.
16. Thompson T, Evans W. Paradoxical embolism. Q J Med 23:135, 1930.
17. Seward JB, Tajik AJ, Hagler DJ, Ritter DG. Peripheral venous contrast echocardiography. Am J Cardiol 39:202, 1977.
18. Valdes-Cruz LM, Pieroni DR, Roland JA, Varghese PJ. Echocardiographic detection of intracardiac right-to-left shunts following peripheral vein injections. Circulation 54:558, 1976.
19. Kremkau FW, Gramiak R, Carstensen EL, Shaf PM, Kramer DH. Ultrasonic detection of cavitation at catheter tips. Am J Roentgenol 110:177, 1970.
20. Banas JS Jr, Meister SG, Gazzaniga AB, O'Conner NE, Haynes FW, Dalen JE. A simple technique for detecting small defects in the atrial septum. Am J Cardiol 28:467, 1971.
21. Miller R, Jordon R, Parker R, Edwards J. Thromboembolism in acute and healed myocardial infarction—systemic and pulmonary arterial occlusion. Circulation 6:7, 1952.
22. Biller J, Johnson MR, Adams HP Jr, Kerber RE, Toffol GJ, Butler MJ. Echocardiographic evaluation of young adults with nonhemorrhagic cerebral infarction. Stroke 17:608, 1986.
23. Biller J, Adams HP Jr, Johnson MR, Kerber RE, Toffol GJ. Paradoxical cerebral embolism: Eight cases. Neurology 36:1356, 1986.
24. Caplan LR, Hier DB, D'Cruz I. Cerebral embolism in the Michael Reese Stroke Registry. Stroke 14:530, 1983.
25. Lechat PH, Mas JL, Lascault G, et al. Prevalence of patent foramen ovale in patients with stroke. N Engl J Med 318:1148, 1988.
26. Lynch JJ, Schuchard GH, Gross ChM, Wann LS. Prevalence of right-to-left atrial shunting in a healthy population: Detection by Valsalva maneuver contrast echocardiography. Am J Cardiol 53:1478, 1984.
27. Schluter M, Langenstein BA, Polster J, et al. Transesophageal cross sectional echocardiography with a phased array transducer system. Technique and initial clinical results. Br Heart J 48:67, 1982.
28. Thier W, Schluter M, Kremer G, et al. Transoesophageale zweidimensionale Echokardiographie: Bessere Darstellung intraatrialer Strukturen. Dtsch Med Wochenschr 108:1903, 1983.
29. AbuRahma AF, Lucente FC, Boland JP. Paradoxical embolism: An underestimated entity—a plea for comprehensive work-up. J Cardiovasc Surg 31:685, 1990.

41

Optimal Treatment of Intermittent Claudication: Role of Conservative Measures, Drugs, Angioplasty, Atherectomy, and Operation

ANTHONY D. WHITTEMORE, M.D.

Most patients with intermittent claudication—the mildest manifestation of lower extremity arterial occlusive disease—remain stable for years and warrant no specific therapy other than reduction of risk factors and surveillance for systemic complications of atherosclerotic cardiovascular disease. For the 20% of patients who become significantly disabled, however, a number of options are now available for palliation.[1,2]

EXERCISE

Lower extremity exercise therapy has been the mainstay of conservative management for intermittent claudication, particularly when the condition is of recent onset. The potential mechanisms underlying reported benefits include the development of altered walking techniques, improved muscle strength, increased pain tolerance and therefore a longer total walking distance, improved rheologic characteristics with reduction in viscosity, and improved oxidative metabolism. Improved pain-free and absolute walking distances are probably not attributable to enhanced collateral arterial supply to the effected extremity.

A thorough evaluation by Radack and Wyderski[3] of 84 studies addressing the efficacy of exercise therapy revealed only five controlled clinical trials that qualified for quantitative analysis. These authors concluded after appropriate meta-analysis that regularly supervised exercise programs improved patients' pain-free and maximal walking distances by approximately 85% compared with those of untreated control subjects. This benefit was usually apparent within 3 months of the initiation of the program, following which patients with claudication remained unchanged or improved unpredictably. In a more recent study, Hiatt et al.[4] documented a 123% increase in peak walking time and a 165% increase in pain-free walking time during a 3-month exercise program compared with only a 20% increase in peak time for untreated control subjects. It therefore seems reasonable to initiate conservative management of claudication with a regularly supervised exercise program, including 30 minutes daily of leg exercise, in conjunction with additional conservative measures, which will be described next. Such regular exercise should not require patients to continue to walk through the point at which they develop discomfort, since edematous muscles may cause discomfort sufficient to discourage individuals from pursuing this regimen.

SMOKING CESSATION

Cigarette smoking has been associated with the progression of systemic atherosclerosis as well as an increased incidence of adverse outcomes following reconstructive surgery. In the Framingham study,[5] intermittent claudication was significantly more prevalent in cigarette smokers, and the relationship was dose dependent. The difference between smokers and nonsmokers was even more significant when additional cardiovascular risk factors were present. Radack and Wyderski,[3] in their exhaustive review, were able to identify only two controlled clinical trials that addressed the relationship between smoking cessation and intermittent claudication. Neither study provided statistically valid conclusions; thus most of the evidence derives from epidemiologic studies of the natural progression of peripheral vascular atherosclerosis and the deleterious effects of the continued use of tobacco following reconstructive arterial surgery. Nevertheless, it is clear that smoking is a cardiovascular risk factor that should be eliminated in patients with intermittent claudication. It may be important to emphasize to our patients that smoking cessation may not in and of itself improve walking distance but that they can expect overall systemic benefits.

PHARMACOLOGIC MANAGEMENT

Although a wide variety of agents have been advocated and used for the treatment of intermittent claudication, few if any have demonstrated convincing efficacy from prospective, double-blinded, crossover trials with adequate lead-in time. Antithrombotic therapy for patients with intermittent claudication seeks to prevent thrombotic occlusion of antecedent atherosclerotic lesions and to maintain patency of resulting compensatory collateral vessels.[6] Tyclopidine, one of the more recent antiplatelet agents, in European trials demonstrated symptomatic relief with resultant increased walking distances; these conclusions are yet to be widely substantiated.[7] A similar but more potent antiplatelet agent, clopidogrel, is also under study in multicenter trials at present. Although evidence is meager that symptoms of intermittent claudication can be effectively palliated with antithrombotic therapy alone, intermittent claudication remains a most significant marker for systemic atherosclerosis. As such, antithrombotic therapy should be included in the management of these patients as both aspirin and Tyclopidine have been shown to reduce the incidence of cardiovascular events. Aspirin, in a maximal dose of 325 mg, significantly reduces mortality from myocardial infarction and the incidence of nonfatal myocardial infarction and stroke, as demonstrated in an exhaustive meta-analysis from the Antiplatelet Trialist Collaboration.[8]

Several vasodilator drugs have also been advocated and include nitrates, β-adrenergic agonists (nylidrin), α-adrenergic antagonists (tolazoline), isoxsuprine, and cyclandelate.[9] Since intramuscular arterioles are usually maximally dilated beyond the proximal stenotic lesion during exercise, perfusion pressure generally falls distal to the stenosis in patients with intermittent claudication, further potentiating vasodilatation and negating any potential benefit of pharmacologically induced vasodilatation. Seratonin antagonists such as ketanserin have also been advocated as a means of increasing collateral blood flow during exercise, but a recent multicenter trial failed to substantiate such a benefit.[10] Based on in vitro studies of blood from claudicants that demonstrate diminished erythrocyte deformability, hemorrheologic agents have been advocated, pentoxifylline being the most recently and widely studied. In addition to enhancing erythrocyte deformability, pentoxifylline has also been shown to diminish hyperviscosity and platelet hyperreactivity, thereby improving skeletal muscle oxygen tension at rest. Whether or not such benefits occur in vivo in the claudicant remains to be substantiated, since well-controlled, prospective, double-blinded crossover trials are lacking.[11] Radack and Wyderski[3] reviewed 12 trials that met their criteria, and only seven proved sufficient for determination of maximal walking distance and only five for pain-free walking distance. The efficacy of pentoxifylline proved extremely variable, negating significant differences from controls. Thus the efficacy of pentoxifylline remains to be determined. Ethylenediaminetetraacetate (EDTA) has been enthusiastically if not evangelically proposed to induce regression of atherosclerotic lesions by binding and removing calcium salts. Nephrotoxicity remains a significant disadvantage, and appropriate placebo controlled studies have not been carried out.[12]

Two relatively recent additions to the pharmacologic armamentarium for intermittent claudication include L-carnitine and cylostazol. L-carnitine increases in the intracellular deposition of energy rich substrates, facilitating the mitochondrial utilization of long-chain fatty acids, which become more readily available during periods of exercise. Although multiple rigorously controlled trials have not been published, one study randomized 20 patients to receive either placebo or L-carnitine for 3 weeks, then crossed over for the final 3 weeks. L-carnitine significantly improved patients' walking capacity in contrast to those given a placebo.[13]

Cylostazol, a phosphodiesterase inhibitor, increases intracellular cyclic adenosine monophosphate and is a potent vasodilator and antiplatelet agent. A recent multicenter trial demonstrated a 40% increase in pain-free and maximal walking distance among patients with moderate claudication, but its use is associated with an equal incidence of adverse gastrointestinal effects.[14] Since the overall benefits of this drug are not comparable to those of an exercise program, its use remains questionable.

Conservative therapy for patients with intermittent claudication should probably consist of a regularly supervised exercise program of at least 3 months' duration, a rigorous attempt at smoking cessation, and daily aspirin. The addition of pentoxifylline remains of controversial value, and the efficacy of either cylostozol or L-carnitine await more extensive evaluation. In addition, recent evidence suggests that rigorous management of hyperlipidemia may facilitate plaque regression and significantly reduce the incidence of coronary deaths.[15,16]

INTERVENTION FOR INTERMITTENT CLAUDICATION

The decision to intervene with an invasive technique for intermittent claudication is fraught with philosophical and judgmental issues. While few surgeons would advocate arterial reconstruction for claudication that was causing relatively minor inconvenience to the patient regarding recreational activities, most surgeons would proceed if the degree of claudication were truly disabling, threatening the patient's job security or ability to carry out essential daily activities. Today the decision to intervene is made at an earlier stage of the disease process than in years past largely because of the efficacy of percutaneous transluminal angioplasty, with its reduced morbidity, and the marked improvement in both morbidity and outcome of conventional arterial reconstruction.

Percutaneous Transluminal Angioplasty

Percutaneous transluminal angioplasty (PTA) for atherosclerotic lesions of the lower extremity has achieved an initial success rate approaching 90% in properly selected individuals and longer term 5-year patency rates ranging from 50% to 60% overall.[17] Important variables influencing patency include indication, site, and extent of lesion and whether the responsible lesion is stenotic or occlusive. Five-year patency rates as high as 75% have been reported for localized short-segment lesions in patients with claudication with proximal common iliac stenoses. In contrast, balloon angioplasty for infrainguinal lesions indicated for limb salvage provides much lower patency rates (approximately 30%). Although PTA for proximal common iliac stenosis has become the procedure of choice when applicable, angioplasty for more distal infrainguinal lesions remains controversial. Our experience with 126 infrainguinal balloon angioplasty procedures at Brigham and Women's Hospital included 72 (57%) indicated for disabling claudication.[18] The majority of these limbs (68%) had two or three distal runoff vessels in continuity and 92% of lesions were stenotic. There were no deaths, nonfatal systemic morbidity occurred in a single patient (1.3%), and the mean ankle/brachial index increased from 0.61 to 0.85 following successful PTA. The 5-year patency rate, as evidenced by maintenance of both hemodynamic and symptomatic improvement without further intervention, was 58%. No limb was lost among these patients.

Atherectomy

Evaluation of the efficacy of the four atherectomy devices currently available remains an onerous task largely because of the lack of standard reporting techniques and heterogeneity of patient populations. In most series, atherectomy was performed for limb-threatening ischemia, but a variable number of claudicants are frequently included as well. Patients with single as well as multiple lesions and with lesions of variable length are often included in the same studies, adjunctive balloon angioplasty is often required, initial technical failures are frequently excluded from longer term patency statistics, and criteria for both initial success and ultimate patency vary considerably. While the technical success rate remains high (ranging from 67% to 99%), for both rotary and directional atherectomy devices, the early restenosis rate remains high, with 2-year patencies varying from 19% with the Auth Rotablator and 37% with the Kensey atherectomy device (which requires adjunctive balloon angioplasty) to a high of 81% with the Simpson directional atherectomy device (Atherocath).[19] It is clear that lesions that are most amenable to atherectomy are also those which are effectively treated with PTA at far less cost.

Surgical Revascularization

Several surgical options are available for the management of intermittent claudication, depending on the site of arterial occlusion, yet the anticipated results are remarkably similar. Claudication resulting from aortoiliac occlusive disease has been effectively palliated with conventional aortobifemoral bypass in the vast majority of patients, with 5-year patency rates approaching 90%. Similar results may be expected with unilateral iliofemoral bypass. Extra-anatomic reconstruction for claudication has not usually been recommended, since 5-year patency remains suboptimal.

The majority of patients with claudication, however, are so affected on the basis of infrainguinal occlusive disease for which autogenous femoral popliteal reconstruction has been routinely used. In previous years, because graft patency rates associated with infrainguinal reconstruction were suboptimal compared with aortoiliac revascularization, many surgeons were not enthusiastic about femoral popliteal reconstruction for indications other than limb salvage. As results have steadily improved, however, proportionally higher percentages of claudicants are being offered infrainguinal repair. Of four series reported in the recent literature,[20-23] the proportion of patients treated for claudication ranged from 2% to 28%, reflecting variations in both patient populations and individual surgeon's policies.

Of 582 infrainguinal in situ bypasses carried out in our institution during the past decade, 181 (31%) were undertaken for claudication; there were no associated deaths and the 5-year primary patency rate was 77%, with a secondary patency rate of 85%, both sustained throughout the longer 10-year interval.[22] Above-knee autogenous reconstructions were associated with an 80% primary patency rate after 5 years, statistically no different than the 76% below-knee rate. Secondary patency rates at 5 and 10 years were 90% for above-knee reconstructions, significantly higher than the 83% associated with below-knee reconstructions. Interestingly, men sustained a significantly higher patency rate at 10 years (88%) than women (74%). Thus without mortality or observed limb loss in this group, results comparable to proximal aortoiliac reconstruction have been achieved and justify infrainguinal reconstruction for disabling claudication.

Of the total group of 181 bypasses carried out for claudication, 57 involved autogenous reconstructions with the distal anastomosis located at the tibial or peroneal level.[24] Again, the 5-year primary patency rate was 74% and secondary patency rates at both 5 and 10 years were 81%. While it has been well established that autogenous infrainguinal bypass is associated with superior results when compared with prosthetic bypass in most situations, considerable interest remains in the above-knee prosthetic bypass used in an effort to preserve the ipsilateral greater saphenous vein for more distal reconstruction should it prove necessary at a later time. Two recent such series document disparate results: the first reported a 57% 5-year patency rate, which declined to 31% after 10 years[25]; the second documented a 68% primary patency rate, sustained for 8 years.[26] Even under the best of circumstances, however, prosthetic grafts do not provide results comparable to autogenous vein grafts in the above-knee location for claudication, which in our experience is associated with an 80% primary patency rate and 90% secondary patency rate sustained for 10 years.

REFERENCES

1. Boyd AM. The natural course of arteriosclerosis of lower extremities. Angiology 11:10-14, 1960.
2. McDaniel MD, Cronenwett JL. Basic data related to the natural history of intermittent claudication. Ann Vasc Surg 3:273-277, 1989.
3. Radack K, Wyderski RJ. Conservative management of intermittent claudication. Ann Intern Med 113:135-146, 1990.
4. Hiatt WR, Regensteiner JG, Hargarten ME, et al. Benefit of exercise conditioning for patients with peripheral arterial disease. Circulation 81:602-609, 1990.
5. Kannel WB, McGee DL. Update on some epidemiologic features of intermittent claudication: The Framingham study. J Am Geriatr Soc 33:13-17, 1985.
6. Claggett GP, Graor RA, Salzman EW. Antithrombotic therapy in peripheral arterial occlusive disease. Chest 102 (Suppl):516S-528S, 1992.
7. Balsano F, Coccheri S, Libretti A, et al. Ticlopidine in the treatment of intermittent claudication: A 21-month double-blind trial. J Lab Clin Med 114:84-91, 1989.
8. Antiplatelet Trialists Collaboration. Collaborative overview of randomized trials of antiplatelet therapy. I. Prevention of death, myocardial infarction, and stroke by prolonged antiplatelet therapy in various categories of patients. BMJ 308:81-106, 1994.
9. Coffman JD, Mannick JA. Failure of vasodilator drugs in atherosclerosis obliterans. Ann Intern Med 76:35-59, 1982.
10. Prevention of Atherosclerotic Complications with Ketanserin Claudication Substudy Investigators. Randomized placebo-controlled, double-blind trial of ketanserin in claudicants: Changes in claudication distance and ankle systolic pressure. Circulation 80:1544-1548, 1989.
11. Lindëgarde F, Jelnes R, Björkman NN, et al. Conservative drug treatment in patients with moderately severe chronic occlusive peripheral arterial disease. Circulation 80:1549-1556, 1989.
12. Lamar CP. Chelation endarterectomy for occlusive atherosclerosis. J Am Geriatr Soc 14:272-294, 1966.
13. Brevetti G, Charello M, Ferulano G, et al. Increases in walking distance in patients with peripheral vascular disease treated with L-carnitine: A double-blind, crossover study. Circulation 77:767-773, 1988.
14. Dawson DL, Cutler BS, Meissner M, et al. Cilostazol improves walking performance in patients with intermittent claudication: Results of a randomized, double-blind, placebo-controlled study. J Vasc Surg 1995 (in press).
15. Blankenhorn DH, Azen SP, Crawford DW, et al. Effects of Colestipol-niacin therapy on human femoral atherosclerosis. Circulation 83:438-447, 1991.
16. Scandinavian Simvastin Survival Study. Lancet 344:1383-1389, 1994.

17. Johnston KW, Rae M, Hogg-Johnston SA, et al. Five-year results of a prospective study of percutaneous transluminal angioplasty. Ann Surg 206:403-413, 1987.
18. Hunink MGM, Donaldson MC, Meyerowitz MF, et al. Risk and benefits of femoropopliteal percutaneous balloon angioplasty. J Vasc Surg 17:32-41, 1993.
19. Ahn SS, Eton D, Moore WS. Endovascular surgery for peripheral arterial occlusive disease: A critical review. Ann Surg 216:3-16, 1992.
20. Leather RP, Shah DM, Chang BB, et al. Resurrection of the in situ saphenous vein bypass. Ann Surg 208:435-442, 1988.
21. Taylor LM, Edwards JM, Porter JM. Present status of reversed vein bypass grafting: 5-year results of a modern series. J Vasc Surg 11:193-206, 1990.
22. Donaldson MC, Mannick JA, Whittemore AD. Femoral-distal bypass with in situ greater saphenous vein: Long-term results using the Mills valvulotome. Ann Surg 213:457-465, 1991.
23. Bergamini TM, Towne JB, Bandyk DF, et al. Experience with in situ saphenous vein bypasses during 1981 to 1989: Determinant factors of long-term patency. J Vasc Surg 13:137-149, 1991.
24. Conte MS, Belkin M, Donaldson MC, et al. Femorotibial bypass for claudication: Do results justify an aggressive approach? J Vasc Surg 21:873-881, 1995.
25. Rosenthal D, Evans D, McKinsey J, et al. Prosthetic above-knee femoropopliteal bypass for intermittent claudication. J Cardiovasc Surg 31:462-468, 1990.
26. Quinones-Baldrich WJ, Prego AA, Ucelay-Gomez R, et al. Long-term results of infrainguinal revascularization with polytetrafluoroethylene: A ten-year experience. J Vasc Surg 16:209-217, 1992.

42

Avoiding Infrainguinal Bypass Wound Complications in Renal Failure Patients: Should Grafts Be Tunneled Subfascially or Subcutaneously?

JONATHAN P. GERTLER, M.D., JAN D. BLANKENSTEIJN, M.D., Ph.D., and WILLIAM M. ABBOTT, M.D.

Revascularization is clearly the treatment of choice for limb-threatening ischemia, and increasing technical sophistication has led to limb salvage in situations previously deemed irreparable. This aggressive stance toward revascularization has led to the understanding that subsets of high-risk patients, including patients with diabetes, isolated tibial runoffs, pedal grafts, and so on, can be successfully treated and amputation thus averted.

Patients with end-stage renal disease (ESRD) have been identified as a particularly difficult group of patients in whom limb salvage is necessary. Because of their many comorbid conditions and unfavorable anatomy for revascularization procedures, some authors have recommended primary amputation for ESRD patients with extensive ulceration or gangrene and have also identified higher perioperative morbidity and mortality in this group. Increased perioperative complications have also been identified in patients with mild chronic renal insufficiency (CRI). Despite these data, however, most recent series have advocated an aggressive approach to patients with limb ischemia who have significant renal disease.

Although there are many aspects to morbidity and mortality in ESRD and CRI, wound healing and infection are prominent among them. The recent enthusiasm for in situ vein grafting in difficult distal situations might need to be tempered in CRI and ESRD patients, based on reports of increased wound complications using the in situ technique in this setting. On our own service, we anecdotally noted several serious complications from breakdown of subcutaneous wounds overlying in situ vein grafts and therefore decided to review our own and others' experience more closely.

Using the vascular registry of the the Division of Vascular Surgery at Massachusetts General Hospital, we were able to identify 129 patients with known renal disease who had undergone an infrainguinal bypass graft. For the purposes of the study, CRI was defined as an elevation in serum creatinine over 2.0 mg/dl for at least 6 months before the procedure. Patients who had undergone kidney transplantation were not excluded if they met these criteria. Emergency operations for acute ischemia were excluded from analysis, and only operations performed for tissue loss or well-documented ischemic rest pain were included. Forty-two patients who underwent 47 infrainguinal bypass procedures met the above criteria and constitute the study population.

All demographic data including risk factor analysis and presentation category were classified and graded according to the standards suggested by the Ad Hoc Committee on Reporting Standards for Lower Extremity Ischemia of the SVS/NA-ISCVS. Wound infections were classified as superficial or deep surgical site infection (SSI) according to the Centers for Disease Control (CDC) 1992 guidelines. The criteria for these two types of SSI are identified below.

Criteria for superficial SSI	Criteria for deep SSI
Purulent drainage from incision, organisms identified	Purulent drainage from fascia/muscle layer
Local pain, tenderness, swelling, erythema, heat	Deliberate opening of deep incision for temperature >38° C and pain, tenderness, swelling, erythema, heat

Only infections that occur within 30 days of an incision are considered SSIs by CDC guidelines. However, if a permanent, nonautogenous graft is used, any infection at any time will be considered an SSI. To further clarify the patients' response, we applied the time frame suggested by the United Kingdom Surgical Infection Study Group: early (less than 30 days), intermediate (30 to 90 days), and late (more than 90 days).

To delineate the role of graft location, patients were classified into two groups. Group I included patients with grafts that were completely or predominantly subcutaneous, whereas patients whose grafts were positioned in anatomic or subfascial planes were enrolled in group II.

Given the multiple influences on wound healing, a statistical model was developed to isolate the effect of graft location on wound complications in ESRD and CRI patients. Twelve possible covariables to wound healing entered into a stepwise logistic regression analysis: age, gender, immunosuppression, diabetes, graft material, duration of surgery, presence of distal infection, creatinine value, level of distal anastomosis, coronary artery disease, risk factor score, and graft location. Continuous covariables were analyzed with the Mann-Whitney test and discrete variables with the Fisher's exact test. Patency, salvage, and survival rates were assessed by life-table analysis (Kaplan-Meier) and compared with a matched group of similar age and gender from the general population. All analysis was two tailed, and $p<.05$ was considered significant.

Twenty-eight men and 14 women were identified, with a mean age of 71 years (range, 25 to 93). All patients received antibiotic perioperative prophylaxis, usually with cephalosporin. A longitudinal, continuous incision was used for all vein harvest regardless of in situ, reversed, or translocated techniques. The graft location was predominantly subcutaneous in 21 limbs (group I) with in situ vein grafts in 17, reversed vein grafts in two, and two composite PTFE-vein grafts used. In the remaining 26 grafts, which constituted group II, positioned in the subfascial or anatomic plane, there were 12 vein grafts and 14 prosthetic grafts (13 PTFE, one Dacron). Nineteen of the 21 distal anastomoses in group I were below-knee, compared with 16 of 26 in group II. Demographic and perioperative data are listed in Table 1.

The SSIs are detailed in Table 2. In group I, seven early, one intermediate, and one late infection were found (9 of 21; 43%). In three of these situations the graft was exposed, and two

Table 1 Demographic and perioperative data

Parameter	Group I (subcutaneous)	Group II (subfascial)
Patients	20	22
Male/female ratio	13:7	15:7
Median age	76.5	68.5
Preoperative limb status (rest pain:tissue loss)	5:16	7:19
Median risk factor score	8.0	9.0
Median duration CRI (months)	36	54
Immunosuppression (yes:no)	0:21	4:22
Median creatinine (mg/dl)	2.9	3.1
Graft material (vein:prosthetic)	19:2	12:14
Median duration of surgery (hr)	4.5	4.25

patients required graft removal. In contrast, only two early and one intermediate SSI were found in group II ($p = .02$ vs. group I). In group I the thigh was involved in five of nine cases, whereas there was one thigh involvement in group II. The groin was involved three times in each group. Four reoperations for infectious complications were necessary in group I, none in group II ($p = .03$). Of the three SSIs in group II, all occurred in immunosuppressed patients (4 of 26 patients).

Multivariate analysis, using the twelve covariables to wound healing previously noted, failed to reveal any factor other than superficial location of the graft as a predictor of wound infection. Relative risk for superficial location of the graft was 11.6 ($p<.01$). Interestingly, univariate analysis demonstrated that the age of the patient was inversely associated with infection risk. Separate analysis of infection risk when only autogenous grafts in both groups were included for review demonstrated that superficial graft location was still a significant risk factor.

Primary patency and salvage rates for all 47 grafts in the study are shown in Fig. 1, and overall survival for groups I and II is given in Fig. 2. Comparing survival of patients with SSIs to those without revealed a highly significant difference of 60% vs. 94% at 1 year ($p = .01$).

The purpose of our patient review was to determine whether subcutaneous graft position,

Table 2 Details of surgical site infections

SSI level	SSI locus	Group	Infected/exposed graft	Bacteriology	Preoperative tissue loss	Treatment
Superficial	Groin	I	No/no	SAu	No	Local care
Superficial	Thigh	I	No/no	PAe, EnC	Yes	Debridement
Deep	Thigh	I	Yes/yes	PAe, CNS, CF, CAlb	No	Graft excision
Superficial	Groin	I	No/no	NA	NA	Antibiotics
Superficial	Knee	I	No/no	NA	NA	Local care
Superficial	Groin/calf	I	No/no	SAu	No	Local care
Deep	Calf	I	No/yes	GCS, SAu	Yes	Debridement
Deep	Groin, thigh	I	Yes/yes	Eco, CNS	Yes	Above-knee amputation
Superficial	Thigh	I	No/no	PAe, SAu	Yes	Antibiotics
Deep	Groin	II	Yes/no	ECo, SAu	Yes	Local care Died
Deep	Groin	II	No/no	NA	NA	Local care
Superficial	Thigh	II	No/no	SAu, EnC	Yes	Antibiotics

CAlb = *Candida albicans*; CF = *Citrobacter freundii*, CNS = *coagulase negative staphylococcus*; ECo = *Eschericia coli*; EnC = *Enterococcus*, GCS = *Group C Staphylococcus*; NA = not available; PAe = *Pseudomonas aeruginosa*; SAu = *Staphylococcus aureus*.

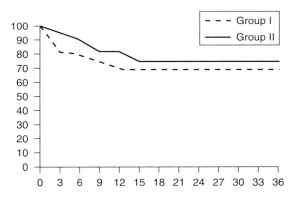

Fig. 1 Patency of grafts for groups I and II.

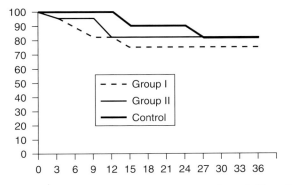

Fig. 2 Life-table survival for groups I and II and control group.

which is of apparent advantage in regard to in situ technique in distal revascularization, might be detrimental in certain subgroups of patients. Our results demonstrate that the wound infection rate is indeed higher when a subcutaneous graft position is used in patients with CRI. A 43% wound infection rate was found in group I (subcutaneous) vs. 12% in the anatomically placed group II grafts. Although 90% of the bypasses in group I were vein grafts, compared with 42% in group II, analysis without prosthetic grafts being included in either group still demonstrates a significant difference. If the patients with immunosuppression as a confounding factor in group II are excluded, the statistical difference between the groups becomes even more pronounced (42%, group I vs. 0%, group II).

In a retrospective review, despite similarity of techniques among surgeons in our division as well as close patient demographics, a multitude of covariables to proper healing are likely involved. Nonetheless, multiple logistical regression clearly demonstrated an independent effect for subcutaneous grafts on SSIs. Surprisingly, an inverse relationship to age was also discerned. This may reflect more aggressive multisystem disease, poorer nutrition, or the role of immunosuppression on the appearance of wound infections. Risk factor scores in patients under 70 years of age were higher, with a statistically significant difference in mean scores when compared with those over 70 years of age (8.0 vs. 6.0; $p = .02$). This tends to support overall debilitation in the young patients selected for this study. Clearly, this is an issue that cannot be resolved retrospectively.

Many of the infections observed in these patients were of consequence only with respect to length of hospital stay and the need for long-term wound care. It should be recognized, however, that despite the classification of a superficial skin infection, a subcutaneous graft is clearly at risk of thrombosis or disruption in this setting. Thus the combination of a greater propensity for wound infection if a subcutaneous graft is used and the immediate risk to life and limb that such a graft poses provides a compelling reason to avoid this approach in renal disease patients unless no other adequate route or approach is feasible. In this setting, a semiclosed or endovascular technique for bypass should be strongly considered.

Explanations for the findings are possible on several theoretical bases that merit further investigation. All wounds disrupt lymphatic flow and drainage, regardless of whether they were from vein harvest alone or for creation of an in situ graft. The presence of a pulsatile graft may alter lymphatic flow and/or wound healing in a way not present without such movement, and this should be studied further. Other plausible explanations must include selection bias for in situ grafting based on anatomic findings on angiography or explantation as well as the degree of distal wound necrosis or contamination. The patient's predisposition to infection because of nutritional factors, skin condition, medications, and vascular anatomy must also be considered.

We reviewed six similar reports describing 275 bypasses in 222 CRI patients. The primary patency rate was 75%, the salvage rate 82%, and the survival rate 53% at 2 years in these studies. Our 2-year patency and salvage rates were similar, at 77% and 76%, respectively, and our survival rate was higher at 79%. All of these data support an aggressive stance toward infrainguinal revascularization in patients with CRI.

The data reviewed and presented in this and other reports are limited by small numbers and retrospective analysis. Yet the findings and the previous anecdotal experience that inspired the study are sufficiently compelling to influence our current approach to infrainguinal bypass in renal failure patients—or indeed in any patient in whom wound healing problems might prove more difficult than usual. We would currently recommend the preferential use of anatomically placed grafts in these patients to avoid superficial breakdown and subsequent catastrophic involvement of an adjacent autogenous or prosthetic vascular graft.

REFERENCES

1. Edwards JM, Taylor LM Jr, Porter JM. Limb salvage in end stage renal disease (ESRD): Comparison of modern results in patients with and without ESRD. Arch Surg 123:1164-1168, 1988.
2. Chang BB, Paty PSK, Shah DM, et al. Results of infrainguinal bypass for limb salvage in patients with end stage renal disease. Surgery 108:742-747, 1990.
3. Harrington EB, Harrington ME, Schanzer H, et al. End stage renal disease— is infrainguinal limb revascularization justified? J Vasc Surg 12:691-695, 1990.
4. Sanchez LA, Goldsmith J, Rivers SP, et al. Limb salvage surgery in end stage renal disease—is it worthwhile? J Cardiovasc Surg 33:344-348, 1992.
5. Whittemore AD, Donaldson MC, Mannick JA. Infrainguinal reconstruction for patients with chronic renal insufficiency. J Vasc Surg 17:32-41, 1993.
6. Drutz DJ, Murphy AL. Altered cell-mediated immunity and its relation to infection susceptibility in patients with uremia. Dial Transplant 8:320-370, 1979.

43

Value and Limitations of Percutaneous Transluminal Angioplasty, Stents, and Lytic Agents for Aortoiliac Disease

KENNETH WAYNE JOHNSTON, M.D., F.R.C.S.(C)

Radiologic interventional procedures have offered important new alternative methods of management for the patients with iliac arterial occlusive disease. Early in the history of the treatment of peripheral arterial occlusive disease, the only alternatives were surgery for patients with severe symptoms and the complications of arterial occlusive disease, or conservative therapy for patients who had minor symptoms. The introduction of interventional radiologic procedures has offered patients with intermediate symptoms an alternative form of therapy. Moreover, it has replaced surgery in some cases and conservative therapy in others.

Over the last 15 years, with the development of new interventional technologies, the proponents of new therapies have often failed to critically evaluate the benefits, risks, and cost implications of their new techniques. I will review the current role of percutaneous transluminal angioplasty (PTA), stents, and fibrinolytic therapy for the management of iliac artery occlusive disease.

PERCUTANEOUS TRANSLUMINAL ANGIOPLASTY

A recent reanalysis of the results of the University of Toronto series of PTA has been published and is summarized in this section.[1] The Toronto series is a large prospective descriptive series of the results of PTA that overcomes some of the methodologic criticisms of other studies: objective noninvasive criteria were used in addition to clinical criteria, to define success; the series represents a consecutive study of patients having PTA; contemporary statistical methods were used; and follow-up was nearly complete.

Methods

As detailed in our previous report,[2] the PTA was considered a success if the clinical symptoms improved by at least one grade (i.e., asymptomatic, mild claudication, disabling claudication, ischemic night pain or rest pain, or ulceration or gangrene) and the ankle/brachial pressure ratio, Doppler waveforms, and/or treadmill exercise improved.

The long-term results were calculated by the Kaplan-Meier method, and the Cox proportional hazards model was used for multivariate analysis to determine the factors associated with late success of PTA.

Results

The 667 procedures involving PTA of the iliac arteries were reanalyzed. The overall results using Kaplan-Meier life-table analysis for all iliac PTAs are presented in Fig. 1. Technical failure occurred in 23 of 664 (3.5%) of the PTAs and was more common ($p < .001$) if the artery was occluded (15 of 83 = 18.1%) vs. stenosed (8 of

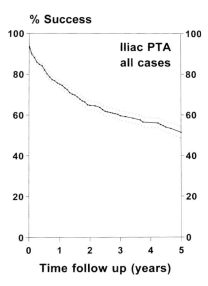

Fig. 1 Life-table analysis for all iliac PTAs.

581 = 1.4%). Thus the data are presented separately for the results of PTA of iliac occlusions and stenoses.

Iliac Occlusions. For the 82 iliac artery occlusions (including the 15 PTAs that failed for technical reasons), the cumulative percent success versus time of follow-up to 3 years, calculated by the Kaplan-Meier method, was as follows: at 1 month, 75.6 ± 4.7%; at 1 year, 59.8 ± 5.5%; at 2 years, 52.8 ± 5.9%; and at 3 years, 48.0 ± 6.3%. Of the variables analyzed, only the number of sites dilated (i.e., one site vs. two or more) was related to late success of the procedure ($p = .04$). For PTA of an iliac occlusion at one site, initial success was 80.3 ± 4.7% vs. 45.5 ± 15.0% if an iliac occlusion and a tandem lesion were dilated at the same time. The late success rate for PTA of an iliac occlusion, predicted from Cox regression, is 66% at 3 years if a single lesion was dilated and 17% if tandem lesions were dilated.

If the 15 cases that were technical failures were excluded, the success rate at 1 month was 91.0 ± 3.5%; at 1 year, 73.2 ± 5.6%; at 2 years, 64.7 ± 6.4%; and at 3 years, 58.8 ± 7.1%.

Iliac Stenoses. For all iliac artery stenoses, the success rates at 1 month were 95.9 ± 0.8%; at 1 year, 77.2 ± 1.8%; at 2 years, 66.5 ± 2.2%; at 3 years, 61.2 ± 2.4%; at 4 years, 57.8 ± 2.6%; at 5 years 54.0 ± 2.9%; and at 6 years 50.0 ± 3.5%. There were only 1.4% (8 of 584) technical failures in this group.

Common Iliac Stenosis. For the common iliac PTAs (n = 313) the success rate at 1 month was 97.1 ± 0.9%; at 1 year, 81.1 ± 2.3%; at 2 years, 70.6 ± 2.9%; at 3 years, 67.8 ± 3.0%; at 4 years, 64.9 ± 3.3%; at 5 years, 60.2 ± 4.0%; and at 6 years, 52.0 ± 5.7%. None of the recorded variables were of statistical significance in predicting the long-term success of the procedure.

External Iliac Stenosis. For PTA of the external iliac artery (n = 209) the success rate at 1 month was 95.2 ± 1.5%; at 1 year, 74.1 ± 3.2%; at 2 years, 62.0 ± 3.8%; at 3 years, 51.0 ± 4.4%; and at 4 years, 48.4 ± 4.5%. By Cox regression analysis, the gender of the patient proved to be a significant predictor of late success: the predicted 3-year success for men was 57% and for women 34%.

Common and External Iliac Stenoses. For PTAs of both common and external iliac stenoses (n = 58), the success rate at 1 month was 92.4 ± 3.7%, at 1 year 67.6 ± 6.6%, at 2 years 59.7 ± 7.2%, at 3 years 59.7 ± 7.2%, and at 4 years 51.6 ± 8.2%. By Cox regression analysis, the runoff was a predictor of late success: for good runoff (i.e., femoral popliteal stenosis <50%), the predicted 3 year success rate was 73% and for poor runoff (i.e., femoral popliteal stenosis ≥50% or occlusion) 30%.

Results Reported in Other Series

The following series also reported results using objective criteria and the life-table analysis method. Wilson et al.[3] used clinical and objective noninvasive criteria to evaluate success and reported a success rate of 89% at 1 month, 78% at 1 year, 74% at 2 years, 67% at 3 years, and 62% at 4 years. Although exact criteria for success were not defined, Tegtmeyer et al.[4] treated 340 aortoiliac lesions and reported an initial success rate of 95% and a cumulative success at 6 years of 85%. Ten patients who were lost to follow-up were excluded from the analysis, and it is not clear if follow-up was current at the end of the study. Van Andel et al.[5] reported an angiographic and clinical success at 14 days of 95%. For those with good runoff, the 6-year patency rate was 86%. Gallino et al.[6] reported a cumulative patency of 90% at 1 year, 89% at 2 years, 89% at 3 years, 88% at 4 years, and 87% at 5 years. Kumpe and Jones[7] reported an initial success rate of 96%, and of the technical successes, 88% were clinically improved and 60% had an objective improvement of distal pressure. When the technical successes were assessed by thigh–brachial pressure index, the 2- and 3-year success rates were 82%. For those who had a technically successful iliac PTA, Spence et al.[8] reported 1-, 2-, and 3-year success rates of 93%, 82%, and 79%. Kadir et al.[9] had an initial technical success of 96% (135 of 141) and a cumulative patency rate of 91% at 1 year and 89% at 3 years.

Complications

In the Toronto series, serious complications were recorded in 3.9% of patients; death in 0.3%; operation was necessary in 1.0% (false aneurysm in 0.1%, ischemia in 0.9%); and hospital discharge was delayed in 2.6% (large hematoma that required transfusion or observation in 1.9% or ischemia that was treated conservatively in 0.7%). As expected, complications were more frequent following PTA of an iliac occlusion than of a stenosis.

In other series of iliac PTA, the complication rates were similar. Kadir et al.[9] had four significant complications in 141 aortoiliac angioplasties (3.5%): two required blood transfusion and two required surgery to remove embolic occlusions. Tegtmeyer et al.[4] reported 15 significant complications in the dilatation of 340 aortoiliac lesions in 200 patients (a patient complication rate of 7.5%): four significant hematomas, one pseudoaneurysm, three arterial thromboses, one iliac rupture, two distal emboli requiring surgical removal, and four with exacerbation of renal failure. Surgical procedures were required in 1.5% of patients. Schoop et al.[10] observed six thrombotic complications in 138 iliac dilatations: three required surgery, two were clinically worse, and one was unchanged.

Consequences of Technical Failure

For the cases that were a technical failure, serious complications were not common. Following failure of PTA of iliac occlusions (n = 15), 7% developed ischemia that did not require emergency surgery, and subsequently 40% of these patients had no further treatment, 52% had surgery, and 7% had an amputation. Following failure of PTA of an iliac stenosis (n = 8), 13% required emergency operation, 13% died of a ruptured iliac artery, and 13% had extravasation of contrast material that was of no clinical consequence. Subsequently 42% had no treatment, 29% repeat PTA, and 29% underwent surgery.

Comparison of PTA to Surgery and Conservative Treatment

The success rates reported in the Toronto series are lower than reported by several other series. The explanation lies in the differences in criteria for success, completeness of follow-up, and methods of data analysis. Direct comparison of the results of PTA and surgery for iliac artery occlusive disease is not possible, because PTA is most often carried out for the treatment of patients with localized arterial stenoses or occlusions, and surgery is often performed because of limb-threatening ischemia and not claudication resulting from more extensive arterial occlusive disease.

However, there is one prospective randomized study that compares PTA and surgery. Wilson et al.[3] reported 76 male patients who were randomly allocated to have aortoiliac surgery and 81 to iliac PTA. The overall cumulative long-term success rate favored surgery (81% vs. 62% at 3 years). The observed differences between surgery and PTA were statistically significant (p = .037) mainly because of the higher early failure rate of PTA rather than late failures. If only those cases that had a technically successful PTA were analyzed, then PTA and surgery had similar long-term success rates. In considering the role of PTA, it seems justified to exclude early failures in the analysis, since a failed PTA does not seem to increase the risk of limb loss[11] or subsequent surgical failure rate.[4] Thus, based on the data from the study by Wilson et al.,[3] for patients who are candidates for either PTA or surgery, since both methods have similar long-term results, in general, PTA is preferred. Note, however, that to be eligible for the study reported by Wilson et al.,[3] all patients had to be candidates for PTA. As a consequence, the incidence of claudication was much higher than would be expected in a normal population of patients with iliac arterial occlusive disease.

Summary of Indications for PTA

The Toronto study has identified that the chance of late success of a PTA is based on the severity of the lesion, the site of the iliac lesion, and other significant variables.[1] Table 1 and Fig. 2 summarize our results at 3 years. For iliac occlusions, late results are good if only one site is dilated. In contrast, the results are poor if an iliac occlusion and a tandem lesion are dilated. PTA of common iliac stenoses yields excellent early and late results. PTA of external iliac stenoses is associated with a good long-term success rate in men but a poor success rate in women. PTA of both common and external iliac stenoses has a

Table 1 Comparison of 3-year results based on severity of lesion, site of PTA, and other significant variables

Severity of stenosis	Site	Other variables	3-year success (%)
Occlusion	Iliac	1 site	66*
		>1 site	17*
Stenosis	Common iliac		68†
	External iliac	Male	57*
		Female	34*
	Both common and external iliac	Good runoff	73*
		Poor runoff	30*

*Cox regression estimate.
†Kaplan-Meier estimate.

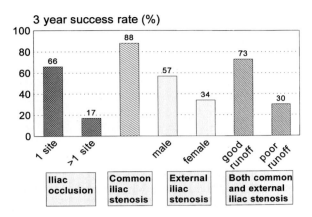

Fig. 2 Results for iliac PTA for the significant groups. The Cox proportional hazards model was used to predict the 3-year success rate.

good success rate in patients with good runoff (less than 50% femoropopliteal stenosis) but not when the runoff is poor (≥50% femoropopliteal stenosis or occlusion). Thus iliac PTA has an important role in the management of patients with arterial occlusive disease and should be considered if the chances of long-term success are good.

The Society of Cardiovascular and Interventional Radiology[12] has identified other factors that should be considered in the selection of the patient for PTA of the iliac artery. The patient's symptoms should be significant and not improved with maximum conservative therapy. Comorbid factors must be carefully evaluated in deciding for or against the procedure. The angiographic characteristics of the lesion may be of prognostic value, specifically, its length, the degree of calcification, the presence of a stenosis vs. an occlusion, and associated aneurysmal or occlusive disease.

STENTS

The possibility of using a stent to improve patency following recanalization was first suggested by Dotter and Judkins.[13] They proposed that "the use of an ... endovascular ... splint could maintain an adequate false lumen" once a channel is created across an occluded arterial segment. Further, they suggested that an "open coil construction" would permit rapid tissue ingrowth and hence the formation of a "new, firmly anchored, autogenous lining surface."

Extensive experience with the use of PTA identified three main causes of failure: (1) inadequate recanalization, (2) the development of intimal hyperplasia, and (3) progression of atherosclerosis. The development of stents has been stimulated by the attempt to prevent these causes of early and late failure following PTA.

Principles of Stents

Becker[14] has summarized the principles underlying the use of stents for iliac artery disease. Stents can be categorized into three general types: balloon-expandable, self-expanding (mechanical), and thermal-expanding. The Palmaz balloon-expandable stent is widely used in North America. It is a metallic device with staggered slots in the wall to permit expansion by an underlying angioplasty balloon. Self-expanding mechanical stents maintain arterial dilatation when they are unloaded from a constraining delivery catheter. Thermal-expanding stents resume their innate size and configuration at body temperature.

The ideal characteristics of an intravascular stent have been tabulated by Becker,[14] and the most important are summarized as follows. The stent must be biocompatible, must be resistant to thrombosis, and should induce minimal neointimal hyperplasia. Several mechanical characteristics are important to permit versatile use. The profile must be low and yet a large expansion permitted. Ideally, it should exhibit longitudinal flexibility to minimize the mechanical trauma that a stiff stent would produce at its ends during arterial pulsation. It must be radiopaque and easily delivered and deployed with a catheter system. Low cost is important, since several stents may have to be used in each case.

Indications

The rationale for the use of stents in the management of patients having PTA of the iliac arteries is based on efforts to improve the early and late patency rates, as discussed in the following sections.

To Prevent Early Failure of PTA. From a purely technical point of view, there are two good indications for using stents to prevent early failure of an iliac PTA. "Elastic recoil" may be observed following balloon deflation and is usually predictive of a poor result. Following PTA, a dissection occurs in approximately 4.5% of cases.[15] When extensive dissection is present, it seems rational that the use of stents will prevent further dissection, reduce intraluminal debris, and reduce turbulent flow and as a consequence may improve early patency rates.

To Prevent Late Failure of PTA. Although it has been suggested that a stent may be indicated when the hemodynamic result is not satisfactory, the data from the Toronto series of PTA did not show a relationship between the residual pressure gradient across the stenosis and the long-term success rate except when the gradient was very large.[2] Thus a small residual gradient without evidence of elastic recoil or a dissection is not likely a primary indication. PTA of an iliac occlusion has been suggested as an indication for the use of a stent; however, the series by Palmaz et al.[16] did not show a statistical difference in success rates between iliac stenoses and occlusions with the use of stents. Indications for using a stent to improve late success rates after PTA are unproved at this time. Although it has been suggested that they may reduce the incidence of intimal hyperplasia, the evidence for this is lacking, and indeed they may incite the intimal fibrocellular proliferative process. Further, it is difficult to understand how a stent could reduce the progression of atherosclerosis. Palmaz et al.[16] noted a 5% per year incidence of proximal or distal progression of atherosclerosis, and this would not be prevented by the use of a localized stent at the site of a stenosis. The suggestion that multiple stents should be placed along the entire iliac segment to prevent recurrent atherosclerotic narrowing requires careful evaluation.

Results

Palmaz Series. Several published series have identified the possible roles of stents in the management of arterial occlusive disease,[17-29] but most are small series from one center. The multicenter trial using the Palmaz stent provides descriptive results of this technique in 486 patients who underwent 587 procedures.[16] "Clinical benefit" was obtained in 91% at 1 year, 84% at 2 years, and 69% at 3.6 years. Unfortunately, when this study is evaluated against the expected reporting characteristics for a good series, there are several potential shortcomings. The report does not indicate whether the data were evaluated by the "intention to treat." Although angiograms were obtained, no consistent objective end point was used in the evaluation of the results represented in the paper. The life-table analysis is unclear as to how many patients were lost to follow-up and whether the follow-up was current for all patients at the time of analysis. There were, however, defined entry and exclusion criteria. Thus the results provide some basis for comparison with other series, but it is difficult to determine whether the data can be generalized.

Comparison to Toronto Series. Direct comparison between the Palmaz multicenter series of PTA and stents and the Toronto series of PTA only is difficult because of the differences in design and analysis of the descriptive studies; however, the comparison provides some insight on the benefits and risks of the procedures. Table 2 and Fig. 3 summarize the results. As analyzed, all cases in the Palmaz series were considered an initial success. Analysis of the Toronto data was based on the intention to treat, and all technical and early failures were included, giving an initial

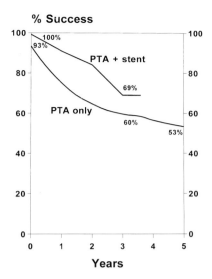

Fig. 3 Comparison of Toronto series of PTA and Palmaz multicenter series of PTA and stent.

Table 2 Comparison of results of PTA plus Palmaz stent and the Toronto series of PTA only

	PTA only (Toronto series)[1,2]	PTA and stent[16]
Number of centers	1 center	Multicenter
Number of cases	587 procedures	662 procedures
Criteria of success	Clinical and objective vascular laboratory measurements	Clinical
Initial success	93%	100%
3-year success rate	60%	69%

success rate of 93%. In Palmaz' series, patients having PTA and a stent had a 69% clinical success rate at 3 years, compared with patients having PTA only, who had a 60% clinical and objective vascular laboratory success rate at 3 years. Note that the 9% improvement in 3-year results with the addition of a stent may be explained by the 7% higher initial success rate, which appears to be the result of exclusion of technical and early failures in Palmaz' series.

In Table 3, the complication rates of PTA plus Palmaz stent are compared with the complications reported in the Toronto series of PTA only. In general, the use of a stent is associated with a higher complication rate.

Randomized Prospective Results. Richter et al.[30] presented the preliminary results of a prospective randomized study comparing balloon angioplasty and stent for iliac artery stenoses and occlusions in an abstract form. As of October 1, 1994, no detailed report of the results has been published. Table 4 summarizes the results from the abstract. The interim data show a clear benefit to the use of stents in the management of iliac disease; however, a final conclusion on the validity of the study and its generalizability must await detailed publication.

Summary of Indications for Stents

In summary, stents appear to have a role in the management of lesions that demonstrate "elastic recoil" after PTA or when extensive dissection occurs. The justification for using stents to improve the long-term results remains unclear. In contrast to the Toronto series of PTA, a large multicenter study of PTA and stents does not show significantly improved long-term success rates, and indeed the complication rate is higher. An ongoing randomized prospective study will provide important information on the role of stents. Publication of the results is eagerly awaited.

LYTIC AGENTS FOR THE MANAGEMENT OF ILIAC ARTERY OCCLUSION

McNamara and Bomberger[31] noted that fibrinolytic therapy for the management of thrombosed iliac arteries resulted in clot lysis and demonstration of an underlying iliac stenosis that may be amenable to balloon angioplasty. The following sections review the methods and results of this approach.

Table 3 Comparison of complications of PTA plus Palmaz stent and the Toronto series of PTA only

	PTA and stent[16]	PTA only (Toronto series)[1,2]
Death	1.9	0.3
Groin hematoma		
Small		2.7
Large		1.9
Severity not specified	1.6	0.0
Bleeding		
Operation required		0.0
No operation		0.0
Treatment not specified	1.9	
Retroperitoneal	0.4	
Arteriovenous fistula		
Operation required		0.1
Treatment not specified	1.6	0.0
Acute ischemia		
Operation required		0.9
Conservative treatment		0.7
Treatment not specified	1.4	0.0
Distal embolization	1.2	0.4
Renal failure	0.8	0.0
Dissection	0.4	1.0
Extravasation or intramural	0.2	0.1
Other	0.2	0.1
Dislodgement of stent	0.8	

Table 4 Interim results of a randomized prospective study comparing PTA with PTA plus stents for the management of iliac artery occlusive disease

	PTA (n = 114) (%)	Stent (n = 112) (%)
Technical success	90.4	98.2
Initial clinical success	88.6	98.2
Additional surgery or intervention	14.9	15.8
Angiographic success at 5 years	64.6	94.6
Clinical success at 5 years	69.7	92.7

Methods

DeMaioribus et al.[32] described their current technique in detail: 240,000 units of urokinase are injected into the thrombus by the pulsed spray technique, and 240,000 units per hour are administered until lysis occurs. Then 60,000 to 120,000 units per hour is given, along with heparin. Serial angiograms are performed to monitor the progress, and the patient is carefully evaluated for bleeding and the severity of ischemia. In patients with acute ischemia, the limb must be viable, since 12 to 18 hours of infusion may be necessary to obtain lysis. Other contraindications include recent surgery, active peptic ulcer disease, recent stroke, or an underlying bleeding diathesis.

In summary, reported experience with fibrinolysis for opening occluded iliac arteries is limited but offers an acceptable alternative for managing patients with localized disease or for patients with significant comorbid conditions that may contraindicate surgery.

Results

DeMaioribus et al.[32] reported 12 patients with iliac artery occlusion who had 15 courses of fibrinolysis. Seven of the 12 were successful after PTA, four had incomplete lysis and femorofemoral crossover grafts were performed, and one amputation was necessary in a patient with a protein-S deficiency. Beck et al.,[33] from the University of Freiburg, Germany, reported a large series of 4750 PTAs between 1978 and 1987. From this group, lysis of iliac artery thrombosis was carried out in 12 cases. Sixty-six percent were technical successes and overall 50% were late successes.

Summary of Indications

Chronic iliac artery thrombosis or acute thrombosis with a viable limb can be treated with fibrinolysis. After opening the artery, PTA of the underlying stenosis may be possible. Larger series of patients are required in order to establish the role of this approach in managing patients with iliac occlusions.

CONCLUSIONS

Iliac PTA has an important role in the management of patients with arterial occlusive disease and should be considered if the chances of long-term success are good: an iliac artery occlusion that is localized to one site, a common iliac stenosis, an external iliac stenosis in a man, or PTA of both common and external iliac artery stenoses if the runoff is good. The adjunctive use of a stent appears justified if the artery exhibits "elastic recoil" or an extensive dissection results from the PTA; however, improvement of the long-term results by inhibiting intimal hyperplasia or reducing the progression of atherosclerosis or providing a better initial hemodynamic result has not been proven by current publications but may be established when the results of an ongoing prospective controlled study are available. Urokinase is useful for opening an iliac artery occlusion and permitting PTA of the underlying stenosis; however, publication of a large series to demonstrate long term results is not available.

I wish to thank Ms. P. Purdy for secretarial assistance.

REFERENCES

1. Johnston KW. Iliac arteries: Reanalysis of results of balloon angioplasty. Intervent Radiol 186:207-212, 1993.
2. Johnston KW, Rae M, Hogg-Johnston SA, Colapinto RF, Walker PM, Baird RJ, Sniderman KW, Kalman PG. Five-year results of a prospective study of percutaneous transluminal angioplasty. Ann Surg 206:403-413, 1987.
3. Wilson SE, Wolf GL, Cross AP. Percutaneous transluminal angioplasty versus operation for peripheral arteriosclerosis. J Vasc Surg 9:1-9, 1989.
4. Tegtmeyer CJ, Hartwell GD, Selby JB, Robertson R Jr, Kron IL, Tribble CG. Results and complications of angioplasty in aortoiliac disease. Circulation 83(Suppl 2):I53–I60, 1991.
5. Van Andel GJ, Van Erp WF, Krepel VM, Breslau PJ. Percutaneous transluminal dilatation of the iliac artery: Long-term results. Radiology 156:321-323, 1985.
6. Gallino A, Mahler F, Probst P, Nachbur B. Percutaneous transluminal angioplasty of the arteries of the lower limbs: A five-year follow-up. Circulation 70:619-623, 1984.
7. Kumpe DA, Jones DN. Percutaneous transluminal angioplasty; Radiologic viewpoint. Appl Radiol 11:29-40, 1982.
8. Spence RK, Freiman DB, Gatenby R, Hobbs CL, Barker CF, Berkowitz HD, Roberts B, McClean G, Oleaga J, Ring EJ. Long-term results of transluminal angioplasty of the iliac and femoral arteries. Arch Surg 116:1377-1386, 1981.
9. Kadir S, White RI Jr, Kaufman SL, Barth KH, Williams GM, Burdick JF, O'Mara CS, Smith GW, Stonesifer GL Jr, Ernst CB, Minken SL. Long-term results of aortoiliac angioplasty. Surgery 94:10-14, 1983.
10. Schoop W, Levy H, Cappius G. Early and late results of PTD in iliac stenosis. In Zeitler E, Gruntzig A, Schoop W, eds. Percutaneous Vascular Recanalization. Berlin: Springer-Verlag, 1978, pp 111-117.
11. Morin J-F, Johnston KW, Rae M. Improvement after successful percutaneous transluminal dilatation treatment of occlusive peripheral arterial disease. Surg Gynecol Obstet 163:453-457, 1986.
12. Standards of Practice Committee of the Society of Cardiovascular and Interventional Radiology. Guidelines for percutaneous transluminal angioplasty. Radiology 177:619, 1990.
13. Dotter CT, Judkins MP. Transluminal treatment of arteriosclerotic obstruction: Description of a new technique and a preliminary report of its applications. Circulation 30:654, 1964.

14. Becker GJ. Intravascular stents: General principles and status of lower-extremity arterial applications. Circulation 83(Suppl I):I-122–I-136, 1991.
15. Becker GJ, Palmaz JC, Rees CR, Ehrman KO, Lalka SG, Dalsing MC, Cikrit DF, McLean GK, Burke DR, Richter GM, et al. Angioplasty-induced dissections in human iliac arteries: Management with Palmaz balloon-expandable intraluminal stents. Radiology 176:31-38, 1990.
16. Palmaz JC, Laborde JC, Rivera FJ, Encarnacion CE, Lutz JD, Moss JG. Stenting of the iliac arteries with the Palmaz stent: Experience from a multicenter trial. Cardiovasc Intervent Radiol 15:291-297, 1992.
17. Williams JB, Watts PW, Nguyen VA, Peterson CL. Balloon angioplasty with intraluminal stenting as the initial treatment modality in aorto-iliac occlusive disease. Am J Surg 168:202-204, 1994.
18. Criado FJ, Queral LA, Patten P, Valentin W. The role of endovascular therapy in lower extremity revascularization. Lessons learned and current strategies. Int Angiol 12:221-230, 1993.
19. Hausegger KA, Cragg AH, Lammer J, Lafer M, Fluckiger F, Klein GE, Sternthal MH, Pilger E. Iliac artery stent placement: Clinical experience with a nitinol stent. Radiology 190:199-202, 1994.
20. Dyet JF, Shaw JW, Cook AM, Nicholson AA. The use of the Wallstent in aortoiliac vascular disease. Clin Radiol 48:227-231, 1993.
21. Blum U, Gabelman A, Redecker M, Noldge G, Dornberg W, Grosser G, Heiss W, Langer M. Percutaneous recanalization of iliac artery occlusions: Results of a prospective study. Radiology 189:536-540, 1993.
22. Zeitler E, Beyer-Enke S, Rompel O. Indications and results after Strecker-stent-application in iliac and SFA. Int Angiol 12:152-161, 1993.
23. Strecker EP, Hagen B, Liermann D, Schneider B, Wolf HR, Wambsganns J. Iliac and femoropopliteal vascular occlusive disease treated with flexible tantalum stents. Cardiovasc Intervent Radiol 16:158-164, 1993.
24. Kidney D, Murphy J, Malloy M. Balloon-expandable intravascular stents in atherosclerotic iliac artery stenosis: Preliminary experience. Clin Radiol 47:189-192, 1993.
25. Liermann D, Strecker EP, Peters J. The Strecker stent: Indications and results in iliac and femoropopliteal arteries. Cardiovasc Intervent Radiol 15:298-305, 1992.
26. Vorwerk D, Gunther RW. Stent placement in iliac arterial lesions: Three years of clinical experience with the Wallstent. Cardiovasc Intervent Radiol 15:285-290, 1992.
27. Hausegger KA, Lammer J, Hagen B, Fluckiger F, Lafer M, Klein GE, Pilger E. Iliac artery stenting—clinical experience with the Palmaz stent, Wallstent, and Strecker stent. Acta Radiol 33:292-296, 1992.
28. Kichikawa K, Uchida H, Yoshioka T, Maeda M, Nishimine K, Kubota Y, Sakaguchi S, Ohishi H, Iwasaki S. Iliac artery stenosis and occlusion: Preliminary results of treatment with Gianturco expandable metallic stents. Radiology 177:799-802, 1990.
29. Vorwerk D, Guenther RW. Mechanical revascularization of occluded iliac arteries with use of self-expandable endoprostheses. Radiology 175:411-415, 1990.
30. Richter GL, Roeren T, Noeldge G, Landwehr P, Allenberg JR, Kauffman GW. Initial long-term results of a randomized five-year study: Iliac stent. Vasa Suppl 35:192-193, 1992.
31. McNamara TO, Bomberger RA. Factors affecting initial and 6-month patency rates after intraarterial thrombolysis with high dose urokinase. Am J Surg 152:709-712, 1986.
32. DeMaioribus CA, Mills JL, Fugitani RM, Taylor SM, Joseph AE. A reevaluation of intraarterial thrombolytic therapy for acute lower extremity ischemia. J Vasc Surg 17:888-895, 1993.
33. Beck AH, Muhe A, Ostheim W, Heiss W, Hasler K. Long-term results of percutaneous transluminal angioplasty: A study of 4750 dilatations and local lyses. Eur J Vasc Surg 3:245-252, 1989.

SECTION V

Noninvasive and Less Invasive Diagnostic and Therapeutic Modalities

This section examines noninvasive and less invasive diagnostic and therapeutic modalities. A chapter on vascular laboratory funding and reimbursement is included along with chapters relating to controversies regarding low-dose heparin and oral anticoagulation for patients undergoing vascular surgery. An update on pneumatic tourniquet occlusion techniques for infrainguinal bypass is also included.

44

Vascular Laboratory Funding and Reimbursement: Present Status and Future Directions

J. DENNIS BAKER, M.D.

In the 1980s the field of noninvasive vascular testing grew rapidly. Technologic improvements, particularly in duplex scanning, expanded the scope of examinations that could be performed. Although at one time noninvasive testing had been performed by some vascular surgeons and a few radiologists with a special interest in ultrasound, the increased demand for noninvasive tests resulted in the establishment of many centers to perform these examinations. Initially the balance between costs and reimbursement meant that most centers functioned well fiscally and some made substantial profits. In the early 1990s, however, this situation was drastically changed when the pressures to contain the growing costs of medical care resulted in substantial cutbacks in reimbursement for all types of services, including noninvasive testing.

TYPES OF VASCULAR LABORATORIES

In past years, it was possible to consider most laboratories as being similar in terms of access to patients, adequate reimbursement, and external controls. However, this conceptual framework is no longer valid, and the specific nature of each laboratory is important in considering how it will be affected by threats, present and future. The specific business structure and its relation to clinical practice are important factors in defining how each laboratory will be affected by the policies of the payor. The following are categories that are relevant to reimbursement and regulation.

Institution Based. An institution-based laboratory is typically within the hospital setting, a health maintenance organization (HMO), or a large group practice. Such a laboratory is usually owned and operated by the institution. The physicians associated with the laboratory may derive part of their income based on their activity in the laboratory or, if they are on a salary, their work may simply be considered part of their overall job. Interpretation services may be billed by the institution (as part of a global charge) or individually by the physicians.

Office Based. The office-based laboratory is the typical arrangement provided by physicians in office practices; the laboratory is owned and operated by the practice. Originally the majority of office-based testing was performed by vascular surgeons, but increasingly it may be performed by other specialists, including neurologists and cardiologists. In this type of setting a large proportion of patients tested are generated by the office practice itself, with relatively few being referred by outside physicians solely for the purpose of having noninvasive testing.

Free-Standing Laboratories Dedicated to Vascular Testing. Such facilities have often been created by vascular surgeons to separate testing services from a specific doctor's practice. In some settings there is a need for complete separation of the invasive testing from the practice of a surgeon or a group of surgeons. Often this need arises when there are competing individuals or groups of physicians and when the practices are not sufficiently large to support an office-based laboratory. It is common for some or all of the physicians who refer patients to the laboratory to have a financial interest in the business.

Free-Standing Multipurpose Testing Centers. Most frequently these are practices in which vascular testing is only a fraction of the overall operation. Typically these centers provide a wide range of patient examinations that, in addition to peripheral arterial evaluation, may include general radiology, angiography, CT and MR scanning, and noninvasive cardiology. Most often this type of center is under the direction of radiologists.

Mobile Facilities. There are two variations on the mobile concept: (1) A self-contained laboratory in a truck or van or (2) a system in which equipment is carried to various sites so that testing can be conducted within an existing facility. Either type of mobile laboratory usually performs testing for a doctor's office, a clinic, or, in some cases, a hospital. Some mobile operations are extensions of a standard fixed-base operation, allowing services to be provided conveniently in remote locations. In other situations the mobile testing is a variation on the theme of the free-standing laboratory, as discussed earlier.

POLICIES AND ISSUES AFFECTING VASCULAR LABORATORIES

In recent years a significant concern of managers of vascular laboratories has been the cutbacks in reimbursement rates for both technical and professional services; however, these reductions are only a part of the problem. Some of the other important issues facing laboratories will be discussed next.

Reduction in Reimbursement Rates

In January 1992 the Medicare fee schedule implemented for the first time a uniform approach to reimbursement across the country. Gone was the "usual, customary, and reasonable" approach, which had been used by Medicare carriers for many years. It was replaced by the Resource-Based Relative Value Scale (RBRVS). (It should be noted that only the physician work relative value units are resource based. The components for practice and malpractice insurance costs are still based on historic charges.)

For most services the drastic cutbacks brought about by the new Medicare fee schedule have been in place for several years. Noninvasive testing is included in the new payment structure. Depending on the reimbursement rates under the earlier "usual, customary, and reasonable" system, payments for physiologic tests were not much affected. On the other hand, there was a significant cutback in the payments for the different duplex scanning procedures, with reimbursement down an average of 38% compared with 1991 levels, before the fee schedule was introduced.[1] Since a substantial proportion of testing is performed on Medicare patients, the impact on laboratory income has been significant.

Although health insurance companies had been considering broad-based reductions in levels of reimbursements, little had been done until the implementation of the Medicare RBRVS program in 1992. A number of carriers as well as HMOs are revising their own fee schedules downward to the point that they are similar to Medicare rates. It is likely that further changes will be instituted by private health care programs. In turn, this will result in further reductions in payments for vascular laboratory work.

Changes in Allowed Indications for Testing

For many years insurance carriers have limited the indications for which noninvasive tests will be reimbursed. In an attempt to reduce costs, carriers are becoming even more restrictive on the clinical situations in which tests can be carried out. The Medicare legislation does not permit most types of screening tests, and vascular testing is included in this ban. Some of the Medicare carriers have tried to further limit testing by expanding the definitions of a screening test. As noted in *Providers' News* of Medicare Services, "In general, noninvasive studies of the arterial system are to be utilized when invasive correction is contemplated but not to follow noninvasive medical treatment regimens. The latter may be followed with physical findings and/or progression or relief of signs and/or symptoms. Screening of the asymptomatic patient is not covered by Medicare."[2] Another approach is to provide more specific definitions of medical necessity. "Noninvasive peripheral arterial examinations, performed to establish the level and/or degree of arterial occlusive disease, are medically necessary if (1) significant signs and/or symptoms of limb ischemia are present *and* (2) the patient is a candidate for invasive therapeutic procedures. . . . It is not medically necessary to proceed beyond the physical examination for minor signs and symptoms such as hair loss, absence of a single pulse, relative coolness of the foot, shiny thin skin or lack of toe nail growth unless related signs and/or symptoms are present which are severe enough to require possible invasive intervention."[2]

One of the great frustrations faced by directors and administrators of vascular laboratories is the lack of consistency in policies on acceptable indications and testing frequency between the different Medicare carriers. Now that the Health Care Financing Administration (HCFA) has developed a nationwide pricing structure, most physicians assume that the agency dictates the uniform payment policies. Actually, the individual carriers have great latitude in establishing these policies, so there is considerable variability in what tests can be covered. In rare situations, a National Coverage Policy Decision can be issued that mandates the exact approach to be used by all carriers. An example of this mechanism is the decision to deny payment for all photoplethysmography. However, the convoluted administrative process required to produce a National Coverage Policy Decision limits the use of this tactic. In an attempt to achieve more uniformity in payment for vascular testing, a subcommittee of the Medicare Carrier Medical Directors was formed in late 1992. This group sought recommendations from physicians and others involved with laboratories and developed a set of guidelines. Unfortunately, their paper was only a recommendation to the carriers, and to date only some of the carriers have actually implemented the model policies. One can only hope that the future will bring more uniform policies.

In the past, screening for appropriate indications was based on the paperwork submitted. The change to electronic claim submission has meant that the laboratory had the option of justifying the tests performed for special indications, thus providing more complete documentation of medical necessity. The more specific definitions of medical necessity and exclusions often cannot be determined from a single diagnosis code, which usually results in a denied claim.

Medicare has served notice that it will be making increasing use of postpayment reviews to monitor the appropriateness of submitted claims: "It is the responsibility of the provider to ensure the medical necessity of procedures and to maintain a record for post-payment audit."[2] Unlike in the past, when a laboratory simply received no payment for denied claims, claims can now be denied after payment has been made. The insurance carrier can choose to review claims for appropriateness of payment, and if the laboratory does not have records to document the appropriate indications for performing a certain test, a refund will be required for all tests for which documentation is inadequate or missing. In practice, a refund is not usually required, but the amount is deducted from future payments. At present it appears that carriers are making only limited use of postpayment audits; however, it is certain that this practice will be expanded in the future. At present I have no information regarding postpayment audits by private programs, but it is prudent to assume that as in other issues, they will follow the lead of the Medicare program. All laboratories should be certain that their permanent records clearly identify the exact indication for each examination performed.

All involved with vascular testing should clearly understand that Medicare holds the provider (i.e., the laboratory) responsible for determining that an examination is performed for an appropriate indication. This means that the fact that a physician orders a test is not sufficient justification for performing (or at least for billing for) the service. Many laboratory directors have complained that they cannot refuse to perform a test ordered by a referring physician; however, laboratories are going to have to take one of three paths: (1) to educate referring physicians regarding appropriate (covered) indications for different tests, (2) refuse to perform inappropriate tests, or (3) perform inappropriate tests to satisfy the referring physician but not bill for these services.

Decreasing Workload

A number of laboratories are experiencing a decrease in patients referred for vascular testing. This has resulted, at least in part, from a change in referral patterns. Increasingly, physicians have had to join HMOs and other types of contracted care systems. The contracts define the referral patterns, so many internists can no longer send patients to the vascular surgeons they used in the past. In addition, the contracts may ban or severely limit the types of testing that can be ordered as part of the patient's workup. Currently, it is not unusual to have to secure authorization from a "gatekeeper" to obtain a carotid duplex scan of a patient. Under these pressures, free-standing facilities may be seeing a decrease in patients, whereas institution-based vascular laboratories may not be significantly affected.

Contracting Potential

Increasingly, various medical services are covered under fixed-cost contracts with HMOs or other providers. Patients enrolled in these programs are limited to using facilities holding contracts. Although there have not been many cases in which there is a limitation on the vascular laboratories that can be used by patients, it is likely that this will occur increasingly. Institution-based laboratories may be able to acquire patients through arrangements made by the institution as a whole. On the other hand, it is currently difficult for office-based or free-standing laboratories to obtain contracts. Since vascular testing represents a minute portion of medical services required by an HMO, there is little incentive for the organization to make efforts to seek such contracts. The exception to this may be the vascular laboratory within a radiology department. The large volume of work provided by the entire service may allow it to obtain a contract.

Self-Referral Legislation

Federal legislation bans a physician from referring Medicare or Medicaid patients to any facility in which that physician has a financial interest. This legislation came about as a protest against the growing practice of referring patients to imaging centers owned by the physicians. The current legislation, informally known as Starke II, specifically includes ultrasound services under the prohibition, so vascular laboratories are definitely affected. It is likely that any major federal health care reform will extend the scope of the prohibition to include participants in other health care programs.

Self-referral bans are also being passed at the state level. In 1994 the California legislature passed a bill banning self-referral. Unlike the federal legislation, this prohibition is not limited to Medicare and Medicaid patients but applies to all patients. It appears that California is preparing to enforce this ruling: as part of the license renewal process physicians are required to list all entities in which they (or their immediate family) have a financial interest.

Physicians will have to follow developments in this area carefully. It is not clear how compliance will be determined. The approach now used in California may be used in other states to develop a database to aid in monitoring compliance.

Current regulations specifically exclude from the prohibition any testing performed within an office or a group practice. Clearly, legislators did not want to confront the medical establishment on what physicians do within their practices. The biggest problem will occur with free-standing laboratories set up by vascular surgeons (and often other specialists). To avoid violations, which carry serious penalties, physicians with financial interests in a facility will either have to end this relationship or stop referring the patients covered by the rules. An important gray area may concern the office-based laboratory, which for economic or other reasons has been set up as an entity separate from the office practice, usually with a different provider number. It is likely that this may not be considered part of the office practice and so will fall under the self-referral ban. It may be necessary for laboratories to change status officially and be incorporated into the physician's office or group practice, thus billing with the same provider number.

The many changes in reimbursement for vascular testing are eroding the income of many laboratories. Additionally, the many pressures toward health care reform are redefining patterns of practice and referral. To date few facilities have been forced to close, but many are foundering. A careful understanding of changes in reimbursement policies, the effects of contracts, and the erosion of traditional referral patterns is essential if a vascular laboratory is to survive the storm.

REFERENCES

1. Baker JD. Costs of duplex scanning and the impact of the changes in Medicare reimbursement. J Vasc Surg 18:702-707, 1993.
2. Providers' News. Baton Rouge, La.: Medicare Services, April 1993, pp 1.12-1.16.

45

Controversies Regarding Low-Dose Heparin Regimens

F. WILLIAM BLAISDELL, M.D., and JOHN T. OWINGS, M.D.

Although the anticoagulant heparin was discovered by McLean[1] in 1916 and subsequently introduced into clinical practice by Murray et al.[2] in 1936, the nature of heparin's actions and appropriate dosage still remains unclear. Considerable controversy exists regarding the advantages and disadvantages of the various low-dose regimens now advocated for thromboembolism prophylaxis. These include (1) the standard low-dose heparin regimen, 5000 units of subcutaneous heparin two to three times a day[3,4]; (2) adjusted-dose heparin, sufficient subcutaneous or intravenous heparin to raise the partial thromboplastin time 2 to 5 seconds above normal[5]; and (3) low-molecular-weight heparin, 30 mg subcutaneously twice daily without monitoring.[6-8]

BACKGROUND

In 1939 Brinkhous[9] demonstrated that the anticoagulant activity of heparin was markedly augmented by a plasma cofactor. This cofactor was named antithrombin III by Abildgaard[10] in 1968. It is now understood that heparin, in normal patients, potentiates the antithrombotic effects of antithrombin III and that heparin itself is only a weak antithrombin.[4,7,11] Although antithrombin III acts at multiple sites on the clotting cascade, its primary mechanism of action is to neutralize activated factor X at the final common pathway of coagulation.[12] The recognition of heparin's ability to potentiate the action of antithrombin III suggested that doses of heparin lower than those used therapeutically might be effective for thromboembolism prophylaxis in surgical patients and carry less risk of hemorrhage than the conventional therapeutic doses.

Kakkar's international study[4] of thromboembolism prophylaxis in hip surgery in 1975 gave credibility to the use of low-dose heparin prophylaxis in surgical patients.[13] In this series, a double-blind randomized international trial in which more than 4000 patients were studied, a control placebo-treated group was compared with one in which 5000 units of heparin was administered subcutaneously twice daily, starting before surgery and continuing for 3 days postoperatively. Sixteen patients in the control group and two in the treated group died of pulmonary embolism; 32 patients in the control and 11 in the treated group developed clinical evidence of deep venous thrombosis (DVT). The bleeding incidence was the same in both groups, giving credibility to the argument that low dosages of heparin were safe and effective.

THE CONTROVERSY

In 1979 Wessler and Gitel,[14] experienced hematologists, expressed skepticism regarding the universal benefit of low-dose heparin and stated, "Despite conflicting claims, low-dose heparin regimens are presently believed to be of limited value in open prostatectomy and in major orthopedic procedures, especially repairs of femoral fractures and reconstructive operations on the hip and knee. Inadequate data are available on prophylaxis for emergency surgery or trauma. A low-dose heparin regimen is also considered inadequate for patients undergoing operation during an active thrombotic process."

Hampson et al.,[15] in 1974, performed a prospective placebo-controlled study of the efficacy of standard low-dose heparin for preventing DVT in patients undergoing hip replacement. He found that although the mean time to the occurrence of DVT was longer in the patients on heparin, there was no significant difference in the incidence between the heparin and control groups. The authors observed that previous trials, which concluded by day 10, likely missed a significant number of thrombi. From this they concluded that "... heparin 5000 units three times daily has no effect on the frequency or extent of postoperative thrombi."

We and others have also found that low-dose heparin prophylaxis appeared to be inadequate in preventing thrombotic complications in trauma patients and after certain major surgical operations.[16,17] Ruiz et al.[18] recently raised a more alarming note. He studied 100 consecutive trauma patients in a nonrandomized fashion, 50 of whom received 5000 units of subcutaneous heparin every 12 hours and the remainder who received no DVT prophylaxis. Although the patients treated with heparin had more risk factors for thromboembolism, the results were remarkable. Fourteen (28%) of 50 patients receiving heparin developed DVT; only one patient (2%) of the 50 who did not receive heparin developed DVT. He concluded that patients who were at increased risk for DVT are better served with either increased doses of heparin or alternative forms of DVT prophylaxis.

Wille-Jorgensen and Ott[19] noted that despite prophylaxis with low-dose heparin, postoperative thromboembolism still occurred in 10% of patients undergoing abdominal operations. They found by multiple logistic regression that age, body mass index, preoperative hemoglobin concentration, and colorectal operations contributed to the prediction of failure for low-dose heparin prophylaxis and that gender, malignant lesions, previous thromboembolism, hypertension, diabetes mellitus, and varicose veins did not.

The reasons for the reported failures of standard low-dose heparin may relate to a marked variation in the availability of the cofactor antithrombin III. Miller et al.,[20] in a study of 50 consecutive trauma admissions, found that more than 60% of all adult trauma patients had low antithrombin III levels at some time during their hospitalization and that low antithrombin III levels correlated with the severity of injury. This finding was confirmed at our institution in a study by Owings et al.,[21] who prospectively evaluated 154 severely injured patients (mean Injury Severity Score, 23) and found that 61% had antithrombin III levels below normal (normal range, 80% to 120%). We found the risk factors for decreased antithrombin III activity to be the same as those previously published for thromboembolism.[22] Low antithrombin III levels were found to be associated with DVT and disseminated intravascular coagulation (DIC). This caused us to conclude that unmonitored thromboembolism prophylaxis using the antithrombin III potentiator, heparin, would likely result in a significant failure rate because those patients for whom prophylaxis was intended lacked adequate amounts of antithrombin III.

Damus and Wallace[23] had noted that antithrombin III levels are low in liver disease, sepsis, and DIC. In an atherosclerosis risk study of 15,800 middle-aged men and women, Conlan et al.[24] reported that antithrombin III levels were significantly higher in women than in men and in blacks than in whites. Antithrombin III levels decreased with age in men but increased in age with women. They concluded that antithrombin III levels as well as other risk factors must be considered when evaluating patients for prophylaxis for arterial thrombosis.

It has become clear that an increased thrombotic tendency can be anticipated in patients who have decreased antithrombin III levels. Factors associated with decreased levels of antithrombin III include congenital deficiency, advanced age, liver disease, nephrotic syndrome, sepsis, major trauma, DIC, and L-asparaginase therapy. Low levels are seen in sick and injured patients and those with preexisting, acquired, or congenital antithrombin III deficiency. All of these patients benefit little or not at all from standard low-dose heparin prophylaxis.

ADJUSTED-DOSE HEPARIN CONCEPT

Leyvraz et al.[5] pointed out that the efficacy of fixed doses of 5000 units of heparin injected subcutaneously every 8 or 12 hours has been disappointing in many clinical settings when objective techniques such as phlebography were used to detect DVT. They noted that individual responses to fixed doses of heparin varied greatly. They tested the hypothesis that dosage adjustment of subcutaneous heparin to produce an activated partial thromboplastin time (aPTT) in the high-normal range might result in greater reduction of postoperative thrombosis than fixed-dose heparin. In 79 patients undergoing elective hip arthroplasty, one group received a fixed dose of 3500 units of heparin subcutaneously every 8 hours for 7 days. Thirty-nine percent of these patients developed DVT as diagnosed by venography. A second group was given the same initial dose, but the dose was subsequently adjusted to keep the aPTT between 35 and 36 seconds from the day of operation to the seventh postoperative day. These patients needed progressively more heparin to maintain the aPTT time in the prescribed range. Only 13% of these patients developed venographic evidence of DVT. The bleeding complications were identical in the two groups. Leyvraz et al. subsequently advised giving sufficient heparin to raise the aPTT 2 to 5 seconds above the upper limit of normal.

Green et al.[25] compared adjusted-dose heparin with conventional-dose heparin in patients with spinal cord injury and found a much lower incidence of DVT in the group receiving adjusted-dose heparin. Hirsh,[26] in a review of the results of studies on low-dose vs. adjusted-dose heparin, found a postoperative incidence of DVT from 25% to 35% with low-dose and 12% to 15% with adjusted-dose heparin. As a result adjusted-dose heparin was widely accepted as the most appropriate means of using heparin for thromboembolism prophylaxis.

LOW-MOLECULAR-WEIGHT HEPARIN

Recently the literature has been flooded with articles advocating the use of low-molecular-weight heparin for clotting prophylaxis.[6-8,27-31] Unfractionated heparin is basically a dirty compound consisting of components with marked variation in molecular weight. Because the mechanism of action of heparin is based on its ability to potentiate the activity of antithrombin III, the demonstration that low-molecular-weight fractions of heparin have a much higher content of the pentasaccharide segment responsible for this potentiation suggested that this would be an ideal drug for thromboembolism prophylaxis. As a result the pharmaceutical industry, using depolymerization, fractionation, and/or other chemical processes, has succeeded in developing a number of different low-molecular-weight fractions from parent unfractionated heparin. As the heparin was broken down into its low-molecular-weight fractions, however, it lost its ability to prolong the aPTT.[11] This led to the hope that the bleeding complications would be lessened while the antithrombotic benefit would be retained.

The primary problem with the use of low-molecular-weight heparin has been an inability to document the effect of a given dose except through measurement of its ex vivo antifactor Xa activity.[11,27,32] There are serious questions, however, as to whether this test accurately reflects the activity of this drug.[33] There are two primary reasons for these questions. First, the relative contribution of antifactor IIa and Xa activity varies between different low-molecular-weight preparations; hence measuring only the antifactor Xa activity may underestimate the effects of those with a higher non–antifactor Xa effect. Second, when an experimental model of thrombosis is used, protection from thrombosis with low-molecular-weight heparin continues after the ex vivo antifactor Xa activity has decreased. The inability of most laboratories to monitor the effect of low-molecular-weight heparin on a practical basis has restricted its use to low-dose prophylaxis in the United States.

A theoretical advantage of low-molecular-weight heparins, in addition to improved anti-Xa activity, is their more prolonged duration of action.[11,28] A reduced binding of low-molecular-weight heparin to plasma proteins and endothelial cells is thought to contribute to their longer plasma half-life, which is two to four times longer than standard heparin at therapeutic doses.[7] Initially it was thought that perhaps one subcutaneous 40 to 60 mg dose every 24 hours would be adequate for thromboembolism prophylaxis; however, clinical studies of low-molecular-weight heparin have shown that the single-dose regimen was not as effective as standard-dose heparin and doses twice daily are required to provide equivalent protection.[8,28]

Another theoretical advantage of using low-molecular-weight heparin was the potential for a reduced risk of bleeding. Experimentally the hemorrhagic effects of standard heparins and low-molecular-weight heparins have been compared in a variety of animal models. In most of these studies, standard heparin appeared to be associated with more bleeding at an equivalent antithrombotic effect than low-molcular-weight heparins.[11] This, however, has not proved to be the case clinically, since almost all comparative clinical studies have showed no difference in the incidence of bleeding between standard heparin and low-molecular-weight heparin.[28,29,32,34,35] The balance of evidence clearly points out that the two types of heparin are comparable in terms of hemorrhagic complications.

The final theoretical advantage of low-molecular-weight heparin prophylaxis was that it was less likely to be associated with heparin-induced thrombocytopenia.[7,11,36] Warkentin et al.[37] noted that heparin-induced thrombocytopenia occurred in 9 of 332 patients who received unfractionated heparin and in none of 303 patients receiving low-molecular-weight heparin. Eight of the nine patients with heparin-induced thrombocytopenia had one or more thrombotic events (venous in seven and arterial in one), and the incidence of heparin-dependent immunoglobulin G antibodies was higher among patients who received unfractionated heparin (7.8%) than among patients who received low-molecular-weight heparin (2%). Even though this difference may seem significant, the current *Physicians' Desk Reference* suggests that the occurrence of thrombocytopenia following the administration of low-molecular-weight heparin is 2% vs. 3% for unfractionated heparin, a trivial difference.[38] Unfortunately, if a patient has been previously sensitized with unfractionated heparin, the low-molecular-weight heparins have an 80% to 100% risk of cross reactivity.[39] Because of this, patients with heparin-induced thrombocytopenia who require continued anticoagulation should not be treated with low-molecular-weight heparins. These patients may be treated with either direct thrombin inhibitors or heparinoids (soon to be released in the United States).

CONTROVERSY REGARDING THE VARIOUS HEPARIN REGIMENS

Because low-molecular-weight heparin offered the promise of being more effective, with prolonged action and less risk of bleeding and platelet-induced thrombocytopenia, it has been promoted with enthusiasm. However, as just noted, its theoretical benefits have not been realized clinically. This drug is expensive because of its cost of purification, and it is still dependent on the presence of antithrombin III for its activity. Those advocating use of low-molecular-weight heparin suggest that it is more effective than standard low-dose heparin.[7,28,30] Although low-molecular-weight heparin is expensive, the lack of monitoring results in costs comparable to those of an adjusted-dose heparin regimen with a daily aPTT.[7]

A fundamental problem with most of the low-molecular-weight heparin studies is that they compared standard low-dose unfractionated heparin with low-molecular-weight heparin. Leyvraz et al.[5] in 1983 demonstrated the clear superiority of adjusted-dose heparin over standard low-dose heparin. Since the original publication of Leyvraz et al., adjusted-dose heparin has been the regimen of choice for thromboembolism prophylaxis in most centers including our own.

Kakkar et al.[35] recently reported a multicenter trial in which low-molecular-weight heparin was compared with standard low-dose heparin in more than 3000 patients undergoing major abdominal surgery. The purpose of the study was to evaluate the incidence of bleeding between the two groups. Strikingly, the incidence of DVT and pulmonary embolism was no different between the two groups. Although there were fewer minor bleeding events (wound hematomas) in the low-molecular-weight heparin group, there was no difference in the incidence of major bleeding events.

Clagett et al.,[34] in their summary of current series, provide information on the effectiveness of various regimens of thromboembolism prophylaxis. This is one of the few reports that compares adjusted-dose heparin with low-molecular-weight heparin. Their series reviewed comparative data on adjusted-dose heparin and low-molecular-weight heparin for the prevention of DVT after elective hip replacement. Their summary found the incidence of DVT to be 50% for untreated control subjects, 34% for low-dose heparin, 16% for low-molecular-weight heparin, and 11% for adjusted-dose heparin.

Using volunteers, Bendetowicz et al.[27] determined plasma levels from 1 to 24 hours after subcutaneous injection of 5000 international units of unfractionated heparin with 40 mg of low-molecular-weight heparin (n = 12 for each type). Levels were calculated for antithrombin and anti-Xa activity using the specific activities of the materials injected. They concluded that the only functional difference between low-molecular-weight heparin and unfractionated heparin is the much higher bioavailability of the former. They surmised that when unfractionated heparin is given subcutaneously, it is primarily the low molecular component that reaches the circulation, that is, a fraction similar to that found with low-molecular-weight heparin. In theory, increasing the dose of subcutaneous unfractionated heparin in the standard-dose heparin regimen would provide equivalent results to those of low-molecular-weight heparin.

CONCLUSION

It can be concluded from a review of the literature that in most patients the difference between low-molecular-weight heparin and adjusted unfractionated heparin is minimal. The incidence of complications in both regimens is small, and so far there are no randomized series that demonstrate a clinically significant difference between them. There are theoretical advantages and disadvantages to each (Table 1). The primary advantages of low-molecular-weight heparins are that the incidence of thrombocytopenia is probably slightly lower than with adjusted-dose unfractionated heparin and monitoring is not used. The primary disadvantages are that it

Table 1 Low-dose heparin regimens

Regimen	Advantages	Disadvantages
Standard low-dose heparin (5000 units subcutaneously bid or tid)	Safe, inexpensive No monitoring needed	Not effective in antithrombin III–depleted patients Platelet aggregation 3%-6%
Adjusted dose heparin (5000 units subcutaneously or intravenously, then adjusted to raise aPTT 2 to 5 seconds above normal)	Safe Automatically adjusted for heparin-refractory patients	Monitoring required Platelet aggregation 3%-6%
Low-molecular-weight heparin	No monitoring needed Less risk of platelet depletion	Expensive Monitoring not possible Not effective in antithrombin III–depleted patients

is difficult if not impossible to monitor the effect of low-molecular-weight heparin, and the drug is still quite expensive.

From the standpoint of prophylaxis in normal patients, with normal antithrombin III levels, all heparin regimens are probably equally effective.[5,39-45] The increased cost of low-molecular-weight heparin is balanced by the nonutilization of monitoring. However, patients who are at the highest risk for clotting or who actually have ongoing low-grade clotting, such as those with major trauma, sepsis, ischemic tissue, or shock, should be assumed to have low or depleted antithrombin III levels. Under these circumstances, the standard low-dose heparin and low-molecular-weight heparin regimens are not only ineffective but may actually increase the clotting tendency. This is likely because low doses of heparin tend to produce platelet aggregation and in so doing may increase thromboembolic complications.[11,18,34,44] Adjusted-dose standard heparin may result in more effective prophylaxis because dosage is increased until an antithrombotic effect is manifested. Because it is difficult, without measuring antithrombin III levels, to determine the group of patients that would benefit from adjusted-dose heparin, we conclude that adjusted-dose heparin should remain the prophylactic method of choice.[46]

REFERENCES

1. McLean J. The thromboplastic action of cephalin. Am J Physiol 41:250-257, 1916.
2. Murray DWG, Jaques LB, Perrett TE, et al. Heparin and vascular occlusion. Can Med Assoc J 35:621-622, 1936.
3. Kakkar VV, Corrigan T, Spindler J, et al. Efficacy of low doses of heparin in prevention of deep-vein thrombosis after major surgery. A double-blind, randomized trial. Lancet 15:101-106, 1972.
4. Kakkar VV. Prevention of fatal postoperative pulmonary embolism by low doses of heparin: An international multicenter trial. Lancet 2:45-51, 1975.
5. Leyvraz PF, Richard J, Bachmann F, et al. Adjusted versus fixed-dose subcutaneous heparin in the prevention of deep-vein thrombosis after total hip replacement. N Engl J Med 309:954-958, 1983.
6. Leyvraz PF, Bachmann F, Hoek J, et al. Prevention of deep vein thrombosis after hip replacement: Randomized comparison between unfractionated heparin and low molecular weight heparin. BMJ 303:543-548, 1991.
7. Hirsh J, Levine MN. Low molecular weight heparin. Blood 79:1-17, 1992.
8. Menzin J, Richner R, Huse D, et al. Prevention of deep-vein thrombosis following total hip replacement surgery with enoxaparin versus unfractionated heparin: A pharmacoeconomic evaluation. Ann Pharmacother 28:271-275, 1994.
9. Brinkhous KM. The inhibition of blood clotting. An unidentified substance which acts in conjunction with heparin. Am J Physiol 125:683-687, 1939.
10. Abildgaard U. Highly purified antithrombin 3 with heparin cofactor activity prepared by disc electrophoresis. Scand J Clin Lab Invest 21:89-91, 1968.
11. Bounameaux H, ed. Low-Molecular-Weight Heparins in Prophylaxis and Therapy of Thromboembolic Diseases. New York: Marcel Dekker, 1994, p 323.
12. Demers C, Henderson P, Blajchman MA, et al. An antithrombin III assay based on factor Xa inhibition provides a more reliable test to identify congenital antithrombin III deficiency than an assay based on thrombin inhibition. Thromb Haemost 69:231-235, 1993.
13. Kakkar VV, Corrigan TP, Fossard DP, et al. Prevention of fatal postoperative pulmonary embolism by low doses of heparin. Lancet 1:567-569, 1977.
14. Wessler S, Gitel SN. Heparin: New concepts relative to clinical use. Blood 53:525-544, 1979.
15. Hampson WG, Harris FC, Lucas HK, et al. Failure of low-dose heparin to prevent deep-vein thrombosis after hip replacement arthroplasty. Lancet 1:795-797, 1974.
16. Blaisdell FW. Prevention of deep vein thrombosis. Surgery 83:243-244, 1978.
17. Gruber UF, Duckert F, Fridrich R, et al. Prevention of postoperative thromboembolism by dextran 40, low doses of heparin, or xantinol nicotinate. Lancet 1:207-210, 1977.

18. Ruiz AJ, Hill SL, Berry RE. Heparin, deep venous thrombosis, and trauma patients. Am J Surg 162:159-162, 1991.
19. Wille-Jorgensen P, Ott P. Predicting failure of low-dose prophylactic heparin in general surgical procedures. Surg Gynecol Obstet 171:126-130, 1990.
20. Miller RS, Weatherford DA, Stein D, et al. Antithrombin III and trauma patients: Factors that determine low levels. J Trauma 37:442-445, 1994.
21. Owings JT, Bagley M, Gosselin R, et al. Effects of critical injury on plasma antithrombin activity: Low antithrombin levels are associated with thromboembolic complications. J Trauma (in press).
22. Geerts WH, Code KI, Jay RM, et al. A prospective study of venous thromboembolism after major trauma. N Engl J Med 331:1601-1606, 1994.
23. Damus PS, Wallace GA. Immunologic measurement of antithrombin III-heparin cofactor and alpha 2 macroglobulin in disseminated intravascular coagulation and hepatic failure coagulopathy. Thromb Res 6:27-38, 1975.
24. Conlan MG, Folsom AR, Finch A, et al. Antithrombin III: Associations with age, race, sex and cardiovascular disease risk factors. Thromb Haemost 72:551-556, 1994.
25. Green D, Lee MY, Ito VY, et al. Fixed- vs adjusted-dose heparin in the prophylaxis of thromboembolism in spinal cord injury. JAMA 260:1255-1258, 1988.
26. Hirsh J. Heparin. N Engl J Med 324:1565-1574, 1991.
27. Bendetowicz AV, Beguin S, Caplain H, Hemker HC. Pharmacokinetics and pharmacodynamics of a low molecular weight heparin (enoxaparin) after subcutaneous injection: Comparison with unfractionated heparin—a three-way crossover study in human volunteers. Thromb Haemost 71:305-313, 1994.
28. Colwell CW Jr, Spiro TE, Trowbridge AA, et al. Use of enoxaparin, a low-molecular-weight heparin, and unfractionated heparin for the prevention of deep venous thrombosis after elective hip replacement: A clinical trial comparing efficacy and safety. J Bone Joint Surg 76:3-14, 1994.
29. Hull RD, Raskob GE, Pineo GF, et al. Subcutaneous low-molecular-weight heparin compared with continuous intravenous heparin in the treatment of proximal vein thrombosis. N Engl J Med 326:975-982, 1992.
30. Thomas DP. Prevention of post-operative thrombosis by low molecular weight heparin in patients undergoing hip replacement. Thromb Haemost 67:491-493, 1992.
31. Turpie AG, Levine MN, Hirsh J, et al. A randomized controlled trial of a low-molecular-weight heparin (enoxaparin) to prevent deep-vein thrombosis in patients undergoing elective hip surgery. N Engl J Med 315:925-929, 1986.
32. Boneu B. Low molecular weight heparin therapy: Is monitoring needed? Thromb Haemost 72:330-334, 1994.
33. Fareed J, Hoppensteadt D, Walenga JM. Low molecular weight heparin in the management of thrombotic disorders. In Fareed J, ed. Low Molecular Weight Heparin in the Prophylaxis and Treatment of Thrombotic Disorders. Chicago: Loyola University Press, 1994, pp 233-241.
34. Clagett GP, Anderson FA Jr, Levine MN, et al. Prevention of venous thromboembolism. Chest 102:391S-407S, 1992.
35. Kakkar VV, Cohen AT, Edmonson RA, et al. Low molecular weight versus standard heparin for prevention of venous thromboembolism after major abdominal surgery. Lancet 341:259-265, 1993.
36. Aster RH. Heparin-induced thrombocytopenia and thrombosis. N Engl J Med 332:1374-1376, 1995.
37. Warkentin TE, Levine MN, Hirsh J, et al. Heparin-induced thrombocytopenia in patients treated with low-molecular-weight heparin or unfractionated heparin. N Engl J Med 332:1330-1335, 1995.
38. The Physicians' Desk Reference Guide to Prescription Drugs, 2nd ed. Montvale, N.J.: Medical Economics Data, 1994, pp 1853-1854.
39. Greinacher A, Michels I, Mueller-Eckhardt C. Heparin-associated thrombocytopenia: The antibody is not heparin specific. Thromb Haemost 67:545-549, 1992.
40. Collins R, Scrimgeour A, Yusuf S, Peto R. Reduction in fatal pulmonary embolism and venous thrombosis by perioperative administration of subcutaneous heparin. Overview of results of randomized trials in general, orthopedic and urologic surgery. N Engl J Med 318:1162-1173, 1988.
41. Eriksson BI, Kalebo P, Anthymyr BA, et al. Prevention of deep-vein thrombosis and pulmonary embolism after total hip replacement. Comparison of low-molecular-weight heparin and unfractionated heparin. J Bone Joint Surg 73:484-493, 1991.
42. Morris GK, Henry AP, Preston BJ. Prevention of deep-vein thrombosis by low-dose heparin in patients undergoing total hip replacement. Lancet 2:797-800, 1974.
43. Planes A, Vochelle N, Mazas F, et al. Prevention of postoperative venous thrombosis: A randomized trial comparing unfractionated heparin with low molecular weight heparin in patients undergoing total hip replacement. Thromb Haemost 60:407-410, 1988.
44. Taberner DA, Poller L, Thomson JM, Lemon G, Weighill FJ. Randomized study of adjusted versus fixed low dose heparin prophylaxis of deep vein thrombosis in hip surgery. Br J Surg 76:933-935, 1989.
45. Thomas DP, Merton RE. A low molecular weight heparin compared with unfractionated heparin. Thromb Res 28:343-350, 1982.
46. Owings JT, Blaisdell FW. Low-dose heparin thromboembolism prophylaxis. Arch Surg (in press).

46

Are Oral Anticoagulants Indicated in Vascular Surgical Patients? Do They Increase Graft Patency and Do They Lower the Death Rate?

MARCO J.D. TANGELDER, M.D., ALE ALGRA, M.D., Ph.D., and BERT C. EIKELBOOM, M.D., Ph.D.

Symptomatic peripheral vascular disease occurs in 2% to 3% of men and in 1% of women at 50 to 65 years of age.[1] Considering the natural course of atherosclerotic disease leading to peripheral vascular stenosis, stabilization or even improvement of clinical course during conservative management can be seen in about 70% to 80% of cases; in 20% to 30% of patients, disease tends to worsen; and less than 10% will undergo surgery for amputation of the lower extremity. During a 14-year follow-up of patients with peripheral vascular disease, Kannel et al.[2] found the cardiovascular morbidity and mortality rate to be much higher as compared with controls, and the risk of death was at least twice as high. The natural course of peripheral vascular disease seems to be rather benign. The principal hazard for patients with claudication appears to derive from an increased propensity to cardiovascular morbidity and mortality rather than from the consequences of impaired blood flow to the limbs.

The number of vascular reconstructions is increasing in patients with severe ischemia of the lower extremity, and failure of bypass grafts, especially in the first year, remains problematic. In previous decades most of the attention was concentrated on technical refinements of techniques and materials; in the last few years, there has been a shift of attention toward the use of antithrombotic therapy to increase patency of vascular bypass grafts. There have been many studies in experimental animals as well as clinical trials with a view to increasing knowledge of the effects of antithrombotic agents on bypass grafts.

In this chapter we will discuss the evidence currently available concerning the efficacy of oral anticoagulants and platelet aggregating inhibitors with regard to graft patency, cardiovascular and cerebrovascular disease, and death from all causes in patients suffering from peripheral occlusive vascular disease.

ANTITHROMBOTIC THERAPY

If patients with femoropopliteal or femorocrural bypasses are not treated with antithrombotic drugs, 28% to 45% of their bypass grafts will occlude in the first year and most of the vascular reconstructions will fail early after operation.[3-6] Graft failure within the first year is usually caused by early thrombotic occlusion, perianastomotic intimal hyperplasia with or without complicating thrombotic occlusion superimposed on the intimal hyperplasia, and fibrotic organization of the thrombus.[7,8] Failure in subsequent years is usually caused by the progression of atherosclerotic disease.[8,9] Intimal hyperplasia resulting in luminal narrowing is—both in vein and in prosthetic grafts—caused by activated platelet–mediated release of smooth muscle cell mitogens and fibroblast proliferation. Consequently, in vein grafts the process can be diffuse,[10] whereas in vascular prostheses intimal hyperplasia occurs at anastomoses.

The goal of antithrombotic therapy is prevention or delay of the thrombotic process, intimal hyperplasia, and the atherosclerotic process. Based on their working mechanisms, there are three types of antithrombotics: anticoagulants, platelet aggregation inhibitors, and thrombolytics. In this chapter we will discuss only oral anticoagulants (coumarin derivatives [OAC]) and a platelet inhibitor (acetylsalicylic acid [ASA]). The working mechanism of coumarin is based on competition with vitamin K, which has a similar structure. Administration of coumarin derivatives results in the production of dysfunctional forms of vitamin K–dependent clotting factors II, VII, IX, and X in the liver. In this way they inhibit the production of thrombin, which results in a reduced conversion of fibrinogen into fibrin, which is indispensable for the formation of thrombus. Thrombin is also a potent platelet activator, so its inhibition also results in reduced platelet aggregation. The effect of coumarin derivatives starts only after 1 or 2 days and is complete after 5 days, because the circulating clotting factors are not influenced. The decreased production of thrombin is obvious only after these factors are depleted.

ASA irreversibly inhibits cyclo-oxygenase activity in platelets by acetylation and thus inhibits thromboxane A_2 synthesis, which is responsible for platelet aggregation, vasoconstriction, and release of other aggregating agents.[11-14] Through inhibition of the same enzyme prostacyclin (prostaglandin I_2), production in endothelial cells is diminished.[15,16] Prostacyclin is not only a powerful inhibitor of platelet adhesion and aggregation but also a vasodilator.[13,15,17] Prostacyclin synthesis, however, is not irreversibly influenced by ASA, and a high dose is required to attain an effect.[18,19] The optimal dose of ASA to achieve the most favorable prostacyclin/thromboxane A_2 balance is still unclear, but low-dose ASA therapy might be more effective.[20-24]

There have been many studies to determine whether antiplatelet therapies can reduce intimal hyperplasia. Despite many studies in experimental animals suggesting that this is so,[25-30] other studies have failed to show any significant effect.[31-33] In studies concerning humans, indications are that it is doubtful that antiplatelet therapy can reduce intimal hyperplasia.[34,35]

Because of the inhibitory effect of OAC on the clotting system and of ASA on platelet deposition, both agents can delay the occlusive process. However, it remains unclear which method is the most effective, not only in preventing graft occlusion, but also in reducing progression of cardiovascular and cerebrovascular disease and in lowering death rates from vascular disease.

EFFECTS ON PATENCY

The role of OAC in preventing peripheral bypass graft occlusion is not quite clear. Two small studies in the 1960s suggested that OAC did not improve the patency of peripheral vascular reconstructions.[36,37] Kretschmer et al.[38] were not able to evince any statistically significant effect of postoperative treatment with OAC in a more recent retrospective analysis of a clinical series. However, the interim results of a prospective trial showed that OAC favorably influenced graft patency in patients suffering from severe ischemia.[38] In addition, the results of this clinical trial, in which 119 patients were randomized in an OAC group and a control group, showed a nonsignificant 36% decrease of graft occlusions in the group treated with OAC during a 5-year follow-up.[39] Patients in this study were followed for an additional 5 years. A total of 130 patients were included in the trial. Presently there is a significant 44% reduction of graft occlusions, as well as a significant 70% decline of number of amputations compared with the control group (Table 1).[40]

Many animal and clinical studies have been done to evaluate the effects of antiplatelet therapy on the patency of femoropopliteal or femorocrural bypasses. Recently the Antiplatelet Trialists' Collaboration[41] demonstrated, in an overview of 10 studies concerning bypass grafts and one study concerning endarterectomy in the lower extremities, an overall odds reduction of graft occlusion of 38% in patients who were treated with platelet inhibitors. ASA dosage ranged from 600 to 1500 mg daily. In the overview of all antiplatelet studies, neither direct nor indirect comparisons of the effects of (or the combination of) different regimens (aspirin, dipyridamole, sulphinpyrazone, ticlopidine, and suloctidil) on vascular patency provided good evidence that one antiplatelet regimen studied was more effective than the other, nor that the point of time at which treatment was started made any difference. The benefits of antiplatelet therapy in preventing vascular bypass graft occlusion and vascular events outweigh any risk of bleeding complications. After March 1990, the closing date of the overview mentioned, two additional randomized trials concerning antiplatelet therapy and peripheral bypass patency were published, although the first one was also mentioned in the overview by the Antiplatelet Trialists' Collaboration.[41] McCollum et al.[6] demonstrated by intention-to-treat analysis in a placebo-controlled double-blind trial with 549 patients that ASA, 300 mg, plus dipyridamole,

Table 1 Overview of trials comparing different antithrombotic regimens in vascular surgical patients

Trial	No. of patients in follow-up	Regimen	Graft material	Patency rate	Best regimen for progression of disease	Survival
Kretschmer et al.[39]	119	OAC vs. P	Vein	OAC	—	OAC*
Kretschmer et al.[40]	130	OAC vs. P	Vein	OAC*	—	OAC*
De Smit and Van Urk[46]	300	OAC vs. P	—	—	OAC*	—
APT[41]	26-549	PI vs. PI or P	Vein, prosthetic	PI*	PI	PI
McCollum et al.[6]	549	ASA + D vs. P	Vein	ASA + D*	ASA + D*	ASA + D*
Franks et al.[42]	145	ASA + D vs. P				
D'Addato et al.[43]	113	ASA + D vs. I				
Hess et al.[47]	199	ASA vs. ASA + D vs. P	—	—	ASA + D*	—
Schneider et al.[44]	91	OAC vs. ASA	Vein	OAC*	—	—
Edmondson et al.[45]	200	H vs. ASA + D	Vein, prosthetic	H†	—	—

ASA = acetylsalicylic acid; APT = Antiplatelet Trialists' Collaboration; D = dipyridamole; H = low-molecular-weight heparin; I = indobufen; OAC = oral anticoagulants; P = placebo; PI = platelet inhibitors.
*Significant.
†Significant in patients undergoing salvage surgery.

150 mg, twice daily had no significant influence on the patency of femoropopliteal vein bypasses and on bleeding complications during the mean 3-year follow-up. However, in an on-treatment subgroup analysis of this population, in which patients with and without detectable concentration serum salicylate were compared, there was a significant difference in graft patency in favor of the treated group.[42] Finally, D'Addato et al.[43] failed to demonstrate a significant difference in patency rate for ASA, 900 mg daily, plus dipyridamole, 225 mg daily, versus indobufen, 400 mg daily, during a 1-year follow-up of 113 patients who received a polytetrafluoroethylene femoropopliteal bypass graft. Given the conclusions of all antiplatelet studies, the regimen of first choice is ASA, probably in a lower dose than has been used in studies so far.

It remains to be seen whether preference should be given to OAC or ASA for prevention of occlusions after peripheral bypass surgery. There has been only one small trial that compared the effectiveness of OAC with ASA in 91 patients who underwent femoropopliteal venous bypass surgery.[44] This study suggested better patency in the group of patients allocated to OAC after a 2-year follow-up.

In a recent trial 200 patients were randomized for postoperative treatment with either a daily injection of 2500 IU of low-molecular-weight heparin subcutaneously or 300 mg aspirin with 100 mg dipyridamole every 8 hours for 3 months. Patients were stratified for indications for reconstruction; during the 1-year follow-up, a better graft patency was shown for the heparin-treated group.[45] This benefit was significant in patients who underwent surgery for critical limb ischemia, and there was no benefit in patients having surgery for claudication.

EFFECTS ON PROGRESSION OF DISEASE

There are indications that OAC and ASA could delay the progression of peripheral occlusive arterial disease. In a placebo-controlled randomized study in which 300 patients, either medically or surgically treated, were recruited, De Smit and Van Urk[46] demonstrated highly significant beneficial effects of long-term treatment with OAC during the 5-year follow-up. The surgically treated group consisted of patients who had undergone central vascular reconstructions (aortoiliac endarterectomy, aortoiliac and aortofemoral bypasses) only. Not only was the risk of progression of atherosclerotic lesions in peripheral vascular disease, as assessed by Doppler exercise test, reduced sixfold ($p \leq .0001$) in patients treated with OAC, but also progression of general vascular disease was delayed compared with the placebo-treated group. When the progression rates of cerebrovascular, cardiovascular, and peripheral vascular disease were combined, the 5-year progression rate was reduced from 29% in patients treated with a placebo to 9% in patients treated with fenprocoumon ($p \leq .0001$). The risk of bleeding complications appeared to be very moderate.

In a trial in which 240 patients were randomized to aspirin, aspirin plus dipyridamole, or a matching placebo control group, the progression of peripheral occlusive arterial disease was studied.[47] An on-treatment analysis of angiograms of 199 patients in the 2-year follow-up showed that the natural course of peripheral arterial disease can be slowed with long-term treatment with a combination of ASA and dipyridamole, which was superior to treatment with ASA alone. Although the study by McCollum et al.[6] demonstrated that antiplatelet therapy had some (but no significant) influence on femoropopliteal vein patency, the trial showed a significant reduction of number of subsequent vascular events (myocardial infarction plus stroke) by just over 30% in patients with peripheral vascular disease.

There is no trial available in which the efficacy of OAC is compared with ASA to study the potential delaying effects on the atherosclerotic process.

EFFECTS ON DEATH RATES

Although the previously mentioned study by De Smit and Van Urk[46] showed a striking reduction of peripheral and general vascular disease progression, they failed to demonstrate a significant beneficial effect of OAC treatment in reduction of mortality rate compared with the placebo group. Kretschmer et al.[39,40] could only show a significantly better graft patency after 10 years' follow-up in the earlier mentioned trials, but the group treated with OAC had, after both 5 and 10 years' follow-up, a significantly higher probability of survival, irrespective of graft performance.

The overview by the Antiplatelet Trialists' Collaboration of patients who had a peripheral artery revascularization procedure suggested that antiplatelet therapy for a couple of years in 1000 such patients might prevent several dozen major vascular events (i.e., myocardial infarction, stroke, or vascular death).[48] However, the number of events was too low to reach statistical significance. McCollum's antiplatelet study[6] showed an overall reduction in mortality rate of 13%, which also failed to reach statistical significance.

Hence it remains unclear whether OAC and ASA can lower death rates in patients after peripheral vascular reconstructions and with which treatment the most favorable results are achieved.

OAC OR ASA?

Considering all studies concerning treatment of vascular surgical patients with OAC or ASA to prevent graft occlusion, vascular events, and death, placebo-controlled studies are no longer justified. In a clinical trial in which 1-year angiographic vein graft patency after aortocoronary bypass surgery was assessed, no significant differences in occlusion rates of distal anastomoses were noticed among patients given aspirin, 50 mg daily (15%), aspirin, 50 mg daily plus dipyridamole 200 mg twice daily (11%), and OAC target range, 2.8 to 4.8 international normalized ratio (INR) (13%).[49] Clinical events, as assessed by the incidence of myocardial infarction, thrombosis, major bleeding, or death, occurred most often in the aspirin-plus-dipyridamole group; however, because of the small number of events during the 1-year follow-up, no statistical differences were observed among the three treatment groups. In view of the anatomic and physiologic differences between coronary and peripheral bypasses, and considering the differences between the patients receiving these two types of bypass grafts, it is not correct to extrapolate these findings to patients after femoropopliteal or femorocrural bypass grafting. No reliable randomized study comparing the effects of OAC with ASA in patients after femoropopliteal or femorocrural bypass surgery has been published to date. Patients with peripheral vascular occlusive disease do have a higher risk of fatal and nonfatal myocardial and cerebral infarction[2,50]; therefore a study concerning all these facets is of great importance. In the United States a prospective clinical trial has started, comparing the benefits of low-dose Warfarin, target INR range 2.0 to 3.0, plus ASA, 325 mg daily, to ASA 325 mg daily only after peripheral vascular reconstruction. This Veterans Affairs cooperative trial will study the occurrence of thrombosis of the arterial reconstruction, amputation, stroke, myocardial infarction, and death during a 6-year follow-up period.

To sort out the inconclusive data concerning the optimal treatment to prevent occlusion of bypasses and cardiovascular and cerebrovascular events and death after peripheral bypass surgery, the Dutch BOA trial was begun in

1995. (The acronym stands for prevention of occlusion after peripheral bypass surgery with oral anticoagulants or acetylsalicylic acid.) Over a 2-year period 2700 patients undergoing femoropopliteal or femorocrural bypass surgery will be included in this prospective, nonblinded, controlled clinical multicenter trial. Patients will be randomized in treatment with OAC (fenprocoumon); target INR range is 3.0 to 4.5 or 80 mg ASA (carbaspirin calcium, 100 mg) daily. Fenprocoumon is a long-acting OAC-like warfarin (7 to 14 days) with a maximum effect after 48 to 72 hours. The mean follow-up is 2 years (minimum 1 year; maximum 3 years). The primary end point of the study will be occlusion of the bypass, and clinical evaluation of the ischemic leg will be assessed. Secondary end points are death, stroke, myocardial infarction, vascular intervention, amputation, and major bleeding. With the Dutch BOA trial we hope to find a clear answer to the question: which is the best treatment for prevention of graft occlusion and vascular events and death in this group of vascular surgical patients?

CONCLUSION

Patients after peripheral vascular surgery are not only threatened by the risk of severe ischemia of the lower extremity but also by the general consequences of vascular disease from atherosclerotic origins. Cardiovascular and cerebrovascular disease and death occur far more often in such patients. Despite excellent operative techniques and materials, bypass grafts still fail as a result of thrombus formation, intimal hyperplasia, and, in the long-term, the continuing atherosclerotic process.

OAC and ASA might delay these occlusive processes in human arteries and in bypass grafts, respectively, by inhibiting the clotting system and platelet aggregation. After many studies the benefits of platelet inhibitors are clear and widely recognized. The role of OAC is less frequently studied and thus less clear, although there is evidence that OAC not only improves graft patency but also reduces vascular disease progression and mortality. Trials comparing treatment modalities with placebo are no longer justified. Hence there is a need for a prospective trial in which patients are randomly allocated to treatment with either OAC or ASA. To determine which of these two treatments is preferable, two different studies, a VA cooperative trial and the Dutch BOA trial, are in progress.

REFERENCES

1. Boobis LH, Bell PR. Can drugs help patients with lower limb ischaemia? Br J Surg 69:S-17–S-23, 1982.
2. Kannel WB, Skimmer JJ Jr, Schwartz MJ, Shurtleff D. Intermittent claudication. Incidence in the Framingham study. Circulation 41:875-883, 1970.
3. Szilagyi DE, Hageman JA, Smith RF, Elliot JP, Brown F, Dietz P. Autogenous vein grafting femoropopliteal atherosclerosis: The limits of its effectiveness. Surgery 86:836-851, 1979.
4. Kacoyanis GP, Wittemore AD, Couch NP, Mannick JA. Femorotibial and femoroperoneal bypass vein graft. A 15-year experience. Arch Surg 116:1529-1534, 1981.
5. Kretschmer G, Wenzl E, Wagner O, Polterauer P, Ehringer H, Minar E, Schemper M. Influence of anticoagulant treatment in preventing graft occlusion following saphenous vein bypass for femoropopliteal occlusive disease. Br J Surg 73:689-692, 1986.
6. McCollum C, Alexander C, Kenchington G, Franks PJ, Greenhalgh R. Antiplatelet drugs in femoropopliteal vein bypasses: A multicenter study. J Vasc Surg 13:150-162, 1991.
7. Fuster V, Chesebro JH. Coronary artery bypass grafting. A model for the understanding of the progression of atherosclerotic disease and the role of pharmacological intervention. In Neri Serneri GG, McGiff JC, Paoletti R, Born GVR, eds. Advances in Prostaglandin, Thromboxane and Leukotriene Research, vol 13. New York: Raven Press, 1985, pp 286-299.
8. Taylor RS, McFarland RJ, Cox MI. An investigation into the cause of failure of PTFE grafts. Eur J Vasc Surg 1:335-343, 1987.
9. Fuster V. Role of platelets in the development of atherosclerotic disease and possible interference with platelet inhibitor drugs. Scand J Haematol 27(Suppl 38):1, 1981.
10. Szilagyi DE, Elliot JP, Hageman JH, et al. Biologic fate of autogenous vein implants as arterial substitutes: Clinical, angiographic and histopathologic observations in femoropopliteal operations for atherosclerosis. Ann Surg 178:232-246, 1973.
11. Smith JB, Willis AL. Aspirin selectively inhibits prostaglandin production in human platelets. Nature 231:235-237, 1971.
12. Roth GJ, Majerus PW. The mechanism of the effect of aspirin on human platelets. I. Acetylation of a particulate fraction protein. J Clin Invest 56:624-632, 1975.
13. Roth GJ, Stanford N, Majerus PW. Acetylation of prostaglandin synthase by aspirin. Proc Natl Acad Sci USA 72:3073-3076, 1975.
14. Hamberg M, Svensson J, Samuelsson B. A new group of biologically active compounds derived from prostaglandin endoperoxides. Proc Natl Acad Sci USA 72:2994-2998, 1975.
15. Moncada J, Higgs EA, Vane RJ. Human arterial and venous tissue generates prostacyclin, a potent inhibitor of platelet aggregation. Lancet 1:18-21, 1977.
16. Burch JW, Baenziger NL, Stanford N, Majerus PW. Sensitivity of fatty acid cyclooxygenase from human aorta to acetylation of aspirin. Proc Natl Acad Sci USA 75:5181-5184, 1978.
17. Moncada S, Gryglewski R, Bunting S, Vane JR. An enzyme isolated from arteries transforms prostaglandin endoperoxides to an unstable substance that inhibits platelet aggregation. Nature 263:663-665, 1976.
18. Pedersen AK, Fitzgerald GA. Dose-related kinetics of

aspirin: Presystemic acetylation of platelet cyclooxygenase. N Engl J Med 311:1206-1211, 1984.
19. McLeod LJ, Roberts MS, Cossum PA, Vial JH. The effect of different doses of some acetylsalicylic acid formulations on platelet function and bleeding times in healthy subjects. Scand J Haematol 36:379-384, 1986.
20. Weksler BB, Pett SB, Alonso D, Richter RC, Stelzer P, Subramanian V, Tack-Goldman K, Gay WA Jr. Differential inhibition by aspirin of vascular and platelet prostaglandin synthesis in atherosclerotic patients. N Engl J Med 308:800-805, 1983.
21. Patrignani P, Filabozzi P, Patrono C. Selective cumulative inhibition of platelet thromboxane production by low-dose aspirin in healthy subjects. J Clin Invest 69:1366-1372, 1982.
22. Prestom FE, Whipps S, Jackson CA, French AJ, Wyld PJ, Stoddard CJ. Inhibition of prostacyclin and platelet thromboxane A_2 after low-dose aspirin. N Engl J Med 304:76-79, 1981.
23. Hanley SP, Cockbill SR, Bevan J, Heptinstall S. Differential inhibition by low-dose aspirin of human venous prostacyclin synthesis and platelet thromboxane synthesis. Lancet 1:969-971, 1981.
24. Masotti G, Pogessi L, Galant G, Abbate R. Differential inhibition of prostacyclin production and platelet aggregation by aspirin. Lancet 2:1213-1216, 1979.
25. Hirko MK, McShannic JR, Schmidt SP, Sharp WV, Evancho MM, Sims RL, Siebert JD. Pharmacologic modulation of intimal hyperplasia in canine vein interposition grafts. J Vasc Surg 17:877-887, 1993.
26. Volker W, Faber V. Aspirin reduces the growth of medial and neointimal thickenings in balloon-injured rat carotid arteries. Stroke 21(Suppl 12):IV-44-IV-45, 1990.
27. Hagen PO, Wang ZG, Mikat EM, Hackel DB. Antiplatelet therapy reduces aortic intimal hyperplasia distal to small-diameter vascular prostheses (PTFE) in nonhuman primates. Ann Surg 195:328-339, 1982.
28. McCann RL, Hagen PO, Fuchs JCA. Aspirin and dipyridamole decrease intimal hyperplasia in experimental vein grafts. Ann Surg 191:238-243, 1980.
29. Metke MP, Lie JT, Fuster V, Josa M, Kaye MP. Reduction of intimal thickening in canine coronary bypass vein grafts with dipyridamole and aspirin. Am J Cardiol 43:1144-1148, 1979.
30. Oblath RW, Buckley FO Jr, Green RM, Schwartz SI, DeWeese JA. Prevention of platelet aggregation and adherence to prosthetic vascular grafts by aspirin and dipyridamole. Surgery 84:37-44, 1978.
31. Bearn PE, Moffa C, Seddon AM, Bulls H, Marston A, Fox B, McCollum CN. The effect of platelet inhibitory therapy on prosthetic graft maturation. Int J Exp Pathol 74:1-8, 1993.
32. Bomberger RA, DePalma RJ, Ambrose TA, Manalo P. Aspirin and dipyridamole inhibit endothelial healing. Arch Surg 117:1459-1464, 1982.
33. Clowes AW, Karnovsky MJ. Failure of certain antiplatelet drugs to affect myointimal thickening following arterial injury. Lab Invest 36:452-458, 1977.
34. Clowes AW. The role of aspirin in enhancing arterial graft patency. J Vasc Surg 3:381-385, 1986.
35. Fuster V, Chesebro JH. Role of platelets and platelet inhibitors in aortocoronary artery vein-graft disease. Circulation 73:227-232, 1986.
36. Ashton F, Slaney G, Raines AJH. Femoro-popliteal arterial obstructions: Late results of Teflon prostheses and arterial homografts. Br Med J 2:1149-1152, 1962.
37. Evans G, Irvin WT. Long term arterial graft patency in relation to platelet adhesiveness, biochemical factors, and anticoagulant therapy. Lancet 2:353-355, 1966.
38. Kretschmer G, Wenzl E, Piza E, Polterauer P, Ehringer H, Minar E, Schemper M. The influence of anticoagulant treatment on the probability of function in femoropopliteal vein bypass surgery: Analysis of a clinical series (1970 to 1985) and interim evaluation of a controlled clinical trial. Surgery 102:453-459, 1987.
39. Kretschmer G, Schemper M, Ehringer H, Wenzl E, Polterauer P, Marcosi L, Minar E. Influence on postoperative anticoagulant treatment on patient survival after femoropopliteal vein bypass surgery. Lancet 1:797-799, 1988.
40. Kretschmer G, Herbst F, Prager M, Sautner T, Wenzl E, Berlakovich GA, Zekert F, Marosi L, Schemper M. A decade of oral anticoagulant treatment to maintain autologous vein grafts for femoropopliteal atherosclerosis. Arch Surg 127:1112-1115, 1992.
41. Antiplatelet Trialists' Collaboration. Collaborative overview of randomised trials of antiplatelet therapy. II. Maintenance of vascular graft or arterial patency by antiplatelet therapy. Br Med J 308:159-168, 1994.
42. Franks PJ, Sian M, Kenchington GF, Alexander CE, Powell JT and the Femoro-popliteal Bypass Trial Participants. Aspirin usage and its influence on femoropopliteal vein graft patency. Eur J Vasc Surg 6:185-188, 1992.
43. D'Addato M, Curti T, Bertini D, Donini I, Ferrero R, Fiorani P, Pellegrino F, Vecchioni R, Visconti W, Zinicola N. Indobufen vs. acetyl salicylic acid plus dipyridamole in long term patency after femoropopliteal bypass. Int Angiol 11:106-112, 1992.
44. Schneider E, Brunner U, Bollinger A. Medikamentöse Rezidivprophilaxe nach fermoro-propliatealer Arterienrekonstruktion. Angio 2:73-77, 1979.
45. Edmondson RA, Cohen AT, Das SK, Wagner MB, Kakkar VV. Low-molecular weight heparin versus aspirin and dipyridamole after femoropopliteal bypass grafting. Lancet 344:914-918, 1994.
46. De Smit P, Van Urk H. The effect of long-term treatment with oral anticoagulants in patients with peripheral vascular disease. In Tilsner V, Mathias FR, eds. Arterielle Verschlusskrankheit und blutgerinnung. Basel: Editioner (Roche), 1988, pp 211-216.
47. Hess H, Mietaschk A, Deichsel G. Drug-induced inhibition of platelet function delays progression of peripheral occlusive arterial disease. A prospective double-blind arteriographically controlled trial. Lancet 1:415-419, 1985.
48. Antiplatelet Trialists' Collaboration. Collaborative overview of randomised trials of antiplatelet therapy. I. Prevention of death, myocardial infarction, and stroke by prolonged antiplatelet therapy in various categories of patients. Br Med J 308:81-106, 1994.
49. Van der Meer J, Hillege HL, Kootstra GJ, Ascoop CAPL, Mulder BJM, Pfisterer M, van Gilst WH, Lie KI, for the CABADAS Research Group of the interuniversity Cardiology Institute of the Netherlands. Prevention of one-year-vein-graft occlusion after aortocoronary-bypass surgery: A comparison of low-dose aspirin, low-dose aspirin plus dipyridamole, and oral anticoagulants. Lancet 342:257-264, 1993.
50. Clagett GP. Antithrombotic therapy for lower extremity bypass. J Vasc Surg 15:873-875, 1992.

47

Vascular Applications of Pneumatic Tourniquet Occlusion Techniques

STANLEY O. SNYDER, Jr., M.D.

Vascular applications for pneumatic tourniquet techniques have been slow to evolve despite their utilization for orthopedic procedures for more than 300 years. In 1979 Scheinin and Lindfors[1] used tourniquet occlusion for a popliteal aneurysm repair, but it was the report of 40 cases of popliteal and tibial reconstructions by Bernhard et al.[2] in 1980 that began to popularize the technique. Vascular surgeons slowly began to embrace and expand the tourniquet concept, but it was not until the reports of Collier[3] in 1992 and Wagner et al.[4] in 1993 that large series began to evolve.

ADVANTAGES

Multiple vascular investigators have documented evidence of intimal denudation and medial arterial wall clamp–related trauma.[5-9] Tourniquet use eliminates clamp-related trauma, decreases the vessel dissection required at the distal anastomotic site, and improves both the visualization and operative mobility of the vessel at the distal anastomotic site. Eliminating clamp trauma and subsequent endothelial damage should decrease the incidence of stenosis at the perianastomotic region, and the dissection requires exposure of only the anterior wall of the vessel without requiring control of the collateral side branches present. This limited dissection is similar to techniques used by cardiac surgeons for coronary revascularization procedures.

APPLICATIONS

Tourniquet occlusion can be beneficial in a variety of vascular procedures, at the discretion of the operative surgeon. Difficult tibial bypasses, pedal bypasses, and "redo" procedures are aided most by limiting the dissection required and avoiding clamp trauma to small and often calcified vessels. The below-knee popliteal artery is also more accessible when clamps are not required. The option is available to perform both the proximal and distal anastomosis under tourniquet occlusion when proximal inflow is at the popliteal (or tibial) level, but the surgeon must use greater care in selecting the conduit length and alignment to prevent kinking or twisting. The tourniquet is especially effective for localized procedures such as short-segment endarterectomy and repair or bypass of vein graft stenosis.

Hemodialysis access procedures of the upper extremities can be facilitated by use of a tourniquet. The limited dissection is helpful for autogenous radiocephalic and brachiocephalic fistulas but is even more beneficial for prosthetic graft fistula placement, where more vessel dissection and clamping is required. The removal of an infected prosthetic graft is particularly aided by this technique, since difficult redo dissection is avoided and primary or vein patch closure of the artery is facilitated by precise suture placement without the vessel walls being distorted by clamps. (NOTE: Esmarch bandaging technique is not recommended for septic cases, and 1 or 2 minutes of limb elevation before tourniquet inflation and acceptance of some venous oozing is required.)

TECHNIQUE

For lower extremity procedures a cuff of appropriate length, width, and shape is placed on the mid- or (more commonly) the distal thigh. Although curved cuffs allow a lower inflation pressure, in clinical practice a straight 4-inch cuff of sufficient length is most often used. Four-inch cuffs are the standard width for most adult legs, but a wider one may be required for obese or extremely large patients. For upper extremity procedures a 3-inch cuff is usually placed above the elbow. Several layers of cotton cast padding are applied to cushion the extremity at the site of tourniquet inflation. Clinical studies by Pedowitz[10] recommend minimal tourniquet inflation pressures, defined as the arterial occlusion pressure plus 50 mm Hg. This ranges from 145 to 270 mm Hg in the upper extremity and from 160 to 280 mm Hg in the lower extremity. In practice, 250 mm Hg in the upper extremity and 275 mm Hg in the lower extremity are usually effective and safe for the short occlusion intervals required for vascular anastomosis. Precise Esmarch bandaging techniques to completely exsanguinate the extremity are required at both levels. Venous oozing that persists after tourniquet inflation is almost invariably secondary to incomplete limb exsanguination rather than inadequate cuff inflation pressures. A theoretical concern about an inability to compress calcified vessels almost never occurs, because the distal superficial femoral artery is almost always chronically occluded in vascular cases, and the resultant collateral vessels are easily compressible. Most orthopedic procedures are done without heparinization, but in vascular cases routine heparinization techniques are used with special attention to *appropriate heparin levels at the time of tourniquet inflation.*

For in situ distal bypass procedures the proximal anastomosis is completed first and the venous valves are ablated. An adventitial stitch is placed between the distal vein and the leg fascia to prevent twisting of the vein during application of the Esmarch bandage. The tourniquet can be used for both proximal and distal anastomosis when the graft origin is below the distal thigh, but extra care is required to achieve appropriate graft length and to avoid misalignment, since the graft does not distend before the distal anastomosis is performed.

For upper extremity autogenous hemodialysis procedures, the vein is transected after Esmarch and tourniquet inflation, but should be marked for proper alignment before tourniquet inflation. Prosthetic grafts are tunneled and aligned before tourniquet inflation. The option for both initial vessel dissection and anastomotic techniques under the tourniquet is available, but this prolongs tourniquet inflation time, requires experience with ischemic anatomic dissection, and may limit the venous outflow selection process for hemodialysis procedures.

RESEARCH

The advantages of a bloodless field are obvious, but the potential exists for ischemic or compression damage to muscle or nerves. The majority of research in this field has been done by orthopedists, with special emphasis by hand surgeons. The tourniquet cuff pressure required depends on multiple variables: systolic blood pressure, limb circumference, limb shape and local anatomy, vascular status, and tourniquet width and cuff design all play a role. Curved cuffs of appropriate size require less pressure than do straight cuffs. Wider cuffs require less pressure and are less likely to cause local pressure damage to nerves and muscles.

Multiple physiologic effects can be measured,[11-14] and complete nerve conduction block has been observed with 15 to 45 minutes of tourniquet inflation. However, with tourniquet inflation times of less than 2 hours, baseline distal nerve conductions are restored within 30 minutes of cuff deflation. The muscle intracellular pH and tissue oxygenation decrease within 30 minutes of tourniquet inflation, but metabolic recovery occurs within 5 to 10 minutes after 1 hour of ischemia and 5 to 20 minutes after 2 hours of ischemia. Technetium-99m pyrophosphate uptake studies used as a measure of physiologic tissue injury are positive after 1 hour of ischemia, but histologic studies reveal no evidence of significant muscle necrosis with ischemia times of less than 2 hours and cuff inflation pressures of less than 250 mm Hg.[11] Heparin reduces the potential for ischemic and reperfusion injury, although the cause of this protective effect is unclear. Anticoagulant, antiplatelet, and anti-inflammatory properties have all been proposed.[15] Tourniquet times longer than 2 hours may be associated with irreversible muscle and nerve histologic changes, with inconsistent recovery of function noted after 4-hour ischemic periods.[11] Reperfusion injury with leukocyte-mediated superoxide radical formation occurs. Intraneural edema formation with persistent tissue ischemia and subsequent nerve degeneration is hypothesized to occur secondary to mechanical deformation, causing direct endothelial disruption with increase protein permeability and mast cell accumulation as well as superoxide radical formation.[10] Although not relevant to most vascular applications, interposing a 5-minute reperfusion interval between 1½-hour ischemic intervals will extend the total tourniquet time allowed to 3 hours without significant tissue damage. The vascular applications described above rarely require even 1 hour of tourniquet time and the post-tourniquet syndrome described as tissue edema, stiffness, pallor, weakness without paralysis, and subjective numbness of the extremity without objective anesthesia virtually never occurs.[16] In 1931

Eckhoff and Lond,[17] in a paper paradoxically entitled "Tourniquet paralysis—a plea for the extended use of the pneumatic tourniquet," stated that they "had no knowledge of ischemic contracture following the use of a tourniquet," and during many hundreds of operations they "used this tourniquet for every operation on the forearm and hand without regret."

CONCLUSION

Pneumatic tourniquet application facilitates many vascular procedures by minimizing the dissection required, improving anastomotic mobilization and visualization, and eliminating the potential for clamp-related trauma. The primary learning curve is related to proper sizing and anatomic "fit" for the tourniquet cuff and conscientious limb exsanguination with the Esmarch bandage. The cuff inflation pressure should be kept under 300 mm Hg, and the ischemic interval should be minimized and kept under 2 hours in all cases, if possible. The potential for additional applications of this technique can be expanded at the discretion and imagination of the individual surgeon once he or she becomes convinced of its utility. My recommendation is to try it— I think you'll like it.

REFERENCES

1. Scheinin TM, Lindfors O. Simplified repair of popliteal aneurysms. J Cardiovasc Surg 20:189-192, 1979.
2. Bernhard VM, Clark HB, Towne JB. Pneumatic tourniquet as a substitute for vascular clamps in distal bypass surgery. Surgery 87:709-713, 1980.
3. Collier PE. Atraumatic vascular anastomoses using a tourniquet. Ann Vasc Surg 6:34-37, 1992.
4. Wagner WH, Treiman RL, Cossman DV, et al. Tourniquet occlusion technique for tibial artery reconstruction. J Vasc Surg 18:637-647, 1993.
5. Manship LL, Moore WM, Bynoe R, et al. Different endothelial injuries caused by vascular clamps and vessel loops. II. Atherosclerotic vessels. Am Surg 7:401-406, 1985.
6. Coelho JC, Sigel B, Flanigan DP, et al. Arteriographic and ultrasonic evaluation of vascular clamp injuries using an in vitro human experimental model. Surg Gynecol Obstet 155:506-512, 1982.
7. Barone GW, Conerly JM, Farley PC, et al. Assessing clamp-related vascular injuries by measurement of associated vascular dysfunction. Surgery 105:465-471, 1989.
8. Henson GF, Rob CG. A comparative study of the effects of different arterial clamps on the vessel wall. Br J Surg 182:561-564, 1956.
9. DePalma RG, Chidi CC, et al. Pathogenesis and prevention of trauma-provoked atheromas. Surgery 82:429-437, 1977.
10. Pedowitz RA. The clinical problem. Acta Othop Scand 62:1-33, 1991.
11. Chervu A, Moore WS, Homsher E, et al. Differential recovery of skeletal muscle and peripheral nerve function after ischemia and reperfusion. J Surg Res 47:12-19, 1989.
12. Pedowitz RA, Gershuni DH, Schmidt AH, et al. Muscle injury beneath and distal to a pneumatic tourniquet: A quantitative animal study of effects of tourniquet pressure and duration. J Hand Surg 16A:610-621, 1991.
13. Hurst LN, Weiglein O, Brown WF, Campbell GJ. The pneumatic tourniquet: A biomechanical and electrophysiological study. Plast Reconstr Surg 67:648-652, 1981.
14. Pedowitz RA, Friden J, Thornell LE. Skeletal muscle injury induced by a pneumatic tourniquet: An enzyme and immunohistochemical study in rabbits. J Surg Res 52:243-250, 1992.
15. Wright JG, Kerr JC, Valeri CR, et al. Heparin decreases ischemia-reperfusion injury in isolated canine gracilis model. Arch Surg 123:470-472, 1988.
16. Sapega AA, Heppenstall RB, Chance B, et al. Optimizing tourniquet application and release times in extremity surgery. J Bone Joint Surg 67-A:303-314, 1985.
17. Eckhoff NL, Lond MS. Tourniquet paralysis. Lancet 2:343-345, 1931.

SECTION VI

Carotid and Vertebral Surgery

This section provides an update on the progress of the North American Symptomatic Carotid Endarterectomy Trial and its recent findings and also includes chapters relating to various technical and other aspects of carotid surgery.

48

The Ongoing Progress of NASCET

H.J.M. BARNETT, M.D., and HEATHER E. MELDRUM, B.A.

The North American Symptomatic Carotid Endarterectomy Trial (NASCET)[1] has been randomizing patients affected with focal symptoms of the retina or hemisphere since December 1987. The patients have been required to accept preliminary investigation by selective arteriography demonstrating that their symptoms were related to a stenosis of the appropriate carotid artery. In February 1991, the "Stopping Rules" of the trial were applied when, after accruing only 659 patients with 70% or greater degrees of stenosis, it was determined that carotid endarterectomy was beneficial for this group.[2] The majority of those in the medical arm who had survived free of major stroke were willing to accept endarterectomy.

Two other randomized studies have concluded that patients with severe stenosis benefit from carotid endarterectomy.[3,4] NASCET has continued to randomize patients with symptoms associated with <70% stenosis, measured by the NASCET method, including central arteriographic review and use of a jeweler's loupe to ensure that no patients with ≥70% stenosis were included in the ongoing phase.[5] The report from the Clinical Advisory issued by the National Institute of Neurologic Disorders and Stroke (NINDS) indicating benefit from endarterectomy for patients with a 60% to 99% stenosis but without symptoms[6] has led to a close analysis of the data accumulating in the NASCET trial and gathered by the European Carotid Surgery Trial (ECST) to ensure that it is ethical to randomize patients into the "moderate" phase of NASCET. This report concerns the present status of these trials in light of the preliminary Asymptomatic Carotid Atherosclerosis Study (ACAS) disclosures.

EVIDENCE TO DATE ABOUT THE "MODERATE" PATIENT

Two multicenter studies have randomized large numbers of patients with symptoms associated with <70% stenosis to determine whether patients who receive best medical care plus endarterectomy do better than those who receive best medical care alone. The ECST[3] ceased accrual of patients with moderate stenosis in 1994 and has been analyzing the results in 2200 patients. The authors have been told that no benefit has been observed, which, after 4.5 years of average follow-up, establishes that surgical treatment is superior to medical care alone when the stenosis is <70% by the ECST method of measure (C. Warlow, personal communication, 1995).

The Stopping Rules of NASCET[1] have continued to require a regularly scheduled confidential analysis that compares the outcome events of ipsilateral stroke, ipsilateral stroke and death, any stroke or death for the 1850 patients randomized to date into NASCET, half of whom are in the surgical arm (927) and half of whom (923) are in the medical arm. The investigators (which include the authors) are not privy to the details of these analyses. We are told the following: in light of the analysis conducted at the time of finalizing this document (April 1995), there is no benefit yet to be claimed for surgical treatment over medical therapy; that this analysis involves more than 450 outcome events in the 1850 patients followed for an average of 3 years; that separate analysis of those in each decile of patients below the seventh (60% to 69%, 50% to 59%, 40% to 49%, 30% to 39%, and less than 30%) are not as yet indicating benefit for endarterectomy.

This lack of benefit cannot be interpreted as a final conclusion. The length of follow-up planned for the study is for an average of 5 years for each patient, and the numbers of patients required in our sample size calculation is 2100 patients.

Failure to be able to claim benefit with the analyses from these two trials has been explained to all collaborators in NASCET and to the NINDS-appointed Monitoring Committee. There is unanimous agreement among all those associated with this study that NASCET must continue until it completes its accrual and predetermined 5-year follow-up or until a positive result is detected by the Stopping Rules analyses.

EVIDENCE FOR THE IMPORTANCE OF THE DEGREE OF STENOSIS IN THE NASCET AND ECST TRIALS

Reports from several surgical case studies and, more precisely, from the observations of several prospective studies conducted over periods ranging from 4 to 16 years and involving large numbers of asymptomatic patients, offer good evidence that the prognostic significance of the higher (75% to 80%+) degrees of stenosis are considerably worse than for patients with <75% stenosis.[7-9]

NASCET data from subgroup analysis determined a distinct prognostic worsening in the medical group between the patients symptomatic at 70% to 79% stenosis (annual risk of ipsilateral stroke) compared with those patients with 90% to 99% stenosis (annual risk of stroke).[2] There was a corresponding increase, in absolute terms, in surgical benefit from 12% in the 70% to 79% group to 26% in the 90% to 99% group.

The results favoring surgery published by ECST investigators were less striking than the benefit demonstrated by NASCET. The medical patients in the European trial fared better than those in NASCET. Believing that it was probable that the importance of severity of stenosis was the main contributor to this differential, the NASCET and ECST investigators collaborated to remeasure the arteriograms so that all were done by the NASCET Stenosis Index. By removing from the ECST calculation the 45% of the patients who were <70% (and who were thus measured as approximately 60% to 69% by NASCET measure), analyses of the two studies yielded results that were no longer disparate (Fig. 1).[10] A separate analysis of the patients who are in the ECST report but are considered "high moderate" by the NASCET measurement has been done, and no benefit for endarterectomy had been detected for this group as of March 1995 (C. Warlow, personal communication, 1995).

The hazard rates in NASCET have been found to be closely tied to the percentage of stenosis by decile, not only in the overall group of patients with severe disease but also strikingly in the subgroup of patients with overt ulceration on the arterial image (Fig. 2).[11] In the subgroup of patients who had only retinal events at entry compared with those with hemispheric events only at entry, there is a strong trend toward increased likelihood of stroke in the higher grades of stenosis[12] (Fig. 3). Hemisphere events carried a twofold risk of stroke compared to patients with retinal events only.

A recent publication, based on prospective follow-up of the patients from ECST with asymptomatic disease on the contralateral side to that which was symptomatic and led to their randomization in that study, has found a low risk of stroke at an average follow-up of 4.5 years.[13] The risk increased as the degree of stenosis increased (Fig. 4). From the 2295 patients with varying degrees of asymptomatic disease, they concluded the following: "Given their low stroke risks, the potential benefit of endarterectomy for asymptomatic patients is small. Population screening is not justified." NASCET has been making observations on a similar group of patients. Preliminary analyses confirm the observations and conclusions made by the ECST observers. In both of these studies the numbers of patients are too small for analyses to be reported as definitively conclusive. The confidence intervals are too wide.

CONCLUSION

The hard data from ECST and NASCET, based on more than 900 outcome events of stroke and death, do not provide a rationale for subjecting symptomatic patients with <70% stenosis to endarterectomy. Longer follow-up from ECST and further acquisition of patients in NASCET may alter this judgment. In both studies the analyses are ongoing in all deciles below 70%, and at the time of writing the disappointing results apply to those between 60% to 69%, as well as to the lower degrees of stenosis.

It is possible that the analyses will indicate that the degree of stenosis, compiled with the other vascular risk profile data, will indicate that a patient with a "high moderate" (60% to 69%) stenosis will benefit, whereas a patient with the same degree of stenosis and a low vascular profile may best be treated medically. All this is speculation, and in this era of evidence-based medicine must await the conclusion of randomized clinical trials.

The stenosis-based prognostic differential reported in the "other asymptomatic side" in ECST

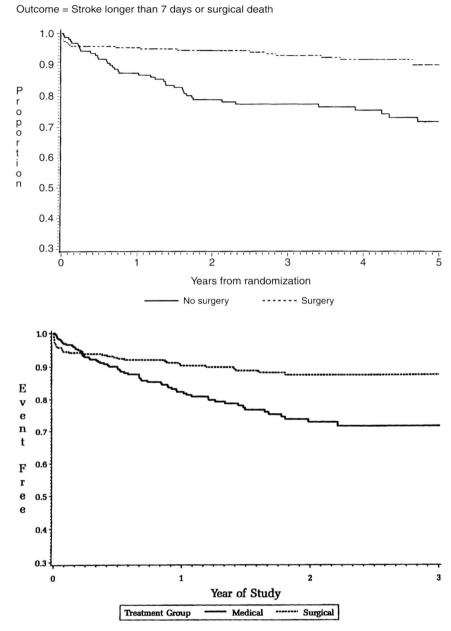

Fig. 1 Preliminary analysis of angiograms of patients randomized in ECST suggests that 82% stenosis measured using the ECST method is approximately equivalent to 70% stenosis measured using the NASCET method. ECST results have been reanalyzed for ECST patients with >82% stenosis by the ECST method. The survival curves for ECST *(top panel)* and those previously published by NASCET *(bottom panel)* look remarkably similar. Stroke risk at 2 years in the medical groups range from 20% to 25% and a "crossover" point in both studies occurs at about 3 months. (Modified from Barnett HJM, Warlow CP. Carotid endarterectomy and the measurement of stenosis. Stroke 24:1281-1284, 1993.)

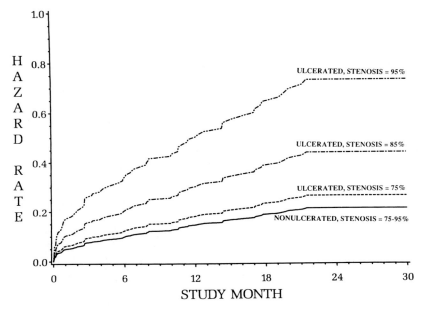

Fig. 2 Cumulative hazard curves showing risk (hazard rate) of any ipsilateral stroke for medically treated nonulcerated and ulcerated patients with 75% to 95% stenosis. The nonulcerated patients are represented by only one curve because the cumulative hazards are identical at all degrees of stenosis. (From Eliasziw M, Streifler JY, Fox AJ, Hachinski VC, Ferguson GG, Barnett HJM for the North American Symptomatic Carotid Endarterectomy Trial. Significance of plaque ulceration in symptomatic patients with high-grade carotid stenosis. Stroke 25:304-308, 1994.)

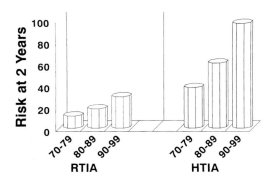

Fig. 3 The risk of ipsilateral ischemic stroke occurring in patients symptomatic from severe stenosis who presented with only retinal events (RTIA) was less (17% at 2 years) than for those who presented with only hemisphere events (HTIA), in whom it reached 44% at 2 years. All patients were in the medical arm of the NASCET study. The risk increased by subgroup analysis as the degree of stenosis increased. (From Barnett HJM, Meldrum HE. Update on carotid endarterectomy. Curr Opin Cardiol 10:511-516, 1995.)

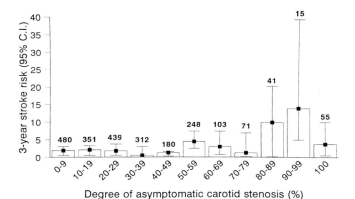

Fig. 4 Kaplan-Meier 3-year estimates (95% CI) of risk of stroke lasting longer than 7 days in distribution of asymptomatic artery. The risk increased with the decile of stenosis. (From The European Carotid Surgery Trialists' Collaborative Group. Risk of stroke in the distribution of an asymptomatic carotid artery. Lancet 345:209-212, 1995.)

and the same findings in the early NASCET observations are in contrast to the ACAS observations. This study reports no differential in the deciles starting at ≥60% to 69% and ending with a combined higher combination of deciles (80% to 99%).[6] (By utilizing Doppler alone, it was not possible for the investigators to distinguish between the results from those patients with the higher and the lower degrees of stenosis.) This is a major disappointment in ACAS, because it contradicts all previous evidence about the importance of the higher degrees of stenosis.

REFERENCES

1. North American Symptomatic Carotid Endarterectomy Trial (NASCET) Steering Committee. North American Symptomatic Carotid Endarterectomy Trial: Methods, patient characteristics, and progress. Stroke 22:711-720, 1991.
2. North American Symptomatic Carotid Endarterectomy Trial Collaborators. Beneficial effect of carotid endarterectomy in symptomatic patients with high-grade carotid stenosis. N Engl J Med 325:445-453, 1991.
3. European Carotid Surgery Trialists' Collaborative Group. MRC European Carotid Surgery Trial: Interim results for symptomatic patients with severe (70-99%) or with mild (0-29%) carotid stenosis. Lancet 337:1235-1243, 1991.
4. Mayberg MR, Wilson SE, Yatsu F, Weiss DG, Messian L, Hershey L, Colling C, Eskridge J, Deykin D, Winn HR, for the Veterans Affairs Cooperative Studies Program 309 Trialist Group. Carotid endarterectomy and prevention of cerebral ischemia in symptomatic carotid stenosis. JAMA 266:3289-3294, 1991.
5. Fox AJ. How to measure carotid stenosis. Radiology 186:316-318, 1993.
6. Special report. Clinical advisory: Carotid endarterectomy for patients with asymptomatic internal carotid artery stenosis. Stroke 25:2523-2524, 1994.
7. Hennerici M, Hulsbomer HB, Hefter H, Lammerts D, Rautenberg W. Natural history of asymptomatic extracranial arterial disease: Results of a long-term prospective study. Brain 110:777-791, 1987.
8. Norris JW, Zhu CZ, Bornstein NM, Chambers BR. Vascular risks of asymptomatic carotid stenosis. Stroke 22:1485-1490, 1991.
9. Shanik GD, Moore DJ, Leahy A, Grouden MC, Colgan MP. Asymptomatic carotid stenosis: A benign lesion? Eur J Vasc Surg 6:10-15, 1992.
10. Barnett HJM, Warlow CP. Carotid endarterectomy and the measurement of stenosis. Stroke 24:1281-1284, 1993.
11. Eliasziw M, Streifler JY, Fox AJ, Hachinski VC, Ferguson GG, Barnett HJM for the North American Symptomatic Carotid Endarterectomy Trial. Significance of plaque ulceration in symptomatic patients with high-grade carotid stenosis. Stroke 25:304-308, 1994.
12. Streifler JY, Eliasziw M, Benavente OR, Harbison JW, Hachinski VC, Barnett HJM, Simard D for the North American Symptomatic Carotid Endarterectomy Trial. The risk of stroke in patients with first-ever retinal vs. hemispheric transient ischemic attacks and high-grade carotid stenosis. Arch Neurol 52:246-249, 1995.
13. The European Carotid Surgery Trialists' Collaborative Group. Risk of stroke in the distribution of an asymptomatic carotid artery. Lancet 345:209-212, 1995.

49

Carotid Endarterectomy in Symptomatic and Asymptomatic Patients Over 80 Years of Age: Indications and Results

BRUCE A. PERLER, M.D.

Carotid endarterectomy (CEA) is the most frequently performed peripheral vascular operation in the United States. In the mid-1980s approximately 100,000 procedures were being performed annually at a cost of well over $1 billion.[1,2] Because of the rapid growth in the number of procedures performed, its associated costs, and isolated reports of excessive operative morbidity, CEA has been intensely scrutinized and challenged by some.[3,4] However, recent randomized prospective multicenter clinical trials have firmly established the safety and efficacy of CEA in the management of patients with symptomatic and asymptomatic atherosclerotic disease at the carotid bifurcation.[5,6]

The frequency with which CEA is performed is not surprising when one considers that its sole purpose is to prevent stroke, a prevalent, highly morbid, and extremely expensive health care problem in this country. An estimated 500,000 new strokes occur per year, as many as 40% are fatal, and atherosclerotic carotid bifurcation disease is one of the most frequent causes of these strokes.[7] There are about 2 million stroke survivors in this country, and rehabilitation can be protracted and expensive. Approximately 40% of stroke survivors require specialized nursing services after they recover from the acute event, and 10% require extended inpatient care.[8] It is estimated that stroke may cost nearly $20 billion annually.[9]

It seems clear from this evidence that CEA should be a highly cost-effective approach to the problem of stroke for a significant percentage of cases, and both the North American Symptomatic Carotid Endarterectomy Trial (NASCET) and the Asymptomatic Carotid Atherosclerosis Study (ACAS) have provided objective evidence to support this proposition.[5,6] On the other hand, some controversy persists and important questions remain unanswered. For example, although the role of CEA in the management of patients with cerebrovascular disease is more widely accepted today in general, there continue to be reservations expressed about its performance in the very elderly. This chapter will address this important issue.

DEMOGRAPHIC CONSIDERATIONS: HOW OLD IS TOO OLD FOR CAROTID ENDARTERECTOMY?

At a time of increasing pressure for health care cost containment in this country, determining how old is too old for a patient to undergo CEA is an especially important question to address for several reasons. First, the elderly represent the fastest growing segment of the population of the United States. The average life expectancy of a 65-year-old individual is 15 years, for a 75-year-old it is 10, and for an 80-year-old it is approximately seven years.[10] There are currently approximately 25 million people in this country between the ages of 65 and 85, and it is projected that by the year 2025 that group will increase to 58 million individuals, and at least 34 million will be older than 75 years of age.[11] Approximately 40% of our population will survive to age 80.[12] From a financial perspective, it seems clear that the elderly will consume a disproportionate fraction of our health care resources.

Second, cerebrovascular disease is essentially a disease of the older segments of our population. In fact, the incidence of stroke increases almost exponentially with age.[13] The annual stroke incidence per 100,000 individuals increases from 262 among individuals between the ages of 55 and 64 to nearly 1400 among individuals between 75 and 84 years of age. The stroke incidence is nearly 2% among individuals 85 years of age and older (Table 1). Third, the morbidity and mortality of stroke increases dramatically with advancing age. Approximately two thirds of individuals less than 75 years of age who experience a stroke

Table 1 Stroke incidence by age

Age	Strokes/100,000 (%)
55-64	262
65-74	582
75-84	1382
85+	1824

survive and are alive 6 months later, whereas only about half of those between the ages of 75 and 84 survive and are alive 6 months after the event. Among individuals over the age of 85, the likelihood of surviving 6 months is approximately 33%.[13] From an economic standpoint, it has been conservatively estimated that the cost of stroke among individuals over the age of 80 is at least $3 billion per year.[14,15]

Operative Risks

It would seem from these observations that CEA would potentially be most efficacious in the very elderly patient population; namely, those at greatest risk of ischemic cerebral infarction. Yet it is that very segment of the population in whom performance of this operation has been most controversial and its performance most restricted.[2] Essentially, there has been a long-standing perception that the inherent risks of this operation are significantly increased in very elderly patients. This attitude was reflected in the results of a survey conducted among 40 primary care physicians in Georgia: 28% said they would not refer an octogenarian for CEA, and 35% predicted that the operative mortality would be 15% among this demographic group.[14]

This pessimistic attitude may not be limited to nonsurgical specialists. Indeed, although the hallmark contributions of NASCET and ACAS are well recognized, one might reasonably question whether the findings and operative indications defined in these investigations are truly applicable to the very elderly patient population, since both studies included only patients under the age of 80. In fact, the mean ages of patients in NASCET and ACAS were 64 and 67, respectively.[5,6]

Part of the skepticism with respect to performing this operation on the very elderly may be based on isolated reports that have documented suboptimal surgical results. For example, the Rand Corporation reviewed the performance of CEA on 1302 Medicare patients in three geographic areas in 1981. The operative mortality was 3.4% and the perioperative stroke rate was 6.4%.[16,17] In a more recent study, the records of 2089 Medicare patients who underwent CEA in New England in 1984 and 1985 were reviewed. Operative mortality increased significantly with age. Specifically, it was 1.1% for those between 65 and 69 years of age, 2% for those between 70 and 74, 3.2% for those between 75 and 79, and 4.7% for those older than 80 years of age. In other words, patients over the age of 80 experienced a fourfold increased risk of operative mortality.[2] However, other large community-wide studies have failed to document increased operative risk among older patients.[18,19] Nevertheless, there are at least two important pathologic considerations that may differentiate the very elderly from the younger patient population undergoing CEA.

PATHOLOGIC CONSIDERATIONS

The association between carotid atherosclerosis and coronary artery disease is well recognized.[20] Further, the incidence of coronary disease increases with age. Therefore one can anticipate that a significant percentage of very elderly patients undergoing CEA harbor coronary artery disease, and in many patients this disease is silent because of their sedentary lifestyles. The prevalence of coronary artery disease in this patient population is largely responsible for the somewhat poorer long-term survival of patients over the age of 80 who undergo CEA when compared with age-matched control subjects.[21] One may therefore logically anticipate a somewhat higher incidence of cardiac complications among very elderly patients who undergo CEA when compared with younger patients.[21-25] Perioperative dysrhythmias are especially prevalent in this patient population.[21] Nevertheless, contemporary experience demonstrates that with careful preoperative preparation, modern anesthetic management, and careful postoperative monitoring, this increased incidence of significant coronary artery disease has not adversely affected outcome among very elderly patients undergoing CEA.

Another pathologic consideration among very elderly patients who present with significant carotid bifurcation disease is the increased prevalence of significant intracerebral lesions when compared with younger operative candidates. Specifically, it has been reported that the incidence of significant intracranial arterial oc-

Table 2 Results of CEA in the elderly

Institution (yr)	Minimum age	No. of cases	No. >80 years (%)	CVA (%)	Death (%)
Hospital Saint Joseph (1985)	75	76	17	2.6	1.3
Georgia Baptist (1986)	80	90	100	5.6	2.2
University of Rochester (1986)	75	77	NA	3.9	0
Creighton University (1988)	80	90	100	1.1	2.2
University of Missouri (1990)	75	125	29	0	0.8
University of Bordeaux (1991)	75	81	NA	6.1	3.7
Cedars-Sinai (1992)	80	183	100	1.7	1.6
Johns Hopkins (1994)	75	63	29	4.8	0

Data compiled from References 14, 21, 22, 24, 25, 33-35.
NA = not available.

clusive disease may be nearly fivefold higher in patients over the age of 80 who undergo CEA when compared with younger individuals.[14,26] Traditionally, there have been two reservations about performing CEA in the presence of significant tandem lesions. First, there was concern that significant siphon disease would predispose to early thrombosis of the endarterectomy site.[27-29] Also, it was assumed that siphon lesions would be responsible for persistent or recurrent symptoms in a significant percentage of cases.[30] However, a growing clinical experience suggests that CEA may be performed safely in the presence of significant siphon disease.[31,32] Furthermore, while the potential adverse impact of siphon disease may be most important in the very elderly, the preponderance of evidence suggests that CEA in appropriately selected patients is safe and markedly improves their long-term prognosis when compared with patients managed medically.[14,33]

CLINICAL EXPERIENCE

More than a decade ago there was considerable skepticism within the medical community with respect to the safety and efficacy of CEA in general. In fact, a great deal of this concern related to isolated reports citing excessive operative risk. Typically, these analyses included large numbers of surgeons among whom there was considerable variability in operative volume and experience.[1] Over the last decade, however, a growing clinical experience with CEA has clearly established its efficacy when performed by experienced surgeons; recent multicenter randomized trials have confirmed this clinical impression.

I suggest that a similar process has influenced the perception of some with respect to the advisability of performing CEA on very elderly patients. Specifically, less favorable outcomes among elderly patients undergoing CEA have been noted when the operation has been performed by those with limited experience with the procedure. For example, in a large study of Medicare patients undergoing CEA, operative mortality was roughly threefold higher in hospitals in which less than 40 CEAs were performed per year.[2] It is axiomatic that surgical experience, like surgical indications, will influence operative results.

However, the preponderance of evidence reported over the last decade does not support the contention that advanced age adversely affects the outcome of CEA (Table 2). The definition of "elderly" has been either 75 or 80 years of age in most studies and is obviously arbitrary. The basic implication of these reports, however, is that the fundamental indications for CEA should not be influenced by the age of the patient, even among those over the age of 80.

In one report, for example, 90 octogenarians underwent CEA over an 8-year period. Perioperative strokes occurred in five patients (5.6%), resulting in two deaths (2.2%). All five strokes occurred in patients with severe intracranial disease.[14] The benefit of CEA in this patient population became apparent during long-term follow-up: strokes occurred in only 2% of operated patients but in 16% of a matched group of octogenarians who did not undergo CEA.[14] In the largest series of octogenarians undergoing CEA reported to date, 183 patients underwent operation with a combined perioperative stroke and mortality rate of 3.3% (see Table 2), which was no different than the 3.5% stroke and mortality rate experienced by younger patients at this institution.[34] This experience is comparable to the perioperative stroke and mortality rate of 3.3% among 90 octogenarians and nonagenarians reported by Schultz et al.[21]

Other reports including patients with a minimum age of 75 undergoing CEA have also documented excellent results (see Table 2). For example, Courbier et al.[33] reported a combined stroke and mortality rate of 3.9% among 76 patients, of whom 17% were over the age of 80. In a more recent study from the University of Missouri, 125 patients with a minimum age of 75 underwent CEA with no operative strokes and one (0.8%) death. More than a quarter of these patients were older than 80 years of age.[25] Furthermore, the 7-year incidence of freedom from stroke was 80%,[25] confirming other studies that suggest that CEA among the elderly clearly improves the long-term prognosis of this patient population.[14,35]

THE JOHNS HOPKINS EXPERIENCE
Patients

The Johns Hopkins experience further supports the performance of CEA, irrespective of patient age. Over a 12-year period, 63 CEA procedures were performed on 59 elderly patients including three patients who underwent bilateral procedures and one who underwent operation on the same vessel twice. The number of CEAs performed on elderly patients increased dramatically during the latter portion of the study period; in fact, nearly half of these procedures were performed during the last 30 months.[22] Whether reflecting the aging of the population, greater acceptance of CEA in the management of cerebrovascular disease by the medical community in general, or other factors, an increasing number of elderly patients with operable carotid disease are being referred, as others have noted.[36]

The patients ranged from 75 to 92 years of age (mean, 79 years); 17 (29%) were older than 80 years of age. The indications for operation included previous ipsilateral stroke in 16 (25%), hemispheric transient ischemic attacks (TIAs) in 25 (40%), amaurosis fugax in three (5%), non-hemispheric symptoms in seven (11%), and asymptomatic carotid stenoses in 12 (19%) cases. The operated internal carotid artery (ICA) was more than 50% stenotic in all cases, more than 70% stenotic in 90%, and more than 90% stenotic in 61% of cases. The operated vessel was at least 80% stenotic in all asymptomatic cases. The contralateral ICA was completely occluded in 20% of the cases. All operations were performed with the patient under general anesthesia, and shunts were used in 49 cases (78%).

Results

There were no operative deaths, and perioperative strokes occurred in three cases (4.8%). Two of these patients made a complete recovery; the third patient was left with a moderate motor deficit but has lived at home for nearly 5 years. One of the strokes was most likely secondary to a cardiac embolus to the posterior circulation, and another was the result of postendarterectomy cerebral hemorrhage. The other stroke appeared secondary to an embolus from the endarterectomy site. One stroke (6%) occurred among the 16 patients undergoing operation for prior stroke, and the other two (4%) among the 25 patients with a history of hemispheric TIAs. No strokes occurred among patients undergoing operation for amaurosis fugax, nonhemispheric symptoms, or asymptomatic carotid stenoses. Only one stroke (6%) occurred among the 17 patients over the age of 80.

As noted previously, coronary disease is especially prevalent in elderly patients with carotid disease. However, major cardiac complications occurred in only five cases (7.9%). Two (3.2%) postoperative myocardial infarctions occurred, without further sequelae. This incidence is comparable to the rate of myocardial infarction experienced by younger operative candidates.[23] Two patients (3.2%) experienced dysrhythmias, including one case of atrial fibrillation managed medically and a bradyarrhythmia caused by a malfunctioning pacemaker that was replaced. One patient (1.6%) developed rest angina postoperatively and underwent cardiac catheterization and successful coronary balloon angioplasty.

However, justifying a potentially risky surgical intervention for the manifestations of an incurable disease such as arteriosclerosis in patients with limited life expectancy requires more than performing the procedure with an acceptable degree of safety; one should also demonstrate that the intervention conveys long-term benefit. The Hopkins experience has clearly satisfied that prerequisite. This patient population has been followed for 1 to 122 months (mean, 27.4 months); there have been no fatal strokes. Six deaths have occurred as a result of cardiac disease (four), malignancy (one), and unknown cause (one), yielding survival of 80% at 5-years' and 52% at 10-years' follow-up. Two nonfatal strokes have occurred at 23 and 50 months, yielding stroke-free survival of 85% at 4-years', 68% at 5-years', and 42% at 10-years' follow-up. Cumulative freedom from stroke was 90% at 4-years' and 80% at 5- and 10-years' follow-up. Although it is somewhat difficult to truly quantitate the impact of an operation on the patient's quality of life, this experience, like others,[14,25] demonstrates that CEA provides excellent long-term stroke prevention among elderly patients.

HOW OLD IS TOO OLD FOR CEA?

The fastest growing segment of our population are individuals over the age of 75, and it is expected that 40% of our population will survive to age 80. The rapidly aging demographic contour of our society mandates that we change the way in which therapeutic decisions are made. Specifically, clinicians must overcome long-standing prejudices with respect to the importance of age in formulating those clinical judgments. Since the oldest individuals are at greatest risk of stroke, the management of cerebrovascular disease is a critical issue in which to examine the influence of age on outcome.

Unquestionably, surgical indications must continue to be considered on an individual basis. However, the preponderance of evidence available suggests that advanced age should not be considered the sole determining contraindication to performing CEA if the patient otherwise has appropriate surgical indications. Specifically, a history of stroke, hemispheric TIAs, or amaurosis fugax in the setting of a high-grade ipsilateral carotid stenosis are strong indications for CEA. Although NASCET has to this point demonstrated surgical efficacy only when stenosis is 70% or greater,[5] in the absence of other potential causes and a 50% or greater carotid lesion, I would recommend surgery. Since there is an increased prevalence of intracranial arteriosclerotic disease in the very elderly patient population with carotid bifurcation disease, one should be more circumspect about performing CEA for nonhemispheric symptoms. Although the presence of tandem lesions may not substantially increase the short-term operative risk, one may anticipate a greater likelihood of persistent or recurrent symptomatology.

Finally, what about the 92-year-old patient with an asymptomatic carotid stenosis who is living independently? How old is too old for CEA? Although it may be somewhat premature to recommend CEA for the nonagenarian with a 60% unilateral stenosis on the basis of ACAS,[6] when one considers that more than 100,000 strokes occur per year among asymptomatic patients, the impact of stroke is most devastating among the very elderly, and the relatively healthy 92-year-old has several years of life expectancy, that 92-year-old patient is probably not too old for CEA, assuming that the stenosis is high grade and that there is not more severe carotid siphon disease.

Ultimately, it is the goal of the health care provider "to postpone chronic illness, to maintain vigor, and to slow social and psychological involution."[37] The performance of CEA, by preventing stroke, is consistent with that goal. Advanced age should be viewed as an identifier of those who could most benefit from the procedure, rather than a contraindication to its performance.[38]

REFERENCES

1. Grotta JC. Current medical and surgical therapy for cerebrovascular disease. N Engl J Med 317:1505-1516, 1987.
2. Fisher ES, Malenka DJ, Solomon NA, et al. Risk of carotid endarterectomy in the elderly. Am J Public Health 79:1617-1620, 1989.
3. Warlow C. Carotid endarterectomy: Does it work? Stroke 15:1068-1076, 1984.
4. Dyken ML. Carotid endarterectomy studies: A glimmering of science. Stroke 17:355-357, 1986.
5. North American Symptomatic Carotid Endarterectomy Trial Collaborators. Beneficial effect of carotid endarterectomy in symptomatic patients with high-grade carotid stenosis. N Engl J Med 325:445-453, 1991.
6. Executive Committee for the Asymptomatic Carotid Atherosclerosis Study. Endarterectomy for asymptomatic carotid artery stenosis. JAMA 273:1421-1428, 1995.
7. Timsit SG, Sacco RL, Mohr JP, et al. Early clinical differentiation of cerebral infarction from severe atherosclerotic stenosis and cardioembolism. Stroke 23:486-491, 1992.
8. Donayre CE, Wilson SE, Hobson RW II. Extracranial carotid artery occlusive disease. In Veith FJ, Hobson RW, Williams RA, Wilson SE, eds. Vascular Surgery. Principles and Practice, 2nd ed. New York: McGraw Hill, 1994, pp 649-664.
9. Mitsias P, Welch KMA. Medical therapy for transient ischemic attacks and ischemic stroke. In Ernst CB, Stanley JC, eds. Current Therapy in Vascular Surgery, 3rd ed. St. Louis: Mosby, 1995, pp 24-29.
10. Harbrecht PJ, Ahmad W, Garrison N, et al. Influence of age on the management of abdominal aortic aneurysm. Am Surg 48:93-97, 1982.
11. U.S. Bureau of the Census. Current population reports. 922:25, 1980.
12. Treiman RL, Levine KA, Cohen JL, Cossman DV, Foran RF, Levin PM. Aneurysmectomy in the octogenarian: A study of morbidity and quality of survival. Am J Surg 144:194-197, 1982.

13. Robins M, Baum HM. Natural survey of stroke incidence. Stroke 121(Suppl 1):45-47, 1981.
14. Rosenthal D, Rudderman RH, Jones DH, et al. Carotid endarterectomy in the octogenarian. Is it appropriate? J Vasc Surg 3:782-787, 1986.
15. Thompson JE, Talkington CM. Carotid surgery for cerebral ischemia. Surg Clin North Am 59:539-553, 1979.
16. Trout HH III. Carotid endarterectomy: Despite the NASCET report, the controversy is not over. J Vasc Surg 14:565-566, 1991.
17. Winslow CM, Solomon DH, Chassin MR, et al. The appropriateness of carotid endarterectomy. N Engl J Med 318:721-727, 1984.
18. Brott T, Thalinger K. The practice of carotid endarterectomy in a large metropolitan area. Stroke 15:950-955, 1984.
19. Plecha FR, Bertin VJ, Plecha EJ, et al. The results of vascular surgery in patients 75 years of age and older: An analysis of 3259 cases. J Vasc Surg 2:761-764, 1985.
20. Hertzer NR, Beven EG, Young JR, et al. Incidental asymptomatic carotid bruits in patients scheduled for peripheral vascular reconstruction: Results of cerebral and coronary angiography. Surgery 96:535-543, 1984.
21. Schultz RD, Sterpetti AV, Feldhaus RJ. Carotid endarterectomy in octogenarians and nonogenarians. Surg Gynecol Obstet 166:245-251, 1988.
22. Perler BA, Williams GM. Carotid endarterectomy in the very elderly: Is it worthwhile? Surgery 116:479-483, 1994.
23. Perler BA, Burdick JF, Williams GM. Does contralateral internal carotid occlusion increase the risk of carotid endarterectomy? A ten-year experience. J Vasc Surg 16:347-353, 1992.
24. Ouriel K, Penn TE, Ricotta JJ, et al. Carotid endarterectomy in the elderly patient. Surg Gynecol Obstet 162:334-336, 1986.
25. Pinkerton JA Jr, Gholkav VR. Should patient age be a consideration in carotid endarterectomy? J Vasc Surg 11:650-658, 1990.
26. Rosenthal D, Zeichner WD, Lamis PA, et al. Neurologic deficit after carotid endarterectomy: Pathogenesis and management. Surgery 94:776-780, 1983.
27. Day AL, Rhoton AL, Quisling RG. Resolving siphon stenosis following endarterectomy. Stroke 11:278-281, 1980.
28. Hugenholz H, Elgie RG. Carotid thromboendarterectomy: A reappraisal. Criteria for patient selection. J Neurosurg 16:705-730, 1959.
29. Sundt TM, Sandok BA, Whisnant JP. Carotid endarterectomy. Complications and preoperative assessment of risk. Mayo Clin Proc 50:301-306, 1975.
30. Lord RSA. Relevance of siphon stenosis and intracranial aneurysms to results of carotid endarterectomy. In Ernst CB, Stanley JC, eds. Current Therapy in Vascular Surgery, 2nd ed. Philadelphia: BC Decker, 1991, pp 94-100.
31. Roederer GO, Langlois YE, Chan ARW, et al. Is siphon disease important in predicting the outcome of carotid endarterectomy? Arch Surg 118:1177-1181, 1983.
32. Lord RSA, Raj TB, Graham AR. Carotid endarterectomy, siphon stenosis, collateral hemispheric pressure, and perioperative cerebral infarction. J Vasc Surg 6:391-397, 1987.
33. Courbier R, Ferdani M, Reggi M. Carotid stenosis. Surgery after 75 years. Int Angiol 4:295-299, 1985.
34. Trieman RL, Wagner WH, Foran RF, et al. Carotid endarterectomy in the elderly. Ann Vasc Surg 6:321-324, 1992.
35. Rogues XF, Baudet EM, Clerc F. Results of carotid endarterectomy in patients 75 years of age and older. J Cardiovasc Surg 32:726-731, 1991.
36. Benhamou AC, Kieffer E, Tricot JF, et al. Carotid artery surgery in patients over 70 years of age. Int Surg 66:199-202, 1981.
37. Fries JF. Aging, natural death, and the compression of morbidity. N Engl J Med 303:130-135, 1980.
38. Perler BA. Vascular disease. Surg Clin North Am 74:199-216, 1994.

50

To Shunt or Not to Shunt? To Patch or Not to Patch?

JONATHAN B. TOWNE, M.D.

THE SHUNT

The necessity for protecting the cerebrum during carotid endarterectomy remains one of the controversies in carotid artery surgery. Surgeons who perform carotid endarterectomy with regional or local anesthesia can easily determine the need for using an intraoperative shunt by noting the patient's response to test clamping. Hafner and Evans,[1] reporting a series of 12,000 procedures done with the patient under local anesthesia, noted a 9% prevalence of patients who required a shunt. As would be expected, patients with contralateral carotid artery occlusion or severe stenosis were more likely to require a shunt than patients with unilateral lesions (30% compared with 5%).

Surgeons who perform a carotid endarterectomy with the patient under general anesthesia follow one of three methods: routine shunting, selective shunting, and shunting only in rare instances. Of surgeons who routinely use a shunt, only the technical mastery of shunt insertion and removal and performance of endarterectomy with the shunt in place are required. The chief proponent of this technique has been Jesse Thompson, who has reported outstanding results.[2] The advantages of routine use of intraluminal shunts are that it allows an unhurried approach to the carotid endarterectomy so that a meticulous procedure can be performed without time constraints. One variation of this technique that I use is to perform the arteriotomy and complete the endarterectomy, including evaluation of the distal intimal break point in the internal carotid artery, tacking it if necessary, and then inserting the shunt. This rarely takes more than 4 minutes, an interval generally regarded as safe in preventing any neurologic sequelae. After the shunt is inserted, the external carotid artery endarterectomy can be performed, since the position of the shunt does not affect it. If the remaining artery following endarterectomy is thin and small, the shunt can aid in the closure of the vessel, making it easier to visualize and precisely place the sutures. Shortcomings associated with use of the shunt that have never been accurately quantitated include the following: (1) Dislodgement of proximal debris in the common carotid artery can occur during shunt placement, with subsequent embolization through the shunt. In 20 years of performing carotid artery surgery with routine shunting, I have observed this twice. This can be minimized through careful attention to the presence of occlusive disease in the common carotid artery proximal to the typical site for an arteriotomy. (2) Injury to the distal internal carotid endothelium can also occur. The intima can be "snowplowed" and intimal flaps potentially can be created that are difficult to detect intraoperatively, which can lead to thrombosis of the internal carotid artery. To avoid this complication, the surgeon must take care not to insert a shunt that is too large for the artery. I prefer the use of straight shunts and rarely use a shunt greater than 10 mm in diameter. In small internal carotid arteries, I use an 8 mm shunt.

Surgeons who use selective shunting determine its need through a variety of techniques; the most common are intraoperative EEG monitoring and measurement of carotid stump pressure.

Intraoperative EEG

A number of authors have used the EEG to determine the need for intraoperative placement of a carotid shunt. This technique requires the equipment to obtain readable EEG tracings and staff who are knowledgeable enough to follow the patient and detect any changes. Callow[3] has reported excellent results from this technique. The significance of EEG changes is occasionally difficult to evaluate: on occasion, EEG changes can persist throughout the procedure, but the patient awakes without having suffered any neurologic sequelae. The chief shortcoming of

EEG monitoring is the level of expertise necessary to evaluate the patient intraoperatively.

Carotid Stump Pressure

To avoid some of the problems associated with continuous EEG, some investigators have attempted to use carotid stump pressures to select patients for shunting during carotid procedures. Most have selected a carotid stump pressure of 50 to 55 mm Hg as a level below which shunting should be performed,[4,5] whereas Moore et al.[6] have set 25 mm/Hg as the critical level. The stump pressure is obtained by inserting a 19-gauge needle into the carotid artery following clamping of the external and common carotid artery. Since there is no flow, the pressure in the distal internal carotid artery equalizes in the carotid bulb and an accurate stump pressure can be obtained.

There is no question that the lower the stump pressure, the greater the need for cerebral protection. However, there are several caveats: first, the fact that the level of the stump pressure is directly related to the systemic blood pressure; if there is a decrease in blood pressure following measurement of the stump pressure, the stump pressure could be significantly affected and the patient who had previously had an adequate stump pressure could have a dangerously low stump pressure. Second, some authors have demonstrated that even in the presence of an adequate stump pressure, EEG changes can occur. Baker et al.[7] demonstrated that in approximately 7% of all patients and 20% of patients with coexistent symptoms of vertebral basilar insufficiency or a history of an old completed stroke, EEG changes can occur despite a stump pressure of 50 mm Hg or more. Hafner and Evans,[1] in their series of procedures performed using local anesthesia, found that of 125 patients with cerebral stump pressures from 0 to 25 mm Hg, only 45% required a shunt.

The chief proponent of performing carotid endarterectomy without a shunt is William Baker. The very large series with excellent results reported by Baker et al.[8] demonstrated that the procedure can be done without a shunt in the vast majority of patients. However, careful perusal of the data of Baker et al. demonstrates that in the presence of significant contralateral stenosis and/or occlusion, the patient is probably best served by placement of an indwelling shunt.

The difficulty in ascertaining the need for cerebral protection during carotid endarterectomy is that most studies do not or are not able to give a definite etiologic cause of strokes when they occur. If a patient develops a stroke secondary to an internal carotid artery occlusion as a result of an endarterectomy that has been poorly performed technically, the type of cerebral protection that was or was not used is not at fault. When the causes of perioperative stroke are analyzed in most series, technical error in the performance of endarterectomy remains the principal cause of neurologic deficits.[9] The surgeon should choose the technique and approach to cerebral protection that allow the most precise, accurate technical repair.

THE PATCH

The role of patching during carotid artery reconstruction addresses two potential problems: (1) the most significant is an attempt to improve the technical result of the endarterectomy reconstruction and minimize technical complications of the repair, many of which will result in perioperative stroke; and (2) the effect, if any, that patching the internal carotid artery has on the subsequent recurrence of stenosis in the repaired artery during the follow-up period. Most authors agree that in a small carotid artery in which there are technical difficulties, particularly at the internal carotid artery end of the arteriotomy, closing with a patch can help to avoid a stricture. This often occurs when making a linear arteriotomy; there are lateral tears at the apex in the internal carotid artery, so that it is difficult to avoid a narrowing during closure of the arteriotomy. Also, in patients who have a thickened intima that extends well up toward the base of the brain, patching can smooth this transition zone from the endarterectomized vessel to the residual vessel beyond. Likewise, in patients who have kinks or elongated arteries, patching is a way to help maintain the lumen and prevent postoperative occlusion.

The role of patching when there are no technical problems remains controversial. As with all topics in vascular surgery, there are positive and negative aspects to whatever technique is used. The chief proponents of patching are Hertzer et al.[10] at the Cleveland Clinic. In a consecutive series of 801 patients who underwent 917 primary carotid endarterectomies, a marked reduction of neurologic morbidity and mortality was noted in patients who had a closure of the carotid repair with an autogenous patch. In the vein patch group the incidence of ischemic strokes was 0.7% compared with 3.1% in the group without patches. Routine postoperative angiography demonstrated occlusions in 0.5% of the vein patch vessels compared with 3.1% of the nonpatched vessels, supporting the thesis of Hertzer et al. that excellent results of carotid endarterectomy could actually be made better by the routine use of patching. However, this study was not prospectively randomized. Eikelboom et al.[11] of The Netherlands reported a randomized prospective study of 129 consecutive patients undergoing carotid procedures who were allocated between primary closure and saphenous vein patching. These patients were prospectively evaluated in the postoperative period with duplex scanning at 3, 6, and 12 months. A 21% recurrent stenosis after primary closure was noted, compared with 3.5% in patients with patch closures. They also noted that recurrent stenosis was higher in women (24%) compared with men (7.5%). In women stenosis recurred in 55% who underwent primary closure, compared with 11% in men. Only 5% of the men with a patch closure had recurrent stenosis; none of the 14 women with patch closures did. The perioperative stroke rate was not significantly different in the two groups. Clagett et al.[12] randomized 152 carotid procedures between vein patch closure and primary closure in a Veteran's Administration Hospital study. They excluded patients who had an internal carotid artery (ICA) diameter of less than 5 mm, arteriotomy extending more than 3 cm beyond the origin of the ICA, or a tortuous and/or kinked ICA. Patients who received an obligatory vein patch constituted 20% of their cases. As in the study of Eikelboom et al., differences in perioperative morbidity were not significant between patients who had undergone primary closure and those with obligatory vein patch closures. They noted recurrent disease in 12.9% of the patients having saphenous vein patch closure compared with 1.7% of those with primary closures. Most of these involved moderate stenosis, and all but one were limited to the carotid bulb, suggesting that the increased size of the artery led to layering of thrombus, resulting in the stenosis. In a study of 461 carotid procedures, Kinney et al.[13] noted the importance of avoiding residual flow abnormalities at the conclusion of the carotid endarterectomy. Duplex scanning was conducted during the operative procedures on all these patients. By life-table analysis, the prevalence of greater than 50% diameter-reducing ICA stenosis or occlusion was increased in patients with residual flow abnormalities. More important was that in patients with normal intraoperative flow studies, a significantly lower rate of late ipsilateral stroke occurred compared with the remaining patient cohort. This study suggests that it is important to achieve a normal hemodynamic result at operation. If a patch is required to accomplish this, then it contributes to the procedure. Our frequency of patching has increased from a range of 1% to 2% of cases to 50% to 60%, coincident with the intraoperative evaluation with duplex scanning. However, in series that have perioperative stroke rates in the 1% to 2% range, it is difficult to demonstrate any significant improvement with changes of technique because of the large numbers necessary to show any statistical difference.

Several other issues must be considered in regard to patching. There is a tendency to make patches too big, and a bulbous patch may result in thrombus layering, much as it does in an abdominal aortic aneurysm. Approximately 1% of saphenous vein patches rupture spontaneously in the perioperative period. This is a lethal event that is difficult if not impossible to predict. When a fabric prosthesis is used, there is approximately a 0.5% to 1% incidence of infection. Although it seldom occurs, it is difficult to treat and can result in significant late morbidity.

As in our consideration of cerebral protection, the most important element in performing a carotid endarterectomy is a precise anatomic and hemodynamic repair. There is no substitute for technical excellence, and to the extent that any individual case requires patching to improve the hemodynamic or technical result, this should be done. Obviously, on large vessels in which repair can be done carefully and the distal end point well controlled, there probably is no need for patching. However, when there are potential problems with the internal carotid artery break point, small vessels, kinked vessels, or there have been some technical problems during the endarterectomy, the surgeon should not hesitate to perform a patch— being careful not to make it too large.

REFERENCES

1. Hafner CO, Evans WE. Carotid endarterectomy with local anesthesia: Results and advantages. J Vasc Surg 7:232-239, 1988.
2. Thompson JE, Talkington CM. Carotid endarterectomy. Ann Surg 184:1-15, 1976.

3. Callow AD. An overview of the stroke problem in the carotid territory. Am J Surg 140:181-191, 1980.
4. Hays RJ, Levinson SA, Wylie EJ. Intraoperative measurement of carotid back pressure as a guide to operative management for carotid endarterectomy. Surgery 72:953-960, 1972.
5. Hobson RW, Wright CB, Sublett JW, et al. Carotid artery back pressure and endarterectomy under regional anesthesia. Arch Surg 109:682-687, 1974.
6. Moore WS, Yee JM, Hall AD. Collateral blood pressure: An index of tolerance to temporary occlusion. Arch Surg 106:520-523, 1973.
7. Baker JD, Gluecklich B, Watson CW, Marcus E, Kamat V, Callow AD. An evaluation of electroencephalographic monitoring for carotid study. Surgery 78:787-794, 1975.
8. Baker WH, Littooy FN, Hayes AC, Dorner DB, Stubbs D. Carotid endarterectomy without a shunt: The control series. J Vasc Surg 1:50-56, 1984.
9. Towne JB, Weiss DG, Hobson RE II. First phase report of cooperative Veterans Administration asymptomatic carotid stenosis study-operative morbidity and mortality. J Vasc Surg 11:252-259, 1990.
10. Hertzer NR, Beven EG, O'Hara PJ, Krajewski LP. A prospective study of vein patch angioplasty during carotid endarterectomy. Ann Surg 206:628-635, 1987.
11. Eikelboom BC, Ackerstaff RGA, Hoeneveld H, Ludwig JW, Teeuwen C, Vermeulen FEE, Welten RJT. Benefits of carotid patching: A randomized study. J Vasc Surg 7:240-247, 1988.
12. Clagett GP, Patterson CB, Fisher DF Jr, Fry RE, Eidt JF, Humble TH, Fry WJ. Vein patch versus primary closure for carotid endarterectomy. J Vasc Surg 9:213-223, 1989.
13. Kinney EV, Seabrook GR, Kinney LY, Bandyk DF, Towne JB. The importance of intraoperative detection of residual flow abnormalities after carotid endarterectomy. J Vasc Surg 17:912-922, 1993.

51

Adjunctive Techniques for the Management of Difficult Carotid Artery Endarterectomies

PATRICK J. LAMPARELLO, M.D., and THOMAS S. RILES, M.D.

Stroke continues to be the third leading cause of death in the United States in addition to being responsible for major disability among survivors.[1] The mortality rate from stroke has decreased, and this has led to an increased prevalence of disability, which adds immeasurably to the cost of health care. There are currently two million surviving stroke victims in the United States. In nearly half of these survivors the strokes occurred in the distribution of the carotid artery and may have been related to carotid artery bifurcation disease.[2] Most of the infarctions are associated with atherosclerotic plaque in the bifurcation of the common carotid artery. The timely identification of patients with carotid bifurcation disease who are at risk for stroke provides the opportunity to perform carotid endarterectomy as a means of stroke prevention.[3] Carotid artery endarterectomy has been offered as a means of stroke prevention for the past 40 years. It has been used with increasing frequency and is currently being performed at a rate of approximately 100,000 operations annually.[4]

Rapid advancements have been made in surgery for carotid artery stenosis, following the pioneering efforts of the first generation of vascular surgeons. The risks of surgery in patients with occlusions and major deficits have been recognized.[5] Initially intraoperative shunting was advocated to protect the brain during the period of carotid artery occlusion.[6] Some surgeons prefer to use local anesthesia with monitoring of the patient's neurologic function,[7] whereas others use general anesthesia with monitoring and protection of cerebral function. Various methods of endarterectomy and closure of the arteriotomy have been evaluated including primary closure, closure with a Dacron patch, and closure with a saphenous vein patch graft.

Although controversy continues regarding methods of closure and cerebral monitoring and protection, the results of surgery are continually improving. Most large centers specializing in extracranial carotid artery surgery report perioperative stroke and morbidity rates in the range of 1% to 2%.[8] Although the approach and technical aspects of carotid artery endarterectomy are taught and discussed as a set technique, the simple fact is that no one technique is suitable for every carotid operation. Variations in the anatomy, the pathologic findings, the medical condition of the patient, and the physiology of blood flow to the brain dictate that the surgeon possess a variety of skills to address the unusual and the unexpected. In terms of the patient's well-being, the surgeon's ability to use a variation of an otherwise standard approach can mean the difference between a perioperative stroke and a successful outcome. Broadening of the surgeon's skills can mean the difference between a 5% and a 2% complication rate. Learning adjunctive techniques for the management of difficult carotid artery endarterectomies allows the surgeon to deal with these occasional unexpected problems.

ANESTHESIA AND MONITORING

For years surgeons have argued about the benefit of general as opposed to local anesthesia with various monitoring techniques for cerebral protection. Although an exhaustive list of treatment options is outside the scope of this chapter, some observations are necessary.

Currently carotid artery endarterectomies are performed under either general or regional cervical block anesthesia. We favor cervical block anesthesia because it allows us to monitor and evaluate the patient while the carotid artery is clamped. We place a shunt if the patient exhibits signs of cerebral ischemia, which usually manifests as changes in mental status or paralysis of the contralateral limb. In some situations, for example, in the patient who has had a cerebral infarction, we consider shunting mandatory.

Surgeons who perform carotid artery endarterectomies with the use of general anesthesia either place shunts selectively or routinely. Surgeons who use selective shunting usually base their decision on criteria from various assessment methods, which include intraoperative electroencephalographic (EEG) monitoring.[9] Recently this technique has been performed by means of spectral array electrodes that are housed in a cap worn by the patient. The device obviates the need for an EEG technician. Another method of assessment is obtaining carotid artery stump pressure[10]; however, we have found that carotid artery stump pressure is a static and sometimes unreliable measurement. Nevertheless, surgeons who have achieved acceptable morbidity and mortality rates favor this method. There is also a group of surgeons who decide whether to place a shunt only after reviewing the patient's clinical status and angiographic findings.[11] As mentioned previously, most surgeons currently favor use of a shunt in the patient who has had a cerebral infarction. Also, there is ample evidence to support the use of a mandatory shunt in the patient with contralateral carotid artery occlusion.[11] Last, some surgeons place a shunt in every patient routinely. The only drawback to this approach is that occasionally the shunt is difficult to place because of the small size of the internal carotid artery or the high degree of carotid artery plaque. Sometimes the shunt is cumbersome and it can become a hindrance during the carotid artery endarterectomy, making it difficult for the surgeon to perform an optimal endarterectomy procedure.[12]

Regional cervical block anesthesia is appropriate for some patients with severe coronary artery disease. Our data indicate that the risks of cardiac complications and myocardial infarction are lessened with cervical block anesthesia.[13] Patients who are extremely anxious or unable to lie flat and cannot tolerate being conscious during carotid artery endarterectomy are considered candidates for general anesthesia.

WHAT MAKES A CAROTID ARTERY ENDARTERECTOMY DIFFICULT?

The following factors have been implicated that can make carotid artery endarterectomy difficult to perform: unusual anatomy of the carotid artery, carotid artery disease, previous surgery, previous radiation to the neck area, problems associated with shunting, and associated medical conditions.

Unusual Carotid Artery Anatomy

Perhaps the two most difficult anatomic problems faced by the vascular surgeon are high carotid bifurcation and redundant carotid artery. In high carotid bifurcation, mobilization of the hypoglossal nerve, division of the digastric tendon, and in some cases removal of the styloid process provide access to the upper reaches of the internal carotid artery. If the styloid process must be removed, the surgeon must be aware of the location of the glossopharyngeal cranial nerve.[14] Injury to this nerve results in severe complications that can be lethal because of the patient's inability to swallow and subsequent problems with pulmonary secretions and resultant aspiration pneumonia. A preoperative angiogram allows the surgeon to plan for a high carotid artery bifurcation. Magnetic resonance angiography (MRA), however, does not show the landmarks commonly used in the preoperative location and evaluation of carotid artery bifurcation. Therefore the vascular surgeon must always be prepared to deal with a high carotid bifurcation at the time of surgery.

Redundancy or excessive tortuosity of the carotid artery can be managed by a variety of techniques. These include reimplantation of the internal carotid artery into a lower segment of the common carotid artery and resection of the redundant segment of the carotid artery.[15] At New York University we prefer to perform a plication of the internal carotid artery. This procedure has been described previously and consists of shortening the posterior wall of the internal carotid artery after the endarterectomy is performed, thereby making it the appropriate length.[16] The plication procedure is performed by placing sutures in the long axis of the vessel and spacing the passage of the needle through the arterial wall as much as a few centimeters, depending on the amount of shortening required. The sutures are tied to the outside of the vessel and a routine carotid patch procedure is performed. It should be noted, however, that plication cannot be performed without carotid patching. Doing so can cause thrombosis of the carotid artery. In our failure to correct the tortuous or redundant carotid artery is a significant cause of postoperative internal carotid artery thrombosis. In our experience this procedure is necessary in approximately 25% of patients.

Another anatomic difficulty is a small internal carotid artery. This problem often becomes apparent on preoperative angiography if it is performed. However, if the preoperative evaluation consists of only duplex scanning and MRA, the condition may not be detected until the carotid endarterectomy is performed. If cervical block anesthesia is used, there is ample opportunity to evaluate the small internal carotid artery and devise an alternate treatment plan. If mandatory shunting or general anesthesia is employed, however, routine placement of the carotid shunt in a timely fashion may not be possible.

The internal carotid artery may be small for a number of reasons. For example, high-grade carotid artery plaque may prevent build up of pressure sufficient to maintain the artery at its normal caliber. When this is the case gentle dilatation using coronary dilators will restore the lumen to its normal size. Dilatation requires extreme caution, however, because use of a dilator that is too large or performing the procedure in too vigorous a manner can lead to internal carotid artery dissection and possible surgical complications. If the internal carotid artery is scarred, the surgeon will have to resort to reconstruction using a patch technique.

Another problem is severe arthritis of the neck. Most vascular operations are performed in the elderly, and thus there is a significant prevalence of inflammation and arthritis of the neck in this group of patients. The patient with cervical arthritis may be unable to adequately extend the neck or turn the head during surgery. The surgeon's operative skills are thus taxed with regard to appropriate positioning of the patient for carotid artery surgery. One advantage of using local anesthesia is that the patient's neck is not hyperextended, thereby avoiding the potential for neurologic injury. If the patient is awake, the surgeon can perform the carotid artery endarterectomy by supporting the patient's head and appropriately turning the table.

Carotid Artery Disease

In carotid artery endarterectomy, plaque must be removed to its end point in the internal carotid artery. Indeed, the focal distribution of the atherosclerotic plaque is the foundation for its surgical removal by carotid artery endarterectomy. On occasion the carotid plaque extends higher into the internal carotid artery than usual, and a higher dissection of the internal carotid artery is required to reach the plaque end point. There is a distinct advantage to performing the surgery under cervical block anesthesia in this situation since shunt placement can be difficult in the carotid artery with high plaque. Knowing that the patient is neurologically intact during dissection and carotid clamping allows the surgeon more time to dissect the carotid artery distal to the plaque and reach an appropriate end point.

The following steps are useful in exposing the upper internal carotid artery.[17] The standard incision is extended posterior to the ear and appropriate retractors are placed. The digastric muscle is then divided. The entire hypoglossal nerve is mobilized and retracted medially. This includes the two small vessels to the sternocleidomastoid muscle, which must be ligated and divided. If further exposure of the internal carotid artery is needed, the styloid process and attached muscle are palpated and removed with a rongeur. During removal of the styloid process, the glossopharyngeal nerve must be identified and protected.[14] By following these techniques we have been able to accomplish dissection of the high internal carotid artery and perform the appropriate carotid artery endarterectomy. In our practice we have not found it necessary to dislocate the jaw, but the surgeon should be prepared to do this should it become necessary.

Another problem associated with carotid disease is extensive atherosclerosis of the common carotid artery. Proximal carotid artery disease can be identified on either preoperative angiogram or duplex scan. If severe stenosis is present at the origin of the common carotid arteries, either an extra-anatomic procedure in the neck, such as a subclavian to carotid artery bypass,[18] or an inline bypass from the aorta must be performed.[19] These are obviously planned for before the carotid artery endarterectomy is performed. If the plaque extends proximally in the common carotid artery, the artery can be dissected free by continuing in the normal plane of dissection to the level of the sternal notch. Usually the plaque in the common carotid artery does not extend proximal to the omohyoid muscle. By dividing this muscle and using appropriate retraction, proximal control is obtained.

Previous Surgery or Radiation

With the increasing frequency of carotid artery endarterectomy and a recurrence rate of approximately 1% to 2%, many vascular surgeons are finding it necessary to perform "redo" carotid surgery.[20] A review of the first operation with attention to any unusual details, such as an extremely high or redundant carotid artery, can make the second or redo operation easier. We have developed the following techniques for dealing with redo carotid artery surgery. We perform cerebral angiography in these patients. The information that is gained from the angiogram, including nuances of anatomy that may not be apparent on MRA, are helpful to the surgeon at the time of redo carotid surgery.[21]

Redo carotid surgery involves proximal dissection to control the common carotid artery. A plane is developed between the jugular vein and the carotid artery. This also allows development of a plane between the vagus nerve and the carotid artery and jugular vein, thereby preventing injury while permitting identification of the vagus nerve. Dissection is continued until the internal carotid artery is located. Further dissection in this area, particularly if the hypoglossal nerve has already been mobilized and retracted medially, allows the surgeon to gain control of the internal carotid artery distal to the area of surgery. Early clamping of the internal carotid artery is performed to prevent embolization and possible neurologic deficits. A frequent cause of endarterectomy failure is recurrent atherosclerosis. Studies indicate that an interposition graft should be considered for the second operation.[20] The patient who requires a redo endarterectomy may eventually need a third carotid operation. Various techniques are used to maintain flow to the external carotid artery, or the artery can be ligated.

Radiation to the neck and previous radical neck surgery are significant problems in carotid artery surgery. Often the initial dissection proceeds more readily than usual because much of the neck contents have already been removed. The usual procedure is to develop flaps over the carotid artery and then perform a standard carotid endarterectomy with appropriate vascular control. After the reconstruction, a dermal graft is used to provide tissue coverage between the skin incision and the vascular reconstruction. If side effects resulting from radiation to the neck are severe and scar tissue is significant, coverage of the carotid reconstruction is performed with a myocutaneous rotational flap based on the pectoralis major muscle. If severe panarteritis is noted, consideration is given at the time of carotid reconstruction to the use of an in-line vein graft to replace the carotid artery bifurcation.[22]

Tracheostomy also presents technical problems. In the acute situation, performance of a tracheostomy in proximity to a carotid artery reconstruction is contraindicated because of the risk of infection with dehiscence of the vascular reconstruction. Every attempt must be made to prevent this. Patients who have a chronic tracheostomy with adherence of the tissues have a slightly increased risk of infection with carotid artery endarterectomy. If the usual precautions are taken, carotid artery surgery can be satisfactorily performed.

Problems Encountered During Shunting

As mentioned previously, a high carotid bifurcation or an unusually long plaque in the internal carotid artery can lead to problems during shunting. Cervical block anesthesia is advantageous because with the patient awake the surgeon can perform a more distal dissection after the arteriotomy without the need for quick placement of a shunt. If general anesthesia is used, a preoperative carotid angiogram is necessary to determine how high the plaque actually extends before a shunt is placed. Many types of shunts are available; the vascular surgeon should be familiar with all of them because some are more amenable to particular anatomic situations. At New York University our standard practice is to use the outlying Javid shunt. If the diameter of the distal internal carotid artery is too small to allow placement of the shunt, then one of the inlying silicone rubber shunts is used because they are available in various sizes. On occasion, extremely high control of the internal carotid artery is impossible so intraluminal control must be achieved instead. This is performed by means of a Fogarty balloon catheter in the awake patient, knowing that the patient is tolerating distal internal carotid artery occlusion. Sometimes a Pruitt-Inahara shunt is used in this situation. There are problems with the flow rates through this shunt, and one patient suffered a stroke because flow through the Pruitt-Inahara shunt was inadequate.[23]

Associated Medical Conditions

The patient requiring carotid artery endarterectomy often has associated medical conditions such as coronary artery atherosclerosis. Preoperatively every potential carotid endarterectomy patient receives a cardiologic consultation. If the patient has a history of previous myocardial disease or has symptomatic coronary artery disease, additional tests including coronary angiography may be performed. Routine stress testing is not performed if the patient has no cardiac symptoms. Our postoperative cardiac morbidity rate indicates that this approach is quite acceptable. It should be noted that performing carotid artery endarterectomy under cervical block anesthesia, with the likelihood of decreased cardiac stress, may be partly responsible for this low morbidity.[13]

CONCLUSION

Carotid disease can take many forms of presentation which vary depending on the particular characteristics of the patient. The more skills and techniques that the vascular surgeon has available to address these problems, the better the outcome will be for these patients.

REFERENCES

1. McDowell FH, Caplin LR, eds. Cerebral Vascular Survey Report 1985. For the National Institute of Neurological Communicative Disorders and Stroke. Bethesda, Md.: National Institutes of Health, Public Health Service, 1985.
2. Mohr JPK, Caplin LR, Melski JW, et al. The Harvard Cooperative Stroke Registry: A prospective registry. Neurology 28:754-762, 1978.
3. NASCET Collaborators. Beneficial effect of carotid endarterectomy in symptomatic patients with high grade carotid stenosis. N Engl J Med 325:445-453, 1991.
4. Ernst CB, Rutkow IM, Cleveland RJ, et al. Vascular surgery in the United States. J Vasc Surg 6:611-621, 1987.
5. Crawford ES. Hemodynamic alterations in patients with cerebral arterial insufficiency before and after operation. Surgery 48:76-81, 1960.
6. Thompson JE, Austin DJ. Surgical treatment of arteriosclerotic occlusions of the carotid artery in the neck. Surgery 51:74-77, 1962.
7. Murphy F, McCubbin DA. Carotid endarterectomy: A long-term follow-up study. J Neurosurg 23:156-159, 1965.
8. Riles TS. The roles and risks of carotid endarterectomy. In Stroke Symposium Proceedings. New York: Excerpta Medica, 1990, pp 30-42.
9. Whittemore AD, Kaufman JL, Kohler TR, et al. Routine electroencephalographic monitoring during carotid endarterectomy. Ann Surg 197:707-711, 1983.
10. Archie JP Jr. Technique and clinical results of carotid stump pressure to determine selective shunting during carotid endarterectomy. J Vasc Surg 13:319-324, 1991.
11. Cherry KJ, Roland CF, Hallett JW, et al. Stump pressure, the contralateral carotid artery, and electroencephalographic changes. Am J Surg 162:185-190, 1991.
12. Sundt TM Jr, Eversold MJ, Sharbrough FW, et al. The risk benefit ratio of intraoperative shunting during carotid endarterectomy: Relevancy to operative and postoperative results and complications. Ann Surg 203:196-201, 1986.
13. Pasternack PF, Grossi EA, Baumann GF, et al. Silent myocardial ischemia during peripheral vascular surgery. J Cardiovasc Surg 30(Suppl):19-24, 1989.
14. Rosenbloom MR, Friedman SG, Lamparello PJ, et al. Glossopharangeal nerve injury complicating carotid endarterectomy. J Vasc Surg 5:464-471, 1987.
15. Sundt TM Jr. Occlusive Cerebrovascular Disease: Diagnosis and Surgical Management. Philadelphia: WB Saunders, 1987.
16. Imparato AM. Surgery for extracranial cerebrovascular insufficiency. In Ransahoff J, ed. Modern Techniques in Neurosurgery 14. Armonk, N.Y.: Futura Publishing, 1980.
17. Mock CN, Lilly MP, McRae RG, Carney WI Jr. Selection of the approach to the distal internal carotid artery from the second cervical vertebrae to the base of the skull. J Vasc Surg 13:846-853, 1991.
18. Perler BA, Williams GM. Carotid-subclavian bypass: A decade of experience. J Vasc Surg 12:716-722, 1990.
19. Reul GJ, Jacobs MJHM, Gregoric ID, et al. Innominate artery occlusive disease: Surgical approach and long-term results. J Vasc Surg 14:405-412, 1991.
20. Gagne PJ, Riles TS, Jacobowitz GR, et al. Long-term follow-up of patients undergoing reoperation for recurrent carotid artery disease. J Vasc Surg 18:991-998, 1993.
21. Riles TS, Eidelman EM, Litt AW, et al. Comparison of magnetic resonance angiography, conventional angiography and Duplex scanning. Stroke 23:341-346, 1992.
22. Hurley JJ, Nordestgaard AG, Woods JJ Jr, et al. Carotid endarterectomy with vein patch angioplasty for radiation induced symptomatic carotid atherosclerosis [abst]. J Vasc Surg 14:419A, 1991.
23. Grossi EA, Giangola G, Parish MA, et al. Differences of flow rates in carotid shunts: Consequences in cerebral perfusion. Ann Vasc Surg 7:39-43, 1993.

52

Nd:YAG Laser Ablation of Carotid Endarterectomy Flaps

MILTON SLOCUM, M.D., PAUL W. HUMPHREY, M.D., and DONALD SILVER, M.D.

A vascular surgeon will eventually encounter a carotid plaque that does not break off cleanly during an endarterectomy. The surgeon may elect to extend the opening of the internal carotid artery and attempt to find a point at which the flap breaks off cleanly or may elect to secure the flap with continuous or interrupted fine sutures. Occasionally the plaque will not break off cleanly at the higher level and the flap must be secured at that frequently difficult-to-reach point with sutures. The occasional difficulty in securing such a flap with sutures, particularly at the distal level, and the rough edges left by the suture-secured flap prompted a search for a better method to secure the distal carotid endarterectomy flap.

McGuff et al.[1] were among the first to evaluate the effect of laser energy on arteriosclerotic plaques in the abdominal aorta and coronary arteries. Since 1963 lasers have been used for arteriovenous anastomoses,[2-5] arterial repair,[6-8] endarterectomy,[9-11] and transluminal angioplasty and laser balloon-assisted angioplasty.[12-15] Despite the promise of the laser, the results from these studies have been relatively unsatisfactory, leading Becker to note in *Vascular Surgery* in 1994 that "lasers came and went between the last edition of this textbook and the current one."[16] Becker also noted, "It will not be surprising if further development of new laser technologies does eventually lead to a clinically useful device." We were encouraged by the report of Eugene et al.[17] of 10 carotid endarterectomies using the argon open beam laser. They noted that the laser beam was used to transect the plaque and that the distal end point was welded in place. They also noted that there were no perforations and that there was no residual thermal injury and good cerebral blood flow.

We first attempted to weld canine carotid endarterectomy flaps with an open beam CO_2 laser but were unsuccessful. We were unable to control the thermal injury and encountered excessive scarring and vascular perforations. With the acquisition of an Nd:YAG laser (Surgical Laser Technologies, Inc., Oaks, Pa.), we had an instrument that permitted precise application through its frosted sapphire tip and permitted control of the amounts of energy delivered. Consequently, we initiated a series of animal studies to evaluate the Nd:YAG laser for securing distal endarterectomy flaps.

CANINE STUDIES

The Nd:YAG laser used in our canine and subsequent clinical studies had a wavelength of 1964 nm. The TCRH-7 fiber with a handpiece and the GRP-6 frosted sapphire tip were used to control the transmission of laser energy.

Both carotid arteries and both femoral arteries in 12 dogs were isolated, and a longitudinal arteriotomy was made in each vessel. A transverse posterior incision was then made in the open artery and a 3 mm distally based flap of intima and media was created. In the left-sided vessels, two to three 7-0 polypropylene sutures were used to repair the "endarterectomy flap." In the right-sided vessels, the Nd:YAG laser, with a 5 W continuous power setting, was used to "weld" the flaps. The time required for flap repair in both procedures was measured. All arteriotomies were irrigated with heparinized saline solution and closed with running 6-0 polypropylene sutures.

At the chosen interval after operation (7 days or 28 days), each artery was subjected to duplex scanning to evaluate patency and search for the presence of stenosis, aneurysm, intimal flap, or turbulent flow. The arteries were then ligated, excised, and prepared for histologic study.

A third group of arteries was used to evaluate the immediate effects of laser welding. Eight arteries in two dogs were subjected to laser welding of the prepared "endarterectomy" flaps.

Two minutes after blood flow was reestablished, the arteries were excised and subjected to histologic evaluation.

The results of these canine studies revealed that Nd:YAG laser repair required much less time than suture repair of intimal flaps (25 seconds vs. 135 seconds, respectively; p <.04). The mean (±SEM) energy used to perform welding of the flaps was 125 ± 19 joules.

Duplex scanning immediately before excision of the arteries revealed no difference between the two types of repairs in either the common carotid or common femoral arteries. All arteries were patent without stenoses, intimal flaps, or turbulence.

Histologic study of the eight laser-repaired flaps, excised 2 minutes after restoration of flow, revealed no microvascular flaps. There was no evidence of carbonaceous deposition in the area of flap repair. There was evidence of intimal thermal injury, but no evidence of thermal injury in the media or adventitia. Histologic evaluation of the arteries removed 7 days after endarterectomy and repair revealed two microvascular flaps in the suture-repaired arteries and one in the laser-repaired arteries. The amounts of scarring, medial proliferation, the type and amount of inflammation, subintimal hemorrhage, and pigment (hemosiderin) deposition were minimal or similar for the two types of repair.

Histologic evaluation of the arteries 28 days after endarterectomy repair revealed one microvascular flap in the suture-repaired vessel and no flaps in the laser-repaired vessels. The amounts of subintimal fibroplastic proliferation, scarring, inflammation, subintimal hemorrhage, and pigment deposition were similar for the laser- and suture-repaired flaps.

HUMAN STUDIES

Since completion of the animal studies, we have encountered 16 patients whose 18 endarterectomies resulted in loose, rough, irregular distal endarterectomy end points. It was felt that suture control of the endarterectomy flaps would be difficult or would leave a more thickened end point than was desired. The contact Nd:YAG laser was used to ablate these flaps. The laser was set at a 5 W continuous power, and the sapphire tip was used to deliver the power. Completion arteriograms were performed on all patients.

Welding of the 18 residual endarterectomy flaps in the 16 patients took 3 to 6 seconds (15 to 30 joules). The completion intraoperative arteriogram showed normal results in each of the 18 arteries welded with the Nd:YAG laser. Thirteen of these 18 were closed with a polytetrafluoroethylene patch. There were no perioperative cerebral ischemic events. Clinical follow-up ranges to 24 months (mean, 7.3 months). Thirteen patients have had follow-up duplex examinations (1 to 24 months; mean, 7.3 months). The scans have not demonstrated evidence of stenosis or abnormality in the area of repair. Two patients died 4 months and 8 months after carotid endarterectomy from unrelated disease (myocardial infarction and metastatic lung cancer).

DISCUSSION

Electron microscopy of laser arterial welds revealed that the collagen fibrils lose their periodicity, increase in caliber, and split into fine fibrillary substructures. These fibrils, although they remain individually recognizable, are not separated as in controls but are closely interdigitated with one another. This interdigitation of collagen fibrils appears to be the basis of the laser weld.[18] Application of lasers to arteries has not been shown to accelerate atherosclerotic progression at the laser site.[19]

At present the laser is most commonly employed in vascular reconstructions through laser-assisted balloon angioplasty. The limitations of the laser in recanalizing obstructed vessels were well described by Ahn.[20]

The Nd:YAG laser used in this study emits light in the near-infrared region of the electromagnetic spectrum at 1064 nm. In the contact Nd:YAG laser system, laser energy is transmitted through a fiberoptic cable to a sapphire tip that is heated by this energy. The heated tip, 0.6 mm in diameter, allows precise vaporization of contacted tissue. Potential advantages of this type of delivery system include a focused, even distribution of laser energy and the absence of beam dispersion.[21] The contact laser produces local thermal damage that is limited by the small tip and the energy applied through the tip. Thermal damage can be limited by applying low energy for short periods to the tissue being "treated." In our study, with laser power set at 5 W, the tip was "stroked" across the endarterectomy flap for up to 6 seconds, with a maximum of 30 joules of laser energy used per repair. The laser-repaired arteries in this study and in studies reported by others healed with minimal inflammatory responses.[19]

It has been reported that contact laser endarterectomies have a higher injury rate (perforation, deeper level of injury) and less secure end points than do free-beam laser endarterectomies.[11] Our study revealed that the transition from media to intima was smooth, and there were no perforations. Another disadvantage of the contact delivery system that has been reported by some investigators is the heated contact tip sticking to the treated tissues, thus causing increased injury and rough end points.[11] We have not found this to be a problem.

The duplex scanning, gross anatomic, and histologic healing characteristics were essentially the same for the canine laser-repaired and suture-repaired intimal flaps at both 7 and 28 days. The laser-repaired endarterectomy flaps, which were studied 2 minutes after flow was restored, revealed no thermal damage in the media or in the adventitia. The group of arteries studied 7 days postoperatively revealed one less microscopic intimal flap and less subintimal fibroblastic intimal proliferation in the laser-repaired group. The only histologic differences in the group of arteries studied 28 days postoperatively was the persistence of one flap in a suture-repaired artery; none was present in the laser-repaired arteries. The healing characteristics, as determined by duplex scanning and gross and histologic studies, were similar, if not slightly better, in the laser-repaired canine arteries at 7 and 28 days when compared with the suture-repaired arteries.

Shortly after the completion of the animal studies, we operated on a patient whose distal carotid endarterectomy proceeded quite high and left an irregular flap that would have been very difficult to secure with sutures. The laser was used to smooth and seal the flap, converting a difficult situation to a safe one. The laser has subsequently been used on 16 additional patients. These 16 patients had 18 carotid endarterectomy end points that were ragged or that demonstrated persistent flaps. Three of the 18 arteries also had very distal end points that, because of the limited anatomic exposure, would have been difficult to secure with sutures. The laser in all cases successfully tapered the edges and sealed the endarterectomy flap to the vessel wall. Inspection and completion angiograms revealed a smooth transition from the endarterectomy site to the undisturbed distal vessel. None of the patients has experienced transient ischemic attacks, a stroke, recurrent stenosis, or occlusion.

Laser repair of endarterectomy flaps seems to be superior to suture repair for several reasons. Laser ablation of the endarterectomy flaps in very high carotid locations is technically much easier than suture repair. Laser energy rapidly seals the intima to the media, producing flaps that are secure histologically and have less subintimal fibroblastic intimal proliferation than suture repair. The transition from the endarterectomy surface to the native intima is smoother and therefore hemodynamically superior. For these reasons, we believe that the use of the laser for securing the cephalad end point after carotid endarterectomy is an important, safe, and effective addition to the armamentarium of the vascular surgeon. Laser welding is becoming our preferred method for securing the distal carotid endarterectomy flap, and we anticipate that this modality will be similarly effective in other arteries.

REFERENCES

1. McGuff PE, Bushnell D, Soroff H, Deterling R. Studies of the surgical applications of laser (light amplification by stimulated emission of radiation). Surg Forum 14:143-145, 1963.
2. Shapiro S, Sartorius C, Sanders S, Clark S. Microvascular end-to-side arterial anastomosis using the Nd:YAG laser. Neurosurgery 25:584-589, 1989.
3. McCarthy WJ, Hartz R, Yao J, Sottiurai V, Kwaan H, Michaelis L. Vascular anastomoses with laser energy. J Vasc Surg 3:32-41, 1986.
4. Gennaro M, Ascer E, Mohan C, Wang S. A comparison of CO_2 laser–assisted venous anastomoses and conventional suture techniques: Patency, aneurysm formation, and histologic differences. J Vasc Surg 14:605-613, 1991.
5. Frazier O, Shehab SA, Radovancevic B, McAllister H, Parnis S. Laser-assisted anastomosis of large-diameter vessels with the carbon dioxide laser. J Thorac Cardiovasc Surg 96:454-456, 1988.
6. White R, Kopchok G, Donayre C, Abergel RP, et al. Comparison of laser-welded and sutured arteriotomies. Arch Surg 121:1133-1135, 1986.
7. White R, Abergel RP, Lyons R, et al. Biological effects of laser welding on vascular healing. Lasers Surg Med 6:137-141, 1986.
8. Zelt DT, LaMuraglia GM, L'Italien GJ, et al. Arterial laser welding with a 1.9 micrometer Raman-shifted laser. J Vasc Surg 15:1025-1031, 1992.
9. Eugene J, McColgan S, Pollock ME, Hammer-Wilson M, Moore-Jeffries EW, Berns M. Experimental arteriosclerosis treated by conventional and laser endarterectomy. J Surg Res 39:31-38, 1985.

10. Eugene J, Ott RA, Baribeau Y, McColgan S, Berns MW, Mason GR. Initial trial of argon ion laser endarterectomy for peripheral vascular disease. Arch Surg 125:1007-1011, 1990.
11. Baribeau Y, Eugene J, Firestein SL, Hammer-Wilson M, Berns MW. Comparison of contact and free beam laser endarterectomy. J Surg Res 48:127-133, 1990.
12. Turnbull IW, Bannister CM. Can laser angioplasty replace carotid endarterectomy in the management of nonstenotic atheromatous disease of the carotid bifurcation? Surg Neurol 38:73-76, 1992.
13. Fleisher H, Thompson B, McCowan T, Ferris E, Reifsteck J, Barnes R. Human percutaneous laser angioplasty. Patient selection criteria and early results. Am J Surg 154:666-670, 1987.
14. Lorenzi G, Domanin M, Constantini A. PTA and laser-assisted PTA combined with simultaneous surgical revascularization. J Cardiovasc Surg 32:456-462, 1991.
15. Geschwind H, Blair J, Mongkolsmai D, et al. Development and experimental application of contact probe catheter for laser angioplasty. J Am Coll Cardiol 9:101-107, 1987.
16. Becker GJ. Limitations of peripheral angioplasty and the role of new devices. In Rutherford RB, ed. Vascular Surgery, 4th ed. Philadelphia: WB Saunders, 1994, pp 369-394.
17. Eugene J, Ott RA, Nudelman KL, et al. Initial clinical evaluation of carotid artery laser endarterectomy. J Vasc Surg 12:499-503, 1990.
18. Schober R, Ulrich F, Sander T, Durselen H, Hessel S. Laser-induced alteration of collagen substructure allows microsurgical tissue welding. Science 232:1421-1422, 1986.
19. Abela GS, Crea F, Seeger JM, et al. The healing process in normal canine arteries and in atherosclerotic monkey arteries after transluminal laser irradiation. Am J Cardiol 56:983-988, 1985.
20. Ahn S. Endovascular surgery. In Moore W, ed. Vascular Surgery: A Comprehensive Review, 4th ed. Philadelphia: WB Saunders, 1993, pp 275-299.
21. Faught WE, Lawrence PF. Vascular applications of lasers. Surg Clin North Am 72:681-704, 1992.

53

Indications and Optimal Techniques for Carotid Shortening During Carotid Endarterectomy

KELLIE A. COYLE, M.D., J.D., and ROBERT B. SMITH III, M.D.

Carotid kinks and coils are found in as many as 16% to 34% of the adult population.[1] Anatomic variants may range from gentle sigmoid curves to abrupt angulations and significant redundancies. Examples are shown in Figs. 1 and 2.

The cause of carotid kinks and angulations has not been fully delineated. However, it has been suggested that coils are frequently congenital, secondary to a failure of straightening of the initially coiled artery with descent of the fetal heart, whereas kinks and redundancies may be acquired and are more often found in association with atherosclerotic carotid disease.[2-4] More acute angulations may create distorted flow patterns, thereby accelerating development of atherosclerotic disease in the proximal vessel. Conversely, it has been suggested that atherosclerotic disease itself causes weakening and thinning of the arterial wall, which may predispose the vessel to kinking. Additionally, athero-

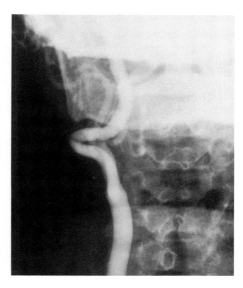

Fig. 1 Arteriogram demonstrating kink of the right internal carotid artery.

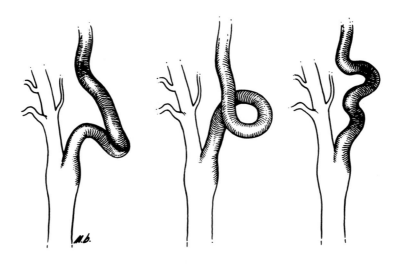

Fig. 2 Internal carotid kink, loop, and sigmoid-shaped redundancy.

sclerotic plaque may act as a stent for the artery, with redundancies becoming more apparent once the plaque is removed.

INDICATIONS FOR SHORTENING

Although the natural history of these variants is not well known, it has been suggested that abnormal kinking may cause cerebrovascular symptoms or accelerate atherosclerosis because of resulting abnormal flow patterns.[5,6] Acute angulations may compromise the vessel lumen, thereby impeding or preventing flow. For these reasons, attention has been directed toward the repair of such abnormalities encountered during carotid endarterectomy for atherosclerotic disease. Because the benefit of any shortening procedure is considered by some to be theoretical, it is important that the shortening procedure not impose added morbidity over that of the carotid endarterectomy.

It is difficult to attribute symptoms to abnormal kinking of the carotid artery, particularly when this condition coexists with significant atherosclerotic disease. Some observers have related positional changes involving kinks and redundancies to the occurrence of symptoms when an acute angulation may be accentuated by extending or rotating the neck.[5,7-10] Intuitively, severe angulations that compromise the vessel lumen could produce cerebrovascular symptoms, especially in the early postoperative period when patients seem at greatest risk for thrombosis of the endarterectomy site or cerebral emboli.

Certainly, where carotid redundancy is responsible for symptomatology, repair is appropriate. In cases where carotid kinking coexists with or is unmasked by carotid disease and carotid endarterectomy, it seems reasonable to straighten the vessel at the time of carotid endarterectomy. Certainly, when severe angulation appears to compromise the vessel lumen, repair is appropriate. Justification is stronger where it can be demonstrated that carotid shortening poses no additional perioperative or postoperative risk.

SHORTENING TECHNIQUES

The first successful operation to correct cerebrovascular symptoms caused by internal carotid artery kinking was an arteriopexy to the sternocleidomastoid muscle performed by Riser et al.[11] in 1951. This straightening procedure actually preceded the first carotid endarterectomy by 3 years. Hsu and Kisten[12] reported resection of a portion of the internal carotid artery in 1956. This method, with simple reanastomosis of the transected ends, continues to be a popular method of carotid shortening. Collins et al.[13] reported a variant of this technique in association with carotid endarterectomy in which, following resection of a portion of the internal carotid artery, the back wall was repaired with an end-to-end transverse anastomosis and the anterior longitudinal arteriotomy was closed with a saphenous vein or Dacron patch. Smith et al.[14] described a similar technique in three cases; however, a segment of the endarterectomized internal carotid artery was used as the patch material. Hamann[15] and Chino,[16] in two separate series, described shortening of the redundant vessel by transecting the internal carotid artery and reimplanting it onto the carotid bulb. Resection of a portion of the common carotid artery has been reported as an alternative technique of carotid shortening.[5,7] Quattlebaum et al.[7] reported a series of 149 procedures for carotid shortening; 106 of these involved resection of the carotid bifurcation with end-to-end anastomosis of the common to the internal carotid artery. Simpler techniques of arteriopexy or tacking the vessel to the surrounding structures have been used, and a method of transverse eversion suture plication was described by Archie.[17] In his group of patients, transverse eversion plication shortening of endarterectomized internal carotid segments was performed before patch angioplasty to prevent kinking following the repair.

In our own series a variety of techniques have been used based on the caliber and mobility of the vessel as well as the location and extent of the angulation or kink. Techniques of shortening by means of internal or common carotid artery resection or by reimplantation of the internal carotid artery onto the carotid bulb are similar to those reported by others. In all cases carotid endarterectomy was performed first by way of a longitudinal arteriotomy with an indwelling shunt. In 25 cases we elected to use a technique wherein, after longitudinal arteriotomy and endarterectomy, the internal carotid artery is transected obliquely at its origin, and the mobilized internal carotid artery is then rotated 180 degrees, advanced, and sutured onto the arteriotomy as an in situ patch. This technique is demonstrated in Fig. 3.

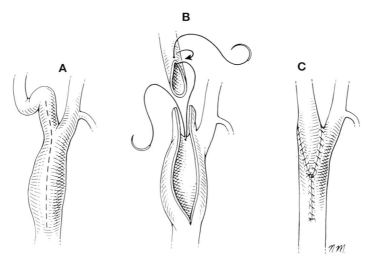

Fig. 3 Technique of internal carotid shortening. **A,** Endarterectomy is performed through a longitudinal arteriotomy. **B,** The internal carotid is transected obliquely at its origin, then rotated 180 degrees before reanastomosis. **C,** Completed anastomosis with previous back wall of the internal carotid advanced onto the arteriotomy as an in situ patch.

CURRENT STUDY

To evaluate the effect on perioperative morbidity and mortality of adding a shortening procedure to carotid endarterectomy, we retrospectively reviewed all carotid endarterectomies performed by the vascular and cardiovascular services at Emory University Hospital between January 1983 and December 1992.[18] During this 10-year period, a total of 1072 carotid endarterectomies were performed. Cases in which a shortening procedure was performed in conjunction with carotid endarterectomy were selected as the subject of this study.

All patients were evaluated preoperatively with four-vessel arch arteriography. Among the study group undergoing concomitant shortening procedures, the average degree of stenosis on the operated side was 80.2%. No patient was operated on solely to repair a carotid kink or coil. Sixteen patients (15%) had contralateral internal carotid artery occlusion. Twenty-eight procedures (26.2%) were performed with the patient under general anesthesia with electroencephalographic monitoring; 79 (73.8%) were performed with the patient under local anesthesia with monitoring by serial neurologic evaluation. Intraluminal shunts were used in 94% of cases. Ten individuals (9.3%) underwent adjunctive surgical procedures (coronary artery bypass in eight patients) either during the same anesthesia or the same hospitalization as carotid endarterectomy. The decision to perform concomitant carotid shortening was made by the operating surgeon at the time of the procedure, based on anticipated excessive redundancy or potential kinking if not corrected. This determination can often be anticipated based on the vascular anatomy of the preoperative arteriogram.

RESULTS

One hundred seven (10%) of the 1072 patients who underwent carotid endarterectomy during the 10-year study period underwent a concomitant shortening procedure. The age range among this group was 47 to 89 years, with an average age of 71 years. There were 53 female and 54 male patients (1:1).

Associated risk factors included hypertension in 79.4%, diabetes mellitus in 19.6%, coronary artery disease in 69.2%, and significant smoking history in 64.5%. Table 1 compares the comorbid characteristics of the study group with those of 965 patients undergoing carotid endarterectomy without carotid shortening during the same time period. Indications for carotid endarterectomy in the subgroup were transient ischemic attacks in 28.0%, previous ipsilateral stroke in 17.6%, amaurosis fugax in 7.5%, and high-grade

Table 1 Comorbid characteristics of patients undergoing endarterectomy

	With shortening (n = 107)	Without shortening (n = 965)
Hypertension	85 (79.4%)	599 (62.1%)
Diabetes mellitus	21 (19.6%)	204 (21.1%)
Coronary artery disease	74 (69.2%)	590 (61.1%)
Smoking history	69 (64.5%)	703 (72.8%)

Table 2 Indications for carotid endarterectomy

	With shortening (n = 107)	Without shortening (n = 965)
Asymptomatic stenosis	50 (46.7%)	440 (45.6%)
Transient ischemic attacks	30 (28.0%)	270 (28.0%)
Cerebrovascular accident	19 (17.6%)	144 (14.9%)
Amaurosis fugax	8 (7.5%)	106 (11.0%)
Vascular tinnitus	0 (0.0%)	5 (0.5%)

Table 3 Complications following carotid endarterectomy

	With shortening (n = 107)	Without shortening (n = 965)
Stroke	1 (0.9%)	25 (2.6%)
Death	2 (1.9%)	15 (1.6%)
Stroke and death	3 (2.7%)	40 (4.1%)
Transient ischemic attacks	2 (1.9%)	20 (2.1%)
Myocardial infarction	0 (0.0%)	9 (0.9%)
Hematoma	7 (6.5%)	35 (3.6%)

asymptomatic stenosis in 46.7%. Table 2 depicts the indications for carotid endarterectomy among the study and control groups.

Carotid shortening procedures were performed using one of the techniques previously described. In 48 patients a segment of the common carotid artery was resected with end-to-end anastomosis, restoring continuity at the level of the arteriotomy. Thirty patients underwent resection of a portion of the internal carotid artery with an end-to-end anastomosis at the distal extent of the arteriotomy. Four individuals had transection of the internal carotid artery with reimplantation onto the carotid bulb. In 25 cases the internal carotid artery was transected obliquely, rotated 180 degrees, and advanced onto the arteriotomy (see Fig. 3).

The combined 30-day mortality and stroke morbidity for patients undergoing carotid shortening procedures in conjunction with endarterectomy was 2.7%, with two deaths and one stroke. One death occurred in a 72-year-old woman as a result of a postoperative stroke. The other death occurred in a 73-year-old woman 4 days after carotid endarterectomy, during coronary artery bypass surgery. Table 3 compares postoperative complications for the study group with those of the control group.

Long-term follow-up data were available for 101 (96%) of 105 patients who survived endarterectomy, at a range of 1 to 10 years postoperatively and an average of 43 months. Seventy-four patients were still alive and 27 were deceased. Late deaths were attributed to cardiac disease in 14 patients, malignancy in three, and unknown causes in seven. Renal failure, a gunshot wound, and a contralateral stroke each accounted for one death. During the follow-up period, there were no ipsilateral strokes or recurrent symptoms referable to the operated side, although five contralateral strokes occurred. Carotid duplex scan data available on 46 patients at an average of 37 months postoperatively demonstrated a normal artery in 69.6% of patients, mild stenosis (<50%) in 6.5%, and moderate stenosis (50% to 79%) in 23.9%. No duplex scan was reported to show severe stenosis (>80%) or ipsilateral internal carotid occlusion. No patient has required ipsilateral carotid reoperation during the follow-up period.

DISCUSSION

The natural history of carotid redundancies and angulations is unclear; therefore the advantages of surgical correction are in part theoretical. Multiple techniques have been described to straighten the redundant carotid artery, with good anatomic results. Justification of the procedure, however, requires the avoidance of additional morbidity and mortality. If the shortening step results in improved long-term patency and avoidance of reoperation, its value to the patient is even more obvious.

In the current series the addition of carotid shortening procedures to carotid endarterectomy did not increase stroke morbidity or mortality. The combined 30-day stroke and death rate of 2.7% among those undergoing concomitant

Table 4 Complications following carotid endarterectomy with conjunctive shortening

Series	No. of patients	Stroke	Death	Stroke and death
Quattlebaum et al. (1973)[7]	153	—	7	—
Smith et al. (1986)[14]	3	0	0	0
Chino (1987)[16]	4	0	0	0
Poindexter et al. (1987)[5]	6	0	0	0
Collins et al. (1991)[13]	19	0	0	0
Archie (1993)[17]	16	—	—	—
Coyle et al. (1995)[18]	107	1	2	3

shortening procedures compared favorably with a rate of 4.1% among patients undergoing carotid endarterectomy without carotid shortening. Other series reporting the outcome of shortening procedures have described similar low complication rates. The stroke and death rates of several recent reports, including the present series, are summarized in Table 4.

During long-term follow-up, carotid shortening was not found to add to late morbidity. Indeed, our own extended follow-up demonstrated no ipsilateral symptoms or ipsilateral carotid occlusion or stenosis greater than 80%. Poindexter et al.[5] also noted no late complications in patients followed for 6 months to 4 years after carotid shortening procedures. At present there are few published data on long-term effects of concomitant carotid shortening. Recurrent stenosis is well known to affect a minority of patients undergoing carotid endarterectomy and in some cases is responsible for symptoms.[19,20] In the current series, long-term follow-up carotid duplex examinations demonstrated normal scans in 70% of patients, mild stenosis in 6%, and moderate stenosis in 24%. In no case did recurrent stenosis become symptomatic or require ipsilateral reoperation. This is similar to other series reporting frequency of recurrent stenosis following endarterectomy alone.[19,21] Although prospective randomized studies comparing carotid endarterectomy with and without carotid shortening procedures have not been done, such comparisons between standard longitudinal arteriotomies and eversion endarterectomy using transverse division of the carotid have been reported. The eversion technique has some anatomic similarity to carotid shortening methods. In two studies by Kieny et al.[22] and Kasprzak and Raithel[23] of 20 and 122 patients, respectively, undergoing eversion endarterectomy, long-term restenosis rates were lower than those found among control patients having standard longitudinal arteriotomy. In a similar report Vanmaele,[24] suggests that lower recurrence rates following eversion endarterectomy result from a lesser diameter reduction after suturing a transverse incision instead of a longitudinal arteriotomy.

Although there are obvious theoretical advantages to the performance of carotid shortening procedures on selected patients, prospective randomized studies have not been performed. The present study suggests that carotid shortening can be done safely in individuals undergoing carotid endarterectomy, with no added short- or long-term morbidity. Based on this preliminary experience, we suggest that carotid shortening procedures may be helpful for selected patients and should be within the abilities of the vascular surgeon.

REFERENCES

1. Cioffi FA, Meduri M, Tomasello F, et al. Kinking and coiling of the internal carotid artery: Clinical-statistical observations and surgical perspectives. J Neurol Surg Sci 19:15-22, 1975.
2. Lochridge SK, Rossi NP. Symptomatic kinked internal carotid artery. J Cardiovasc Surg 21:108-111, 1980.
3. Gray SW, Skandalakis JE. The thoracic aorta. In Embryology for Surgeons, the Embryological Basis for the Treatment of Congenital Defects. Philadelphia: WB Saunders, 1972, pp 809-857.
4. Weibel J, Fields WS. Tortuosity, coiling, and kinking of the internal carotid artery. I. Etiology and radiographic anatomy. Neurology 15:7-11, 1965.
5. Poindexter JM, Patel KR, Clauss RH. Management of kinked extracranial cerebral arteries. J Vasc Surg 6:127-133, 1987.
6. Mukherjee D, Inahara T. Management of the tortuous internal carotid artery. Am J Surg 149:651-655, 1985.
7. Quattlebaum JK, Wade JS, Whiddon CM. Stroke associated with elongation and kinking of the carotid artery: Long-term follow-up. Ann Surg 177:572-579, 1973.
8. Roberts B, Hardesty WH, Holling HE, et al. Studies on extracranial cerebral blood flow. Surgery 56:826-833, 1964.

9. Vannix RS, Joergenson EJ, Carter R. Kinking of the internal carotid artery: Clinical significance and surgical management. Am J Surg 134:82-89, 1977.
10. Stanton PE, McClusky DA, Lamis PA. Hemodynamic assessment and surgical correction of kinking of the internal carotid artery. Surgery 84:793-802, 1978.
11. Riser MM, Gerand J, Ducoudray J, et al. Dolicho internal carotid with vertiginous syndrome. Rev Neurol 85:145-147, 1951.
12. Hsu I, Kisten AD. Buckling of the great vessels. Arch Intern Med 98:712-714, 1956.
13. Collins PS, Orecchia P, Gomez E. A technique for correction of carotid kinks and coils following endarterectomy. Ann Vasc Surg 5:116-120, 1991.
14. Smith BM, Stames VA, Maggart MA. Operative management of the kinked carotid artery. Surg Gynecol Obstet 162:71-72, 1986.
15. Hamann H. Carotid endarterectomy: Prevention of stroke in asymptomatic (Stage I) and symptomatic (Stage II) patients? Thorac Cardiovasc Surg 36:272-275, 1988.
16. Chino ES. A simple method for combined carotid endarterectomy and correction of internal carotid artery kinking. J Vasc Surg 6:197-199, 1987.
17. Archie JP. Carotid endarterectomy with reconstruction techniques tailored to operative findings. J Vasc Surg 17:141-151, 1993.
18. Coyle KA, Smith RB, Chapman RL, et al. Carotid artery shortening: A safe adjunct to carotid endarterectomy. J Vasc Surg 22:257-263, 1995.
19. Nicholls SC, Phillips DJ, Bergelin RO, et al. Carotid endarterectomy: Relation of outcome to early restenosis. J Vasc Surg 2:375-386, 1985.
20. Edwards WH, Edwards WH Jr, Mulherin JL, Martin RS. Recurrent carotid artery stenosis. Ann Surg 209:662-669, 1989.
21. Bernstein EF, Toren S, Dilley RB. Does carotid restenosis predict an increased risk of late symptoms, stroke, or death? Ann Surg 212:629-636, 1990.
22. Kieny R, Seiller C, Petit H. Evolution of carotid restenosis after endarterectomy. Cardiovasc Surg 2:555-560, 1994.
23. Kasprzak PM, Raithel D. Eversionendarteriektomie der A. carotis interna (EEA). Angiology 12:1-8, 1990.
24. Vanmaele RG. Surgery for carotid stenosis: The quest for the ideal technique. Eur J Vasc Surg 7:361-363, 1993.

54

Treatment of Perioperative Neurologic Deficits After Carotid Surgery

WILLIAM H. BAKER, M.D.

The purpose of carotid endarterectomy is to alleviate symptoms and prevent stroke. Unfortunately the operation itself carries a risk of stroke that ideally should be less than 5% and perhaps as low as 1% or 2%. The exact incidence of postoperative stroke is difficult to ascertain. The North American Symptomatic Carotid Endarterectomy Trial (NASCET) had an operative (30-day) stroke rate of 5.5%.[1] The European trial had a higher stroke rate of 7.5% associated with surgery.[2] This latter number would be considered unacceptable by most American standards. Yet both of these figures pale in comparison to those collected in a study from the Rand Institute.[3] After reviewing the records of patients who had undergone carotid endarterectomy, Rand investigators found a 9.8% incidence of postoperative stroke. These distressing statistics were virtually identical in different parts of urban and rural America. These rather high numbers are balanced by the recently reported findings from the Asymptomatic Carotid Atherosclerosis Study.[4] In this study surgeons from 39 centers were preselected on the basis of their past accomplishments.[5] After operating on more than 800 patients, these surgeons achieved a perioperative stroke rate of only 1.2% (2.3% including stroke related to angiography). The preceding wide range of numbers indicates that although the problem may be minimized, even the best surgeons will occasionally encounter a patient who suffers a stroke during the postoperative period following carotid endarterectomy.

There are three general causes of stroke immediately following carotid endarterectomy. Intraoperative embolization may occur at any time during the procedure. The carotid bifurcation, the seat of offending atheroma and oftentimes thrombus, should not be manipulated prior to placement of clamps. The use of a shunt invites emboli of "snowplowed" atheromatous debris, air, or thrombus. As flow is restored, the surgeon must be aware of any potential air or particulate matter that may escape when the internal carotid artery is opened.

Stroke may also occur as a result of intraoperative ischemia. During the operation, clamps are applied to the internal carotid artery, potentially resulting in inadequate blood flow to the ipsilateral cerebral cortex. Some surgeons routinely use a shunt to obviate this problem. Others operate on the awake patient, inserting a shunt only if a neurologic deficit occurs with clamping. Still others rely on electroencephalograms or carotid artery back pressure measurements. Regardless, insertion of the shunt may not be timely or the shunt may inadvertently fail to function during the procedure. Fortunately both of these complications are rare.

Finally, the internal carotid artery may occlude with thrombosis. Thrombosis usually occurs because the end point of the endarterectomy becomes elevated, flow is slowed, and finally thrombus forms to occlude the artery. This process may also occur at the site of internal carotid clamping or along a narrowed closure. Technical difficulties may lead to a slow, prolonged closure and in situ thrombosis may occur within the carotid bulb. Whatever the reason, when thrombosis occurs and flow stops in the internal carotid artery, the ipsilateral cerebral cortex may become ischemic leading to stroke.

PREVENTION

The best way to prevent all of the preceding complications is through technical perfection. The carotid bifurcation should not be manipulated excessively before placement of clamps. "Dissect the patient away the carotid artery" is an excellent dictum. Care must be taken when inserting the shunt to avoid introducing air into the system, as well as snowplowing debris with the ends of the shunt. The distal end point must be carefully inspected and tacked down if necessary. The closure should not compromise the internal carotid artery, and many advocate the liberal use of patches. Prior to restoring flow, the surgeon should make sure that all particulate matter, clot, and air are directed out of the arteriotomy or up the external rather than the internal carotid artery.

After all of the aforementioned technical precautions have been taken, careful inspection of the endarterectomized segment is recommended. The surgeon should always check for a distal pulse and local thrill. Some surgeons rely on intraoperative arteriography. Blaisdell et al.[6] from San Francisco General Hospital, found relatively few internal carotid artery defects but corrected more external carotid artery shelves and retained plaque. Alpert et al.,[7] from New Jersey, employed an ingenious technique that uses dental x-ray film to ensure that closure and endarterectomy are adequate. Others use a hand-held Doppler probe to either listen to or record the peak systolic and end-diastolic frequencies (velocities).[8] Turbulent flow as well as increased frequencies indicate an imperfect technical result. Intraoperative angioscopy is used less frequently.[9]

We have used duplex ultrasonography in the operating room to detect intraoperative imperfections.[10] The duplex scanner from the peripheral vascular laboratory is rolled into the operating room. A 10 mHz probe is inserted into a long sterile plastic sheath. Gel is placed in the sheath to ensure ultrasonic coupling. The wound is irrigated with saline solution and the artery is directly examined. The common carotid artery is first visualized and the flow is recorded. Although step off is always observed between the common carotid retained atheroma and the endarterectomized segment, this should be minimal. By means of color-flow imaging, the peak systolic and end-diastolic frequencies are recorded throughout. Areas of turbulent flow in particular are examined. The black and white image is more useful for identifying small fronds of intima or media that are retained and attached to the endarterectomized segment. Adherent clumps of thrombi can be seen. Every effort is made to visualize the distal end point. Under most conditions this cannot be identified on the duplex monitor. The surgeon will have no problem estimating where the end point should be located in relationship to the end of the closure.

In a 7-year review, we have reopened nine arteries on the basis of this examination. Although one artery was reopened on the basis of high flow alone, a recognizable defect was seen in the other eight. The surgeon should be cautioned that we have seen three postoperative occlusions in patients whose intraoperative duplex findings were normal.

RECOGNITION OF STROKE

The diagnosis of perioperative stroke is based on physical examination findings. In a patient who is neurologically intact preoperatively, this does not present a problem. Patients who have a neurologic deficit preoperatively, however, may awaken with an exacerbation of the preexisting deficit. This phenomenon may occur in a patient awakening from any operation in which general anesthesia is used (e.g., after gallbladder surgery). If, indeed, the magnification of the neurologic deficit is merely caused by the general anesthetic, this deficit will rapidly correct itself and the patient should assume his or her preoperative status within minutes. Thus it is especially important for the operating surgeon to have performed a complete neurologic examination preoperatively. If the surgeon assumes that the patient is neurologically intact, when in fact there is a subtle preoperative neurologic deficit, the patient may be returned to the operating room unnecessarily for reexploration should such a deficit become more pronounced in the postoperative period.

There is one category of patients that I find especially difficult to assess. The patient who develops an occlusion of the surgically treated carotid artery, and who also has a preexisting occlusion of the contralateral common carotid, may merely be "slow to wake up." This patient may not demonstrate a lateralizing neurologic deficit but may have total global ischemia. If, indeed, the anesthesiologist cannot adequately explain such a phenomenon, the artery should be quickly examined either noninvasively in the recovery room or during reexploration in the operating room. There were at least two patients in our series in whom prompt reoperation was not undertaken because the surgeon did not believe there was a neurologic deficit but that the patient was merely slow to wake up.

TREATMENT

The goals of treatment of any post–carotid endarterectomy neurologic deficit are straightforward. If an embolic event has already occurred, the surgeon is helpless to assist the patient. At that point the surgeon may remove the source of the embolus if in fact this source is prone to repeat embolism. The surgeon cannot revive brain that has been damaged as a result of intraoperative ischemia. The surgeon's only hope to help the patient is to find a totally occluded internal carotid artery that can be easily treated with thrombectomy with restoration of flow. If flow can be restored within 1 to 2 hours of the onset of a neurologic deficit, isolated anecdotal reports suggest that many patients will show improvement.[11] Thus when the surgeon finds a patient with a postoperative neurologic deficit, he or she must employ an algorithm that will definitively confirm or deny the existence of an internal carotid artery occlusion and will, in addition, restore blood flow to the internal carotid artery within 1 hour.

STROKE IN THE OPERATING ROOM

Surgeons performing carotid endarterectomies would prefer that all patients awaken while they are still in the operating room so they could be tested neurologically. When a patient awakens with an obvious neurologic deficit, the safest policy is to reexplore the wound. This maneuver usually takes only a few minutes. Once the wound has been examined, the surgeon can state with certainty whether the artery is occluded, thereby blunting any further discussion as to how to proceed.

There are some exceptions to the preceding rule. We have had patients who had prolonged intraoperative cerebral ischemia whose duplex scans were perfectly normal 15 minutes before the discovery of the neurologic deficit. In these cases reexploration of the wound can sometimes be avoided. We have not, as of yet, been mistaken in our assessment, that is, the internal carotid artery was proved to be patent on later duplex or angiographic examinations.

STROKE IN THE RECOVERY ROOM

When postoperative stroke is recognized in the recovery room, after a period during which the patient was neurologically normal, the patient is assumed to have had either an occlusion of the internal carotid artery or an embolic event. These patients should be promptly returned to the operating room. My practice is to obtain a duplex scan only in the middle of the day when such a test can be performed expeditiously. Arteriography should not be performed before the patient is returned to the operating room because this procedure will delay that return by at least 1 hour. Reexploration may restore flow, thus giving the patient a chance for neurologic improvement, and reexploration involves very little risk. In patients who are otherwise unstable, this procedure can be performed under local anesthesia.

TRANSIENT ISCHEMIC ATTACK

The patient who has a postoperative transient ischemic attack is immediately tested for patency of the internal carotid artery. It is assumed that the patient has had an embolic event, but some patients will only have transient symptoms even with total internal carotid artery occlusion. In those patients who have an occlusion, the surgeon must decide whether the condition warrants a return to the operating room. By definition, since the patient has had a transient ischemic attack, he or she is now neurologically normal. Will reexploration, thrombectomy, and restoration of flow be beneficial over time or can this patient tolerate the occlusion and remain neurologically intact? The patient who has tolerated carotid endarterectomy without a shunt, has relatively high internal carotid artery back pressure (>70 mm Hg), and has a widely patent contralateral internal artery and vertebral arteries may actually tolerate the occlusion well if he or she can be protected from embolism in the middle cerebral or anterior cerebral artery. Those patients who have multiple extracranial atherosclerotic lesions and in whom a shunt was required for whatever reason, should probably be returned to the operating room.

Those patients who have a widely patent internal carotid artery are assumed to have had an embolus and are treated with anticoagulation. A CT scan is obtained to rule out intracerebral hemorrhage. An angiogram should be obtained in most instances. If the angiogram is normal, the patient should be maintained on aspirin. If the angiogram is abnormal, the surgeon must make a decision as to how to treat the abnormality.

OPERATIVE PROCEDURE

The patient is expeditiously wheeled into the operating room and the incision area is sprayed. Local anesthesia may be used but I prefer general anesthesia. The sutures are removed, retraction is obtained, and the artery is gently examined. Care must be taken to avoid displacing the thrombus that is located at the carotid bulb. If the distal internal carotid artery is pulsatile, a decision must be made as to whether the artery should be opened. If intraoperative duplex scanning or arteriography is readily available, it may be used in place of reexploration. In my opinion it is preferable to apply clamps, open the artery for direct inspection, insert an indwelling shunt, and then close the artery using a patch angioplasty technique. The onus is on the surgeon to prove the presence or absence of thrombus, and if it is present to remove it.

If, indeed, thrombus is present, a proximal common carotid clamp is applied as is an external carotid artery clamp. No clamp is placed distally on the internal carotid artery. The arteriotomy is reopened and the thrombus is extracted. Back bleeding should force thrombus that is located distally in the internal carotid artery out through the arteriotomy. If a Fogarty catheter is used, it should be inserted only a few centimeters. It should not traverse the carotid siphon. The catheter should be withdrawn by the senior surgeon, taking care not to injure the wall of the artery. If any doubt exists regarding the completeness of the thrombectomy, an operative arteriogram or angioscopy may settle the issue. Once the surgeon is confident that no further thrombus remains, a temporary indwelling shunt is placed so that the duration of ischemia is minimized. The endarterectomy site is inspected to determine the cause of the thrombosis. Any abnormality is appropriately corrected before closing the artery using a patch angioplasty technique. These patients are ordinarily not maintained on heparin in the postoperative period, especially if the neurologic deficit persists.

THE LOYOLA EXPERIENCE

During the past 10 years we have treated 16 cases of postoperative stroke, which represents a neurologic deficit rate of 2.7% (Fig. 1). In addition, we have treated five patients who had transient ischemic attacks. Eight of these events occurred in the immediate postoperative period, 10 within the same hospitalization, and three after discharge but within 30 days of surgery. Of the eight immediate deficits, five were not reexplored and no internal carotid artery occlusions were knowingly missed. Among the three that were explored, no thrombus was found. Four patients had transient ischemic attacks and six additional patients suffered a stroke, which occurred during the same hospitalization after the patient had left the postoperative recovery area. Two of these latter patients had proven occlusions. One of these patients underwent reexploration, albeit more than 2 hours after the onset of symptoms, and his dense hemiparesis did not improve. In the second patient the internal carotid artery occlusion was not recognized in a timely fashion. He did not undergo reexploration and eventually died of neurologic complications.

Three of the five patients who had transient ischemic attacks had normal angiographic findings. One patient who was not studied suffered a stroke many months later. This stroke was not easy to characterize in terms of which hemisphere was involved. One patient who had a transient ischemic attack was found to have a kink of the internal carotid artery on noninvasive testing.

It is of interest that three of our patients had onset of their neurologic postoperative deficits

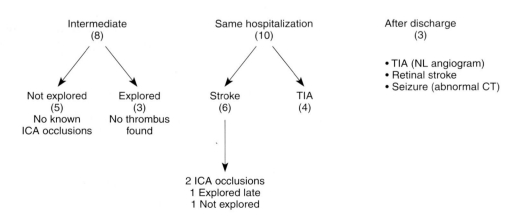

Fig. 1 Post–carotid endarterectomy stroke: Loyola experience.

after they were discharged from the hospital but within 30 days of the operation. One of these patients had a transient ischemic attack but the angiogram showed a normal internal carotid artery. A second patient had a seizure and had an abnormal CT scan that was consistent with the clinical picture. A third patient had a retinal stroke.

DISCUSSION

It is obvious from the preceding experiences that we do not follow all of our dicta. That is, all of our patients do not undergo reexploration. In this limited review we have not knowingly missed any internal carotid occlusions. Those patients who had occluded arteries were not recognized in a timely fashion and thus did not undergo reexploration.

How does this compare with the experiences of other authors? Edwards et al.[12] from Nashville, Tennessee, reported their experience in 1988 (Fig. 2). Of 20 patients who underwent exploratory operations because of postendarterectomy stroke, 12 were found to have thrombosed internal carotid arteries. After flow was restored, nine of these patients recovered with deficit and only three were considered normal. No thrombus was found in eight additional patients. Three of these patients also recovered normally and five were left with some neurologic deficit. Thus, although exploration was undertaken in all patients, it did not seem to make a difference whether thrombosis of the internal carotid artery was indeed found. Restoration of flow of these vessels did not restore neurologic integrity. We have no knowledge of the interval between the onset of symptoms and the restoration of flow.

Courbier and Ferdani[13] from Marseille, France, reported 20 patients who had postoperative thrombosis of the internal carotid artery (Table 1). Of the 12 patients who underwent reexploration and thrombectomy, four died. Only one of eight who were observed without reoperation died. Two of the reoperated patients had a complete neurologic recovery compared to only one of the patients who was only observed. Six patients who underwent reexploration were left with either a mild or a severe deficit compared to five of the patients who were observed. It should be noted that this was not a randomized study, and it may well have been that those patients who had a milder deficit were treated with observation, whereas those who had a more severe deficit were rushed to the operating room. Regardless, reexploration did not yield a noticeable improvement in the status of their patients.

In light of our experience and that of Edwards and Courbier, we propose a slight modification of the current dictum that all patients who suffer a post–carotid endarterectomy stroke must undergo reexploration.

All patients who have a postoperative neurologic deficit or transient ischemic attack must be promptly diagnosed and treated. In this era of postendarterectomy intraoperative assessments such as duplex scanning or arteriography, the surgeon can be somewhat reassured that the artery is indeed open. As before, patients who are neurologically intact when they awaken but later develop a neurologic deficit that does not promptly (within minutes) abate should undergo reexploration. Although in some patients reexploration may be unnecessary, we believe this is the safest policy. All patients who have a known contralateral carotid occlusion and who exhibit signs of a neurologic deficit should undergo reexploration. In my opinion, patients who have bilateral internal carotid artery occlusions fare poorly. Thus the modified algorithm states that all patients in whom internal carotid artery occlusion is suspected should undergo prompt

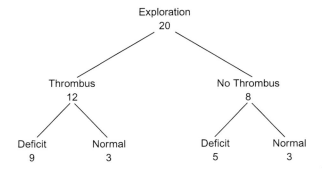

Fig. 2 Postoperative stroke: Data from Nashville, Tennessee.

Table 1 Postoperative thrombosis: Data from Marseille, France

	Reoperation (n = 12)	Observation (n = 8)
Died	4	1
Total recovery	2	1
Mild deficit	3	4
Severe deficit	3	1
Contralateral deficit	—	1

reexploration. However, such an occlusion will not be suspected in all patients.

Nevertheless, if the patient undergoes exploratory surgery, the operation must be performed in a timely fashion. Although some recovery has been noted antecdotally after 1 or 2 hours, restoration of flow within 1 hour is preferable. Since there are reported recoveries with exploration, the surgeon making these decisions regarding patient care should tend toward reexploration rather than procrastinate.

REFERENCES

1. North American Symptomatic Carotid Endarterectomy Trial Collaborators. Beneficial effect of carotid endarterectomy in symptomatic patients with high-grade carotid stenosis. N Engl J Med 325:445-453, 1991.
2. European Carotid Surgery Trialists' Collaborative Group. MRC European carotid surgery trial: Interim results for symptomatic patients with severe (70-99%) or with mild (0-29%) carotid stenosis. Lancet 337:1235-1243, 1991.
3. Winslow CM, Solomon DH, Chasin MR, Kosecoff J, Merrick NJ, Brook RH. The appropriateness of carotid endarterectomy. N Engl J Med 318:721-727, 1988.
4. National Institute of Neurological Disorders and Stroke. Carotid endarterectomy for patients with asymptomatic internal carotid artery stenosis. Clinical Advisory, 1994.
5. Moore WS, Vescera CL, Robertson JT, Baker WH, Howard VJ, Toole JF. Selection process for surgeons in the Asymptomatic Carotid Atherosclerosis Study. Stroke 22:1353-1357, 1991.
6. Blaisdell FW, Lim R Jr, Hall AD. Technical results of carotid endarterectomy: Arteriographic assessment. Am J Surg 114:239-246, 1967.
7. Alpert J, Brener BJ, Parsonnet V, Meisner K, Sadow S, Brief DK, Goldenkranz RJ. Carotid endarterectomy and completion contact arteriography. J Vasc Surg 1:548-554, 1984.
8. Bandyk DF, Kaebnick HW, Adams MB, Towne JB. Turbulence occurring after carotid bifurcation endarterectomy harbinger of residual and recurrent carotid stenosis. J Vasc Surg 7:261-274, 1988.
9. Towne JB, Bernhard VM. Vascular endoscopy: Usable tool or interesting toy. Surgery 82:415-419, 1977.
10. Baker WH, Koustas G, Burke K, Littooy FN, Greisler HP. Intraoperative duplex scanning and late carotid artery stenosis. J Vasc Surg 19:829-833, 1994.
11. Kwann JHM, Connolly JE, Sharefkin JB. Successful management of early stroke after carotid endarterectomy. Ann Surg 190:676-678, 1979.
12. Edwards WH Jr, Jenkins JM, Edwards WH Sr, Mulherin JL Jr. Prevention of stroke during carotid endarterectomy. Am Surg 54:125-128, 1988.
13. Courbier R, Ferdani M. Criteria for immediate reoperation following carotid surgery. In Bergan JJ, Yao JST, eds. Reoperative Arterial Surgery. Orlando: Grune & Stratton, 1986, pp 495-507.

55

Is Carotid-Subclavian Prosthetic Bypass a Durable and Effective Procedure for Subclavian Occlusive Disease? A 22-Year Experience

ROBERT W. BARNES, M.D.

In 1961 Reivich et al.[1] described the association of transient cerebrovascular symptoms and reversed flow in the vertebral artery distal to subclavian artery obstruction, a syndrome termed "subclavian steal" in an editorial[2] accompanying that report. Since that seminal paper, at least 13 different therapeutic alternatives have been suggested for management of this syndrome, as listed in Table 1. Of these many options, carotid-subclavian bypass[3] has been performed most frequently. Subclavian-carotid transposition[4] has been suggested as a more durable procedure but comparative data on patient outcomes are lacking. Recently percutaneous transluminal angioplasty[5] of subclavian artery stenosis has been recommended as a less invasive alternative to surgical intervention for subclavian steal syndrome. Since 1968 carotid-subclavian bypass has been the treatment of choice for subclavian steal syndrome at our medical centers.[6] Vitti et al.[7] have recently reported our long-term experience with this procedure. The purpose of this chapter is to review our extended results with carotid-subclavian bypass, along with those reported in the English literature, to provide a benchmark with which to compare alternative therapeutic approaches for the subclavian steal syndrome.

METHODS

This study constitutes a retrospective review of all patients undergoing carotid-subclavian bypass at the Little Rock VA Medical Center between June 1968 and January 1990. There were 124 patients including 116 men and eight women whose ages ranged from 42 to 78 years with a mean of 57.9. The presenting symptoms are depicted in Table 2. The majority (70%) of

Table 1 Treatment options for subclavian steal syndrome

Procedures
Transthoracic
Endarterectomy ± patch
Bypass graft
Interposition graft
Transcervical
Carotid-subclavian bypass
Subclavian-carotid transposition
Axillary-axillary bypass
Subclavian-subclavian bypass
Endarterectomy ± patch
Vertebral-carotid transposition
Carotid-vertebral anastomosis
Vertebral ligation
Other
Femoroaxillary bypass
Percutaneous transluminal angioplasty
Observation

Table 2 Presenting symptoms

Symptoms	No. (%)
Extremity ischemia (n = 87)	
Weakness	34 (42%)
Claudication	38 (44%)
Acute ischemia	12 (14%)
Vertebrobasilar insufficiency (n = 55)	
Dizziness*	21 (39%)
Drop attacks	15 (28%)
Ataxia	11 (20%)
Vertigo	8 (13%)
Syncope	8 (13%)
Diplopia	6 (11%)

*Dizziness plus arm weakness (n = 8), dizziness plus claudication (n = 7), and dizziness plus drop attacks (n = 6).

patients had symptoms of upper extremity ischemia with or without concomitant cerebrovascular symptoms. Symptoms of vertebrobasilar insufficiency were present in 44% of patients, over half of whom had concomitant upper extremity symptoms. Although dizziness was the most common cerebrovascular symptom, no patient was operated on for dizziness alone. Risk factors common for atherosclerosis included cigarette smoking in 97% of patients, hypertension in 70%, coronary artery disease in 68%, diabetes mellitus in 17%, and hyperlipidemia in 13%.

Arteriographic findings included left subclavian artery obstruction in 99 patients (80%), right subclavian obstruction in 21 (17%), and common carotid obstruction in four (3%). Concomitant ≥50% stenosis of the internal carotid artery was found in 36 patients (29%), which was ipsilateral in 32 patients and contralateral in four.

Indications for operation included upper extremity ischemia alone in 33 patients (27%), upper extremity ischemia with vertebrobasilar insufficiency in 31 (25%), upper extremity ischemia with transient ischemic attacks in 23 (19%), vertebrobasilar insufficiency alone in 24 (19%), and transient ischemic attacks alone in 13 (10%).

Prosthetic material was used for all carotid-subclavian bypasses. During the first portion of this study Dacron was employed in 80 patients (65%), whereas during the latter period polytetrafluoroethylene (Gore-Tex, W.L. Gore & Associates, Flagstaff, Ariz.) prostheses were used in 44 patients (35%). Concomitant carotid endarterectomy was performed for ipsilateral ≥50% stenosis of the internal carotid artery. Antecedent carotid endarterectomy was performed in four patients with contralateral carotid stenosis several weeks prior to carotid-subclavian bypass.

RESULTS
Perioperative (30-day) Period

One patient died of myocardial infarction 3 days after carotid-subclavian bypass, for a perioperative mortality rate of 0.8%. There were 10 postoperative complications (8%) including three myocardial infarctions, one gastrointestinal hemorrhage, one thoracic duct fistula, and five temporary nerve injuries. The latter included injury to the phrenic nerve in two, recurrent laryngeal nerve in two, and marginal mandibular branch of the facial nerve in one. No patient suffered perioperative stroke or transient ischemic attack and there were no early postoperative graft thromboses. All patients were initially relieved of symptoms.

Late Follow-up Period

The long-term results of the initial 64 patients were reported by Thompson et al.[6] Late follow-up of the remaining 60 patients treated between 1975 and 1990 extended from 5 to 176 months with a mean of 91.5 months. There were 22 deaths (37%) including 12 from myocardial infarction or congestive heart failure, five from malignancy, and five from unknown causes. The cumulative patient survival is depicted in Fig. 1 and was 83% at 5 years, 59% at 10 years, and 51% at 15 years. Three grafts occluded at 30,

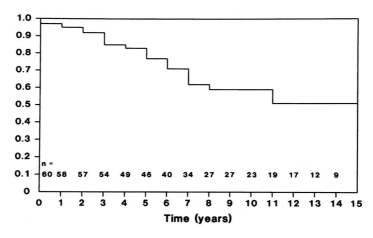

Fig. 1 Cumulative patient survival.

36, and 51 months postoperatively. The cumulative graft patency was 94% at 5, 10, and 15 years after operation (Fig. 2). Recurrent symptoms developed in six patients (10%) between 9 and 66 months after operation. Recurrent symptoms of upper extremity ischemia developed in the three patients with postoperative graft thrombosis. The three remaining patients developed recurrent dizziness despite patent grafts documented by duplex ultrasound evaluation. The cumulative symptom-free survival was 98% at 1 year, 90% at 5 years, and 87% at 10 and 15 years (Fig. 3).

Literature Review

Including the seminal paper on carotid-subclavian bypass by Diethrich et al.[3] in 1967, there have been 27 reports[3,6,8-32] in the English literature that describe unique patients in sufficient detail to provide a comparison with our recent publication.[7] Including our own series, a total of 971 patients have undergone carotid-subclavian bypass, 81% on the left side and 19% on the right. Prosthetic grafts have been used preferentially (82%), with Dacron employed in 62%, polytetrafluoroethylene in 20%, and vein grafts in the remainder (18%). The early postoperative (30-day) results include death in 1.8% of patients, graft thrombosis in 2.2%, and stroke in 1.9%. Late results after a mean follow-up of 50 months include death in 21% of patients, graft thrombosis in 7.8%, stroke in 3.2%, and graft infection in 1.1%. The cumulative late graft patency rates in eight reports ranged from 77% to 100% at 5 years and from 55% to 94% at 10 years.

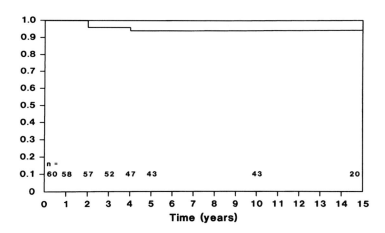

Fig. 2 Cumulative primary graft patency.

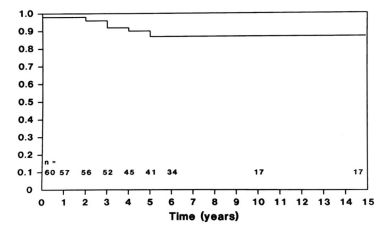

Fig. 3 Cumulative symptom-free survival.

DISCUSSION

Since the initial description of the subclavian steal syndrome nearly 34 years ago, a plethora of therapeutic approaches have been suggested for management of this condition. Initial attempts to control cerebrovascular symptoms by ligation of the vertebral artery[33] carrying reversed flow were soon followed by more direct arterial reconstructive techniques. Transthoracic procedures including endarterectomy or bypass offered correction of the hemodynamic abnormality.[34] However, the morbidity and mortality of these procedures were excessive because of the comorbidity of the patients, especially coronary and pulmonary disease. Extrathoracic procedures were introduced that carried less risk while offering hemodynamic correction and symptom relief. Carotid-subclavian bypass has been the most common method to treat subclavian steal syndrome. Other cervical procedures most frequently recommended include axillary-axillary bypass, subclavian-subclavian bypass, and subclavian-carotid transposition.

Axillary-axillary bypass[35] has the virtue of avoiding the need to clamp the carotid artery and is relatively easy to perform. However, late graft patency rates of this procedure, with the longer bypass conduit, have been inferior to those of carotid-subclavian bypass or subclavian-carotid transposition. Furthermore, the presternal subcutaneous position of the graft occasionally leads to skin erosion and graft infection, and it is an impediment to medial sternotomy for coronary bypass grafting.

Subclavian-subclavian bypass,[36] while involving a shorter conduit than axillary-axillary bypass, is a technically more complicated procedure than axillary-axillary bypass. Furthermore, the passage of the prosthesis across the lower neck may lead to either patient discomfort or cosmetic disturbance. In addition, the late patency rates have been inferior to those reported for carotid-subclavian bypass.

Subclavian-carotid transposition[4] has the appeal of avoiding the need for graft material and only involves a single anastomosis. The reported late patency rates equal or surpass those for carotid-subclavian bypass. However, the procedure is technically more challenging than the other extrathoracic methods of treating subclavian steal syndrome and few centers have reported experience with this procedure. The mobilization of the subclavian artery may lead to kinking of the vertebral artery, and the leading proponent of this procedure[37] admits to the occasional need to transpose the vertebral artery separately onto the carotid artery. Permanent Horner's syndrome is a risk of the procedure.

Our experience with carotid-subclavian bypass for subclavian steal syndrome is the largest reported to date, with cumulative follow-up to 15 years.[7] Our data suggest that this procedure carries a negligible perioperative risk and the potential for long-term relief of symptoms. Caution should be exercised in treating patients with isolated symptoms of dizziness. Although none of our patients had this symptom alone perioperatively, three patients developed recurrent dizziness in the late postoperative period despite patent grafts. The three patients with late postoperative graft thromboses developed recurrent symptoms of upper extremity ischemia. No patients developed early or late postoperative stroke, despite the concomitant or staged performance of carotid endarterectomy in 29% of patients. Our cumulative late graft patency of 94% up to 15 years surpasses that of any other series reported in the literature.

CONCLUSION

More than a dozen interventional procedures have been recommended for the treatment of subclavian steal syndrome since its first description nearly 34 years ago. Carotid-subclavian bypass is currently the most common procedure for managing this condition. Recently percutaneous transluminal angioplasty has been suggested as an alternative to surgical intervention for subclavian steal syndrome. To provide a benchmark for evaluating this procedure, our experience with carotid-subclavian bypass was reviewed over a 22-year period. Of 124 patients treated, the perioperative mortality was 0.8% and there were no strokes or early graft thromboses. Cumulative graft patency was 94% at 5, 10, and 15 years postoperatively and symptom-free survival was 90% at 5 years and 87% at 10 and 15 years follow-up. These results surpass those of most other series of 971 patients reported in the literature over the past 25 years. We conclude that carotid-subclavian bypass remains the procedure of choice for treating patients with the subclavian steal syndrome.

REFERENCES

1. Reivich M, Holling HE, Roberts B, et al. Reversal of blood flow through the vertebral artery and its effect on cerebral circulation. N Engl J Med 265:878-885, 1961.
2. Fisher CM. A new vascular syndrome—"the subclavian steal." N Engl J Med 265:912-913, 1961.
3. Diethrich EB, Garrett HE, Ameriso J, et al. Occlusive disease of the common carotid and subclavian arteries treated by carotid-subclavian bypass. Am J Surg 114:801-808, 1967.
4. Parrott JC. The subclavian steal syndrome. Arch Surg 88:661-664, 1964.
5. Bachman DM, Kim RM. Transluminal dilatation for subclavian steal syndrome. Am J Roentgenol 135:995-996, 1980.
6. Thompson BW, Read RC, Campbell GS. Operative correction of proximal blocks of the subclavian or innominate arteries. J Cardiovasc Surg 21:125-130, 1980.
7. Vitti MJ, Thompson BW, Read RC, et al. Carotid-subclavian bypass: A twenty-two year experience. J Vasc Surg 20:411-418, 1994.
8. Najafi H, Javid H, Ostermiller WE. Carotid bifurcation stenosis and ipsilateral subclavian steal. Arch Surg 99:289-292, 1969.
9. Ewing DD, Campbell DW, Kartchner MM, et al. Subclavian steal syndrome. Vasc Surg 101:155-160, 1970.
10. Schramek A, Hashmonai M, Meir M, et al. The subclavian steal syndrome. Isr J Med Sci 10:596-598, 1970.
11. Wylie EJ, Effeney DJ. Surgery of the aortic arch branches and vertebral arteries. Surg Clin North Am 59:669-680, 1979.
12. Rostad H, Hall RV. Arterial occlusive disease of the upper extremity. Scand J Thorac Cardiovasc Surg 14:223-226, 1980.
13. Luosto R, Ketonen P, Harjola PT, et al. Extrathoracic approach for reconstruction of subclavian and vertebral arteries. Scand J Thorac Cardiovasc Surg 14:227-231, 1980.
14. Raithel D. Our experience of surgery for innominate and subclavian lesions. J Cardiovasc Surg 21:423-430, 1980.
15. Maggisano R, Provan JL. Surgical management of chronic occlusive disease of the aortic arch vessels and vertebral arteries. Can Med Assoc J 124:972-977, 1981.
16. Gerety RL, Andrus CH, May AG, et al. Surgical treatment of occlusive subclavian artery disease. Circulation 64:228-230, 1981.
17. Welling RE, Cranley JJ, Krause RJ, et al. Obliterative arterial disease of the upper extremity. Arch Surg 116:1593-1596, 1981.
18. Vogt DP, Hertzer NR, Phara PJ, et al. Brachiocephalic arterial reconstruction. Ann Surg 196:541-552, 1982.
19. Crawford ES, Stowe GL, Powers RW. Occlusion of the innominate, common carotid, and subclavian arteries: Long-term results of surgical treatment. Surgery 94:781-791, 1983.
20. Harris RW, Andros G, Dulawa LB, et al. Large-vessel arterial occlusive disease in symptomatic upper extremity. Arch Surg 119:1277-1282, 1984.
21. Pasch AR, Schuler JJ, DeVord JR, et al. Subclavian steal despite ipsilateral vertebral occlusion. J Vasc Surg 2:913-916, 1985.
22. Ziomek S, Quiñones-Baldrich WJ, Busuttil RW, et al. The superiority of synthetic arterial grafts over autologous veins in carotid-subclavian bypass. J Vasc Surg 3:140-145, 1986.
23. Mohr LL, Smith LL, Smith DC. Subclavian steal with ipsilateral vertebral artery occlusive disease. J Cardiovasc Surg 27:434-439, 1986.
24. Shifrin EG, Anner H, Romanoff H. Extrathoracic approach in surgical treatment of subclavian steal. Isr J Med Sci 22:567-571, 1986.
25. Ackerman H, Diener HC, Seboldt H, et al. Ultrasonographic follow-up of subclavian stenosis and occlusion: Natural history and surgical treatment. Stroke 19:431-435, 1988.
26. Sterpetti AV, Schultz RD, Farina C, et al. Subclavian artery revascularization: A comparison between carotid-subclavian artery bypass and subclavian-carotid transposition. Surgery 106:624-632, 1989.
27. Perler BA, Williams GM. Carotid-subclavian bypass — a decade of experience. J Vasc Surg 12:716-722, 1990.
28. Kretschmer G, Teleky B, Marosi L, et al. Obliterations of the proximal subclavian artery: To bypass or to anastomose? J Cardiovasc Surg 32:334-339, 1991.
29. Mingoli A, Feldhaus RJ, Farina C, et al. Comparative results of carotid-subclavian bypass and axillo-axillary bypass in patients with symptomatic subclavian disease. Eur J Vasc Surg 6:26-30, 1992.
30. AbuRahma AF, Robinson PA, Khan MZ, et al. Brachiocephalic revascularization: A comparison between carotid-subclavian artery bypass and axilloaxillary artery bypass. Surgery 112:84-91, 1992.
31. Synn AY, Chalmers TA, Sharp WJ, et al. Is there a conduit of preference for a bypass between the carotid and subclavian arteries? Am J Surg 166:157-162, 1993.
32. Smith JM, Koury HI, Hafner CD, et al. Subclavian steal syndrome. J Cardiovasc Surg 35:11-14, 1994.
33. Rob C. Incipient strokes: Technique of surgical therapy. In Millikan CH, Siekert RG, Whisnent JP, eds. Cerebral Vascular Disease. New York: Grune & Stratton, 1961, pp 110-114.
34. DeBakey ME, Crawford ES, Morris GC, et al. Surgical considerations of occlusive disease of the innominate, carotid, subclavian, and vertebral arteries. Ann Surg 154:698-724, 1961.
35. Myers WO. Axillo-axillary bypass graft. JAMA 217:826, 1971.
36. Ehrenfeld WK, Levin SM, Wylie EJ. Venous crossover bypass grafts for arterial insufficiency. Ann Surg 167:287-291, 1968.
37. Edwards WH Jr, Tapper SS, Edwards WH Sr, et al. Subclavian revascularization. Ann Surg 219:673-678, 1994.

56

Revascularization Across the Neck Using the Retropharyngeal Route

RAMON BERGUER, M.D., Ph.D.

The retropharyngeal route is the shortest distance for an arterial bypass that must cross the midline of the neck. The specific indication for this type of reconstruction arises in a patient with severe disease or occlusion of the ipsilateral subclavian and common carotid arteries in whom a standard transthoracic reconstruction is not advisable, usually because of a previous myocardial revascularization, emphysema, or, rarely, extensive calcification of the ascending aorta. When such a patient needs a bypass, of necessity it must originate in the opposite side of the neck. Traditionally, bypasses crossing the midline have been placed subcutaneously in front of the airway. We have described a shorter and more direct route for crossing the neck using the retropharyngeal space in front of the vertebrae, precisely between the pharynx and the lamina prevertebralis.[1,2]

The coincidence of severe ipsilateral common carotid artery (CCA) and subclavian artery (SA) disease and a contraindication for medial sternotomy is rare. In the past 13 years covered by this review, 224 patients have undergone reconstruction of the branches of the aortic arch in our service through a cervical or transthoracic approach. Of these, 16 (7%) underwent a bypass by the retropharyngeal route. In all cases the bypass was from the right (donor) to the left (recipient) side. All patients have been followed with periodic examinations.

Since 1980 we have used a retropharyngeal tunnel in all patients needing revascularization from a vessel on the opposite side of the neck. The CCA and SA on the left side are more commonly affected than their counterparts on the right.[3] In this series 13 patients underwent revascularization of the left CCA or internal carotid artery, two of the left SA, and one of a left vertebral artery (Fig. 1).

When the *donor vessel was the right SA,* it was approached through a standard supraclavicular incision. At the beginning of our experience, we exposed the right SA conventionally in its retroscalene segment (Fig. 2). Later we preferred to isolate the right SA between the scalenusanticus and the brachial plexus—a simpler access that does not require division of the scalenus muscle or isolation of the phrenic nerve. The tunnel through the retropharyngeal space is accessed behind the carotid neurovascular bundle, in front of the transverse processes of the cervical vertebrae.

When the *donor vessel was the right carotid system,* we have used both the CCA and the external carotid artery as source arteries. The retropharyngeal space is entered by dissecting medially over the sympathetic chain and behind the pharynx. The lamina prevertebralis lets the exploring finger slide easily into the virtual space between the vertebrae and the pharynx.

The external carotid artery was chosen as a donor in the patient in whom the left internal carotid artery was to be revascularized using a saphenous vein (Fig. 3). We did not want to interrupt the right internal carotid flow, which in this patient supplied most of the blood to the brain.

On the other side of the neck the recipient artery was exposed through conventional techniques. In one patient the *recipient vessel was the left vertebral artery* in its third segment. If the recipient artery was the *left subclavian artery,* the latter was exposed in its first segment. This required cutting the clavicular insertion of the sternomastoid muscle. The subclavian artery is isolated, divided low in the thoracic inlet and, if needed, cleared up to or including the origin of the vertebral artery by eversion endarterectomy. The retropharyngeal space is completed from the recipient side and the graft is tunneled through it. The anastomosis to the SA is end to end to its

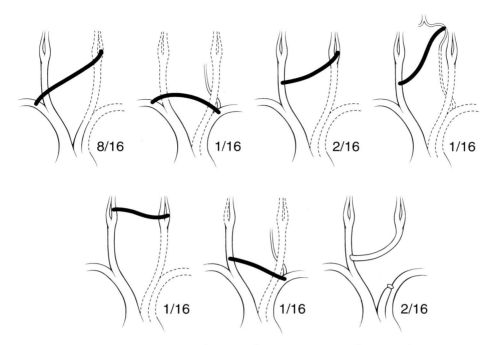

Fig. 1 Schematic diagram of retropharyngeal reconstructions done in this series. (From Berguer R, Gonzalez JA. Revascularization by the retropharyngeal route for extensive disease of the extracranial arteries. J Vasc Surg 19:217-225, 1994.)

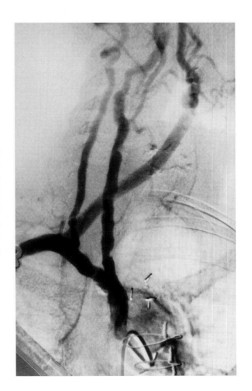

Fig. 2 Retropharyngeal bypass from the second segment of the right SA to the left carotid bifurcation. The left SA and CCA are chronically occluded. The left internal carotid was kept open by retrograde flow from the external carotid artery. This patient had undergone two previous aortocoronary bypass procedures, which contraindicated a direct reconstruction based on the ascending aorta. (From Berguer R, Gonzalez JA. Revascularization by the retropharyngeal route for extensive disease of the extracranial arteries. J Vasc Surg 19:217-225, 1994.)

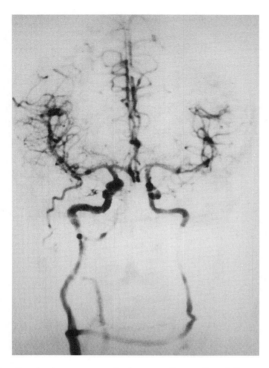

Fig. 3 Autogenous vein bypass from the right external carotid to the left internal carotid artery. (From Berguer R, Gonzalez JA. Revascularization by the retropharyngeal route for extensive disease of the extracranial arteries. J Vasc Surg 19:217-225, 1994.)

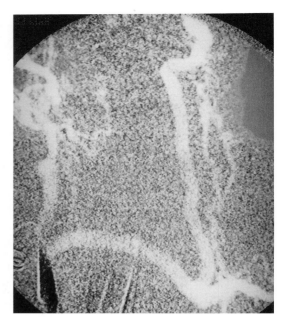

Fig. 4 Retropharyngeal graft from the right to the left SA. Note the distal anastomosisis made end to end to the prevertebral segment of the left SA. (From Berguer R, Gonzalez JA. Revascularization by the retropharyngeal route for extensive disease of the extracranial arteries. J Vasc Surg 19:217-225, 1994.)

prevertebral segment (Fig. 4). Although the situation did not occur in this series, this technique is obviously contraindicated if the patient has had a left internal mammary artery for myocardial revascularization. In such a case we would anastomose the graft to the third segment of the SA.

The *left carotid bifurcation* was the most common recipient side, and it required an endarterectomy in all cases (Fig. 5). The anastomosis was constructed to the posterior aspect of the bulb at the beginning of the series (Fig. 6, *A*). Eventually we changed the technique to a transection of the distal common carotid artery, eversion endarterectomy of the bifurcation, and end-to-end anastomosis of the graft to the distal common carotid artery (Fig. 6, *B*). The latter is easier to construct and does not result in the angulation of the carotid bulb sometimes seen with the former (Fig. 7).

In two cases a lesion originating in the left CCA was corrected by *direct transposition of the common carotid artery to its opposite counterpart* (Fig. 8) without the use of a bypass graft. This

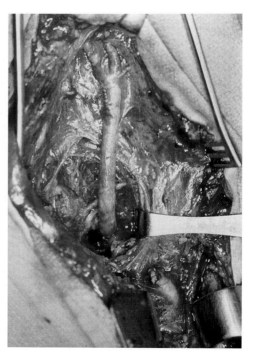

Fig. 5 Left CCA seen transposed to the right CCA through the retropharyngeal tunnel. The left carotid bifurcation has also undergone endarterectomy.

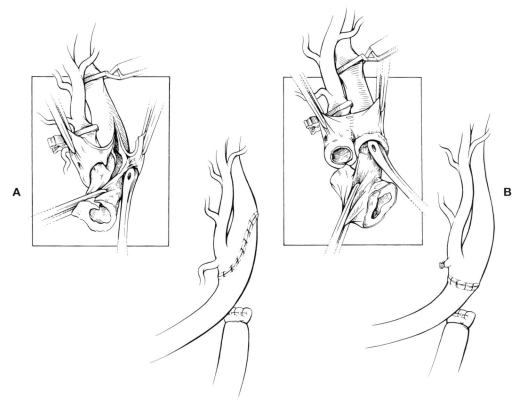

Fig. 6 A, Initial method of combining endarterectomy of the carotid bifurcation and anastomosis of the latter to the retropharyngeal bypass. **B,** Method preferred in the latter part of this study. (From Berguer R, Gonzalez JA. Revascularization by the retropharyngeal route for extensive disease of the extracranial arteries. J Vasc Surg 19:217-225, 1994.)

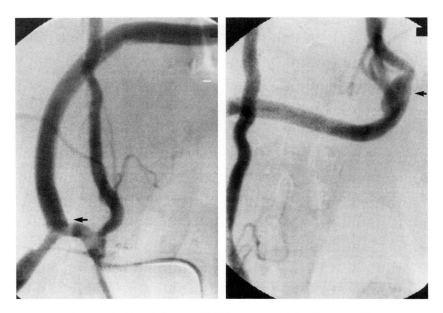

Fig. 7 Right subclavian (left) to left carotid bifurcation (right) bypass. Note some angulation of the internal carotid artery above the bulb (arrows).

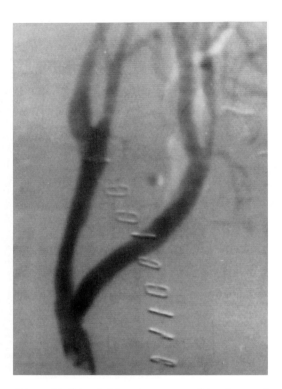

Fig. 8 Direct transposition of left to right common carotid artery using the retropharyngeal route. (From Berguer R, Gonzalez JA. Revascularization by the retropharyngeal route for extensive disease of the extracranial arteries. J Vasc Surg 19:217-225, 1994.)

direct carotid-to-carotid transposition can be done through the short retropharyngeal space because the distance between the two CCAs across this pathway is only 5 cm (Fig. 9). This is perhaps the only instance in which a temporary intraluminal shunt is used while clamping the CCA. Evidently in a CCA-to-CCA transposition flow is simultaneously interrupted in both carotid systems, presenting a serious threat of brain ischemia unless some form of shunting is used.

We use both polytetrafluoroethylene (PTFE) and saphenous vein for bypass material. PTFE is preferred when the recipient vessel is the CCA or the SA. In one case the patient had previously undergone neck radiotherapy, and because the retropharyngeal space felt tight to the tunneling finger, we chose a ringed graft (Fig. 10). We use saphenous vein whenever the recipient vessel is the internal carotid or the vertebral artery (see Fig. 3).

The fact that the patients in this series had severe disease of at least two supra-aortic trunks and a contraindication to sternotomy suggests that this is a high-risk group. Seven of 16 patients (43%) had a history of stroke. Coronary artery disease was present in 69% of these patients. It is interesting that 8 (50%) of 16 patients in this series had had at least one previous carotid endarterectomy, and 5 (31%) of 16 had undergone at least one myocardial revascularization procedure.

COMPLICATIONS

Three complications occurred in our series, all the result of management errors. One patient bled from a subclavian anastomosis in the recovery room and developed massive bilateral neck swelling with acute compromise of the airway requiring emergency cricothyroidotomy. Bleeding was controlled, the anastomosis was properly redone, and the patient remained well for 5 years with a patent graft.

The second complication was a stroke 90

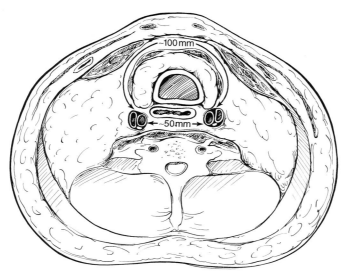

Fig. 9 Diagram of a cross section of the arch illustrating the shorter distance between both CCAs across the prevertebral space. (From Berguer R, Gonzalez JA. Revascularization by the retropharyngeal route for extensive disease of the extracranial arteries. J Vasc Surg 19:217-225, 1994.)

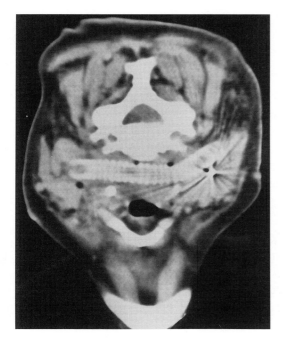

Fig. 10 CT scan of the neck showing a ringed graft across the retropharyngeal space.

minutes after the operation from an inappropriate dose of Labetalol given to control hypertension. The patient suffered a stroke in the hemisphere opposite the recipient artery where she had a chronic occlusion of the internal carotid artery.

The third complication occurred in a patient who underwent a multiple synchronous revascularization procedure consisting of a distal vertebral bypass, an external carotid angioplasty, and a retropharyngeal bypass to the contralateral external carotid artery. This bypass across the neck was done to an external carotid artery on the side where the internal carotid artery was occluded. On routine postoperative arteriography this patient was found to have an occluded retropharyngeal bypass graft, although the other reconstructions were patent. There were no symptoms from the occlusion. Clearly, this bypass to the external carotid artery was a superfluous operation and would have not been done today.

Figs. 11 and 12 show the primary patency and survival rates for these reconstructions. Two patients died during the follow-up interval—one from a cardiac event and the other from an unknown cause. Of the 16 living patients, all

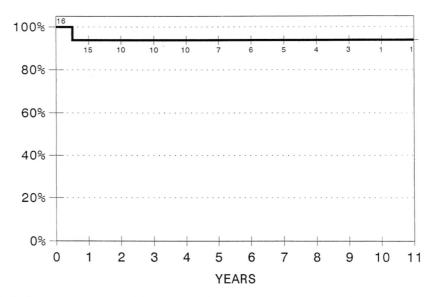

Fig. 11 Primary patency rate for 16 retropharyngeal bypasses. Numbers indicate patients at risk. (From Berguer R, Gonzalez JA. Revascularization by the retropharyngeal route for extensive disease of the extracranial arteries. J Vasc Surg 19:217-225, 1994.)

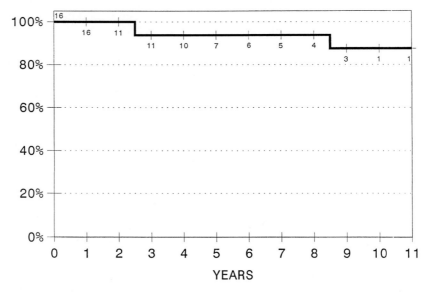

Fig. 12 Survival table for 16 patients undergoing retropharyngeal bypass. Numbers indicate patients at risk. (From Berguer R, Gonzalez JA. Revascularization by the retropharyngeal route for extensive disease of the extracranial arteries. J Vasc Surg 19:217-225, 1994.)

have patent grafts. It is interesting to note that there are two patients in the series with a retropharyngeal vein bypass to the external carotid artery placed as a first step to a superficial temporal artery to middle cerebral artery (STA-MCA) anastomosis. In both patients the retropharyngeal vein bypass and the STA-MCA anastomosis are patent after 8 and 6 years.

The primary patency rate for these retropharyngeal reconstructions has been 94%. Most surprising was the 87% survival in this group of high-risk patients. One is tempted to speculate that such a good survival rate in a patient population at high risk may be the result of the fact that their cerebrovascular reconstructions continue to be patent and one third of them underwent myocardial revascularization procedures.

REFERENCES

1. Berguer R. The short retropharyngeal route for arterial bypass across the neck. Ann Vasc Surg 1:127-129, 1986.
2. Berguer R, Gonzalez JA. Revascularization by the retropharyngeal route for extensive disease of the extracranial arteries. J Vasc Surg 19:217-225, 1994.
3. Hass WK, Fields WS, North RR, et al. Joint study of extracranial arterial occlusion. JAMA 203:961-968, 1968.

SECTION VII

Scientific Findings With Clinical Applications

This section includes chapters on the natural history of moderate carotid artery stenosis, a report on the etiology of paraplegia in thoracoabdominal aneurysm repair, and an update on reversal of atherosclerotic lesions and the natural history of iliac artery aneurysms. Other chapters examine the importance of genetic and biochemical factors in the practical management of aneurysms, present an update on the natural history of intermittent claudication and how to predict when it carries a dire prognosis, and stress the importance of bacteriology in determining the management of infected prosthetic arterial grafts. Also included are chapters that deal with the adaptation of vein grafts to arterialization and bleeding time as a predictor of early PTFE graft failure. Finally, a chapter that relates smoking and fibrinogen levels to vein graft failure appears in this section.

57

Natural History of Moderate Internal Carotid Artery Stenosis in Asymptomatic and Symptomatic Patients

DAVID S. SUMNER, M.D., M. ASHRAF MANSOUR, M.D., and MARK A. MATTOS, M.D.

The North American Symptomatic Carotid Endarterectomy Trial (NASCET)[1] and the European Carotid Surgery Trialists (ECST)[2] studies confirmed the high incidence of stroke in medically treated symptomatic patients with 70% to 99% stenosis of the internal carotid artery (26% at 2 years and 22% at 3 years, respectively). The stroke risk in symptomatic patients with 30% to 69% stenosis is currently under investigation by the NASCET group. In the nonsurgical arm of the Veterans Administration trial, 9.4% of asymptomatic patients with 50% to 99% internal carotid artery stenosis developed an ipsilateral stroke during an average follow-up period of 41 months.[3] Patients with medically managed 60% to 99% internal carotid artery stenosis in the Asymptomatic Carotid Atherosclerosis Study (ACAS) experienced an aggregate stroke risk of 11.0% over a 5-year period.[4] Other studies, however, have shown that the risk of stroke in the subgroup of asymptomatic patients with critically severe stenosis (80% to 99%) is appreciably higher (18% to 19% over a 2-year period).[5,6]

Although these studies provide information concerning the risk of stroke in symptomatic and asymptomatic patients with high-grade stenosis and in asymptomatic patients who present with moderate- to high-grade stenosis, none has specifically addressed the issue of stroke risk in patients with moderate (50% to 79%) internal carotid artery stenosis. Moreover, the effect of disease progression on the development of stroke in this group has been neglected.

Internal carotid artery stenosis in the 50% to 79% range is not uncommon. According to a duplex scan survey conducted by our laboratory at Southern Illinois University School of Medicine, approximately 4% of asymptomatic subjects over 60 years of age have lesions in this range.[7] Based on 1994 estimates, there are 43 million people in the United States in this age group, which means that approximately 1,700,000 people have disease of this magnitude. Moreover, 18% of the internal carotid arteries of patients undergoing arteriography in our institution have stenoses in the 50% to 79% range.

Several questions must be answered. First, is the stroke risk in patients with moderate stenosis less than that in patients with high-grade stenosis? Second, what is the incidence of disease progression and how does progression influence the incidence of stroke? Finally, what is the proper management of patients with moderate stenosis? This article summarizes the results of a retrospective study undertaken to answer these questions.[8]

METHODS

Over a 6-year period, our vascular laboratory registered 1727 patients with 50% to 79% stenosis of the internal carotid artery. Of these, 272 patients who had undergone serial color-flow duplex scans were identified. The average number of follow-up scans was 2.4 per patient (range, 2 to 11). The patients had been followed up for a mean period of 44 ± 15 months (range, 11 to 82 months) and follow-up data were complete in 99% of the subjects. At the time of the initial scan, 142 patients were asymptomatic, 43 had ill-defined nonhemispheric symptoms, and 87 had experienced transient ischemic attacks (TIAs), amaurosis fugax, or mild strokes (cerebrovascular accidents [CVAs]). The three groups did not differ with regard to age or gender distribution. All had the usual risk factors, and with the exception of peripheral vascular disease, which was significantly less frequent in the patients with nonhemispheric symptoms, and atrial fibrillation, which was less common in the asymptomatic patients, there were no major differences between the groups. Clinical end points were new TIAs (deficit lasting less than 24 hours) or CVAs (deficit lasting longer than 24 hours) and death. Patients were censored at the time of carotid endarterectomy.

INCIDENCE OF NEUROLOGIC EVENTS

During follow-up, 20 (23%) of the symptomatic patients (those presenting with TIAs or CVAs), seven (16%) of the patients with nonhemispheric symptoms, and 21 (15%) of the asymptomatic patients developed additional ipsilateral or contralateral localizing neurologic symptoms ($p = .28$). Ipsilateral localizing events (TIAs or CVAs) occurred in 15% of the initially symptomatic patients, 16% of the patients with nonhemispheric symptoms, and 10% of the asymptomatic patients. Ipsilateral strokes occurred in nine (10%) of the symptomatic patients and seven (5%) of the asymptomatic patients. Only one patient (2%) with nonhemispheric symptoms suffered a stroke and this occurred 5 years after entry into the study.

Life-table comparison of ipsilateral ischemic events showed a significantly ($p = .03$) higher cumulative rate in the symptomatic patients (20%) than in the asymptomatic patients (7%) at 2 years (Fig. 1). Cumulative ipsilateral event rates at 4 years were 34% ± 14%, 27% ± 10%, and 17% ± 6% for patients with nonhemispheric symptoms, symptomatic patients, and asymptomatic patients, respectively.

The 4-year cumulative ipsilateral stroke rate in the symptomatic patients was 23% ± 9%, while that in the asymptomatic group was considerably lower, 9% ± 5% (Fig. 2). Mean annual stroke rates were 5.7% and 2.3% in the symptomatic and asymptomatic patients, respectively. None of the patients with nonhemispheric symptoms experienced a stroke within 4 years of the initial study.

Cumulative death rates at 4 years were 37% in symptomatic patients, 40% in patients with nonhemispheric symptoms, and 27% in asymptomatic patients. Fifty percent of the deaths in symptomatic patients and 30% in the asymptomatic group were caused by stroke. Overall, cardiac disease was the most common cause of death (40%).

DISEASE PROGRESSION

Progression to severe stenosis or total occlusion occurred in 16% of the symptomatic patients and patients with nonhemispheric symptoms and in 17% of the asymptomatic patients. Intervals between the initial study and detection of progression were highly variable, ranging from 2 to 61 months (average, 20 ± 14 months) in those internal carotid arteries that developed 80% to 99% stenosis and from 3 to 55 months (average, 28 ± 15 months) in those that became totally occluded.

Two of 10 symptomatic patients whose lesions progressed to 80% to 99% stenosis experienced new TIAs at the time of progression. One of the four symptomatic patients who developed total occlusion suffered a stroke at the time of disease progression and another patient had a stroke after an initially asymptomatic period. No strokes occurred in the patients with nonhemispheric symptoms in conjunction with disease progression (four progressed to 80% to 99% stenosis and three progressed to total occlusion). One patient with nonhemispheric symptoms, however, experienced a TIA at the time of internal carotid artery occlusion.

Of the 21 asymptomatic patients who developed 80% to 99% stenosis, three had ipsilateral TIAs and four developed a stroke. One patient who had a stroke was asymptomatic at the time of progression and another had nonhemispheric symptoms. Two of the three patients whose internal carotid artery occluded suffered a stroke, one following an initially asymptomatic period. Overall, duplex scanning detected disease progression in 19 (79%) of the 24 asymptomatic patients before the artery occluded or the stroke occurred.

Tables 1 and 2 compare the neurologic event

Table 1 Effect of disease progression on incidence of total ipsilateral events (TIA plus CVA)

Initial symptom group	Progression*	Stable disease†	p value
Symptomatic	4 of 14 (29%)	9 of 73 (12%)	.21
Nonhemispheric	1 of 7 (14%)	6 of 36 (17%)	.99
Asymptomatic	9 of 24 (38%)	5 of 118 (4%)	<.0001

*Number of events/number of patients with disease progression.
†Number of events/number of patients with stable disease.

Table 2 Effect of disease progression on incidence of ipsilateral strokes

Initial symptom group	Progression*	Stable disease†	p value
Symptomatic	2 of 14 (14%)	7 of 73 (10%)	.63
Nonhemispheric	0 of 7 (0%)	1 of 36 (3%)	.99
Asymptomatic	6 of 24 (25%)	1 of 118 (1%)	.0001

*Number of strokes/number of patients with disease progression.
†Number of strokes/number of patients with stable disease.

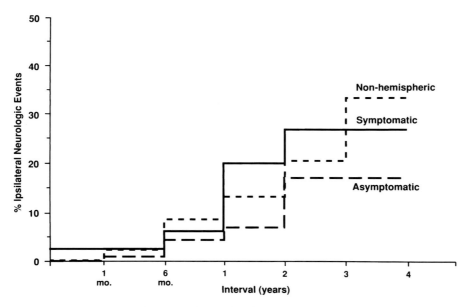

Fig. 1 Cumulative rates of new ipsilateral ischemic neurologic events (TIAs, amaurosis fugax, CVAs) for patients with moderate (50% to 79%) stenoses of the internal carotid artery. Patients are grouped according to their symptoms at initial examination. (From Mansour MA, Mattos MA, Faught WE, et al. The natural history of moderate [50% to 79%] internal carotid artery stenosis in symptomatic, nonhemispheric, and asymptomatic patients. J Vasc Surg 21:346-357, 1995.)

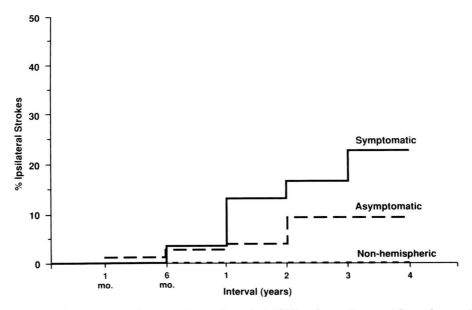

Fig. 2 Cumulative rates of new ipsilateral strokes (CVAs) for patients with moderate (50% to 79%) stenoses of the internal carotid artery. Patients are grouped according to their symptoms at initial examination. (From Mansour MA, Mattos MA, Faught WE, et al. The natural history of moderate [50% to 79%] internal carotid artery stenosis in symptomatic, nonhemispheric, and asymptomatic patients. J Vasc Surg 21:346-357, 1995.)

rates in patients with stable disease with those in patients with disease progression. Although total ipsilateral neurologic events (TIAs and CVAs) were more frequent in symptomatic patients with disease progression (29%) than in symptomatic patients with stable disease (12%), there was relatively little difference in the incidence of stroke (14% vs. 10%). In patients with nonhemispheric symptoms, the presence or absence of disease progression had even less effect on the incidence of ipsilateral neurologic events (14% vs. 17%). In asymptomatic patients, however, ipsilateral neurologic events occurred far more frequently ($p = .00002$) in patients with disease progression (38%) than in patients with stable lesions (4%). Although six (25%) of 24 initially asymptomatic patients with disease progression suffered a stroke, only one (0.9%) of 118 patients with stable disease developed a stroke ($p = .0001$).

RISK FACTORS

Stroke was statistically more frequent ($p = .02$) in symptomatic patients with six or more risk factors (29%) than it was in patients with five or less risk factors (7%). The number of risk factors had less impact on stroke incidence in asymptomatic patients (16% with six or more risk factors, 7% with five or less risk factors; $p = .15$).

MANAGEMENT OF PATIENTS WITH 50% TO 79% INTERNAL CAROTID ARTERY STENOSIS
Symptomatic Patients

Given the limitations of a retrospective review, this study suggests that although the risk of stroke is less in symptomatic patients with moderate (50% to 79%) stenosis than it is in patients with severely stenotic lesions,[1,2] the risk is still appreciable (approximately 6% per year). Patients in this category should be considered seriously for carotid endarterectomy, especially if they have multiple risk factors or advancing disease and the stroke/mortality rate of the surgeon performing the procedure is within advocated guidelines. The cumulative risk of stroke in the medically treated symptomatic patients with 50% to 79% stenosis was compared with that of a group of patients who underwent carotid endarterectomy for TIAs or mild stroke on our vascular surgical service[9] (Fig. 3). Based on this comparison, carotid endarterectomy is projected to confer a definite benefit by 2 years and a 16% stroke reduction rate by 4 years.

Asymptomatic Patients

Our results indicate that medically treated patients who are asymptomatic when they present with moderate internal carotid artery stenosis have a more benign prognosis. The average annual incidence of ipsilateral stroke was only 2.3%, approximately one third of that for patients with localizing symptoms. The 4-year cumulative risk of ipsilateral stroke in this series of asymptomatic patients was compared with that of patients who underwent carotid endarterectomy on our service for severely stenotic asymptomatic disease (Fig. 4).[9] Although a slight benefit is evident by 1 year, the projected stroke reduction rate at 4 years is only 5%. Moreover, six of the seven strokes in the medically treated asymptomatic patients occurred in association with disease progression. If these strokes are subtracted from the cumulative results, the benefits of surgery disappear.

Thus it is difficult to justify carotid endarterectomy in patients with stable asymptomatic 50% to 79% lesions because the apparent risk of stroke is less than 1% over an average follow-up period of 4 years. On the other hand, our results suggest that patients with advancing disease, who have a stroke risk of 25%, should be offered surgical therapy. That disease progression was detected in 79% of the patients in the current series before the internal carotid artery occluded or stroke occurred strongly supports a policy of routine duplex surveillance of asymptomatic patients with 50% to 79% internal carotid artery stenosis.

RELATED REPORTS

In a prospective follow-up study, Johnson et al.,[10] at the University of Washington, found a 7-year cumulative stroke rate of 11% and a 1.6% average annual incidence of stroke in medically treated patients who, at the time of the initial study, were symptom free and had 50% to 79% internal carotid artery stenosis. At 7 years, the cumulative rates of progression to 80% to 99% stenosis and to total occlusion were 27% and 20%, respectively, or approximately 15% and 11% at 4 years. Whereas strokes occurred in only one (1.6%) of 64 patients with stable disease, six (20%) of 30 patients with disease progression suffered a stroke. Except for a somewhat greater incidence of disease progression, these results are remarkably similar to our observations. Johnson et al.[10] concluded that a nonoperative course should be followed in asymptomatic patients with 50% to 79% internal carotid artery stenosis "... because the risk of stroke is so low and probably cannot be matched by operation when the perioperative complications are taken into account."

Although the Veterans Administration study reported equivalent stroke rates of approximately 9% in symptom-free patients with 50% to 75% and 76% to 99% internal carotid artery stenosis, these patients were not followed up for disease progression.[3] It is possible, therefore, that many of the initially moderate stenoses had progressed to a more severe category before strokes occurred.[10] The ACAS cumulative 5-year stroke rate of 11.0% in medically treated symptom-free patients with 60% to 99% stenosis was similar to our 9% 4-year rate for patients

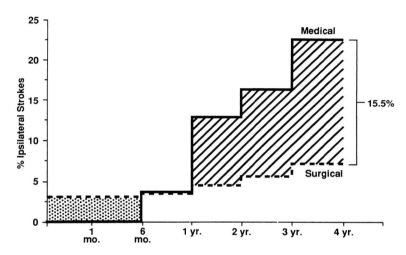

Fig. 3 Comparison of cumulative ipsilateral stroke rates of medically treated patients with symptomatic 50% to 79% internal carotid artery stenoses and ipsilateral stroke rates of symptomatic patients undergoing carotid endarterectomy. Stippled area indicates period in which medically managed patients have superior results and cross-hatched area represents period in which surgical management confers a beneficial effect.

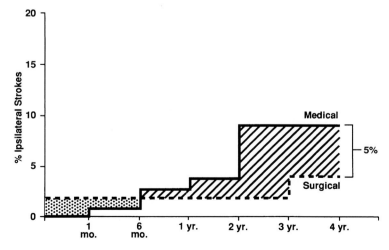

Fig. 4 Comparison of cumulative ipsilateral stroke rates of medically treated patients with asymptomatic 50% to 79% internal carotid artery stenoses and ipsilateral stroke rates of asymptomatic patients undergoing carotid endarterectomy. Stippled area indicates period in which medically managed patients have superior results and cross-hatched area represents period in which surgical management confers a beneficial effect.

with 50% to 79% stenosis.[4] Stroke rates, however, did not appear to correlate with the severity of stenosis; but again no information on disease progression was available.

CONCLUSION

The annual risk of stroke in our study of symptom-free patients presenting with 50% to 79% stenosis of the internal carotid artery was only 2%, whereas in symptomatic patients it was 6%. Over a mean period of 4 years, approximately 16% of the arteries progressed to high-grade stenosis or total occlusion. In symptomatic patients, disease progression had little influence on the incidence of stroke, but the incidence of stroke strongly correlated with the number of risk factors. The incidence of stroke in asymptomatic patients with disease progression was 25%, far higher than the 1% incidence in patients with stable disease. Moreover, color-flow duplex scanning detected disease progression in 79% of asymptomatic patients, before strokes or total occlusion occurred.

In conclusion, asymptomatic patients with moderate carotid artery stenosis do not require surgical intervention as long as their disease remains stable. However, they should have serial duplex scans to detect progression. Carotid endarterectomy should be offered to all asymptomatic patients who develop high-grade stenosis during follow-up and to all symptomatic patients with moderate disease with or without disease progression.

REFERENCES

1. North American Symptomatic Carotid Endarterectomy Trial Collaborators. Beneficial effect of carotid endarterectomy in symptomatic patients with high-grade carotid stenosis. N Engl J Med 325:445-453, 1991.
2. European Carotid Surgery Trialists' Collaborative Group. MRC European carotid surgery trial: Interim results for symptomatic patients with severe (70-99%) or with mild (0-29%) carotid stenosis. Lancet 337:1235-1243, 1991.
3. Hobson RW, Weiss DG, Fields WS, et al. Efficacy of carotid endarterectomy for asymptomatic carotid stenosis. N Engl J Med 328:221-227, 1993.
4. Executive Committee for the Asymptomatic Carotid Atherosclerosis Study. Endarterectomy for asymptomatic carotid artery stenosis. JAMA 273:1421-1428, 1995.
5. Moneta GL, Taylor DC, Nicholls SC, et al. Operative versus nonoperative management of asymptomatic high-grade internal carotid artery stenosis: Improved results with endarterectomy. Stroke 18:1005-1010, 1987.
6. Caracci BF, Zukowski AJ, Hurley JJ, et al. Asymptomatic severe carotid stenosis. J Vasc Surg 9:361-366, 1989.
7. Colgan MP, Strode GR, Sommer JD, et al. Prevalence of asymptomatic disease: Results of duplex scanning in 348 unselected volunteers. J Vasc Surg 8:674-678, 1988.
8. Mansour MA, Mattos MA, Faught WE, et al. The natural history of moderate (50% to 79%) internal carotid artery stenosis in symptomatic, nonhemispheric, and asymptomatic patients. J Vasc Surg 21:346-357, 1995.
9. Mattos MA, Hodgson KJ, Londrey GL, et al. Carotid endarterectomy: Operative risks, recurrent stenosis, and long-term stroke rates in a modern series. J Cardiovasc Surg 33:387-400, 1992.
10. Johnson BF, Verlato F, Bergelin RO, et al. Clinical outcome in patients with mild and moderate carotid artery stenosis. J Vasc Surg 21:120-126, 1995.

58

Natural History of Moderate Carotid Stenosis

D. EUGENE STRANDNESS, Jr., M.D., and BRIAN F. JOHNSON, M.D.

Although carotid bifurcation disease is a common cause of transient ischemic events and strokes, the time scale during which such lesions develop is largely unknown. It has also become fairly well established that it is high-grade stenoses that are of particular danger to the patient. The definition of "high grade" will depend on which study is referred to, but it would appear that lesions that narrow the carotid bulb by less than 50% are less dangerous than those that exceed that limit. Unfortunately, there were no uniform methods used for grading carotid artery lesions, even in the North American Symptomatic Carotid Endarterectomy Trial (NASCET)[1] and the European Carotid Surgery Trial (ECST).[2] In NASCET the internal carotid artery distal to the bulb was taken as the reference "normal" artery, whereas in ECST all the measurements were made from the bulb itself. This has a big effect (particularly for lower grade lesions) in calculating the degree of diameter reduction. For example, a 50% diameter-reducing stenosis in ECST is a 0% stenosis by NASCET criteria. This fact has led and continues to lead to confusion.

Since arteriography does not lend itself to long-term and repeat studies, some other form of evaluation is necessary. In addition, the results of the noninvasive test must provide information that is clinically relevant. There is only one method available at the moment that can fill this bill—ultrasonic duplex scanning. It is also important that the studies of natural history be done at intervals that are likely to permit detection of disease progression when it occurs.

Our own studies of the natural history of carotid disease were first published in 1984.[3] This study showed that it was asymptomatic patients with high-grade lesions (>80% diameter reduction) who were most likely to have an event—a transient ischemic attack (TIA), a stroke, or progression to occlusion of the internal carotid artery. In that first study it also appeared that less severe lesions (<79%) had a much more favorable prognosis. We have continued the study of 232 patients with these moderate to minimal lesions. The results of this study form the basis for this report.

MATERIALS AND METHODS

The long-term follow-up program began at our center in 1979. To qualify for entry into the study, patients had to fulfill the following criteria:
- The patient had to be asymptomatic, their lesion discovered by the presence of a neck bruit.
- The degree of carotid stenosis at the time of entry had to be ≤50% to 79%.
- The patient had had no previous carotid surgery.
- The patient was able to be followed at regular intervals.

For inclusion in this report, the patients had to have at least 180 days of follow-up. The method of study was ultrasonic duplex scanning using peak systolic velocity, end-diastolic velocity, and spectral broadening detected from the site of maximal narrowing. The categories of stenosis to be considered were these:
- Normal
- Less than 50% diameter-reducing stenosis
- 50% to 79% narrowing
- 80% to 99% stenosis
- Total occlusion

It should be noted that the original confirmation studies comparing duplex ultrasound with arteriography used measurements from the bulb, as in the ECST.[2] The follow-up studies were done at 6 months, 1 year, and annually thereafter. At the time of each visit, an extensive health history was taken. No attempt was made to influence treatment in reporting the ultrasound results to the patient's physician. For this analysis, follow-up was terminated if the patient

Table 1 Baseline degree of narrowing, sex distribution, and mean age (N = 232)

	Male age (no.)	Female age (no.)
Baseline disease		
Bilateral <50%	62 (78)	63 (60)
50%-79% and <50%	67 (45)	65 (25)
Bilateral 50%-79%	66 (13)	67 (11)
	(136)	(96)

Table 2 Status of carotid artery at entry

Worst side (%)	Least side (%)	No.
1-15	Normal	5
1-15	1-15	35
16-49	1-15	42
16-49	16-49	56
50-79	1-15	19
50-79	16-49	51
50-79	50-79	24

underwent operation but was continued for those who did not have surgery.

The outcome variables examined were progression of the degree of stenosis and its relationship (if any) to clinical outcome. The mean age, sex distribution, and baseline degree of narrowing in these patients is shown in Table 1. The status of the carotid arteries at the time of the patients' entry into the study are shown in Table 2.

RESULTS

The outcomes for this follow-up study were considered in the following categories.

Progression to 50% to 79% Stenosis. There were 138 patients with a <50% diameter-reducing lesion at entry. Of this group 25 progressed, which resulted in a cumulative progression rate of 21% at 7 years.

Progression to 80% to 99% Stenosis. During follow-up there were 24 patients who progressed to this level of narrowing. For this group there were 20 of 94 with a 50% to 79% lesion at entry and 4 of 138 with a <50% lesion who progressed during the follow-up after 7 years. The rate of progression for the 50% to 79% lesion was 26% ± 6% and 4% ± 3% for the <50% lesions ($p < .01$).

Progression to Total Occlusion. Ten patients during follow-up progressed to a total occlusion. None of these patients was in the <50% category at the time of entry. For those with an initial 50% to 79% lesion, the cumulative rate of progression was 20% after 7 years. The difference between these and the <50% lesions at entry was significant ($p < .01$).

Stroke

Twelve patients had strokes during follow-up. These can be considered in reference to the original findings and its relationship to what happened to these patients' lesions over time. It is important to remember that the strokes developed without prior warning. In addition, the degree of stenosis found at the time of study after the stroke was assumed to be a causative factor in its development. This may or may not be true.

Baseline Disease. Five of the patients who ultimately developed a stroke had a <50% diameter-reducing stenosis at the time of entry into the study. The other seven were in the 50% to 79% category.

Stroke Without Disease Progression. In four of the patients the stroke that occurred developed in the presence of a lesion that did not progress during follow-up. In three of the cases the lesions were in the <50% stenosis range. The strokes occurred at 31, 66, and 68 months after entry into the study. The remaining patient had a stable 50% to 79% lesion. The stroke in this patient developed after 102 months of follow-up.

Stroke With Disease Progression. In this group of eight patients, there were two who progressed from a <50% to a 50% to 79% lesion. There were four who progressed from a 50% to 79% lesion to a >80% stenosis. One of these was discovered at the time of the stroke, with the other three going on to total occlusion and stroke at 1, 2, and 27 months after the initial progression was discovered. There were two patients who at the time of stroke had progressed from a 50% to 79% stenosis to total occlusion without discovered intermediate progression to a 80% to 99% lesion.

Surgical Intervention. Carotid endarterectomy was performed in 27 patients (22 men and five women) 8 to 92 months after entering the study. The degree of stenosis at the time of operation is shown in Table 3. Only 5 (4%) of 138 patients whose initial lesion was <50% underwent endarterectomy, whereas 22 (24%) of 93 of the patients whose initial lesion was in the 50%

Table 3 Degree of stenosis at the time of operation

Operated lesion (%)	Year of follow-up							
	Y1	Y2	Y3	Y4	Y5	Y6	Y7	Y8
<50*	1	1						
50-79*	1	2	2	1	1		1	1
80-99	2	3	3†	1	3	1†	1	2

*Indicates that all patients in these groups were symptomatic.
†Indicates that one patient in each of these groups was symptomatic.

to 79% category underwent carotid surgery. All 11 patients with a <80% stenosis were symptomatic. In the 16 patients who were in the 80% to 99% group, only two had developed symptoms as the basis for operation. There were no deaths, but there was one disabling stroke (3.7%).

DISCUSSION

Some of the controversy surrounding carotid endarterectomy may have been settled. Based on the clinical trials that have reported their results, the one factor that appears to be predictive of outcome is the degree of stenosis. While NASCET and ECST both arrived at the conclusion that it was a 70% or greater diameter-reducing stenosis that was best treated by operation in symptomatic patients, the method used arteriographically to measure the degree of stenosis was entirely different.[1,2] The NASCET group used the internal carotid artery distal to the bulb as the reference (normal) artery, the ECST study used only the bulb itself. A 50% diameter-reducing stenosis in the ECST study would be a 0% stenosis in NASCET. The Veterans Administration Asymptomatic Trial used the method employed by NASCET.[4]

This difference has produced a great deal of confusion about what a 70% stenosis really is and how it should be measured. In our original validation trials of duplex scanning, we used the bulb itself as the only site of estimation. For the study reported here, we have continued to use the same, and the ultrasonic criteria proposed have not changed. Another positive factor in this study is that all studies were done by the same technologist (Ms. Jean Primozich). In our original study published in 1984, we pointed out that a >80% diameter-reducing stenosis was particularly dangerous and when found should be treated by endarterectomy. This policy was followed and continues to be followed in our service.

This is the only study that we are aware of that has been prospective or of this duration. At the time of each follow-up visit, a letter was sent to the treating physician without recommendations as to treatment— either medical or surgical. It is important to realize that none of the clinical trials has presented or will present us with any data on the effects of disease progression on outcome. The NASCET and ECST studies entered the patients at the time they were symptomatic.[1,2] In addition, during follow-up of both arms of the trials—surgery and medical therapy— we are not provided with any data on what changes took place in these patients that led to the events that occurred after randomization. For example, did the strokes that occurred happen with stable high-grade lesions or were they secondary to progression to total occlusion? It is unfortunate that the follow-up studies did not include high-quality duplex scans on a regular basis. These could have provided us with the type of progression data reported here.

Can the results of this study provide any guidelines for our practices? The following observations would appear to be appropriate. (1) Since the lesser lesions (<50%) are not operated on, it will be a rare patient who will sustain a stroke without disease progression. These lesions place the patient at some risk, which might be modified by the use of agents such as aspirin. (2) The patients who are at greatest risk are those that progress into the higher grade category. What do we do with patients who fall into the 50% to 79% group but are asymptomatic? The Veterans Administration trial would suggest that operation is superior to medical therapy for the prevention of TIAs and strokes when taken as combined events.[4] The inclusion of TIAs has been criticized as not being a good end point, since this event does not produce a permanent neurologic deficit at the time of its occurrence. However, it should be noted that in both NASCET and ECST, it was permissible to have a TIA as an entry finding for randomization. (3) The finding of a >80% diameter-reducing stenosis should, in our view, warrant serious consideration for operation.

The follow-up for repeat study can probably safely be done annually, but even then, some strokes will occur that cannot be avoided. However, it is our view that patients who have an occlusion on one side and a 50% to 79% stenosis on the other should be studied every 6 months if operation is not being offered. The risk to the patient with bilateral occlusions of the internal carotid artery is great enough to warrant an aggressive approach in our view.

REFERENCES

1. Beneficial effect of carotid endarterectomy in symptomatic patients with high-grade carotid stenosis. North American Symptomatic Carotid Endarterectomy Trial collaborators. N Engl J Med 325:445-463, 1991.
2. European Carotid Surgery Trialsts' Collaborative Group. MRC European carotid surgery trial: Interim results for symptomatic patients with severe (70-99%) or with mild stenosis. Lancet 337:1235-1243, 1991.
3. Roederer GO, Langlois YE, Jager KA, Primozich JF, Beach KW, Strandness DE Jr. The natural history of carotid arterial disease in asymptomatic patients with cervical bruits. Stroke 15:605-613, 1984.
4. Hobson RW, Weiss DG, Fields WS, et al. Efficacy of carotid endarterectomy for asymptomatic carotid stenosis. N Engl J Med 328:221-227, 1993.

59

Progress in Understanding the Etiology of Paraplegia in Thoracoabdominal Aneurysm Repair: Possible Remedies

G. MELVILLE WILLIAMS, M.D.

In adapting the techniques pioneered by Crawford et al.,[1] progress has been made in the management of patients with thoracoabdominal aneurysms. However, the mortality rate remains high (10%) and paraplegia occurs in 5% to 32% of patients with the most extensive disease. Multisystem organ failure and intraoperative bleeding largely because of the failure of tissues to retain sutures remain the leading causes of death. Paraplegia, although not the most common cause of morbidity, is certainly the one most feared by patient and surgeon alike, and its etiology remains unclear.

THE MECHANISM OF PARAPLEGIA

Although controversy exists regarding *specific* mechanisms of paraplegia, all experts in this field agree that spinal cord ischemia is, at the very least, the triggering event leading to paresis or paraplegia. If the spinal cord were not rendered ischemic at some point during these operations, there would be no paresis.

Anatomy of Spinal Cord Circulation

The spinal cord neurons are nourished by two fairly small posterior spinal arteries and a larger anterior spinal artery. These arteries originate high in the neck from branches of the vertebral artery and may have additional contributions from the costacervical or thyrocervical trunk. Intercostal and lumbar arteries provide a rich network of blood vessels supplying the musculature of the back. Careful and elegant dissections in human specimens generally disclose the existence of two or more radicular arteries that unite with the anterior spinal artery. Adamkiewicz[2] was the first to demonstrate the presence of a sizable contribution to the anterior spinal artery originating from the lower intercostal arteries or upper lumbar arteries. This is currently called the great radicular artery (GRA). A smaller radicular artery originates from upper intercostal vessels and this is termed the thoracic radicular artery. Finally, less well-defined blood vessels originating from the internal iliac or inferior mesenteric artery form a circular artery connecting the anterior and posterior spinal arteries at the terminal end of the spinal cord. It is also possible that some patients have their major intercostal arteries supplied by the internal mammary arteries. This is most likely to occur when mural thrombus slowly occludes the aortic orifices of the intercostal arteries.

Controversy continues regarding the importance of these various contributions because of the following indisputable facts: (1) the GRA is inconsistent in location, originating as a branch of an intercostal artery from T6 to T12 or a lumber artery from L1 to L2'; (2) the GRA is inconsistent in size and may be large or small[3]; (3) the GRA may be absent in patients with fusiform aneurysms and mural thrombus; (4) the thoracic radicular artery is sacrificed commonly without sequelae; and (5) anatomic circumstances account for the consistent observation that the greater the length of aorta repaired, the greater the risk of paresis.

Because of the inconsistencies in size, location, and presence, different investigators report almost divergent outcomes. A recent study from Houston emphasizes the importance of the lower thoracic intercostal arteries.[4] When technical problems did not allow attachment of *patent* intercostal vessels T11 through L1, paresis developed in five of eight patients. When none was patent or all were attached at this level, only 23% and 29%, respectively, of the patients were paretic ($p <.01$). However, the recent report by Acher et al.[5] emphasizes the importance of the blood supply at the terminal end of the spinal cord. These investigators treated 61 patients with cerebrospinal fluid (CSF) drainage and naloxone and did not implant any intercostal or lumbar vessels. All but one patient recovered without neurologic sequelae. In contrast, 11 of 49 patients, some of whom were treated with one or the other of their adjuncts but not both, suffered paresis or paralysis. The best explanation for these findings is that these adjuncts influenced intraoperative ischemia or its secondary effects. Once the inferior blood supply was restored, ischemia ceased. Although this inferior contribution does not appear to be significant in most patients undergoing infrarenal abdominal aneurysm repair, it may enlarge to compensate for the lack of intercostal arteries supplying patients with mural thrombus in descending thoracic aortic aneurysms.

Primary and Secondary Mechanisms

A distinction must be made between the immediate and delayed forms of paralysis or paresis. Patients who awaken unable to move their legs most likely have suffered intraoperative severe ischemia. Evidence to support this statement comes from results of animal experiments and from our experience in humans where spinal cord function was monitored by somatosensory and epidural evoked potentials. When these were lost rapidly (10 to 20 minutes) after aortic occlusion, one patients died before neuromuscular function was assessed and two awoke paraplegic.

It is the delayed form of paresis that emphasizes the importance of the secondary effects of ischemia. Although anastomotic failure may cause delayed paralysis, this is not common and some patients experiencing this complication have had no intercostal arteries attached. Why should a patient with normal lower extremity function become paretic 2 to 5 days later unless the secondary effects of ischemia are extremely significant and influence perfusions of the spinal cord watershed? Results of experiments in animals shed some light; for example, rabbits subjected to shorter periods of ischemia than those causing the immediate form of paralysis have delayed-onset paresis.[6] Consequently, it is likely that the first "hit" is operative ischemia and a variety of secondary causative factors combine to induce the injury.

Secondary Occurrences

Hypotension. In our experience, half of the patients with delayed paresis have had a hypotensive episode in close temporal relationship to the loss of neuromuscular function. In these patients spinal cord perfusion must have been borderline and the fall in pressure reduced perfusion below any compensatory mechanism.

"Overexcitation" Injury. This form of reperfusion injury is unique to the central nervous system.[7] During periods of ischemia, amino acids and other neurotransmitters accumulate. When receptors are expressed at reperfusion, the neurons are injured by overexcitation. The abundance of opiate receptors in the spinal cord has been well recognized, and it has been proposed that opiates and endorphins may contribute to spinal cord injury after trauma or periods of ischemia.[7] Acher et al.,[8] noticing the onset of paresis in two of their patients in association with morphine injections, inoculated both of them with naloxone and both recovered. This finding led them to begin using naloxone and CSF drainage during and for 1 or 2 days following repair of thoracoabdominal aneurysms. Their outcomes are the best reported and may represent a blockade of "excitotoxicity."

THERAPEUTIC STRATEGIES
Limiting Operative Ischemia

Atriofemoral bypass is a simple method that allows perfusion of the aortic segment distal to the site of cross-clamping. Additionally, the left ventricle can be unloaded easily and rapidly, and the use of nitrates, which are known to cause swelling of the central nervous system, can be avoided. Standard sensory evoked potential monitoring has proved to be reliable because the lower extremities are perfused and peripheral nerve conduction is unimpaired. Finally, a heat exchanger can be added to the circuit to accurately control body temperature.

Caution must be exercised when using this approach in patients with atherosclerotic disease of the iliac vessels and in those with aortic dissection. Preliminary arteriography is required to ensure that the viscera, kidneys, and descending thoracic aorta are well supplied through the lumen of the left common femoral artery. We have used this approach in more than 50 patients and have had no complications at the proximal inflow cannulation site in either the atrium or the aorta. However, we lost perfusion to the left leg in one patient who eventually required an above-knee amputation.

Knowledge of the site and size of the GRA also reduces ischemia. For this reason we continue to try to identify the GRA angiographically. When it is identified, we always anastomose the intercos-

Table 1 Application of theory: Recent outcome

Aneurysm type	No.	Deceased	Paraparesis	Walking
Crawford group 2	20	1	2	20
DeBakey type IIIB	10	1	0	10
TOTAL	30	2(6.6%)	2(6.6%)	28

tal pair and no others. When the GRA cannot be identified, we oversew the intercostal arteries if the aorta is diseased or if the vessel has been ruled out angiographically. As a consequence, when uncertainty exists we limit attachment to the unstudied large intercostal or upper lumbar arteries.

Intraoperative Monitoring

We have used motor and sensory evoked potentials to evaluate spinal cord function intraoperatively.[9] Under conditions of 30° to 32° C hyperthermia and sequential reconstruction, we have lost electrical conductivity *only* when the circulation to the legs has also been impaired, for example, during the final graft to aortic anastomosis. Interestingly, this is the time when circulation to the cord from the internal iliac system is reduced. Sensory evoked potentials have always returned after reperfusion. This type of monitoring provides assurance of spinal cord function and a real-time measure of successful revascularization.

Cerebrospinal Fluid Drainage

Thirty-one years ago, Blaisdell and Cooley[10] reported their experimental findings and advocated the use of CSF drainage to ameliorate the effects of high thoracic aortic cross-clamping. The rationale is straightforward. The effect of low inflow pressure and high CSF pressure is to reduce perfusion pressure throughout the spinal cord. By removing CSF, the low inflow pressure associated with cross-clamping is more likely to provide adequate prograde flow in the microcirculation.

Recent clinical reports, although still anecdotal, emphasize dramatically the importance of CSF drainage in patients with delayed-onset paresis. There are currently two reports involving three patients who underwent CSF drainage at the onset of delayed paresis. Large volumes of CSF were drained with complete recovery of neurologic function. This is welcome and badly needed information because it implies that spinal cord swelling within a confined space is important in the pathogenesis of the delayed form as well as the early form of paresis.

Clearly the best documentation of the value of CSF drainage is the report by Acher et al.[5] CSF drainage was necessary to reduce significantly the rates of paraplegia attending repairs of group 2 aneurysms from 26% to 5%. The same held true in our recent experience in that the only two patients among 30 who experienced neurologic deficits were those in whom catheters were nonfunctional intraoperatively. One of these patients had immediate and one had delayed-onset paresis. Fortunately, both have made a nearly complete recovery.

Hypothermia

Naslund et al.[6] presented convincing evidence in the rabbit that moderate hypothermia (30° C) not only ameliorated paralysis associated with 30 minutes of ischemia but eliminated the delayed form of paresis associated with shorter periods of spinal cord ischemia. Clinically profound hypothermic arrest has been used to repair complex arch and descending thoracic aortic aneurysms, and I have been unable to find a report of paraplegia in these patients. Naslund et al. simply allowed their patients' body temperatures to drift and reported low rates of neuromuscular deficit.

We have used a heat exchanger to reduce body temperature to 30° C.[11] After 37 uneventful cases, we encountered a sudden intractable ventricular tachycardia. This dysrhythmia was not controlled until full bypass was instituted and body temperature reached 36° C. The operation was completed without incident. We now lower the body temperature to 32° C and raise it to 37.5° C.

In conclusion, considering only the very highest risk patients (i.e., Crawford group 2 and DeBakey IIIB dissections; Table 1), I believe our approach is sound.

REFERENCES

1. Crawford ES, Crawford JL, Safi HJ, et al. Thoracoabdominal aneurysms: Pre-operative and intraoperative factors determining immediate and long-term results in 605 patients. J Vasc Surg 3:389-404, 1986.
2. Adamkiewicz A. Die Blutgefüsse Ves Menschlichen Rückernmorkes: Die Gefüsse der Ruckenmarksubstanz. Sitz Akad Wiss Wein Math Natur Kluss 84:469, 1882.
3. Williams GM, Perler BA, Burdick JF, et al. Angiographic localization of spinal cord blood supply and its relationship to postoperative paraplegia. J Vasc Surg 13:23-35, 1991.
4. Svensson LG, Hess KR, Coselli JS, Safi HJ. Influence of segmental arteries, extent, and atriofemoral bypass on postoperative paraplegia after thoracoabdominal aortic operations. J Vasc Surg 20:255-262, 1994.
5. Acher CW, Wynn MM, Hoch JR, et al. Combined use of cerebral spinal fluid drainage and naloxone reduces the risk of paraplegia in thoracoabdominal aneurysm repair. J Vasc Surg 19:236-248, 1994.
6. Naslund TC, Hollier LH, Money SR, et al. Protecting the ischemic spinal cord during aortic cross-clamping: The influence of anesthetics and hypothermia. Ann Surg 409-415, 1992.
7. Faden AI, Knoblach S, Mays C, Jacobs TP. Motor dysfunction after spinal cord injury is mediated by opiate receptors. Peptides 6:15-17, 1985.
8. Acher CW, Wynn MM, Archibald J. Naloxone and spinal fluid drainage as adjuncts in the surgical treatment of thoracoabdominal and thoracic aneurysms. Surgery 108:755-762, 1990.
9. Laschinger JC, Owen JH, Rosenbloom M, et al. Direct noninvasive monitoring of spinal cord function during thoracic aortic occlusion: Use of motor evoked potentials. J Vasc Surg 7:161-171, 1988.
10. Blaisdell FW, Cooley DA. The mechanism of paraplegia after temporary thoracic aortic occlusion and its relationship to spinal fluid pressure. Surgery 51:351-355, 1962.
11. Frank SM, Parker SD, Rock P, et al. Moderate hypothermia, with partial bypass and segmental sequential repair for thoracoabdominal aortic aneurysm. J Vasc Surg 19:687-697, 1994.

60

Update on Progress in the Reversal of Atherosclerotic Lesions

ALLAN D. CALLOW, M.D., Ph.D.

Apparently the first clinical evidence that atherosclerotic lesions might regress was provided by observations that the incidence of ischemic heart disease and death was transiently reduced during World War I in countries with severe dietary restrictions. The experience was repeated in World War II, especially in Norway and during the siege of Leningrad.[1-5]

The rationale for clinical trials to study the reversal of atherosclerosis is based on the premise that high lipid levels are associated with a high incidence of cardiovascular disease and on data showing that diet-induced hyperlipidemia in animal models is accompanied by lipid lesions in the arterial wall. A return to the animal's customary low-fat diet is followed by a decrease in these elevated lipid levels and by a reduction in the size of the induced fatty arterial lesions. All but a few animal lesions lack the two features particular to humans: (1) the development of a fibrous cap and (2) accumulation of connective tissue and extracellular matrix within the plaque. The human lesion consists of fatty streak formation, the atherosis, and collagen production, the sclerosis portion of the lesion. The hardened artery loses elasticity and displays reduced production of endothelium-derived relaxing factor (EDRF).[6] The potential for reversal of the sclerotic phase is much less than for the softer atheromatous stage, and when this phase is far advanced, with accompanying calcification, the possibility of reversal is probably nonexistent. Regression of fatty streak lesions and some fibrous lesions has been reported in several monkey models placed on a strict lipid-lowering diet. In spite of these observations, human atherosclerosis was considered to be irreversible, except when it was a consequence of drastic starvation such as that imposed by wartime deprivation and wasting disease. Surgery was the only accepted means of clinical management.

The reluctance to accept opposing viewpoints so often demonstrated in medicine is illustrated by the ignorance of and skepticism directed by the medical establishment against the report by Ost and Stenson[6] in 1967, which detailed the lessening of claudication and improvement in femoral arterial imaging in 31 patients treated with niacin, and was in direct contrast to the femoral computer densitometry artery imaging and autopsy calibration studies of Crawford et al.[7] at the University of Southern California and the Jet Propulsion Laboratory at the California Institute of Technology in 1977; animal model data showing regression of lesions because these lesions were of short duration were also dismissed.[8,9]

With the introduction of lipid-lowering drugs, clinical trials proliferated. In 1993 Klag et al.[10] demonstrated the importance of stabilizing the plaque even if no regression ensued. A total of 1017 men who were students at Johns Hopkins Medical School (mean age, 22 years) were followed for 27 to 42 years to determine their risk of developing cardiovascular disease. At entry the mean serum cholesterol level was 192 mg/dl. During a mean follow-up of 30.5 years, 125 cardiovascular disease events occurred, of which 97 were due to coronary heart disease. A difference in baseline serum cholesterol level of 36 mg/dl—the difference between the twenty-fifth and seventy-fifth percentiles of the baseline cholesterol level in the population—was associated with an increased risk of cardiovascular disease of 1.72, coronary disease of 2.01, and death from cardiovascular disease of 2.02. Furthermore, a difference in the baseline cholesterol level of 36 mg/dl was associated with a significantly increased risk of death of 1.64 before age 50 years.

Prevention of abrupt or gradual worsening of the threatening atherosclerotic lesion is of primary importance. Brown et al.[11] subscribe to the theory that lipid-lowering therapy prevents clinical events by the selective depletion of lipids or "regression" of a relatively small subgroup of lipid-rich plaques that are predisposed to ulceration, rupture, and hemorrhage. In the coronary circulation these are the lesions that account for the majority of clinical events, not the preocclusive stenosis lesion usually identified by vascular surgeons and neurologists as the most threatening in the carotid artery.

A large number of randomized lipid-lowering trials have been reported and many more are underway. The particulars vary but the components are comparable: lipid-lowering drugs, exercise, cessation of smoking, dietary restrictions, and usually repeat coronary arteriograms. End points are normally arteriographic evidence of regression and reduction in the incidence of myocardial events. Based on arteriographic findings, the results are disappointing. Changes in the percentage of stenosis over all the lesions measured per patient were clustered between 0.7% and 2.2%. In the Familial Atherosclerosis Treatment Study (FATS), in which event reduction was 80%, average estimates of disease severity per patient worsened.[12] The lesion progressed by approximately 3% among the control subjects and improved, that is, regressed, by 1% to 2% stenosis among the treated patients; these findings are disappointing and unimpressive by any standard. Expressed in terms of absolute change in arterial narrowing, the difference is miniscule. The minimum diameter of the lumen for control group lesions narrowed progressively by a per-patient average of –0.050 mm over 2.5 years. In the treated group lesions improved (regressed) by +0.024 mm for a treatment-induced difference of 0.074 mm or less than 0.1 mm. Recognizing and interpreting differences this small is taxing to even the sharpest eye.

More encouraging are results in terms of incidence of clinical events. These are usually identified as death, myocardial infarction, and unstable ischemia requiring revascularization. Reduction ranged from 35% to 80%.[12-14] It is estimated that in the coronary circulation not more than 5% of atherosclerotic lesions undergo spontaneous regression, amounting to as much as 10% of the original lesion. However, there is the strong perception that intensive lipid-lowering therapy does reduce the rate of progression approximately fourfold in mild and moderate lesions. This is not the case for advanced lesions.[11] The FATS[12] and the St. Thomas' Atherosclerosis Regression Study (STARS)[14] trials point out the seeming paradox: an average of 1% to 2% regression of stenosis in only 12% of all treated lesions was associated with a reduction of clinical events of 70% to 80%. Theoretically, reducing low-density lipoprotein may lessen the possibility of plaque rupture by decreasing plaque instability. Plaque rupture, fissuring, fracture, and intraplaque hemorrhage all contribute to the conversion of an asymptomatic plaque to a symptomatic one. Foam cell density, the size of the core lipid pool, and "possible cytotoxicity from oxidized low-density lipoprotein"[11] are factors that lessen the stability of the plaque. Plaque size or volume is less a factor in plaque stability and subsequent rupture than plaque composition. Tensile strength of a plaque, its ability to resist hemodynamic stresses that are most marked at branch sites and where most plaques rupture, is affected by proteolysis. Proteolytic enzymes and matrix modulators such as plasminogen activator, urokinase, stromelysin, elastases, and heparinases are now being identified as being released locally by macrophages and other inflammatory cells.[15]

For symptomatic patients the recommended low-density lipoprotein level is 80 mg/dl and the total cholesterol level is 100 mg/dl, values that require a treatment regimen that is extremely difficult to maintain and is rarely achieved without lipid-lowering medication.[16] The Monitored Atherosclerosis Regression Study (MARS) was the first angiographic trial to test the effects of single-drug therapy: the 3-hydroxy-3-methylglutaryl coenzyme A reductase inhibitor lovastatin.[17] Regression was 23% in the lovastatin group compared to 12% in the control group. In the multinational pravastatin study, over a patient observation period of 78 weeks, 16 cases of myocardial infarction or unstable angina occurred vs. two such cases in the pravastatin-treated group. This rapid reduction in clinical events in so short a time, and without a concomitant reduction in atheromatous mass, raises many questions about mechanisms.[18] Most of these questions revolve around the observation that endothelial cell dysfunction occurs in the presence of hyperlipidemia. Endothelial-dependent vasomotor mechanisms are impaired in the atherosclerotic vessel. Endothelial dysfunction is now recognized as one of the earliest and most critical events in atherogenesis.[19] A limited number of human studies have shown that endothelial-dependent relaxation can be restored in association with regression of atherosclerotic lesions.[12,16,20-22] As pointed out by Loscalzo,[23] the benefits of lowering lipid levels with regard to clinical outcome in these patients may not be related solely to the direct regression of lesions but rather to improvements in vascular function—for example, improved endothelial function or a decreased propensity for plaque activation and rupture—for which lesion regression is simply a marker.

The effect of lipid-lowering regimens has been the object of several studies. Utilizing B-mode ultrasonography, the mean maximum far wall intima-medial thickness (IMT) was measured in 919 asymptomatic men and women, 40 to 79 years of age, with early carotid atherosclerosis as defined by B-mode ultrasonography and low-density lipoprotein cholesterol between the sixtieth and ninetieth percentiles. Lovastatin (20 to 40 mg/dl) or its placebo was evaluated in a double-blind randomized clinical trial with factorial design along with warfarin (1 mg/dl) or its placebo. Low-density lipoprotein cholesterol fell 28%, from 156.6 mg/dl at baseline to 113.1 mg/dl at 6 months ($p < .0001$), in the lovastatin-treated groups and was largely unchanged in the lovastatin placebo groups. Among participants receiving warfarin, regression of the mean maximum IMT was seen after 12 months in the lovastatin group compared with the placebo group. The 3-year difference was statistically significant[24] (Figs. 1-4).

The laboratory experimental effort that is underway in the United States and abroad is as impressive as these clinical trials. With increasing frequency, imaginative and thoughtful attempts to halt the atherosclerosis lesion and its consequences are being reported. Molecular biology and molecular genetics are in the forefront. The single-bullet approach is hardly likely to be of much benefit, given the fact that atherosclerosis is a multifactorial disease. Aiming for effective treatment and effective measures for prevention may be like aiming at a moving target. As one risk factor is brought under control, another one, previously unrecognized because it is masked by the power of the first, may become evident. Blankenhorn and Hodis[25] remind us that the florid atherosclerosis of the sinus of Valsalva secondary to tertiary syphilitic aortitis seen prior to World War II commonly produced myocardial infarction and aortic aneurysms. Widespread penicillin treatment caused these advanced forms of atherosclerosis to dis-

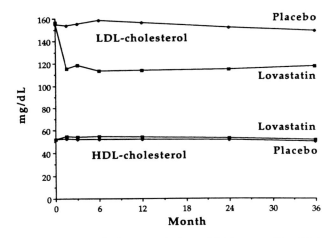

Fig. 1 Graph showing temporal characteristics of intima-media thickness change with colestipol-niacin therapy and placebo over a 48-month period in the CLAS study. (From Blankenhorn DH, Hodis HN. Arterial imaging and atherosclerosis reversal. George Lyman Duff Memorial Lecture. Arterioscler Thromb 14:189, 1994.)

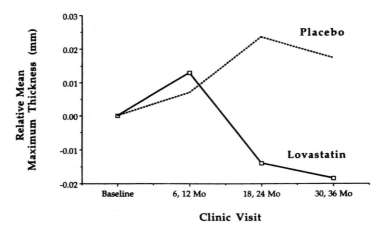

Fig. 2 Graph showing cross-sectional intima-media thickness for the lovastatin and placebo groups, excluding participants assigned to warfarin. (From Furberg CD, Adams HP Jr, Applegate WB, et al. Effect of lovastatin on early carotid atherosclerosis and cardiovascular events for the Asymptomatic Carotid Artery Progression Study [ACAPS]. Circulation 90:1684, 1994.)

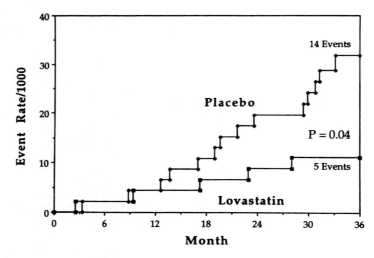

Fig. 3 Graph showing incidence of fatal and nonfatal cardiovascular disease by treatment group. (From Furberg CD, Adams HP Jr, Applegate WB, et al. Effect of lovastatin on early carotid atherosclerosis and cardiovascular events for the Asymptomatic Carotid Artery Progression Study [ACAPS]. Circulation 90:1684, 1994.)

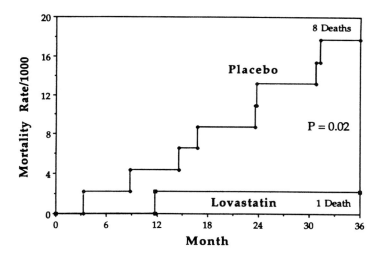

Fig. 4 Graph showing all-cause mortality rates by treatment group. (From Furberg CD, Adams HP Jr, Applegate WB, et al. Effect of lovastatin on early carotid atherosclerosis and cardiovascular events for the Asymptomatic Carotid Artery Progression Study [ACAPS]. Circulation 90:1685, 1994.)

appear. More recently, the MARS and the Cholesterol-Lowering Atherosclerosis Study (CLAS), with their intensive lipid-lowering regimens, demonstrated that when the low-density lipoprotein cholesterol was controlled as a risk factor, triglyceride-rich lipoprotein rose to the fore as a more important risk factor in the progression of the lesion. In all probability the same phenomenon will be repeated when smoking prevalence is reduced, diminishing its strength as a risk factor for atherogenesis.

REFERENCES

1. Malmros H. The relation of nutrition to health: A statistical study of the effect of wartime on arteriosclerosis, cardiosclerosis, tuberculosis and diabetes. Acta Med Scand (Suppl) 246:137-150, 1950.
2. Strom A, Jensen RA. Mortality from circulatory diseases in Norway 1940-1945. Lancet 1:126-129 1951.
3. Brozek J, Wells S, Keys A. Medical aspects of semistarvation and Leningrad siege (1941-1942). Am Rev Soviet Med 4:790, 1946.
4. Schettler G. Cardiovascular diseases during and after World War II: A comparison of the Federal Republic of Germany with other European countries. Prev Med 8:581, 1979.
5. Aschoff L. Lectures in Pathology. New York: Hoeber, 1924.
6. Ost RC, Stenson S. Regression of peripheral atherosclerosis during therapy with high doses of nicotinic acid. Scand J Clin Lab Invest 99:241-245, 1967.
7. Crawford DW, Brooks SH, Selzer RH, et al. Computer densitometry for angiographic assessment of arterial cholesterol content and gross pathology in human atherosclerosis. J Lab Clin Med 89:378-392, 1977.
8. Armstrong ML, Warner ED, Connor WE. Regression of coronary atheromatosis in rhesus monkeys. Circ Res 27:137-150, 1967.
9. Vesselinovitch D, Wissler RW, Fisher-Dzoga K, et al. Regression of atherosclerosis in rabbits. I. Treatment with low-fat diet, hyperoxia and hypolipidemic agents. Atherosclerosis 19:259-275, 1974.
10. Klag MJ, Ford DE, Mead LA, et al. Serum cholesterol in young men and subsequent cardiovascular disease. N Engl J Med 328:318, 1993.
11. Brown BG, Zhao Z-Q, Sacco DE, et al. Lipid lowering and plaque regression: New insights into prevention of plaque disruption and clinical events in coronary disease. Circulation 87:1781-1791, 1993.
12. Brown BG, Albers JJ, Fisher LDF, et al. Regression of coronary artery disease as a result of intensive lipid lowering therapy in men with high levels of apolipoprotein B (Familial Atherosclerosis Treatment Study [FATS]). N Engl J Med 323:1289-1298, 1990.
13. Kane JP, Malloy MJ, Ports TA, et al. Regression of coronary atherosclerosis during treatment of familial hypercholesterolemia with combined drug regimens (UC-SCOR). JAMA 264:3007-3012, 1990.
14. Watts GF, Lewis B, Brunt JNH, et al. Effects on coronary artery disease of lipid-lowering diet, or diet plus cholestyramine, in the St. Thomas' Atherosclerosis Regression Study (STARS). Lancet 339:563-569, 1992.
15. Unemori EN, Bouhana KS, Werb Z. Vectorial secretion of extracellular matrix proteins, matrix-degrading proteinases, and tissue inhibitor of metalloproteinases by endothelial cells. J Biol Chem 265:445-451, 1990.
16. Cashin-Hemphill L, Mack WJ, Pogoda MJ, et al. Beneficial effects of cholesterol-niacin therapy on coronary atherosclerosis (CLAS-II). JAMA 264:3013-3017, 1990.
17. Blankenhorn DH, Azen SP, Kramsch DM, et al. The Monitored Atherosclerosis Regression Study (MARS): Coronary angiographic changes with lovastatin therapy. Ann Intern Med 119:969-976, 1993.

18. The Pravastatin Multinational Study Group for Cardiac Risk Patients: Effects of pravastatin in patients with serum total cholesterol levels from 5.2 to 7.8 mmol/L (200-300 mg/dl) plus two other additional atherosclerotic risk factors. Am J Cardiol 782:1031-1037, 1993.
19. Harrison DG, Armstrong ML, Freiman PC, et al. Restoration of endothelium-dependent relaxation by dietary treatment of atherosclerosis. J Clin Invest 80:1808-1811, 1987.
20. Kramsch DM, Blankenhorn DH. Regression of atherosclerosis: Which components regress and what influences their reversal. Wien Klin Wochenschr 104:2-9, 1992.
21. Creager MA, Cooke JP, Mendelsohn ME, et al. Impaired vasodilation of forearm resistance vessels in hypercholesterolemic humans. J Clin Invest 86:228-234, 1990.
22. Dzau VJ. Pathobiology of atherosclerosis and plaque complications. Am Heart J 128:1330-1304, 1994.
23. Loscalzo J. Regression of coronary atherosclerosis [editorial]. N Engl J Med 323:1337-1339, 1990.
24. Furberg CD, Adams HP Jr, Applegate WB, et al. Effect of lovastatin on early carotid atherosclerosis and cardiovascular events for the Asymptomatic Carotid Artery Progression Study (ACAPS). Circulation 90:1679-1687, 1994.
25. Blankenhorn DH, Hodis HN. Arterial imaging and atherosclerosis reversal. George Lyman Duff Memorial Lecture. Arterioscler Thromb 14:177-192, 1994.

61

Natural History of Iliac Artery Aneurysms: When Should They Be Treated?

PETER F. LAWRENCE, M.D., and JOSE C. ALVES, M.D.

The management of aneurysms of the iliac artery has an illustrious history. The first surgical procedure involving an iliac artery aneurysm was performed by Sir Ashley Cooper in 1817, and the first successful ligation of an aneurysm of the common iliac artery was described by Valentine Moll in 1827. In 1913 McLaren successfully ligated an internal iliac aneurysm secondary to postpartum trauma. Rudolph Matas performed the first successful ligation of the aorta for an associated aortoiliac aneurysm in 1923. Since the 1950s, when prosthetic vascular grafts were developed, arterial aneurysms have been repaired by the graft inclusion technique. Endovascular techniques have been recently reported for repairing iliac aneurysms.

Iliac artery aneurysms occur much less frequently than aortic aneurysms, with isolated iliac aneurysms comprising 1% of the abdominal aortic aneurysm (AAA) incidence; yet they are potentially more lethal because of their deep location in the pelvis. They are difficult to palpate or diagnose even when they rupture, leading to a high mortality rate. Isolated iliac artery aneurysms are usually degenerative or atherosclerotic in etiology (80% to 90%). The remainder are secondary to trauma, caused by fungus, develop postpartum, result from infection, and, rarely, occur as congenital anomalies or as a result of Marfan's syndrome, Ehlers-Danlos syndrome, Takayasu's syndrome, Kawasaki disease, cystic medial necrosis, and spontaneous dissection. Isolated iliac aneurysms are usually asymptomatic (50%) and occur mostly in older patients (during the sixth or seventh decade of life) with a male-female ratio of 6-7:1. There are no large prospective studies describing the natural history of isolated iliac aneurysms; however, indications for surgical repair are well described in many small retrospective series.

There are five types of aneurysms involving the iliac arteries: aortoiliac, common iliac, internal iliac, and external iliac artery aneurysms, and iliac arteriomegaly (Fig. 1). The percentages shown in Fig. 1 correspond to the average incidence of each iliac aneurysm.

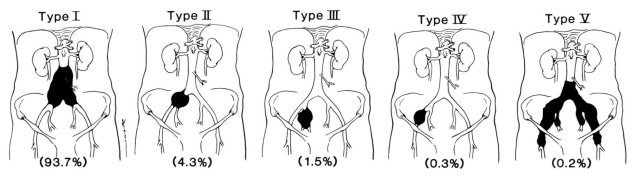

Fig. 1 There are five types of aneurysms involving the iliac arteries. Aortic aneurysm associated with iliac artery aneurysm (type I) represents the largest proportion. The other types represent a small percentage when compared with the incidence of aortoiliac aneurysms.

Table 1 Size criteria for iliac artery aneurysm repair

	Normal diameter (cm)		Aneurysm (cm)	
	Male	Female	Male	Female
Aorta	1.41-2.0	1.19-1.87	>2.6	>2.3
Common iliac artery	1.17-1.23	0.97-1.02	>1.8	>1.5
Internal iliac artery	0.54	0.54	>0.8	>0.8
External iliac artery	0.8	0.6-0.7	>1.2	>1.0

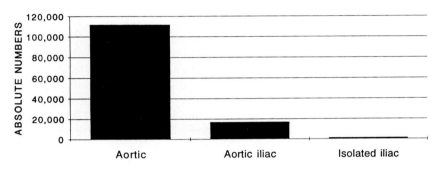

Fig. 2 Number of diagnosed aneurysms per year. In a large epidemiologic study by Lawrence et al.,[3] the estimated number of aortic aneurysms diagnosed in the United States per year is 111,580; aortoiliac aneurysms is 16,737; and isolated iliac aneurysms is 1,115.

SIZE CRITERIA FOR ILIAC ARTERY ANEURYSMS

The Subcommittee on Reporting Standards on Arterial Aneurysms[1] defined an aneurysm as "a permanent localized (i.e., focal) dilation of an artery having at least a 50% increase in diameter compared to the expected normal diameter of the artery in question." Using CT scan for measurement, the range of normal diameter of the common iliac artery in male adults is 1.17 to 1.23 cm (SD = 0.20 cm) (Table 1). The female diameter is 0.97 to 1.02 cm (SD = 0.15 to 0.19 cm). Using arteriography for measurement, the normal diameter for internal iliac arteries in male and female adults is 0.54 cm (SD = 0.15 cm) and for external iliac arteries in male and female adults is 0.8 cm and 0.6 to 0.7 cm, respectively. Consequently, for the average patient, iliac arteries become aneurysmal when the common iliac artery is greater than 1.8 cm in males and greater than 1.5 cm in females; the internal iliac artery is greater than 0.8 cm for both sexes; and the external iliac artery is greater than 1.2 cm in males and greater than 1.0 cm in females. However, most clinical reports define an iliac aneurysm as greater than 2.5 cm in diameter. Another method to determine whether an aneurysm is present is to compare the dilated portion to a normal-sized proximal or distal artery. Even though an arterial dilatation fulfills the criteria for an aneurysm, repair may not be indicated until the aneurysm reaches a larger size and the risk of rupture exceeds the risk of therapy.

AORTOILIAC ANEURYSMS

Iliac artery aneurysms that coexist with infrarenal aortic aneurysms are the most common form of iliac aneurysms.[2] Some authors have reported that up to 40% of patients with AAA have iliac involvement as well; however, a large epidemiologic study[3] indicated that there are approximately 110,000 aortic aneurysms diagnosed per year in the United States, and an additional 17,000 patients with aortoiliac aneurysms, and approximately 1100 with isolated iliac aneurysms (Fig. 2). These studies indicate that aortoiliac aneurysms comprise 10% to 20% of aortic aneurysms. Usually the iliac component is asymptomatic, and indications for repair are similar to those for AAAs without iliac involve-

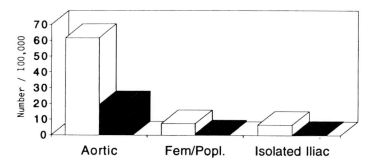

Fig. 3 Incidence of aneurysms in hospitalized patients. In these patients, aortic aneurysms occur eight times more frequently than femoropopliteal and isolated iliac aneurysms, and the incidence in men is much higher than that in women.

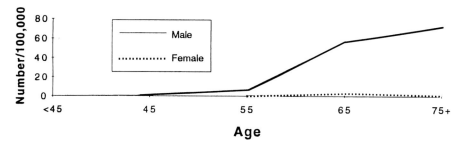

Fig. 4 Isolated iliac artery aneurysms present the same age-specific rates as aortic aneurysms, and the incidence increases significantly when men reach 55 years of age.

ment. Long-term follow-up of AAA repair at Mayo Clinic showed an extremely low incidence of delayed iliac aneurysm formation following tube or bifurcated graft.[4] Provan et al.[5] performed periodic abdominal ultrasound examinations 3 to 5 years postoperatively in 23 patients with tube grafts for AAA. Nine iliac arteries that were enlarged from 1.5 to 3.0 cm at the time of AAA repair remained stable in size. Based on available data, late development of iliac aneurysms after tube graft repair for AAA does not appear to be a major clinical concern as long as the iliac component is less than 3 cm. However, young patients with a long life expectancy should have all aneurysmal disease corrected, including iliac dilatation.

ISOLATED ILIAC ARTERY ANEURYSMS
Incidence

Autopsy studies and clinical reports of isolated iliac aneurysms vary greatly in reported incidence, risk of rupture, and mortality. Brunkwall et al.[6] found seven cases of isolated iliac aneurysms in 26,251 hospital autopsies over a 15-year period for an incidence of 0.03%, including one ruptured iliac aneurysm. Richardson and Greenfield[7] reported that 2.2% of all intraabdominal aneurysms are isolated iliac aneurysms. Minato et al.[8] reported a relative incidence of isolated iliac aneurysms to AAA of 11.7%. In a report of hospitalized patients by Lawrence et al.,[3] the male and female incidence of isolated iliac artery aneurysms in the United States is 6.58/100,000 and 0.26/100,000 per year, respectively (Fig. 3). Additionally, iliac artery aneurysms show the same age-specific rate curve as aortic aneurysms with a marked increase in the slope after 55 years of age, predominantly in men (Fig. 4).

Risk of Rupture

Because isolated iliac artery aneurysms are located in the pelvis, many patients remain undiagnosed until rupture. Based on clinical series, it is reasonable to assume that there is a

Table 2 Isolated iliac aneurysms: Risk of rupture

Author	Mean diameter (cm)	Ruptured (%)
Richardson and Greenfield[7]	5.5	33
Lowry and Kraft[2]	7.5	75
McCready et al.[9]	8.2	58
Schuler and Flanigan[10]	8.5	69

Table 3 Symptoms and physical findings in patients with iliac aneurysms

Symptom or physical finding	Percent
Asymptomatic	50
Gastrointestinal and/or genitourinary symptoms	20-30
Neurogenic symptoms (femoral, obturator, sciatic nerve)	20
Palpable abdominal or rectal mass	35-90 (most ≥70%)
Compression/erosion	30
Lower extremity edema	5
Perianal ecchymosis	Rare
Anal sphincter paralysis	Rare

correlation between size of aneurysm and risk of rupture (Table 2). Lowry and Kraft[2] reported that 75% of their patients presented with ruptured aneurysms with a mean arterial diameter of 7.5 cm. Most studies show a high incidence of ruptured iliac aneurysms. Richardson and Greenfield[7] reported a 33% incidence of rupture; the mean diameter of ruptured iliac aneurysms was 5.5 cm and the smallest aneurysm to rupture was 3.5 cm. It is extremely uncommon for iliac aneurysms smaller than 3 cm to rupture. Like AAAs, iliac aneurysms tend to enlarge predictably with an estimated average expansion rate of 4 mm/yr.[10] The frequency of rupture is similar for common and internal iliac aneurysms, although aneurysms in the common iliac artery occur more often.

Distribution

Seventy percent of isolated iliac aneurysms occur in the common iliac artery (Fig. 5). The reason for this predilection is unknown.[11] Twenty-five to twenty-eight percent of iliac aneurysms are situated in the internal iliac artery.

Multiplicity of iliac artery aneurysms has been reported to range from 30% to 67%, and in 23% of the patients they are bilateral. When iliac aneurysms are single, they are most likely to involve the hypogastric artery, whose anatomic location within the pelvis contributes to late recognition. In the series of Richardson and Greenfield,[7] 12 out of 72 iliac aneurysms involved the internal iliac artery and had a mean diameter of 7.7 cm, although the incidence of rupture was the same as for common iliac artery aneurysms. External iliac aneurysms are rare, occurring in 2% to 5% of isolated iliac aneurysms.

Signs and Symptoms

Half of patients with iliac aneurysms present with symptoms or physical findings related to the aneurysm (Table 3) and symptoms are almost always present in clinical reports of hypogastric artery aneurysms. One third of patients complain of lower abdominal pain, often associated with genitourinary symptoms. One fifth present with gastrointestinal symptoms, 15% have both genitourinary and gastrointestinal symptoms, and 20% develop neurogenic symptoms as a result of compression of the femoral, obturator, or sciatic nerves. Marked leg swelling and congestive heart failure can develop from spontaneous rupture of an iliac artery aneurysm into the adjacent vein, producing an arteriovenous fistula. Renal failure caused by obstruction of the ureter or bladder, ileus resulting from compression of the sigmoid colon or rectum, and ilioenteric fistulas have also been reported.[12]

The average incidence of palpable abdominal or rectal mass prior to rupture is 55%. Five percent of patients present with lower extremity edema resulting from venous compression. Perianal ecchymosis caused by dissection of blood through the retroperitoneal space and anal sphincter paralysis have been reported after rupture of iliac aneurysms but are exceedingly rare. Iliac aneurysms may present with distal embolization, although emboli have not been reported in most series of iliac aneurysm.

Diagnosis

In addition to clinical presentation and physical examination, iliac aneurysms are diagnosed by ultrasound, CT, MRI, and arteriography. There are no large series comparing these different methods for iliac aneurysm diagnosis.

Table 4 Iliac aneurysm results

Author	No.	Elective	Size (cm)	Emergent	Size (cm)	Elective mortality (%)	Ruptured mortality (%)
Lowry and Kraft[2]	8	2	?	6	?	7	52
Minato et al.[8]	16	8	7.0	5	?	0	50
Brunkwall et al.[6]	4	1	?	3	?	0	33
McCready et al.[9]	50	16	4.7	11	8.1	0	57
Richardson and Greenfield[7]	55	26	5.5	18	10.7	11	33
Nachbur et al.[13]	53	38	?	15	?	0	20

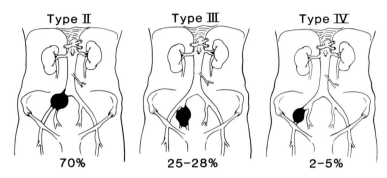

Fig. 5 Distribution of aneurysms. Most isolated iliac artery aneurysms occur in the common iliac artery. Aneurysms of the internal iliac artery have one third the incidence and are lethal because of their deep location. External iliac aneurysms are extremely rare.

Ultrasound, CT, and MRI have the advantage of showing the outer diameter of the vessel and are more accurate in evaluating aneurysm size than arteriography. Although less expensive, ultrasound has the disadvantage of being operator dependent, and intra-abdominal gas may cause difficulty visualizing the internal iliac arteries deep in the pelvis. There is general agreement that arteriography is useful in planning elective repair of iliac aneurysms in the patient who presents with associated lower extremity occlusive disease or to assess the pelvic circulation. CT scan is the technique of choice for detecting enlargement of iliac aneurysms[13] and accurately detects aneurysm leak.

Indications for Treatment

Based on available data, all patients in satisfactory health with isolated iliac artery aneurysms greater than 3 cm in diameter should undergo repair. Asymptomatic fusiform aneurysms less than 3 cm in diameter should be followed conservatively with periodic CT examination. All symptomatic patients need immediate repair, and saccular aneurysms should be repaired regardless of their size as should iliac artery aneurysms presenting with peripheral emboli.

Mortality

Rupture is an important factor determining survival. Mortality with rupture has been consistently reported to be high (Table 4), ranging from 20% to 57%,[9] whereas the mortality rate ranges from 0% to 11% (mean, 3%) when isolated iliac aneurysms undergo elective repair. These data show the importance of clinical suspicion in detecting and repairing iliac aneurysms electively. Nachbur et al.[13] reported a 70% 5-year survival following elective iliac aneurysm repair.

ILIAC ARTERIOMEGALY

Arteriomegaly is defined as "diffuse, nonfocal arterial enlargement involving several arterial segments, with an increase in diameter of greater than 50% by comparison to the expected normal diameter."[1] Reviewing 5771 consecutive aortofemoral angiograms, Hollier et al.[14] reported a 1.6% incidence of patients that met the criteria for arteriomegaly. Out of 430 aneurysms (91 patients), 10 involved the common iliac artery, four involved the internal iliac artery, and one involved the external iliac artery. Because arteriomegaly is rare, there are few data showing the natural history of this disease; surgical repair is indicated in most patients with an aneurysm greater than 3 cm in diameter but is associated with higher morbidity and mortality than surgical treatment of isolated aneurysms.

CONCLUSION

Isolated iliac artery aneurysms are rare, comprising 1% of AAAs; they predominate in men and are often asymptomatic. Iliac aneurysms are usually degenerative in etiology and associated with a high incidence of rupture and mortality if they enlarge (>3 cm) and are not repaired electively. Iliac aneurysms are difficult to palpate and to diagnose because of their deep anatomic location. The best method for detecting and sizing an iliac artery aneurysm is a CT scan. Arteriography is used when occlusive disease is present or if the pelvic circulation needs to be assessed. Asymptomatic fusiform aneurysms less than 3 cm in diameter should be followed with periodic CT scan evaluations, and iliac artery aneurysms greater than 3 cm should be repaired. All patients with symptoms, saccular aneurysms, or distal embolization require surgical repair regardless of the size of the aneurysm.

REFERENCES

1. Subcommittee on Reporting Standards for Arterial Aneurysms, Ad Hoc Committee on Reporting Standards, Society for Vascular Surgery and North American Chapter, International Society for Cardiovascular Surgery. Suggested standards for reporting on arterial aneurysms. J Vasc Surg 13:452-458, 1991.
2. Lowry SF, Kraft R. Isolated aneurysms of the iliac artery. Arch Surg 113:1289-1293, 1978.
3. Lawrence PF, Lorenzo-Rivero S, Lyon JL, et al. The incidence of iliac, femoral, and popliteal artery aneurysms in hospitalized patients. J Vasc Surg 22:409-416, 1995.
4. Plate G, Hollier LA, O'Brien P, et al. Recurrent aneurysms and late complications following repair of abdominal aortic aneurysms. Arch Surg 120:590-594, 1985.
5. Provan JL, Fialkov J, Ameli FM, St. Louis EL. Is tube repair of aortic aneurysm followed by aneurysmal change in the common iliac arteries? Can J Surg 33:394-397, 1990.
6. Brunkwall J, Kauksson H, Bengtsson H, et al. Solitary aneurysms of the iliac arterial system: An estimate of their frequency of occurrence. J Vasc Surg 10:381-384, 1989.
7. Richardson JW, Greenfield LJ. Natural history and management of iliac aneurysms. J Vasc Surg 8:165-171, 1988.
8. Minato N, Itoh T, Natsuaki M, et al. Isolated iliac artery aneurysm and its management. Cardiovasc Surg 2:489-494, 1994.
9. McCready RA, Pairolero PC, Gilmore JC, et al. Isolated iliac artery aneurysms. Surgery 93:688-693, 1983.
10. Schuler JJ, Flanigan DP. Iliac artery aneurysms. In Bergan J, Yao JST, eds. Aneurysms: Diagnosis and Treatment. New York: Grune & Stratton, 1982, p 469.
11. Weimann S, Tauscher Th, Flora G. Isolated iliac artery aneurysms. Ann Vasc Surg 4:297-301, 1990.
12. Conroy KM, Bush RW, Shiota MG, et al. Isolated iliac artery aneurysm causing acute renal obstruction and fatal rectal hemorrhage. J Clin Gastroenterol 18:255-257, 1994.
13. Nachbur BH, Inderbitzi RG, Bar W, et al. Isolated iliac aneurysms. Eur J Vasc Surg 5:375-381, 1991.
14. Hollier LH, Stanson AW, Gloviczki P, et al. Arteriomegaly: Classification and morbid implications of diffuse aneurysmal disease. Surgery 93:700-708, 1983.

62

The Importance of Genetic and Biochemical Factors in the Practical Management of Aneurysms

SANDRA C. CARR, M.D., and WILLIAM H. PEARCE, M.D.

Abdominal aortic aneurysm (AAA) ranks as the thirteenth leading cause of death in the United States and is responsible for approximately 15,000 deaths per year. Several autopsy studies have placed the incidence between 1.8% and 6.6%.[1] There has been a dramatic rise in the age-standardized incidence of death from AAA in the United States, United Kingdom, and Australia.[2] The incidence of symptomatic AAA has increased by more than twofold in the United States, and a similar increase has been documented in western Australia for 1971 through 1981.[1,3] As there has also been an increase in the number of operations for elective aneurysm repair, these mortality statistics likely reflect a true increase in the prevalence of the disease. The rise in death rates from AAA is surprising since both cerebrovascular and coronary artery diseases, which share similar risk factors, have shown significant decreases over the past 10 to 15 years. The increase in AAA disease is thought to be caused partially by improved diagnostic capabilities with increased detection of small asymptomatic aneurysms and partially by the aging of the population. Elective surgical repair of abdominal aortic aneurysm can prevent rupture and is associated with markedly improved survival of these patients. Thus research concerning the mechanisms of aneurysm pathogenesis, dilation, and rupture has the potential to help decrease the death rate of this disease.

AAA is a late-onset disease and most commonly occurs in the fifth to seventh decade of life. The risk factors for AAA are very similar to the known risk factors for atherosclerosis. Known risk factors for AAA include smoking, hypertension, aging, familial clusters, hyperlipidemia, and connective tissue disorders. The two factors most commonly studied are smoking and hypertension. Smoking is the most powerful environmental agent associated with aneurysm formation and death. In an autopsy series, AAAs occurred eight times more frequently among smokers than among nonsmokers.[4] The relative risks of developing an AAA associated with smoking are greater than those found with smoking in coronary artery disease. Hypertension is another risk factor common to both atherosclerosis and aneurysmal disease. Elevated diastolic blood pressure, more so than systolic, has been shown to be an important determinant of death from ruptured AAA. Turk[5] noted that 50% of men with AAA had evidence of hypertension, whereas only 20% of the women in his study were hypertensive, suggesting that other factors, perhaps a genetic component, are more important in this population. Cronenwett et al.[6] noted a 60% incidence of hypertension among patients with AAA. Interestingly, it was the presence of chronic obstructive pulmonary disease, independent of smoking, which was most predictive of aneurysm rupture in this series. Two characteristics—smoking and a proband with AAA at an age of less than 60 years—increase the chance to over 50% of AAA being present in a male sibling. Another factor that is more prominent in aneurysmal disease than in atherosclerosis is the substantial male predominance of the disease. Deaths from AAA rupture occur mainly among men. The male-to-female ratio ranges from about 3:1 in the older age groups to approximately 11:1 in the youngest group. The most striking example of male predominance is in aneurysms associated with popliteal or femoral arteries. These types of aneurysms are very rare in females. AAA is also more common among whites than blacks. White men have a nearly threefold higher incidence than black men and women.

Classically, aneurysmal disease has been thought to be secondary to atherosclerotic degeneration of the abdominal aorta. However, this view has been challenged by several investigators over the past decade who have discovered numerous biochemical, pathologic, epidemiologic, and genetic differences between patients with aneurysms and those with atherosclerotic disease. However, it is still unknown why some patients develop aortic occlusive disease whereas others develop aneurysms. Recently research has been concentrated on the molecular mechanisms of aneurysm formation and on the genetic component of this disease.

BACKGROUND

Over the years, a number of factors have been implicated in the pathogenesis and progression of arterial aneurysms. These factors include physical forces, hemodynamic alterations, and compositional changes in the aneurysm wall. Biochemical research in this area has concentrated on investigating the factors that may be important in weakening of the arterial wall. In 1970, Sumner et al.[7] demonstrated a decrease in collagen and elastin in the aneurysm wall when compared with atherosclerotic aorta. They also demonstrated that collagen and elastin were concentrated in the adventitial layer of the artery. Since then, research has focused on describing factors responsible for altering collagen and elastin in the aneurysm wall.

Elastin is a component of virtually every tissue in the body and plays a critical role in the integrity of tissues such as skin, lung, and aorta. The major catabolic enzyme that degrades elastin is the protease elastase. Elastase activity is modified by the serum antiprotease inhibitor, α-1-antitrypsin, which is responsible for approximately 90% of the total protease inhibitory capacity in serum. The elastin gene is expressed primarily during fetal development and early neonatal life in human fibroblasts and has decreased expression in the adult with increasing age. In the normal adult infrarenal aorta, elastin maintains a relatively constant concentration of 12%.[8] The half-life of elastin is estimated to be approximately 70 years. Both histologic and biochemical analysis of aneurysmal tissue have demonstrated a significant decrease in elastin concentration.[9,10] In AAA tissue, elastin is decreased in concentration, whereas collagen concentration is unchanged or increased slightly. Studies using Northern blot analysis of aneurysm tissue have demonstrated a decrease in elastin mRNA compared with collagen mRNA in aneurysm tissue, suggesting that impaired synthesis of elastin may be contributing to the pathogenesis of AAA.

In addition to a decrease in elastin synthesis, deficient cross-linking of elastin has also been implicated in the formation of aneurysms. Simpson et al.[11] have demonstrated a direct correlation between elastin cross-link concentration and aortic tensile strength. The contribution of decreased elastin in the pathogenesis of aneurysms was further supported by studies by Sandberg et al.,[12] who found that inhibition of lysyl oxidase, an essential enzyme for elastin cross-linking, resulted in aneurysm formation in an animal model. By inducing a state of copper deficiency, lysyl oxidase is inhibited, soluble elastin is prematurely degraded, and aneurysmal dilation occurs.[12] Similarly, the blotchy mouse develops aneurysms because of impaired absorption of copper from the gut, a defect which has been linked to the X chromosome. Lathrogens, which impair elastin cross-link formation, induce dilation and rupture of the aorta in turkeys. Although the mechanism of aneurysm formation in humans is likely more complex, these animal models have demonstrated the reliability of aneurysm production when elastin cross-linking is inhibited. Studies in human aneurysm tissue, however, have failed so far to demonstrate a deficiency of stable cross-links in the mature aneurysmal wall.[13]

Selective catabolism of elastin is thought to be one of a number of possible mechanisms leading to aneurysm formation. The homeostatic balance between elastase and antiprotease may be altered in the aortic wall during aneurysm formation and rupture. Enzymatic activity studies have demonstrated an increase in elastase activity in aneurysm tissue.[9,11,14] The aortic wall elastase to α-1 antitrypsin activity ratio has been shown to be elevated in patients who have undergone elective AAA repair compared with patients with atherosclerotic aortic disease undergoing operation for occlusive disease. Additionally, the levels were noted to be significantly higher in patients undergoing operation for ruptured AAA.[14] Furthermore, patients with aneurysmal disease, compared with those with occlusive aortic disease, have a significantly elevated serum elastolytic activity, especially in those who smoke. It is possible that smoking stimulates circulating proteolytic activity that predisposes to aneurysm formation. Practical applications of this biochemical research include the possibility of developing agents which alter serum proteolytic activity. Drugs that stimulate serum α-1 antitrypsin antiprotease concentration and trypsin inhibitory capacity such as the androgen danazol, have not been used clinically. Synthetic choramethyl ketone elastase inhibitor has been given orally to reduce proteolysis but has not been used to prevent aneurysmal dilation or rupture. These types of agents may be useful in preventing dilation and rupture of aneurysms, especially if diagnosed early.

Studies by Dobrin et al.[15] suggest that wall integrity in arteries depends on intact collagen rather than elastin. They have demonstrated that elastase infusion into an artery results in dilatation, whereas collagenase infusion causes wall rupture.[16] Interstitial collagen types I and III account for 90% of the six collagen types within the aorta, with a predominance of type I collagen. Collagen type I and III molecules consist of α-procollagen chains, which combine to form the fibrillar triple helices. A single gene locus codes for each of these collagen precursors. In Ehlers-Danlos syndrome type IV, a deficiency of collagen type III results in fragile and sometimes aneurysmal arteries. Collagen type III deficiency has also been found in several types of aneurysms, including some previously thought to be "atherosclerotic" aneurysms.[17]

In contrast to elastin, the role of collagen in the pathogenesis of AAA is less well defined. Different investigators have published conflicting reports concerning the changes in collagen within aortic aneurysms. In 1970, Sumner et al.[7] reported a 38% decrease in collagen concentration in the aneurysm adventitia. Since then, others have reported increases in AAA wall collagen. Most of these studies, however, have been based on the use of full-thickness aortic wall.[7,18] These variations in aneurysm wall collagen content may result from differences in aneurysm size, the control artery used, extraction technique, and degree of contamination with mural thrombus. It is thought that collagen synthesis and accumulation may occur as a response to increasing wall tension in the aneurysm as arterial dilatation occurs from loss of elastin. The increase in aneurysmal collagen concentration may also be caused in part by loss of elastin, which creates a more concentrated aortic wall. Although the concentration of collagen may be altered in AAA disease, the ratio of collagen type I to type III is constant in aneurysmal disease.[8]

It appears that active collagen synthesis continues to occur in both normal and diseased aortas. Studies using Northern blot analysis have demonstrated an increase in the gene expression of collagen types I and III in AAA wall compared with normal aorta. Interestingly, collagen types I and III mRNA were found to be greater in aneurysmal and atherosclerotic occlusive aortas, although an excess of collagen accumulation was found only in the occlusive group. This suggests that there may be an increase in proteolytic activity in aneurysms. Busuttil et al.[19] have noted an increase in collagenase activity in aneurysm wall tissue. They also described a significant correlation between aneurysm size and collagenase activity. Type IV collagenase mRNA has also been shown to be increased in AAA tissue.[20] It is thought that changes in collagenase activity may play a role in aneurysm rupture. Swanson et al.[21] described a series of patients with known asymptomatic aneurysms that ruptured within an average of 10 days after surgery for an unrelated condition. Although there is speculation that operative trauma may increase the chance of aneurysm rupture by inducing collagenase activation within the aortic wall, animal studies so far have failed to demonstrate any increase in aortic wall collagenase activity.[22] Potential clinical applications of this research include the possibility of altering collagenase activity in patients with asymptomatic aneurysms that require operation for concomitant coronary or carotid artery disease, or other necessary procedures.

Enzymes that regulate the activity of collagenase may also play a role in aneurysm expansion and rupture. Collagenase, which degrades native triple helical collagen, and gelatinase, which degrades denatured collagen, are both metalloproteases. Not only are the metalloproteases thought to play a pivotal role in aneurysmal disease, but their major inhibitor, tissue inhibitor of metalloprotease (TIMP), may play a role in the matrix degradation underlying aneurysm formation. Studies using Western blot analysis have demonstrated a decrease in TIMP in AAA extract.[23]

Plasmin is another enzyme that directly degrades the extracellular matrix and plays a key role in the activation of metalloproteinases, including collagenase and the metalloelastases. Using gel enzymography, an increase in elastolytic activity at approximately 80 kD has been noted in aneurysm tissue. Immunologic studies have identified this enzyme as plasmin.[24] Further studies will better determine the role of the plasminogen system in aneurysm formation.

INFLAMMATION

It is postulated that the proteases responsible for aneurysm formation are produced or modulated by inflammatory cells and their mediators. The infiltration of mononuclear cells is thought to participate in the early stages of atherosclerosis. Similarly, inflammation has been associated with aneurysmal disease, particularly in the case of inflammatory aneurysms. Using immunohistochemical techniques, it has been shown that AAA has an increase in total inflammatory cell infiltrate compared with atherosclerotic and normal aorta. This inflammatory infiltrate consists of CD-3 positive lymphocytes, CD-11 positive macrophages, and an increase in the CD-4 positive to CD-8 positive lymphocyte ratio.[25] Additionally, acute phase proteins, such as C-reactive protein, α-1 antiprotease, and ceruloplasmin are also elevated in patients with aneurysms, further supporting the presence of an inflammatory process. Furthermore, the signals that attract lymphocytes and monocytes into the aortic wall, such as interleukin-8 and monocyte chemoattractant protein-1, are expressed to a greater extent in conditioned media from explants of AAA compared with explants from either atherosclerotic or normal aortas.[26] The inflammatory process, which is prominent in the adventitia and extends to the media, may provide the proteases responsible for the degradation of the aortic extracellular matrix seen in AAA. This raises the possibility that therapy directed against this inflammatory reaction may have a future role in the practical management of AAA.

GENETIC ASPECTS

In 1977, Clifton[27] reported three male siblings with ruptured AAA and similar blood types, suggesting that there may be a genetic component to the disease. Tilson and Seashore[28] were among the first to describe familial clustering of aneurysms. They studied 50 families exhibiting clustering of AAA in two or more first-order relatives. Several of the families that they studied appeared to have an autosomal dominant pattern of inheritance. Analysis of pedigree patterns suggested that some families appeared to have an X-linked mechanism of inheritance, whereas most of the aneurysms appeared to have a multifactorial pattern. The incidence of popliteal aneurysm appeared to be higher in families in which X-linkage was considered.[29] Other family studies have suggested that the inheritance of AAA is controlled by a major autosomal diallelic locus, with the disease-causing allele being recessive.[30] So far, no common mode of inheritance has been found.

Outside of the less common family cluster of AAA, patients with "atherosclerotic" aneurysms have an unusually high frequency of AAA among other family members. Johansen and Koepsell[31] compared the family histories of 250 patients with AAA with those of 250 control subjects. Among the control subjects, six (2.4%) reported having a first-degree relative with an aneurysm, compared with 48 (19.2%) of the patients with AAA. The diagnosis of AAA in a first-degree relative was associated with a 12-fold increase in risk of an individual developing an AAA. Others have reported a similar incidence.[32,33] Studies have demonstrated that patients with familial AAA were more likely to be female (35% versus 14%). Men with familial AAA tended to be about 5 years younger than female relatives with AAA. Identification of a family with aneurysms and a female member with an aneurysm was strongly correlated with the risk of rupture.[33] In these studies, there was no significant difference between patients with nonfamilial and familial AAA in anatomic extent of disease, multiplicity of aneurysms, associated occlusive disease, or blood type. This genetic research further strongly suggests that AAA may be caused by a genetic defect. It does not, however, contradict the general impression that the development of aneurysms is accelerated by atherosclerosis, hypertension, or other factors. In fact, the higher incidence of AAA among brothers than among sisters of patients with AAA strongly suggests that a secondary component, such as atherosclerosis, also contributes to the disease.

The importance of these genetic studies lies in the identification of risk factors for AAA that might permit discovery of early, asymptomatic aneurysms amenable to elective repair. Screening of the brothers of patients with AAA using ultrasound has provided an incidence of 29%, compared with a prevalence of 5.4% found during screening of unselected men ages 65 to 74 years.[34] In a similar study by Bengtsson et al.,[35] screening 87 asymptomatic siblings of patients with AAA showed that 29% of the brothers and 6% of the sisters had an AAA greater than 2.9 centimeters. Webster et al.[36] also screened 103 first-degree relatives of patients with AAA and found that 13% of the siblings older than 50 years of age had an asymptomatic AAA.

Generalized arteriomegaly, the presence of multiple aneurysms in some patients, and an association with inguinal hernia and emphysema suggest an underlying systemic disorder in connective tissue metabolism in aneurysmal disease.[37] Actually, a small percentage of aneurysms are known to be associated with a proven connective tissue disorder. In Ehlers-Danlos syndrome type IV, the defect consists of decreased or absent production of collagen type III. Similarly, aneurysm formation in Marfan's syndrome is caused by a genetic defect in the fibrillin-1 gene on chromosome 15, resulting in an abnormality of connective tissue.[38] Several studies have suggested that a mutation in the collagen type III gene may be a common cause of some familial aortic aneurysms.[2,39] The role of the collagen type III gene was further strengthened with a family study describing cosegregation of the collagen type III gene with the AAA phenotype.[40] A mutation that converted the codon for glycine at a-1-619 to arginine in collagen type III was found in two members of a family who died of sudden rupture of arterial aneurysms. Further studies in this family identified members who are likely to be prone to develop AAA.[16] In addition to Ehlers-Danlos and Marfan's syndrome variants, congenital aneurysms and the presence of tuberous sclerosis should also be considered when evaluating very young patients with aneurysmal disease. These patients should be carefully examined with skin biopsy and tissue culture, and their family members should be carefully screened.

This research into the genetic basis of AAA is not only interesting, but it also has importance in the practical management of AAA. Identifying early asymptomatic aneurysms would facilitate elective repair. Numerous reports have demonstrated that individuals who undergo elective surgery for repair of AAA have a survival rate of greater than 90% and may have a near-normal life span.[29] In contrast, the mortality rate from ruptured AAA is as high as 80%. Additionally, the hospitalization costs for individuals undergoing elective AAA repair is about one tenth the cost of emergent surgery.[29] For these reasons, screening of patients at greatest risk for development of AAA with elective repair of asymptomatic aneurysms is likely to be cost effective. A DNA diagnostic test for the mutation causing AAA would clearly be of benefit to families in whom such mutations can be identified.

AAA is likely to be genetically heterogeneous (the same phenotype arising from different genotypes), with a multifactorial etiology. The mode of inheritance and the mechanisms of gene-environment interactions remain unknown. It appears that in younger patients the genetic influences predominate, while in older patients environmental factors and aging of the aorta appear to have a greater influence on the development of AAA. At present, the clinical applications of this research are more theoretical than practical. However, better knowledge of the molecular mechanisms responsible for the pathogenesis of aortic aneurysm may be used to alter the disease process or identify patients at risk. The development of diagnostic tests would facilitate early elective repair of aneurysms and prevent the complications of thromboembolism and rupture.

REFERENCES

1. Reilly JM, Tilson MD. Incidence and etiology of abdominal aortic aneurysms. Surg Clin North Am 69:705-711, 1989.
2. Adiseshiah M, MacSweeney STR, Henney AM, Poulter N, Powell JT, Greenhalgh RM. Abdominal aortic aneurysms. Lancet 341:215-220, 1993.
3. Melton L, Bickerstaff L, Hollier L. Changing incidence of AAA: A population based study. Am J Epidemiol 120:379-386, 1984.
4. Auerbach O, Garfinkel L. Atherosclerosis and aneurysm of the aorta in relation to smoking habits and age. Chest 78:805-809, 1980.
5. Turk K. Post-mortem incidence of AAA. Proc R Soc Med 58:869-870, 1965.
6. Cronenwett J, Murphy T, Zelnock G. Actuarial analysis of variables associated with rupture of small AAA. Surgery 98:472-483, 1985.
7. Sumner D, Hokanson D, Strandness D. Stress-strain characteristics and collagen-elastin content of AAA. Surg Gynecol Obstet 130:459-466, 1970.
8. Mesh CL, Baxter BT, Pearce WH, Chisholm RL, McGee GS, Yao JST. Collagen and elastin gene expression in aortic aneurysms. Surgery 112:256-262, 1992.
9. Rizzo RJ, McCarthy WJ, Dixit SN, Lilly MP, Shively VP, Flinn WR, Yao JST. Collagen types and matrix protein content in human abdominal aortic aneurysms. J Vasc Surg 10:365-373, 1989.
10. Campa JS, Greenhalgh RM, Powell JT. Elastin degradation in abdominal aortic aneurysms. Atherosclerosis 65:13-21, 1987.
11. Simpson CF, Boucek RJ, Noble NL. Influence of d-, l- and dl-propranolol and practolol and b-amino proprionitrile-induced aortic rupture in turkeys. Toxicol Appl Pharmacol 38:169-175, 1976.
12. Sandberg LB, Hackett TN, Carnes WH. The solubilization of an elastin-like protein from copper-deficient porcine aorta. Biochem Biophys Acta 181:201-207, 1969.
13. Baxter BT, McGee GS, Shively VP, Drummand IAS, Dixit SN, Yamauchi M, Pearce WH. Elastin content, cross-

links, and mRNA in normal and aneurysmal human aorta. J Vasc Surg 16:192-200, 1992.
14. Cohen JR, Mandell C, Chang JB. Elastin metabolism of the infrarenal aorta. J Vasc Surg 7:210-214, 1988.
15. Dobrin PB, Baker WH, Gley WC. Elastolytic and collagenolytic studies of arteries: Implications for the mechanical properties of aneurysms. Arch Surg 119:405-409, 1984.
16. Campa JS, Greenhalgh RM, Powell JT. Elastin degradation in abdominal aortic aneurysms. Atherosclerosis 65:13-21, 1987.
17. Kuivaniemi H, Tromp G, Prockup DJ. Mutations in collagen genes: Causes of rare and some common diseases in humans. FASEB J 5:2052-2060, 1991.
18. Menashi S, Campa JS, Greenhalgh RM. Collagen in abdominal aortic aneurysms: Typing content, and degradation. J Vasc Surg 6:578-582, 1987.
19. Busuttil RW, Abou-ZamZam AM, Machleder HI. Collagenase activity of the human aorta. Arch Surg 115:1373-1378, 1980.
20. McMillan WD, Patterson BK, Keen RR, Shively VP, Cipollone M, Pearce WH. In situ localization and quantification of mRNA for 92-kD type IV collagenase and its inhibitor in aneurysmal, occlusive, and normal aorta. Arterioscler Thromb Vasc Biol 15:1139-1144, 1994.
21. Swanson RJ, Littooy FN, Hunt TK, Stoney RJ. Laparotomy as a precipitating factor in the rupture of intraabdominal aneurysms. Arch Surg 115:299-304, 1980.
22. Cohen JR, Perry MO, Hariri R, Holt J, Alvarez O. Aortic collagenase activity as affected by laparotomy cecal resection, aortic mobilization, and aortotomy in rats. J Vasc Surg 1:562-565, 1984.
23. Brophy CM, Marks WH, Reilly JM, Tilson MD. Decreased tissue inhibitor of metalloproteinases (TIMP) in abdominal aortic aneurysm tissue: A preliminary report. J Surg Res 50:653-657, 1991.
24. Jean-Claude J, Newman KM, Li H, Gregory AK, Tilson DM. Possible key role for plasmin in the pathogenesis of abdominal aortic aneurysm. Surgery 116:472-478, 1994.
25. Koch AE, Haines GK, Rizzo RJ, Radosevich JA, Pope RM, Robinson PG, Pearce WH. Human abdominal aortic aneurysm: Immunophenotypic analysis suggesting an immune-mediated response. Am J Pathol 137:1199-1213, 1990.
26. Koch AE, Kunkel SL, Pearce WH, Shah MR, Parikh D, Evanoff HL, Haines GK, Burdick MD, Strieter RM. Enhanced production of the chemotactic cytokines interleukin-8 and monocyte chemoattractant protein-1 in human abdominal aortic aneurysm. Am J Pathol 142:1423-1431, 1993.
27. Clifton MA. Familial abdominal aortic aneurysms. Br J Surg 64:765-766, 1977.
28. Tilson DM, Seashore MR. Fifty families with abdominal aortic aneurysms in two or more first-order relatives. Am J Surg 147:551-553, 1984.
29. Tilson DM, Seashore MR. Human genetics of the abdominal aortic aneurysm. Surg Gynecol Obstet 158:129-132, 1984.
30. Kuivaniemi H, Tromp G, Prockop DJ. Genetic causes of aortic aneurysms: Unlearning at least part of what textbooks say. J Clin Invest 88:1441-1444, 1991.
31. Johansen K, Koepsell T. Familial tendency for abdominal aortic aneurysm. JAMA 256:1934-1936, 1986.
32. Norrgard O, Rais O, Angquist KA. Familial occurrence of abdominal aortic aneurysm. Surgery 95:650-656, 1984.
33. Darling RC, Brewster DC, Darling RC, LaMuraglia GM, Moncure AC, Cambria RP, Abbott WM. Are familial abdominal aortic aneurysms different? J Vasc Surg 10:39-43, 1989.
34. Collin J, Walton J. Is abdominal aortic aneurysm familial? Br Med J 299:493, 1989.
35. Bengtsson H, Norrgard O, Angquist KA, Ekberg O, Oberg L, Bergquist D. Ultrasonographic screening of the abdominal aorta among siblings of patients with abdominal aortic aneurysms. Br J Surg 76:589-591, 1989.
36. Webster MW, Ferrell RE, St. Jean PL, Majumder PP, Fugel SR, Steed DL. Ultrasound screening of first-degree relatives of patients with an abdominal aortic aneurysm. J Vasc Surg 13:9-14, 1991.
37. Cannon DJ, Casteal L, Read RC. Abdominal aortic aneurysm, Leriche syndrome, inguinal herniation, and smoking. Arch Surg 119:387-389, 1984.
38. Dietz HC, Cutting GR, Pyeritz RE. Marfan syndrome caused by a recurrent de novo missense mutation in the fibrillin gene. Nature 352:337-339, 1991.
39. McGee GS, Baxter TB, Shively VP, Chisholm R, McCarthy WJ, Flinn WR, Yao JST, Pearce WH. Aneurysm or occlusive disease: Factors determining the clinical course of atherosclerosis of the infrarenal aorta. Surgery 110:370-376, 1991.
40. Kontusaari S, Tromp G, Kuivaniemi H, Romantic A, Prockop DJ. A mutation in the gene for type III collagen in a family with aortic aneurysms. J Clin Invest 86:1465-1473, 1990.

63

Is the Natural History of Intermittent Claudication Worse Than We Thought?

JACK L. CRONENWETT, M.D.

Before the era of arterial reconstruction, the natural history of intermittent claudication (IC) was measured by the number of patients whose condition progressed to the point at which amputation was necessary. Several reports, such as the classic article by Bloor,[1] established that the likelihood of amputation was less than 10% in these patients after 3 to 8 years of follow-up. These observations are the basis for current dogma that IC is a benign disease, because amputation is seldom required. From the perspective of a patient with IC who wants to walk farther, however, amputation is a crude end point. Furthermore, most early studies of IC did not objectively document arterial disease and were performed in an era of shortened life expectancy among patients with atherosclerosis. Thus it is possible that these studies do not reflect the contemporary outcome of IC, especially when viewed from the patients' perspective of symptom progression or reconstruction requirement rather than amputation requirement alone.

For these reasons we analyzed a group of 91 male patients who were followed in a Veterans Administration Medical Center for mild IC.[2] All of these patients had stable IC for at least 6 months. The average age of these patients was 58 years; 88% were white, diabetes mellitus affected 27%, hypertension was present in 62%, and 96% of patients had smoked cigarettes for an average of 60 pack/years. At the time of their initial evaluation 98% of these men exhibited "mild" IC, defined as the ability to walk at least 50 yards without pain. Patients with worse initial symptoms were 2.4 times more likely to be diabetic and 3.1 times more likely to be hypertensive. These patients were followed for a mean duration of 31 months, during which symptom progression and operation requirement were assessed. After this 2.5 years' average follow-up, only 56% of patients could walk at least 50 yards without pain; 44% had progressed to "severe" IC (Fig. 1). This change in walking distance correlated well with patients' subjective assessment of their walking ability. At final follow-up, patients categorized their symptoms as follows: much improved, 2%; improved, 10%; unchanged, 28%; worse, 22%; and much worse, 38%. Thus, after 2.5 years' follow-up, 60% of patients believed that their IC was worse, whereas 40% categorized their IC as unchanged or improved.

Analysis of more objective end points in these patients demonstrated that the mean ankle/brachial index (ABI) decreased from an initial value of 0.63 to a final value of 0.53. The change in ABI was highly correlated with symptom progression. In patients who improved or were unchanged, the ABI did not change (mean, 0.62 to 0.61). In patients who developed worse symptoms during follow-up, however, the mean ABI decreased from 0.65 to 0.47, a highly significant difference ($p < .0001$).

Life-table analysis indicated that the mortality rate of these patients with initially mild IC averaged 4.5% per year during follow-up.[2] Twice this number, 9% per year, required operative intervention because of severe disease progression in their affected leg. Thus 20% (18 of 91) of patients required operative intervention: arterial reconstruction or angioplasty in 16 and amputation in only two. The indications for intervention were evenly distributed among tissue loss, rest pain, and claudication progression that prevented employment. Thus, despite relatively strict criteria for vascular reconstruction, this was required in 9% of patients per year, at a rate that was constant during the first 4 years of follow-up.

Other contemporary reports have also examined the likelihood of progression to critical ischemia in patients with IC. In a group of 257 such patients with IC, followed for a mean duration of 6.5 years, Jelnes et al.[3] found that 7.5% progressed to critical ischemia requiring surgical reconstruction or amputation during the first year and that 2.2% per year developed critical ischemia thereafter. After initially ex-

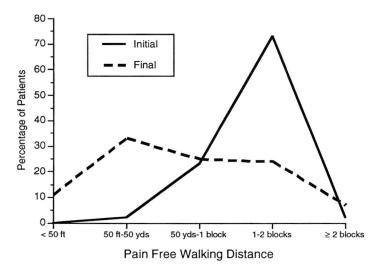

Fig. 1 Symptom progression in 91 men with claudication after 2.5 years' follow-up.[2] Note decrease in walking distance between initial and final assessment. (Based on data from Cronenwett JL, Warner KG, Zelenock GB, et al. Intermittent claudication: Current results of nonoperative management. Arch Surg 119:430-436, 1984.)

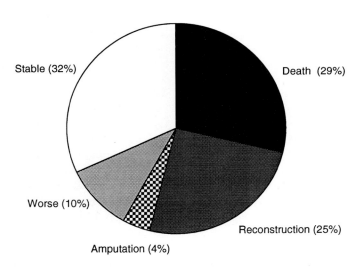

Fig. 2 Estimated 5-year outcome of patients with initially stable claudication. (Based on data from McDaniel MD, Cronenwett JL. Basic data related to the natural history of intermittent claudication. Ann Vasc Surg 3:273-277, 1989.)

cluding patients with severe claudication who were initially selected for operation, Rosenbloom et al.[4] found that 24% of patients with stable IC developed critical ischemia that required operation within 5 years. In a very large study of 1969 patients with IC who were followed as the control group in a drug treatment study, Dormandy and Murray[5] reported the 1-year outcome as follows: 4.3% died, 1.6% required amputation, and 5.6% required arterial reconstruction, yielding a 7.3% rate of progression to critical ischemia during 1 year. Based on these estimates, it appears that the contemporary natural history of IC is worse than we thought based on classic studies performed before the era of surgical reconstruction.

In an attempt to provide a more accurate current estimate of outcome, we recently reviewed this literature to estimate the projected 5-year outcome of patients who present with mild, stable IC (Fig. 2).[6] These results indicate that few patients require amputation, but by conservative estimates, 5% per year will require arterial reconstruction to prevent amputation and 5% per year will die, largely from complications of systemic atherosclerosis. Smoking cessation will reduce this mortality by half, eliminate major amputation, and reduce the operation requirement to less than 2% per year. Unfortunately, diabetes increases the projected annual mortality rate to 10% per year, with a 4% per year annual amputation requirement despite a 7% per year need for arterial reconstruction.[6]

Recognizing that a subgroup of patients who initially present with stable IC will subsequently require arterial reconstruction because of progression to critical ischemia, it would be useful to identify risk factors associated with disease progression. In an attempt to identify such risk factors, we analyzed variables available at the initial evaluation of these patients.[2] Using multivariate techniques, we found that much worse IC progression was independently predicted by continued cigarette smoking, by minimal daily exercise, and by a low initial ABI. Despite the statistical significance of these predictive variables, however, the overall accuracy for determining individual patient outcome was only 63%. The probability of requiring operative intervention in these patients was significantly related to a greater smoking history (in pack/years) and a lower initial ABI. Patients who had smoked at least 40 pack/years had a subsequent operation requirement that was 3.3 times higher than those who had smoked less. This regression analysis resulted in an overall accuracy of 79% for predicting operation requirement. Thus while this study substantiated our clinical belief that exercise, smoking, and initial disease severity (as assessed by ABI) were important predictors of patient outcome, the accuracy of the prediction model was insufficient for clearly identifying future needs. However, we concluded that patients with an initial ABI of less than 0.60 who continue to smoke or have a substantial smoking history warrant more frequent and structured follow-up. Vascular laboratory assessment of disease progression is important because a decrease in the ABI of 0.15 or more during follow-up was associated with an operation requirement 2.5 times greater than that in patients whose ABI remained stable. Thus by initially identifying patients whose ABI is less than 0.60 or patients whose ABI decreases by 0.15 or more during vascular laboratory follow-up, a high-risk group can be identified for more frequent follow-up to prevent late presentation with tissue loss and possible amputation requirement before arterial reconstruction can be accomplished.

Other investigators have also looked at specific risk factors in patients with IC that predict subsequent deterioration. Rosenbloom et al.[4] also found that a low initial ABI predicted the development of critical ischemia, but that a significant decrease in the ABI during follow-up was even more predictive. Jonason and Ringqvist[7] found that cigarette smoking and multilevel occlusive disease best predicted the development of rest pain in patients with initially stable IC. Jelnes et al.[3] emphasized the importance of an initial ankle pressure of less than 70 mm Hg, a toe pressure of less than 40 mm Hg, or an ABI of less than 0.50 in predicting subsequent development of critical ischemia. In their experience patients with an initial ABI greater than 0.70 never required amputation during mean follow-up of 6.5 years. Dormandy and Murray[5] also found that an initial ABI of less than 0.50 predicted a subsequent operation requirement rate 2.3 times higher than patients with an initial ABI greater than 0.50 and found that previous vascular surgery was an important predictor of subsequent deterioration in patients with IC.

Two additional studies have demonstrated the importance of stratifying patients with IC according to initial vascular laboratory criteria to predict the likelihood of deterioration. Gertler et al.[8] followed 51 patients with IC who initially had an ABI of less than 0.50 or a markedly blunted pulse volume recording. Rest pain or tissue loss developed in 29% of these patients, which necessitated vascular reconstruction within 3 years. Further analysis demonstrated that cigarette smoking and hypertension were each associated with a fivefold greater likelihood of intervention in this subgroup. Bowers et al.[9] followed 56 men with stable IC who had an initial toe pressure of 40 mm Hg or less. After a mean follow-up of only 31 months, 19 of these patients (34%) had developed rest pain or tissue loss. In this population, diabetes conferred a threefold higher likelihood of progression to critical ischemia. Both of these studies provide further evidence for the importance of careful follow-up in patients with IC who initially present with more severe disease as indexed by vascular laboratory pressure measurements.

It is important to emphasize that IC is a reliable predictor of systemic risk for atherosclerotic complications, best indicated by the higher than expected mortality of patients with IC. In a recent analysis of 112 patients with stable IC, O'Riordain and O'Donnell[10] reported a 5-year actuarial mortality of 23%. Patients with an initial ABI of less than 0.50 had a 50% mortality, whereas patients whose ABI was greater than 0.50 had only a 16% mortality. This emphasized the association between more severe lower extremity atherosclerosis and generalized atherosclerotic risk, since most (72%) deaths resulted from myocardial infarction or stroke. Of the other variables studied (including age, smoking, hypertension, and sex), only the initial ABI was a statistically significant predictor of survival in patients with IC.[10] Thus in considering the natural history of IC one must focus not only on the extremity but also on the patient as a whole, since the mortality from atherosclerosis is higher than the amputation rate. Hertzer,[11] among others, has emphasized the importance of evaluating and treating underlying cardiac disease in these patients if one undertakes intervention to effect limb salvage.

Given this knowledge of the natural history of patients with IC, one must ask whether this can be modified without surgical or endovascular intervention. Although optimally controlled studies are not available, cessation of cigarette smoking appears to be an important factor, especially during long-term follow-up.[12] There is general agreement that this is the most important risk factor, but it is also the most difficult to modify. In our study we found that patients with a longer history of smoking had a much higher operation rate than those who smoked less and that patients who stopped smoking during follow-up had a substantially lower rate of symptom progression. We also found that major daily exercise was associated with more stable claudication.[2] In 56 patients with IC, Carter et al.[13] found that a structured treadmill exercise program (1 hour three times per week) significantly increased the maximal walking distance from 0.59 to 1.0 km after 3 to 6 months. The optimal target seems to be 30 minutes of exercise per day.[12] The value of a structured exercise program for patients with IC is so well established that a supervised program should be more aggressively prescribed. The optimal program should be supervised, performed regularly for at least 2 months, and be of high intensity.[14] Compliance with the exercise regimen must be assured to achieve a satisfactory outcome. Although a supervised exercise program achieves more predictable, uniform improvement, even exercise at home appears useful.[12] We have found that purchase of a home treadmill by patients with IC promotes better adherence to exercise, especially during winter weather, or in rural areas where travel to a physical therapy program is difficult.

Of the various medications that have been evaluated for the treatment of IC, pentoxifylline (Trental) has achieved the best results. However, in a recent review of the 12 randomized prospective studies concerning this drug, it was concluded that insufficient evidence exists to prove or deny a beneficial effect of pentoxifylline.[12] Although most controlled studies have shown a statistically significant improvement in IC, the maximum benefit has generally been small, ranging from 20% to 35% of the baseline maximal walking distance.[12,15] Given the cost of this therapy, most patients consider such an improvement insufficient. There may be a subgroup of patients who benefit more dramatically, but this is not predictable without testing the medication for at least 1 month. Whether pentoxyfylline offers substantial benefit beyond standard exercise therapy is unproven in the aggregate and requires a patient-specific evaluation.

The benefit of surgery in patients with IC is better established. Lundgren et al.[16] randomized 75 patients to surgical intervention, treadmill exercise training, or a combination of both, and examined the effect on walking distance after 1 year. Initially the mean walking distance in these patients was 200 meters. After 1 year, the percentage of patients with a maximal walking distance of more than 600 meters was 80% after operative treatment, 95% after operative treatment plus exercise training, but only 25% after exercise training alone. These authors emphasized not only the superiority of operative therapy but also the potential morbidity and mortality associated with this intervention. Thus the extent to which arterial reconstruction is recommended for patients with IC depends in large part on the operative risk of the patient, the long-term patency rate of the procedure, and an evaluation of other factors that might limit subsequent walking distance, such as severe cardiopulmonary disease.

The benefit of balloon angioplasty for patients with IC is less well established. In a small study of 36 patients randomized to structured exercise vs. balloon angioplasty, the maximum walking distance increased from 150 to 600 meters after 12 months in the exercise group, whereas no significant increase occurs in the angioplasty group despite an improvement in the ABI.[17] This experience has recently been updated with the report of 56 patients randomized and followed for up to 15 months.[18] A greater functional benefit in terms of maximum walking distance was seen in the exercise group, especially those whose disease was confined to the superficial femoral artery. At long-term follow-up (5 years), neither the exercise group nor the angioplasty group showed significant improvement in walking distance. Thus it appears that a structured exercise program provides a greater short- and medium-term improvement for patients with IC than does balloon angioplasty, although in the long-term no difference was seen, likely because of disease progression. This study raises significant questions about the large number of patients undergoing balloon angioplasty for IC.

Although many studies have been reported concerning the outcome of surgical and endovascular intervention for patients with IC, many of these studies are difficult to directly compare because they may include patients with disease at different levels, different severity of symptoms, and so on. A recent review by Hunnik et al.[19] pooled the data from appropriate series to yield 5-year patency rates for femoral popliteal arterial disease. Unadjusted 5-year patency rates for balloon angioplasty were 45%, for vein bypass surgery 73%, and for PTFE bypass surgery 49%. The results for balloon angioplasty actually varied from 12% to 68% depending on the severity of symptoms and the extent of occlusive disease. Similarly, patency after surgery varied from 33% to 80% depending on the symptom severity and graft type. When considering patients with IC alone, the 5-year primary patency rate for vein bypass surgery was 80%, compared with 35% to 68% for balloon angioplasty, depending on whether the artery was stenotic (best results) or occluded. Finally, the results for PTFE bypass grafting indicated a 5-year patency rate of 75% for claudicating patients when the bypass was above the knee and 65% for below-knee bypasses in these patients. Unfortunately, none of these studies has measured walking improvement, the functional outcome that is significant for patients.

In response to the criticism that contemporary surgeons may be operating too aggressively in patients with IC, Kent et al.[20] have pointed out the efficacy and appropriateness of arterial reconstruction for these patients if practiced with low morbidity and mortality and with good long-term patency. Conte et al.[21] recently suggested that even patients with severe IC who require tibial-level reconstruction are appropriate candidates for surgical treatment, emphasizing, however, that this is a highly selected and small percentage of patients with claudication in which excellent results must be achieved to warrant intervention. Thus for patients with long life expectancy, who do not have other disabling problems, surgeons with excellent operative results can recommend arterial reconstruction for patients with disabling IC. The same criteria must be applied to analyze the potential benefit of endovascular interventions. This decision-making process requires knowledge of the factors that influence the natural history of IC, balanced against a careful evaluation of patient risk. For patients with less severe symptoms, in whom surgical or endovascular intervention is not currently required, careful long-term follow-up with attention to a deteriorating ABI is most important. Modification of risk factors, especially cessation of smoking and encouragement of daily exercise, are important interventions to improve the natural history of IC. Without aggressive attention to risk factor modification, the natural history of patients with IC is likely to continue to be worse than we usually think.

REFERENCES

1. Bloor K. Natural history of arteriosclerosis of the lower extremities. Ann R Coll Surg Engl 28:36-52, 1961.
2. Cronenwett JL, Warner KG, Zelenock GB, et al. Intermittent claudication: Current results of nonoperative management. Arch Surg 119:430-436, 1984.
3. Jelnes R, Gaardsting O, Jensen KH, et al. Fate in intermittent claudication: Outcome and risk factors. BMJ 293:1137-1140, 1986.
4. Rosenbloom MS, Flanigan DP, Schuler JJ, et al. Risk factors affecting the natural history of intermittent claudication. Arch Surg 123:867-870, 1988.
5. Dormandy JA, Murray GD. The fate of the claudicant—a prospective study of 1969 claudicants. Eur J Surg 5:131-133, 1991.
6. McDaniel MD, Cronenwett JL. Basic data related to the natural history of intermittent claudication. Ann Vasc Surg 3:273-277, 1989.
7. Jonason T, Ringqvist I. Factors of prognostic importance for subsequent rest pain in patients with intermittent claudication. Acta Med Scand 218:27-33, 1985.
8. Gertler JP, Headley A, L'Italien G, et al. Claudication in the setting of plethysmographic criteria for resting ischemia: Is surgery justified? Ann Vasc Surg 7:249-253, 1993.

9. Bowers BL, Valentine RJ, Myers SI, Chervu A, Clagett GP. The natural history of patients with claudication with toe pressures of 40 mm Hg or less. J Vasc Surg 18:506-511, 1993.
10. O'Riordain DS, O'Donnell JA. Realistic expectations for the patient with intermittent claudication. Br J Surg 78:861-863, 1991.
11. Hertzer NR. The natural history of peripheral vascular disease. Circulation 83[Suppl I]:I-12–I-19, 1991.
12. Radaek K, Wyderski RJ. Conservative management of intermittent claudication. Ann Intern Med 13:135-146, 1990.
13. Carter SA, Hamel ER, Paterson JM, Snow CJ, Mymin D. Walking ability and ankle systolic pressures: Observations in patients with intermittent claudication in a short-term walking exercise program. J Vasc Surg 10:642-649, 1989.
14. Ernst E, Fialka V. A review of the clinical effectiveness of exercise therapy for intermittent claudication. Arch Intern Med 153:2357-2360, 1993.
15. Lindegärde F, Jelnes R, Björkman H, et al. Conservative drug treatment in patients with moderately severe chronic occlusive peripheral arterial disease. Circulation 80:1549-1556, 1989.
16. Lundgren F, Dahllöf AG, Lundholm K, Scherstén T, Volkmann R. Intermittent claudication—surgical reconstruction or physical training? Ann Surg 209:346-355, 1989.
17. Creasy TS, McMillan PJ, Fletcher EWL, et al. Is percutaneous transluminal angioplasty better than exercise for claudication? Preliminary results from a prospective randomized trial. Eur J Vasc Surg 4:135-140, 1990.
18. Perkins JMT, Collin J, Morris PJ. Exercise training vs. angioplasty for stable claudication. Long and medium term results of a prospective randomized trial. Presented at the Eastern Vascular Surgery Ninth Annual meeting. Anthwarp, Belgium: September 30, 1995.
19. Hunnik MGM, Wong JB, Donaldson MC, et al. Patency results of percutaneous and surgical revascularization for femoropopliteal arterial disease. Med Decis Making 14:71-81, 1994.
20. Kent KG, Donaldson MC, Attinger CE, et al. Femoropopliteal reconstruction for claudication. The risk to life and limb. Arch Surg 123:1196-1198, 1988.
21. Conte MS, Belkin M, Donaldson MC, et al. Femorotibial bypass for claudication: Do results justify an aggressive approach? J Vasc Surg 21:873-881, 1995.

64

Effect of Gram-Positive and Gram-Negative Bacteria on Selective Preservation of Infected Prosthetic Arterial Grafts

KEITH D. CALLIGARO, M.D., FRANK J. VEITH, M.D., MICHAEL L. SCHWARTZ, M.D., MATTHEW J. DOUGHERTY, M.D., and DOMINIC A. DeLAURENTIS, M.D.

Gram-negative bacteria are generally believed to cause more virulent arterial graft infections than gram-positive bacteria.[1-10] Certain characteristics of gram-negative bacteria enable them to resist antibiotics and the host's cellular defense mechanisms.[11] Traditional treatment of *prosthetic* arterial graft infections consists of total graft excision regardless of the type of bacteria responsible for the graft infection.[12-14] However, selective complete graft preservation may be a simpler and better method to treat these infections when certain preexisting criteria exist.[15-18] We tried to determine whether the presence of gram-negative bacteria should be a routine contraindication to attempted graft preservation in these situations.

PATIENTS AND METHODS

We attempted complete graft preservation only when certain criteria were fulfilled. The graft had to be patent, the anastomoses had to be intact, and the patient could not have systemic sepsis. Aerobic and anaerobic wound cultures were obtained from all patients. Appropriate intravenous antibiotics were generally administered for 6 weeks based on the results of the wound cultures. An indwelling central venous catheter was frequently placed in patients who were discharged prior to 6 weeks of hospitalization so that intravenous antibiotics could be administered on an outpatient basis.

An important aspect of our treatment included repeated, aggressive operative wound debridement. Any exudative material on the exposed graft was also carefully debrided. Further debridements were continued until healthy granulation tissue developed in the surrounding soft tissue. Patients were monitored in the intensive care unit until the graft was covered by granulation tissue or until a muscle flap was placed. Until the wound healed or a flap was placed, wet-to-dry dressing changes were performed three times a day with antibiotic or dilute povidone-iodine solution.

When our strategy proved unsuccessful, the infected graft was completely excised. To avoid limb loss in patients who would have developed an ischemic limb following graft removal, a new bypass was placed usually lateral to the infected wound whenever possible. We attempted to perform revascularization prior to graft excision to limit the ischemic period of the threatened limb.[1,16,19,20]

We have followed this protocol at Montefiore Medical Center in New York and Pennsylvania Hospital in Philadelphia for more than 20 years. We analyzed 42 consecutive patients with infected prosthetic arterial grafts treated by complete graft preservation (Table 1). In the majority of cases, the indication for the reconstructive procedure was limb salvage, the infection involved the anastomosis, and the type of prosthetic graft was polytetrafluoroethylene.

Table 1 Type of infected prosthetic arterial graft

Graft	No.
Femorodistal (25)	
Femoropopliteal	18
Femoroinfrapopliteal	7
Aortobifemoral*	5
Iliac-distal*	4
Femoral interposition	4
Femorofemoral crossover	3
Axillofemoral	1

*Infection was confined to the distal limb of these grafts.

Supported by the John F. Connelly Foundation, the James Hilton Manning and Emma Austin Manning Foundation, the Anna S. Brown Trust, and the New York Institute for Vascular Studies.

Twenty-two patients (52%) had undergone at least one previous vascular operation involving the incision that ultimately became infected (range, 1 to 4 operations; mean, 1.8). The 21 male and 21 female patients ranged in age from 38 to 91 years (mean, 64 years).

RESULTS
Patient Survival

This strategy resulted in a 10% in-hospital mortality rate. Four wounds cultured gram-positive bacteria and two cultured gram-negative bacteria. Two patients died of sepsis despite the appearance of wound healing. A third patient required graft excision after the graft thrombosed and died of persistent sepsis despite an open, healing groin wound. The fourth patient died of sepsis after undergoing total graft excision for a nonhealing wound, an above-knee amputation, and finally a hip disarticulation.

Limb Loss

Only one of the surviving patients required a major amputation after hemorrhaging from an infected anastomosis 2 weeks following wound debridement. Lack of an adequate outflow artery precluded a secondary bypass. This wound cultured only gram-negative bacteria.

Wound Healing

Twenty-nine of the wounds in the 38 surviving patients remained healed after long-term follow-up (mean, 3 years; range, 3 months to 18 years). These patients required an average of 26 days (range, 11 to 56 days) of aggressive wound care in the hospital to achieve successful wound healing. Many were discharged within 2 weeks of the initial treatment, especially when muscle flap placement resulted in successful wound healing.

The other nine patients required total graft excision when wound complications developed. Wounds did not heal in seven patients even after as long as 140 days of repeated debridement. Gram-positive bacteria were cultured from six and gram-negative bacteria from two of these seven nonhealing wounds. Two other patients developed delayed anastomotic hemorrhage 2 weeks and 12 months after operative debridement of the infected wound. Both of these wounds cultured only gram-negative bacteria. Twenty-nine surviving patients did not require additional bypasses because their wounds healed successfully with their functioning grafts intact, whereas four patients required a secondary bypass to prevent limb loss, four maintained a viable limb without additional revascularization, and one underwent an above-knee amputation.

Seven of the 42 patients were treated with a rotational muscle flap (2 gracilis, 2 rectus femoris, 1 semimembranous, 1 sartorius, and 1 gastrocnemius). Five wounds healed, one patient required graft excision for persistent sepsis and later died, and one patient required graft excision for a nonhealing wound and survived. Nine other patients required graft excision. The remaining 26 wounds were allowed to heal by delayed secondary intention. In the last few years we have used muscle flaps more frequently.

Bacteriology

Staphylococcus aureus was the most common gram-positive bacteria cultured and *Pseudomonas aeruginosa* was the most common gram-negative bacteria. Gram-positive bacteria were cultured from 33 of the 42 wounds (Table 2) and gram-negative bacteria from 22 wounds (Table 3). Twenty of the 42 wounds cultured only gram-positive bacteria, nine cultured only gram-negative bacteria, and the other 13 wounds cultured both types of organisms. Of the 42 patients with infected prosthetic arterial grafts, the grafts were completely preserved and the wounds healed without complications in 29 survivors for an overall success rate of 69%. A successful outcome was achieved in 73% (16/22) of the wounds that cultured gram-negative bacteria and 70% (23/33) of the wounds that cultured gram-positive bacteria. When *Pseudomonas* was cultured from the wound, only four of nine wounds healed. Therefore a successful outcome was achieved in 92% (12/13) of the patients whose wounds cultured gram-negative bacteria other than *Pseudomonas*. Successful graft preservation in the 22 wounds that cultured gram-negative bacteria did not differ significantly if the wounds cultured only gram-negative bacteria (9 cases) or if both gram-negative and gram-positive organisms were cultured (13 cases). Similarly, the results of treatment of the 33 wounds that cultured gram-positive bacteria did not differ if only gram-positive bacteria (20

Table 2 Bacteriology of 42 infected prosthetic arterial grafts: Gram-positive bacteria cultured from 33 wounds*

Bacteria	No.
Staphylococcus (26)	
aureus	18
epidermidis	8
Streptococcus (13)	
faecalis	8
viridans	3
Group D nonenterococcus	2
Diphtheroides	3
Corynebacterium	2
Clostridium perfringens	2

*Both gram-positive and gram-negative bacteria were cultured from 16 of the 42 wounds, and only gram-positive or only gram-negative bacteria were cultured from the remaining 26 wounds. Many wounds grew more than one species of gram-positive or gram-negative bacteria.

Table 3 Bacteriology of 42 infected prosthetic arterial grafts: Gram-negative bacteria cultured from 22 wounds*

Bacteria	No.
Pseudomonas aeruginosa	9
Proteus mirabilis	6
Bacteroides (5)	
fragilis	4
cloaca	1
Escherichia coli	4
Morganella morganii	2
Serratia marcescens	1
Acinetobacter	1

*Both gram-positive and gram-negative bacteria were cultured from 16 of the 42 wounds, and only gram-positive or only gram-negative bacteria were cultured from the remaining 26 wounds. Many wounds grew more than one species of gram-positive or gram-negative bacteria.

cases) or if both gram-positive bacteria and gram-negative bacteria (13 cases) were cultured.

DISCUSSION

We and others have proposed that selective complete prosthetic graft preservation may represent an improved method of treating infected grafts with lower amputation rates and possibly improved survival.[15-18] A critical question has been the effect of the type of infecting bacteria on the success of this treatment. Traditionally the presence of gram-negative bacteria has been believed to be almost uniformly associated with anastomotic hemorrhage, persistent or recurrent sepsis, and nonhealing wounds if all of the prosthetic material was not excised.[1,9,10,12]

We agree that graft excision is essential for patients with infected grafts accompanied by bleeding, graft occlusion, or systemic sepsis, regardless of the offending organism. If a patient has anastomotic disruption or an occluded graft, and the rest of the graft is uninvolved with infection, then subtotal graft excision may be an acceptable treatment.[15,16,18] As previously mentioned, however, when the graft is patent and intact and the patient is not septic, complete graft preservation can be an easier and more efficacious method of treating infected peripheral prosthetic grafts.[15,16,18] We are not in favor of treating infected intracavitary grafts in this manner because observation of the graft and surrounding wound, and repeated operative debridements, are usually not possible.[15,21] Besides avoiding difficult wound dissections and the possibility of inadvertent hemorrhage, we believe that improved limb salvage is one of the most evident advantages of selective graft preservation. When routine total graft excision is performed, high amputation rates have been reported.[13,14]

This report demonstrates that attempted complete graft preservation was equally likely whether gram-positive or gram-negative bacteria were cultured from the wound. Graft preservation has previously been reported to be successful when gram-positive bacteria were cultured from the wound.[1-3,13] This has recently been shown to be especially true when *Staphylococcus epidermidis* was present.[2,3] In our series *S. aureus* was associated with the most virulent gram-positive infections, and this has been noted in other reports.[22] However, in our series 11 of 18 of wounds that cultured *S. aureus,* either alone or in combination with other bacteria, healed and remained healed. None of the graft infections associated with *S. aureus* resulted in anastomotic disruption.

Gram-negative bacteria are generally considered much more virulent than gram-positive bacteria,[1,2,6-10] but in our series a successful outcome was achieved in the majority of gram-negative infections. We are not completely certain why our results are better compared to most other series, but our improved findings may be due to the prolonged course of appropriate intravenous antibiotics, aggressive wound debridements, and application of graft preservation only in patients who fulfilled the previously mentioned criteria. To the contrary, when *Pseudomonas* was cultured from the wounds, a successful outcome was achieved in fewer than half of our cases. This finding is supported by others who have noted that this organism is particularly virulent and associated with a very high incidence of sepsis and anastomotic disruption. This is probably because *Pseudomonas aeruginosa* has a high adaptability to a wide variety of physical conditions and can survive under adverse conditions. Additionally, its mucoid exopolysaccharide coating represents an adhesion that protects it from host immune factors such as phagocytic cells and antibodies.[11] The organism also is highly resistant to most antibiotics and produces extracellular products such as elastase and alkaline protease, which inhibit phagocytosis and can degrade the arterial wall.[10,11] The endotoxin produced by *Pseudomonas* mediates septic shock, particularly through release of tumor necrosis factor.[11]

Of particular interest was our finding that if *Pseudomonas* was excluded from the analysis of attempted graft preservation, a very successful outcome was achieved when other gram-negative bacteria were cultured from the wounds. These results strongly suggest that infected grafts associated with gram-negative bacteria other than *Pseudomonas* are at least as likely to be successfully managed by complete graft preservation as infected grafts associated with gram-positive bacteria. Other gram-negative bacteria may not be as virulent as *Pseudomonas* because they do not have the characteristics previously mentioned that are associated with *Pseudomonas*.[11]

CONCLUSION

We recommend complete graft preservation if the graft is patent, the anastomoses are intact, the patient does not have systemic sepsis, and cultures of the wound yield gram-positive or gram-negative bacteria other than *Pseudomonas*. If *Pseudomonas* is cultured from the wound, then graft excision is generally recommended. We will continue to assess outcome of graft preservation in the presence of different types of bacteria and determine whether these results extend to larger series of patients.

REFERENCES

1. Geary KJ, Tomkiewicz ZM, Harrison HN, et al. Differential effects of a gram-negative and a gram-positive infection on autogenous and prosthetic grafts. J Vasc Surg 11:339-347, 1990.
2. Bandyk DF, Bergamini TM, Kinney EV, et al. In situ replacement of vascular prostheses infected by bacterial biofilms. J Vasc Surg 13:575-583, 1991.
3. Schmitt DD, Bandyk DF, Pequet AJ, et al. Bacterial adherence to vascular prostheses—A determinant of graft infectivity. J Vasc Surg 3:732-740, 1986.
4. Lorentzen JE, Nielsen OM, Arendrup H, et al. Vascular graft infection: An analysis of sixty-two graft infections in 2411 consecutively implanted synthetic vascular grafts. Surgery 98:81-86, 1985.
5. Bunt TJ. Synthetic vascular graft infections. I. Graft infections. Surgery 6:733-746, 1983.
6. Baltimore RS, Mitchell M. Immunologic investigation of mucoid strains of Pseudomonas aeruginosa. Comparison of susceptibility of opsonic antibody in mucoid and non-mucoid strains. J Infect Dis 141:238-247, 1980.
7. Rotschafer JC, Shikuma LR. Pseudomonas aeruginosa susceptibility in a university hospital: Recognition and treatment. Drug Intell Clin Pharm 20:575-581, 1986.
8. Nicas TI, Iglewski BH. The contribution of exoproducts to virulence of Pseudomonas aeruginosa. Can J Microbiol 31:387-392, 1985.
9. Conn JH, Hardy JD, Chavez CM, et al. Infected arterial grafts: Experience in 22 cases with emphasis on unusual bacteria and techniques. Ann Surg 171:704-714, 1970.
10. Threlkeld MG, Cobbs CG. Infectious disorders of prosthetic valves and intravascular devices. In Mandell GL, ed. Principles and Practice of Infectious Disease, 3rd ed. New York: Churchill Livingstone, 1990, pp 706-715.
11. Pollack M. Pseudomonas aeruginosa. In Mandell GL, ed. Principles and Practice of Infectious Disease, 3rd ed. New York: Churchill Livingstone, 1990, pp 1673-1691.
12. Szilagyi DE, Smith RF, Elliot JP, et al. Infection in arterial reconstruction with synthetic grafts. Ann Surg 176:321-333, 1972.
13. Liekweg WG Jr, Greenfield LJ. Vascular prosthetic infections: Collected experience and results of treatment. Surgery 81:335-342, 1977.
14. Kikta MJ, Goodson SF, Bishara RA, et al. Mortality and limb loss with infected infrainguinal bypass grafts. J Vasc Surg 5:566-571, 1987.
15. Veith FJ. Surgery of the infected aortic graft. In Bergan JJ, Yao JST, eds. Surgery of the Aorta and Its Body Branches. New York: Grune & Stratton, 1979, pp 521-533.
16. Calligaro KD, Veith FJ, Gupta SK, et al. A modified method for management of prosthetic graft infections involving an anastomosis to the common femoral artery. J Vasc Surg 11:485-492, 1990.
17. Kwaan JHM, Connolly JE. Successful management of prosthetic graft infection with continuous povidone-iodine irrigation. Arch Surg 116:716-720, 1981.
18. Samson RH, Veith FJ, Janko GS, et al. A modified classification and approach to the management of infections involving peripheral arterial prosthetic grafts. J Vasc Surg 8:147-153, 1988.

19. Stone KS, Walshaw R, Sugiyama GT, et al. Polytetrafluoroethylene versus autogenous vein grafts for vascular reconstruction in contaminated wounds. Am J Surg 147:692-695, 1984.
20. Shah PM, Ito K, Clauss RH, et al. Expanded microporous polytetrafluoroethylene (PTFE) grafts in contaminated wounds: Experimental and clinical study. J Trauma 23:1030-1033, 1983.
21. Calligaro KD, Veith FJ. Management of the infected aortic graft. Surgery 110:805-813, 1991.
22. Malone JM, Lalka SG, McIntyre KE, et al. The necessity for long-term antibiotic therapy with positive arterial wall cultures. J Vasc Surg 8:262-267, 1988.

Adaptation of Vein Grafts to Arterialization in Infrainguinal Bypasses: Does This Play a Role in Development of Vein Graft Stenoses?

ROBERT M. ZWOLAK, M.D., Ph.D.

When autogenous veins are used as arterial substitutes in the lower extremity circulation, the graft failure rate at 5 years is a disappointing 15% to 40%. In a classic study performed to determine the reasons for lower extremity vein graft failure, Szilagyi et al.[1] correlated arteriographic findings with histologic observations in grafts that underwent reoperation. They estimated that 25% of the structural changes seen on arteriograms were caused by intimal thickening. Although more recent analyses suggest that the overall rate of graft failure is decreasing, the proportion resulting from intimal hyperplasia actually may be increasing as technical causes for failure become less common.[2,3] The unique aspect of vein graft failure is that the maladaptive patency-threatening intimal hyperplasia is superimposed on the series of adaptive events known as "arterialization." Although arterialization is a biologic misnomer, the term is used commonly to describe the adaptive vascular remodeling that occurs following graft placement. Most of what we know about the cellular events that constitute arterialization is based on autopsy studies, evaluations of failed or failing grafts, and data from animal models.[4] Autopsy studies have confirmed that intimal thickening is found in virtually all grafts that remain patent for 1 month after placement, whereas only a small proportion develop lesions thick enough to cause a significant stenosis. Unfortunately, neither the stimuli for adaptive arterialization nor the stimuli for maladaptive intimal hyperplasia in vein grafts have been fully identified. Studies performed in animal models have helped to elucidate the cellular events that occur in adaptive vein graft remodeling. However, the dissimilarities between graft-threatening intimal hyperplasia in humans and the adaptive intimal hyperplasia that develops in animal models further complicate the issues of pathogenesis and successful intervention. The remainder of this chapter will discuss adaptive intimal hyperplasia in experimental vein graft models, adaptive remodeling and maladaptive intimal hyperplasia in human vein grafts, and the differences between humans and animal models. The yet unanswered question of what causes graft-threatening intimal hyperplasia in human grafts will be addressed based on current data.

ADAPTIVE INTIMAL HYPERPLASIA IN EXPERIMENTAL VEIN GRAFTS

Publications attempting to elucidate the mechanism and details of vein graft wall thickening when veins are used for arterial conduits have appeared in the literature since Carrel and Guthrie made the original observation in 1906. Most experiments have been done in rabbits, dogs, and rats. In a study of rabbit vein grafts published several years ago, we found that vein graft placement results in an initial migration of smooth muscle cells to the intima and a subsequent burst of proliferation of these previously quiescent cells.[5] This rapid increase in smooth muscle cell replication occurs during the first week after implantation and then quickly falls (Fig. 1). Accumulation of the smooth muscle cells and extracellular matrix results in thickening of the intima and media. After the first 4 weeks, additional wall thickening in this rabbit model results primarily from matrix production, and most of the remodeling changes are complete by 12 weeks. It is important to note that the changes that occur in this model constitute adaptive remodeling, and at no point is there encroachment on the flow channel. This is also probably true of other animal models, although the diameter of the flow channel is not a parameter that has been measured frequently in other species.

Hemodynamic factors including distending blood pressure and shear stress affect the remodeling that occurs in experimental vein grafts, but

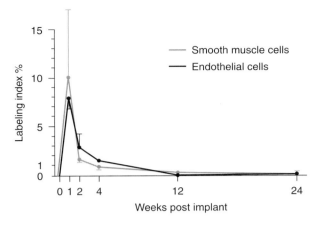

Fig. 1 Smooth muscle cell and endothelial cell thymidine labeling index during the 24 weeks following implantation of jugular vein grafts in the carotid artery in rabbits. The labeling index represents the proportion of cells in the S-phase of the cell cycle. At baseline both cell types are quiescent with indices less than 0.05%. Peak proliferative activity was measured at 1 week with a smooth muscle cell index of 10.28 ± 6.12% and an endothelial index of 8.10 ± 1.20%. The labeling rates decrease to just above basal activity by 12 weeks.

disagreement still exists regarding the exact roles of tissue deformation, wall tension and stress, and shear stress as the stimuli that elicit intimal and medial hyperplasia. The thickness of the intima is the variable most widely studied, and this has been shown by several authors to increase as mean shear stress decreases.[6-9] However, one report provides evidence that variation in shear stress with the cardiac cycle is more closely associated with intimal thickening than mean shear stress.[10] Thickening of the media has been identified in experimental vein grafts in dogs and rabbits, and this is most closely associated with increased circumferential deformation of the vein wall in canine experiments.[5,7,8] In rabbit experiments the total thickness of the vein graft wall (intima plus media) is proportional to the wall tension.[5]

To help define the effect of shear stress in the rabbit vein graft model, we placed bilateral jugular vein grafts in the common carotid arteries of rabbits.[9] We then ligated the external carotid artery outflow on one side, thereby creating a reduction in shear stress through a reduction in blood flow. Flow decreased by approximately 25% and this reduction remained constant throughout the duration of the experiment. The external carotid artery ligation had no impact on blood pressure within the grafts, and in each rabbit the graft with normal flow in the contralateral carotid artery served as a paired, blood pressure–matched control. Thus a reduction in blood flow was the single, cleanly controlled variable in this experiment.

All grafts were harvested with pressure perfusion fixation 1 month after insertion. Grafts with reduced flow were found to have markedly enhanced intimal hyperplasia when compared to grafts with normal blood flow. There was also far more smooth muscle cell proliferation and matrix accumulation in grafts with reduced flow. This resulted in intimal compartments that measured almost 70% thicker than comparable region in grafts with normal flow (Fig. 2). Although the most impressive differences were found in the intima, grafts with low flow also had 15% more medial thickening than control grafts with normal flow. However, to our surprise, the marked additional thickening that occurred in the vein graft walls did not result in a reduction in lumen diameter, and therefore a compensatory upward adjustment in shear stress did not occur. The graft cylinder actually grew somewhat larger in the outward direction as a result of the increased wall thickness.

In this experiment the common carotid arteries just proximal to the vein grafts were also harvested to compare arterial remodeling with vein graft remodeling under normal and reduced-shear circumstances. On the side with reduced flow, the arteries responded in a predictable manner by remodeling to a smaller lumen diameter with an increase in medial thickness. This change resulted in a normalization of shear stress. There was no change in the thickness of the intima, which remained a single layer of endothelial cells. Thus, although both arteries and vein grafts responded to the physiologic stimulus of reduced blood flow with an increase in wall thickness, the mechanism of the response differed substantially (see Fig. 2). We had predicted the increase in wall thickness of the vein grafts as a response to reduced flow, but we were surprised that this was not accompanied by a reduction in the caliber of the flow channel. We postulated that the cellular response to reduced shear in the vein grafts may have been physiologically appropriate, but the structurally limited adventitia of the rabbit jugular vein was inadequate to contain the inward growth.

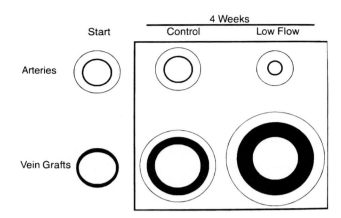

Fig. 2 Diagrammatic representation of architectural changes in rabbit arteries and vein grafts 4 weeks following graft implantation. Control conditions indicate no alteration in the normal carotid artery outflow bed. Low-flow conditions were attained by ligation of the external carotid artery. For arteries the dark inner circle represents the intima. Low flow results in a reduction in the arterial lumen diameter but no change in the thickness of the intima. The arterial media is represented by a clear space outside the intimal ring. Low flow brings about an increase in medial thickness. For vein grafts the initial graft is represented by a virtually invisible intima, and the dark circle is the media. Under normal flow conditions at 4 weeks, both the intima and the media of the vein graft are markedly thickened compared to baseline measurements. The intima is represented by the dark ring and the media by the clear ring. With reduced flow the vein graft intima thickness is 57 ± 12 µm compared to 35 ± 5 µm with normal flow ($p = .05$). The vein graft media is 74 ± 4 µm thick with reduced flow compared to 63 ± 4 µm with normal flow ($p = .02$). Despite increases in intima and media thickness with reduced flow, the lumen of the reduced flow vein graft was equal to that of the normal flow grafts. The increased compartment thickness was accommodated by outward growth of the grafts. (From Galt SW, Zwolak RM, Wagner RJ, Gilberson JJ. Differential response of arteries and vein grafts to blood flow reduction. J Vasc Surg 17:563-570, 1993.)

ADAPTIVE REMODELING AND MALADAPTIVE INTIMAL HYPERPLASIA IN HUMAN VEIN GRAFTS

The relationship between maladaptive intimal thickening in human grafts and the remodeling changes of arterialization remains poorly understood, now more than 20 years after the original observations of Szilagyi et al.[1] If intimal hyperplasia occurs in all vein grafts during arterialization, why does it proceed to the point of forming graft-threatening stenoses in portions of some grafts? Far less is known about intimal hyperplasia at the cellular level in human grafts than in animal models.[4] Some early electron microscopic analyses revealed a predominance of smooth muscle cells and collagen in the thickened intima, with very few fibroblasts, whereas others suggested a predominance of fibroblasts. A recent study employed immunohistochemical techniques with antibodies to smooth muscle cell actin on segments of four multiply thrombectomized vein grafts. The authors identified smooth muscle cells as the primary cell type.[11] This report is arguably the most sophisticated analysis of the cellular composition of failing grafts to date, but more work is needed to firmly establish the cellular makeup of adaptive arterialization and maladaptive stenosis in human vein grafts.

If reduced shear stress increases intimal hyperplasia in animal vein grafts, is there any possibility that maladaptive hyperplastic lesions in human grafts result from low shear stress or perhaps an exaggerated response to low shear? Is arterialization in human vein grafts a response to shear stress? We attempted to determine whether human vein grafts respond to shear stress by retrospectively reviewing duplex ultrasound bypass graft surveillance data.[12] Forty-eight infrainguinal in situ saphenous vein bypass grafts were studied to determine whether a correlation existed between hemodynamic factors and changes in graft diameter during the first year after placement. All grafts had undergone four routine postoperative duplex ultrasound surveillance evaluations, with the initial study completed within 1 week after placement. Grafts that had thrombosed or required surgical revision were excluded from this study, since the object was to determine the response to flow of normally functioning conduits. The duplex studies included measurements of peak systolic velocity and vein diameter, whereas average velocity and volumetric flow rate were determined by validated software algorithms available on the scanner. Shear stress was calculated based on flow rate and graft diameter. For purposes of analysis, these veins were divided into three groups based on the initial diameter determined after placement. The grafts were considered initially small if the below-knee diameter was less than 3.5 mm. Medium diameter was defined as 3.5 to 4 mm, and grafts were categorized as large in diameter if the initial measurement was greater than 4 mm.

The analysis revealed that diameter changes did occur over time in a predictable manner. The small-diameter grafts increased in caliber during the first year, whereas the diameter of large grafts decreased. No change occurred in the medium-sized grafts. When the changes in diameter during the first year were plotted against the initial shear stress, a strong correlation was identified (Fig. 3). The statistical evaluation revealed that grafts with a diameter increase of greater than 10% had significantly higher initial shear stress than grafts with a diameter that decreased by 10% (28.6 ± 3.8 vs. 13.1 ± 1.8 dynes/cm^2, $p < .01$).

The results of this study support the hypothesis that vein grafts remodel to normalize shear stress, and the "target" value of shear stress may equal that for normal arteries, approximately 20 dynes/cm^2. The changes in diameter seen in the human vein grafts were similar to those that occur in human and animal arteries following alterations in shear stress, but they differed substantially from what we observed in the rabbit vein grafts.[9] Since this study was based on duplex ultrasound data, it was impossible to determine whether the changes in lumen diameter occurred as a result of alterations in the intimal or medial compartment of the grafts. Thus we do not know whether the changes in human vein graft diameters were brought about by changes in the media, similar to arteries, or by changes in the intima, as was found in the rabbit

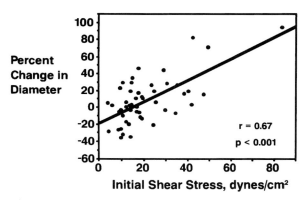

Fig. 3 Linear regression of the percentage change in graft diameter (over a 12-month period) vs. initial shear stress (1 week after bypass). (From Fillinger MF, Cronenwett JL, Besso S, Walsh DB, Zwolak RM. Vein adaptation to the hemodynamic environment of infrainguinal grafts. J Vasc Surg 19:970-979, 1994.)

vein graft experiment. Finally, it is important to point out that the changes in diameter observed in this study constitute an analysis of adaptive change in widely patent grafts rather than an analysis of maladaptive, stenosis-forming intimal hyperplasia.

WHAT DOES CAUSE THE DEVELOPMENT OF VEIN GRAFT STENOSIS?

If arterialization in animal models is an adaptive process that does not cause graft stenosis, and if shear stress in animal models and nonfailing human vein grafts is a stimulus for a controlled series of remodeling events, what causes the uncontrolled maladaptive intimal hyperplasia that leads to graft failure? The following three hypotheses are presented:

1. Perhaps maladaptive lesions occur in veins that were abnormal before grafting.
2. Poor surgical technique may injure normal veins at the time of surgery, inciting a "response to injury" reaction in the graft.
3. Some veins may have an abnormal preexisting proliferative potential when stimulated by arterial levels of shear stress, or other elements of the arterial environment. This might be called "exuberant" arterialization.

Is there evidence to support these theories? Some recent data support the notion that preexisting pathology contributes to late vein graft stenosis. Panetta et al.[13] reviewed 513 infrainguinal saphenous vein arterial bypasses and found 63 cases (12%) in which the surgeon identified the vein as being abnormal during the operation. Abnormal veins were described as thick walled, occluded, recanalized, calcified, or varicose. In 13 cases the findings were diffuse and the vein was not used. In the remaining 50 cases the vein was used despite identification of focal, seemingly acceptable abnormalities. Follow-up in this subgroup revealed a high rate of early graft failure (20%) and an extraordinarily low primary patency rate at 30 months (32%) in vein grafts that contained these abnormal segments. The patency was less than half that seen in undiseased vein grafts. This simple yet original observation serves to support the hypothesis that early thrombosis may be the destiny of veins with even minor preexisting abnormalities.

Marin et al.[14] have extended this analysis by studying the histology of abnormal saphenous veins. Among the many observations noted in this chapter regarding the preoperative status of human saphenous veins were the following findings: (1) a large range of vein wall thicknesses (20 to 360 μm), (2) a substantial variation in the quantity of extracellular matrix, and (3) a significant difference in endothelial and smooth muscle cell histology. Thus these data also support the hypothesis that preexisting venous pathologic conditions may contribute to early stenosis and failure in bypass grafts. The difficulty in the clinical application of these observations lies in identification of the abnormal venous segments at the time of the operation. Ideally, graft-threatening vein segments would be excised while normal segments were included in the bypass. The extra work and additional anastomoses could be justified only if one were confident that truly dangerous segments were being eliminated. Sales et al.[15] have approached these issues by comparing intraoperative angioscopic observations with histology of abnormal veins. These authors identified irregular white plaques during angioscopy that corresponded to sclerotic vein segments seen using light microscopy. As might be predicted, they found the angioscope to be relatively insensitive for the identification of thickened but nonsclerotic vein segments. The authors concluded that angioscopy may identify pre-existing lesions and thereby improve graft patency. However, these are really preliminary findings. Much more work is needed to determine how often a preexisting pathologic condition of saphenous vein is associated with graft failure and how accurate angioscopy is at identifying these abnormal segments.

The hypothesis that poor surgical technique results in late vein graft failure is supported by two relatively early reports, one studying human veins and one studying animal vein grafts. Gundry et al.[16] evaluated remnants of normal human saphenous vein that remained unused following harvest for coronary artery bypass grafting. These veins were traumatized by compression with surgical instruments and by fluid distention at various pressures and temperatures. The degree of intimal injury was then evaluated by scanning electron microscopy. The findings that these manipulations resulted in intimal injury led the authors to recommend the "no-touch" surgical technique for vein graft implantation. However, since only segments of vein and no actual vein grafts were evaluated in this study, the impact of the intimal injury on subsequent graft patency could not be addressed. Adcock et al.[17] studied the impact of vein preparation techniques on canine vein grafts. They compared vein grafts prepared by unmonitored (i.e., high) pressure distention using cold heparinized saline solution with grafts pressurized to a maximum of 100 mm Hg using papaverine-containing heparinized blood maintained at body temperature. They found that the latter "improved" preparation technique resulted in less wall thickening when grafts were excised and measured 10 days after implantation. However, the magnitude of these changes was minimal and no difference in graft patency was reported. Thus the data may show a measurable effect of the preparation technique on wall thickness, but the experiment falls short of proving that differences in vein harvest and preparation techniques affect long-term patency. Since the contribution of suboptimal surgical technique to subsequent intimal hyperplasia and graft failure will never be addressed in humans by a randomized controlled trial, these reports and others like it should lead us to assume the virtue of minimizing vein trauma. However, the quantitative contribution of these efforts to improved long-term patency will almost certainly remain unknown.

The third hypothesis is that of "exuberant" arterialization; that is, do some arteries overreact to the stimuli that bring about adaptive remodeling? It is in this area that the differences between animal vein graft models and human grafts are most apparent. In human vein grafts adaptive remodeling is called arterialization, whereas maladaptive changes causing graft failure are described as intimal hyperplasia. In contrast, the adaptive remodeling in animal graft models is called intimal hyperplasia, a term that accurately describes the histologic changes. Maladaptive intimal hyperplasia leading to graft stenosis virtually never occurs in animal models. Thus, although articles have been published indicating that treatment with marine oils and short peptides limit intimal hyperplasia in animal vein grafts,[18,19] neither of these interventions has prevented graft stenosis, because graft stenosis does not occur in animal models. Rather, the interventions limit the intimal hyperplasia that occurs as part of the adaptive remodeling process. There is no evidence to suggest that these will limit development of human graft stenosis. As an interesting comparison, heparin treatment, which limits smooth muscle cell proliferation in vitro and in injured arteries, has failed to show limitation of adaptive intimal hyperplasia in experimental vein grafts, as noted in two of three recent publications.[20-22] Based on the same logic, it is impossible to predict that heparin would be ineffective in limiting human vein graft stenosis.

CONCLUSION

The relationship between adaptive "arterialization" and maladaptive stenosis formation in human vein grafts is unknown. Evidence exists in humans that adaptive remodeling occurs as a response to normalize shear stress at arterial levels of approximately 20 dynes/cm^2. No data exist to determine whether this adaptive remodeling is accomplished primarily by changes in the medial compartment of the vessel, as in arteries, or primarily by changes in the intima, as occurs in experimental vein grafts. The differences between human saphenous vein grafts and experimental animal vein grafts make direct extrapolations from animals to humans impossible. No good animal model of the human saphenous vein is commonly employed, since the vein wall in experimental models has nowhere near the structural integrity or thickness encountered in humans. This preexisting wall thickness of human saphenous vein is distinctly different from other human superficial veins, for instance, cephalic or basilic veins, and is most likely due to a lifelong adaptive response to gravitational distending pressure in the absence of external support. It may be that the experimental animal grafts are more accurate models of human cephalic or basilic vein grafts. In addition to preexisting wall thickness, the saphenous vein frequently contains preexisting pathology that may contribute more to graft failure than any aspect of adaptive arterialization. Whether angioscopy or any other method can accurately identify these regions pre- or intraoperatively remains to be seen. Likewise, the true pathogenesis of graft-threatening stenosis remains elusive.

REFERENCES

1. Szilagyi DE, Elliott JP, Hageman JH, Smith RF, Dall'olmo CA. Biologic fate of autogenous vein implants as arterial substitutes. Ann Surg 178:232-245, 1973.
2. Bergamini TM, Towne JB, Bandyk DF, Seabrook GR, Schmitt DD. Experience with in situ saphenous vein bypasses during 1981 to 1989: Determinant factors of long-term patency. J Vasc Surg 13:137-149, 1991.
3. Mannick JA. Improved limb salvage from modern infrainguinal artery bypass techniques. Surgery 111:361-362, 1992.
4. Dilley RJ, McGeachie JK, Prendergast FJ. A review of the histologic changes in vein-to-artery grafts, with particular reference to intimal hyperplasia. Arch Surg 123:691-696, 1988.
5. Zwolak RM, Adams MC, Clowes AW. Kinetics of vein graft hyperplasia: Association with tangential stress. J Vasc Surg 5:126-136, 1987.
6. Berguer R, Higgins RF, Reddy DJ. Intimal hyperplasia: An experimental study. Arch Surg 115:332-335, 1980.
7. Dobrin PB, Littooy FN, Endean ED. Mechanical factors predisposing to intimal hyperplasia and medial thickening in autogenous vein grafts. Surgery 105:393-400, 1989.
8. Dobrin PB. On the roles of deformation, tension, and wall stress as critical stimuli eliciting myointimal/medial hyperplasia. J Vasc Surg 15:581-582, 1992.
9. Galt SW, Zwolak RM, Wagner RJ, Gilbertson JJ. Differential response of arteries and vein grafts to blood flow reduction. J Vasc Surg 17:563-570, 1993.
10. Morinaga K, Okadome K, Kuroki M, et al. Effect of wall shear stress on intimal thickening of arterially transplanted autogenous veins in dogs. J Vasc Surg 2:430-433, 1985.
11. Sayers RD, Jones L, Varty K, et al. The histopathology of infrainguinal vein graft stenoses. Eur J Vasc Surg 7:16-20, 1993.
12. Fillinger MF, Cronenwett JL, Besso S, et al. Vein adaptation to the hemodynamic environment of infrainguinal grafts. J Vasc Surg 19:970-979, 1994.
13. Panetta TF, Marin ML, Veith FJ, Goldsmith J, Gordon RE, Jones AM, Schwartz ML, Gupta SK, Wengerter KR. Unsuspected preexisting saphenous vein disease: An unrecognized cause of vein bypass failure. J Vasc Surg 15:102-112, 1992.
14. Marin ML, Gordon RE, Veith FJ, Panetta TF, Sales CM, Wengerter KR. Human greater saphenous vein: Histologic and ultrastructural variation. Cardiovasc Surg 2:56-62, 1994.

15. Sales CM, Marin ML, Veith FJ, Suggs WD, Panetta TF, Wengerter KR, Gordon RE. Saphenous vein angioscopy: A valuable method to detect unsuspected venous disease. J Vasc Surg 18:198-206, 1993.
16. Gundry SR, Jones M, Isihara T, Ferrans VJ. Optimal preparation techniques for human saphenous vein grafts. Surgery 88:785-794, 1980.
17. Adcock GD, Adcock OT, Wheeler JR, et al. Arterialization of reversed autogenous vein grafts: Quantification light and electron microscopy of canine jugular vein grafts harvested and implanted by standard or improved techniques. J Vasc Surg 6:283-295, 1987.
18. Landymore RW, Manku MS, Tan M, et al. Effects of low-dose marine oils on intimal hyperplasia in autologous vein grafts. J Thorac Cardiovasc Surg 98:788-791, 1989.
19. Calcagno D, Conte JV, Howell MH, Foegh ML. Peptide inhibition of neointimal hyperplasia in vein grafts. J Vasc Surg 13:475-479, 1991.
20. Makhoul RG, Davis WS, McCann RL, Hagen PO. Heparin decreases intimal hyperplasia in experimental vein grafts [abst]. Circulation 74(Suppl II):29, 1986.
21. Kohler TR, Kirkman T, Clowes AW. Effect of heparin on adaptation of vein grafts to arterial circulation. Arteriosclerosis 9:523-528, 1989.
22. Cambria RP, Ivarsson BL, Fallon JT, et al. Heparin fails to suppress intimal proliferation in experimental vein grafts. Surgery 111:424-429, 1992.

66

Bleeding Time as a Predictor of Early PTFE Graft Failure: Does It Work and Why?

RICHARD J. FOWL, M.D., KEVIN J. OSE, M.D., JOSEPH E. PALASCAK, M.D., SANDRA J. UHL, R.N., JOHN BLEBEA, M.D., and RICHARD F. KEMPCZINSKI, M.D.

Previous studies have demonstrated that the causes of early failure of expanded polytetrafluoroethylene (PTFE) grafts are multifactorial, including technical errors, poor distal runoff, acute hypotension, hypercoagulopathies, and most commonly progression of distal disease.[1-3] During the past 10 years we have preferentially used PTFE for above-knee femoropopliteal bypass grafts. During this time we identified a group of patients whose grafts occluded within 6 months despite normal intraoperative angiograms and marked improvement in postoperative hemodynamics. Some of these patients underwent successful thrombolytic therapy, and no anatomic explanation for graft failure was discovered. Results of routine coagulation studies in these patients were normal. In contrast, other patients have maintained primary uncomplicated PTFE graft patency beyond 5 years. To determine whether there were any identifiable hemostatic differences that could explain early graft thrombosis, we evaluated the hemostatic profiles of these two groups of patients.

MATERIALS AND METHODS
Patients

We retrospectively reviewed the records of all patients in our computerized vascular registry to identify those who had a femoropopliteal bypass using a PTFE graft. All operations were performed at the University of Cincinnati Medical Center, the Cincinnati Veterans Affairs Medical Center, or The Christ Hospital. We located 19 patients meeting our inclusion and exclusion criteria who agreed to participate in this study. Ten patients met the following inclusion criteria: (1) a PTFE femoropopliteal bypass, (2) increase in postoperative ankle/brachial index (ABI) of more than 0.15 before graft thrombosis,[4] and (3) graft thrombosis within 6 months postoperatively. Nine other patients fulfilled the following inclusion criteria: (1) a PTFE femoropopliteal bypass with documented postoperative hemodynamic improvement, and (2) graft patency maintained for at least 5 years. Patients were excluded for any of the following reasons: (1) chronic renal failure requiring dialysis, (2) chronic anticoagulation, (3) diagnosed hypercoagulable state, or (4) failure to improve the postoperative ABI more than 0.15.

All study participants were interviewed and their medical records reviewed to identify current medications and risk factors for vascular occlusive disease including diabetes mellitus, hypertension, cardiac disease, renal failure, hyperlipidemia, and tobacco use. The operative report, angiography reports, and noninvasive vascular laboratory studies were carefully reviewed.

HEMATOLOGIC EVALUATION

Once a patient was determined to be eligible for the study, blood samples were drawn by personnel from the coagulation laboratory who had no knowledge of the status of the patient's PTFE graft. Assays performed included the following: hemoglobin, hematocrit, white blood cell count, platelet count, sodium, potassium, chloride, carbon dioxide, blood urea nitrogen (BUN), creatinine, template bleeding time, protein C (functional, antigen), protein S functional and antigen (free and total), antithrombin III, Russell's dilute viper venom time, and anticardiolipin antibody (IgG, IgM) for the lupus anticoagulant, prothrombin time (PT), partial thromboplastin time (PTT), thrombin time, fibrinogen, D-dimer, fibrin degradation products, platelet aggregation studies, fibrinolytic profile, and serum viscosity.

The bleeding time was performed using a Surgicutt bleeding time kit (International Technidyne Corporation, Edison, N.J.). A sphygmo-

Supported in part by a grant from W.L. Gore & Associates, Inc.

manometer cuff was placed on the upper arm and inflated to 40 mm Hg pressure. A 5 mm long by 1 mm deep incision was made on the lateral aspect of the volar surface of the forearm. Every 30 seconds the cut was blotted using filter paper until the bleeding stopped, and the time was noted.[5]

Protein C and S levels were determined using an electrophoresis Laurell Rocket technique.[6] Antithrombin III levels were determined using a chromogenic method.[7] Russell's viper venom time was assayed using the method described by Exner et al.[8] Immunoglobulin G and immunoglobulin M assays for anticardiolipin antibodies were performed using the method of Harris et al.[9] Prothrombin time and partial thromboplastin time were measured using a clot-based assay performed on an MLA 1000C photopic instrument (Medical Laboratory Automation, Inc., Pleasantville, N.Y.). Thrombin time was also determined using a clot-based assay performed on an MLA 800 photopic instrument. Fibrinogen was measured with a clot-based assay performed with Clauss methodology using electromechanical instrumentation (Becton-Dickinson Microbiology Systems, Hunt Valley, Md.).[10] D-dimer was assayed with a rapid latex agglutination slide test using mouse monoclonal antibodies.[11] Fibrin degradation products were determined using a rapid latex agglutination slide test using rabbit antihuman fibrinogen.[12] Platelet aggregation studies were performed on a PACKS-4 Aggregometer (Helena Laboratories, Beaumont, Tx.) using platelet agonists epinephrine, adenosine diphosphate, and collagen.[10] Tissue plasminogen activator (tPA) activity, tPA inhibitor activity, α-2-antiplasmin, and plasminogen were assayed using a chromogenic method, and the tPA antigen was assayed by ELISA.[13] Serum viscosity was determined using an Ostwald viscosimeter.[14]

All data were expressed as mean ± standard deviation and entered into a computerized relational database (DataEase, Turnbull, Ct.). Statistical analysis was performed using the two-tailed unpaired Student's t-test with $p \leq .05$ considered as statistically significant. Differences in risk factors between groups was analyzed using Fischer's exact test. This study was reviewed and approved by the University of Cincinnati Institutional Review Board, which monitors all studies involving human subjects.

RESULTS

Ten patients with early (less than 6 months) graft occlusion and nine patients with primary graft patency of over 5 years were evaluated. In each group, all but one patient had above-knee femoropopliteal grafts (FPG) and the other had a below-knee FPG. One patient in each group had an above-knee FPG to an isolated popliteal artery segment. Eight patients with occluded grafts were men, compared with only five men with patent grafts ($p = .52$, Fisher's exact test). The mean age of patients with occluded grafts was 58 ± 16 years (range, 21 to 75 years) compared with 69 ± 9 years (range, 65-83 years) for those with patent grafts ($p = .091$, two-tailed t-test). The mean patency interval for occluded grafts was 4 ± 2 months (range, 3 weeks to 6 months), and the mean patency interval for patent grafts was 88 ± 26 months (range, 60 to 125 months) ($p < .0001$). There was no significant difference in the incidence of any atherosclerotic risk factor between the two groups.

Table 1 summarizes the lower extremity arterial Doppler measurements. There was no significant difference in the preoperative and postoperative ABIs nor in the postoperative change in ABI between the two groups.

Table 2 summarizes the mean values of all but two laboratory tests. There was no significant difference between groups for any of these tests. There was also no significant difference in platelet aggregation between the two groups: five patients had decreased aggregation in each group, three in the early occlusion and two in the patent group had increased aggregation, and one in the occluded group and two with patent grafts had normal aggregation ($p = .57$). One patient did not undergo platelet aggregation studies because of a technical error. Only one patient with a patent graft had a lupus anticoagulant, and none of the patients with occluded grafts had a lupus anticoagulant.

Table 3 summarizes the individual results of bleeding time and PTT for both groups of patients. The difference in the mean bleeding time was highly significant ($p < .0002$). Nine of 10 patients with an occluded graft had a bleeding time of 5.5 minutes or less, and all patients with a patent graft had bleeding times of 5.5 minutes or more. Additionally, all but one patient in each group were taking aspirin when the bleeding times were measured. The mean PTT was higher

Table 1 Ankle/brachial index data

	Preoperative		Postoperative		Postoperative change	
	Occluded	Patent	Occluded	Patent	Occluded	Patent
	0.39	0.53	0.96	1.00	0.57	0.47
	0.58	0.93	0.95	1.10	0.37	0.67
	0.25	0.38	1.00	0.86	0.75	0.48
	0.45	0.18	0.92	0.91	0.47	0.73
	0.21	0.77	0.41	1.10	0.20	0.33
	0.61	0.50	0.97	1.09	0.36	0.59
	0.57	0.31	1.01	0.69	0.44	0.38
	0.47	0.74	0.71	0.96	0.24	0.22
	0.34	0.41	0.78	0.93	0.44	0.52
	0.00		1.06		1.06	
Mean ± SD	0.39 ± 0.19	0.47 ± 0.19	0.83 ± 0.20	0.91 ± 0.16	0.49 ± 0.25	0.44 ± 0.19
	$p = .36$		$p = .68$		$p = .65$	

Occluded = Patients with occluded PTFE grafts; patent = patients with patent PTFE grafts; SD = standard deviation.

Table 2 Measured hematologic parameters (mean ± SD)

Study	Normal values	Occluded	Patent	p Value
Hematocrit	37-52%	41.0 ± 6.3	37.8 ± 6.5	0.20
Platelet count	150-375 × 1000/mm^3	261 ± 80	255 ± 75	0.82
BUN	5-20 mg/dl	15 ± 6	33 ± 26	0.0502
Creatinine	0.7-1.4 mg/dl	1.0 ± 0.3	2.3 ± 2.1	0.07
Prothrombin time	10.3-12.7 sec	11.7 ± 0.5	12.1 ± 0.9	0.20
Thrombin time	24-36 sec	10.8 ± 0.9	11.3 ± 1.0	0.28
Fibrinogen	150-400 mg/dl	345 ± 106	399 ± 150	0.37
Protein C functional	80-140% nl	101 ± 17	101 ± 30	0.77
Protein C antigen	70-150% nl	100 ± 21	93 ± 23	0.40
Protein S free	65-135% nl	94 ± 28	89 ± 25	0.63
Protein S total	70-150% nl	113 ± 34	116 ± 29	0.82
Antithrombin III	80-120% nl	106 ± 20	103 ± 16	0.65
D-dimer	<0.25 µg/ml	0.30 ± 0.1	0.31 ± 0.11	0.83
Liproprotein (a)	<30 mg/dl	25 ± 34	40 ± 35	0.28
Fibrin degradation products	<16 µg/ml	<16	<16	NS
Serum viscosity	1.4-1.8	1.6 ± 0.1	1.6 ± 0.1	0.87
Fibrinolytic profile				
tPA activity	0.11-1.94 IU/ml	0.45 ± 0.27	0.64 ± 0.52	0.31
tPA antigen	3.7-13.7 µg/ml	13.6 ± 7.8	14.6 ± 5.5	0.30
PAI activity	3.5-26.9 IU/ml	13.6 ± 9.3	17.1 ± 18	0.63
α-2 antiplasmin	77-129% nl	107 ± 15	98 ± 14	0.20
Plasminogen	75-133% nl	100 ± 15	94 ± 20	0.44

nl = normal; NS = not significant; occluded = patients with occluded PTFE grafts; PAI = plasminogen activator inhibitor; patent = patients with patent PTFE grafts; SD = standard deviation; sec = seconds; tPA = tissue plasminogen activator.

Table 3 Individual bleeding times and PTTs

	Bleeding time (min) (normal <9.5 min)		PTT (sec) (normal 24-36 sec)	
	Occluded (ASA)	Patent (ASA)	Occluded	Patent
	8.0 (Yes)	15.0 (Yes)	33	44
	5.5 (Yes)	11.5 (Yes)	32	40
	5.0 (Yes)	10.5 (Yes)	30	38
	4.5 (No)	10.0 (Yes)	29	40
	4.0 (Yes)	9.0 (Yes)	28	35
	4.0 (Yes)	8.0 (Yes)	28	32
	3.5 (Yes)	7.0 (Yes)	27	28
	3.0 (Yes)	6.5 (Yes)	27	27
	2.0 (Yes)	5.5 (No)	25	22
	2.0 (Yes)		23	
Mean ± SD	4.2 ± 1.8	9.1 ± 2.9	28 ± 4	33 ± 7.0
	$p = .0002$		$p = .044$	

ASA: (Yes) = patient taking aspirin when bleeding time was measured; (No) = patient not taking aspirin.

in the patients with a patent graft, although there was considerable overlap in individual values between the two groups ($p = .044$).

DISCUSSION

Common causes of PTFE failure include technical error, hypotension, poor runoff, and, most commonly, progression of distal disease as a result of neointimal hyperplasia or atherosclerosis.[1-3] Most PTFE grafts that fail occlude within 1 year.[1,2] Quiñones-Baldrich et al.[2] noted that progression of distal disease was the cause of PTFE graft failure in 42% of their patients. Over half of these patients had neointimal hyperplasia, although it was not considered extensive enough to produce graft failure. They believed graft failure was caused by reduced flow secondary to poor runoff. Ascer et al.[1] found no identifiable cause for graft thrombosis in 30% of patients in their series of 165 failed PTFE grafts. They could not provide a good explanation for failure of these grafts and speculated that hematologic abnormalities may have been responsible. However, measurement of routine coagulation parameters such as antithrombin III, protein C, and protein S levels were not helpful. These authors failed to mention any evaluation of platelet function in their patients.

Hypercoagulable states are more commonly being implicated in graft failure. In one recent report a hypercoagulable state was discovered in 9.5% of patients undergoing a variety of vascular surgical procedures.[15] The most common disorders that cause hypercoagulability are deficiencies of protein C, protein S, antithrombin III, the presence of a lupus anticoagulant, or heparin-induced thrombocytopenia with thrombosis.[16-18] Recently resistance to activated protein C has been shown to be a common hypercoaguable state in patients with deep venous thrombosis.[19] However, the assay for this was not available for the patients in this study. Other less common coagulation abnormalities implicated include abnormalities in the fibrinolytic system and increased levels of coagulation factors V, VIII, and IX.[18] In our study there were no significant differences in levels of protein C, protein S, or antithrombin III between those patients with patent grafts and those who developed early occlusion. There was no difference in the fibrinolytic profiles of the two groups. Assays for lupus anticoagulants (elevated PTT with increased dilute viper venom time) were also not significantly different. We did not measure factor V, VIII, and IX levels, but elevated levels of these factors rarely cause thrombotic states.[18] Since none of our patients were receiving heparin, we did not attempt to detect the presence of heparin antibodies.[17] Therefore none of the commonly identifiable hypercoagulable states could be implicated as the cause of graft failure in our patients.

Bleeding time evaluation has been proposed as (1) a test of platelet function in certain bleeding disorders, (2) a measure of efficacy for various forms of therapy (such as transfusions), and (3) a predictor of abnormal bleeding.[20] Rodgers and Levin[21] recently reviewed 862 articles representing 1321 studies related to bleeding time and its usefulness. In this extensive review the authors noted multiple factors that affect the bleeding time. Factors that increase the bleeding time include variations in the technique, female sex, decreased platelet count, anemia, a multitude of hematologic disorders that cause impaired platelet aggregation (e.g., von Willebrand's syndrome) and others that do not affect platelet function (e.g., dysfibrinogenemia), and uremia. Factors that decrease the bleeding time include increased age, male sex, increased platelet count and hematocrit level, and atherosclerosis. After applying multiple statistical tests to the available data from the literature, the authors found very little proven clinical usefulness for this test. They noted that there was no correlation between bleeding time and platelet count. Although bleeding time is prolonged in disorders with impaired platelet function, it is not necessarily a specific indicator of in vivo platelet function. Deficiencies of coagulation factors, administration of anticoagulants (heparin, coumadin), and anemia will prolong the bleeding time, yet they have no known affect on platelet function. There was also no correlation between bleeding time and the risk of hemorrhage elsewhere in the body. In our study there was no significant difference in platelet count, hematocrit level, age, or sex between our patient groups. All patients had atherosclerosis, and patients were excluded if they had known hematologic disorders that could affect their coagulation system. Therefore none of these factors could account for the marked difference we observed in the bleeding time.

Two factors that have definitely been shown to increase the bleeding time are uremia and aspirin therapy.[22-24] Although there was no statistically significant difference in the BUN levels between our two study groups, there was a very strong trend (mean of 15 ± 6 mg/dl for patients with occluded grafts vs. a mean of 37 ± 27 mg/dl for those with patent grafts; $p = .0502$) that suggests that uremia could have been partly responsible for the longer bleeding times present in the patients with patent grafts. However, two patients with patent grafts had BUN and creatinine values of 60/5.8 mg/dl and 73/6.2 mg/dl (not on dialysis), respectively, which greatly skewed the mean values for the entire group. If these two patients are excluded from the analysis, the remaining seven patients with patent grafts had creatinine values of less than 2.0 mg/dl, and their mean BUN value decreases to 23 ± 20 mg/dl ($p = .24$), but the difference in bleeding time still remains statistically significant (4.2 ± 1.8 minutes vs. 8.6 ± 2.3 minutes; $p = .0004$). Since all but one patient in each group were taking aspirin, there was no difference between groups for this factor. In fact the patients with early graft thrombosis had very short bleeding times despite aspirin therapy, which suggests that aspirin does not clinically affect platelet function in these patients. Although the evidence for its usefulness is controversial, bleeding time has mainly been used to predict the risk for increased bleeding and not to predict an increased risk for thrombosis. Our data suggest that patients who have a bleeding time of 5.5 minutes or less while taking aspirin may be at great risk for early PTFE femoropopliteal graft thrombosis.

The one other test that achieved statistical significance ($p = .044$) between our two study groups was the partial thromboplastin time (PTT). Since the mean PTT value was longer in the patients with patent grafts, some other factor in the intrinsic pathway of the coagulation system could exist that causes these patients to have a more hypocoagulable status than those with early graft thrombosis. However, since patients with graft occlusion had shorter PTTs, this also suggests that they could have low-grade activation of their hemostatic mechanisms that makes them prone to forming thrombus on foreign surface such as PTFE. However, the bleeding time was much more predictive of graft thrombosis because of the highly significant difference in the mean values, and there was little overlap in individual values between groups compared with individual PTTs.

Since platelet function abnormalities do affect the results of bleeding time, a recent study by Saad et al.[25] provides further evidence that platelet function may greatly affect prosthetic graft patency. These investigators evaluated platelet function in a group of 40 patients who underwent 53 femoropopliteal bypass grafts using externally supported Dacron and who were followed for a mean of 50 months. Saad et al. developed a numerically derived platelet aggregation (PA) score based on the platelet count and aggregation pattern. When the PA score remained less than 15 (decreased platelet aggregability), 15 of 16 grafts remained patent. If the PA score was 30 or more (increased platelet aggregability), only two of 17 grafts remained patent. The PA score was more predictive of prolonged graft patency than runoff, since patients with 2- or 3-vessel runoff and a PA score of less than 30 had an 80% 5-year patency rate, but those with good runoff and a PA score of 30 or higher had only a 27% 5-year patency rate ($p = .0001$). Therefore increased platelet aggregability, as reflected by a PA score of 30 or more or by a bleeding time of 5.5 minutes or less, may play a far more important role in determining prosthetic graft patency than has previously been realized. A major advantage for using bleeding times compared with platelet aggregation studies is relative cost effectiveness: a bleeding time evaluation at our institution costs $50, compared with $173 for standard platelet aggregation studies.

Our study suggests that platelet activation, as reflected by a bleeding time of 5.5 minutes or less, may be responsible for some early PTFE femoropopliteal graft thromboses. Aspirin therapy does not seem to correct this abnormality and prolong bleeding time in patients with early graft thrombosis. Based on our data, patients who are being considered for a PTFE femoropopliteal graft should have a bleeding time measured preoperatively. Although all patients with early graft thrombosis had a "normal" bleeding time of less than 9.5 minutes, patients with bleeding times less than 5.5 minutes appear to be at increased risk for infrainguinal PTFE graft failure and every effort should be made to find an autogenous conduit. If others confirm a correlation between decreased bleeding times and early graft thrombosis, this test may become a useful predictor of thrombosis rather than bleeding. Because of the relatively small sample size, further data from a large prospective study must be obtained to confirm these initial observations and to determine what factors decrease bleeding time in patients requiring femoropopliteal graft procedures.

We thank Peg Story, R.N., for her assistance in recruiting patients for the study.

REFERENCES

1. Ascer E, Collier P, Gupta SK, Veith FJ. Reoperation for polytetrafluoroethylene bypass failure: The importance of distal outflow site and operative technique in determining outcome. J Vasc Surg 5:298-310, 1987.
2. Quiñones-Baldrich WJ, Prego A, Ucelay-Gomez R, Vescera CL, Moore WS. Failure of PTFE infrainguinal revascularization: Patterns, management alternatives, and outcome. Ann Vasc Surg 5:163-169, 1991.
3. O'Donnell TF, Mackey W, McCullough JL, et al. Correlation of operative findings with angiographic and noninvasive hemodynamic factors associated with failure of polytetrafluoroethylene grafts. J Vasc Surg 1:136-148, 1984.
4. Rutherford RB, Flanigan DP, Gupta SK, et al. Suggested standards for reports dealing with lower extremity ischemia. J Vasc Surg 4:80-94, 1986.
5. Surgicutt Bleeding Time Kit Instruction Manual. International Technidyne Corporation, Edison, N.J.
6. Comp PC, Nixon RR, Cooper MR, Esson CT. Familial protein S deficiency is associated with recurrent thrombosis. J Clin Invest 74:2082-2088, 1984.
7. Chockley M, Renner JA. An improved clinical assay for antithrombin III (heparin cofactor). Am J Clin Pathol 74:213-217, 1980.
8. Exner T, Papadopoulos G, Koutts J. Use of a simplified dilute Russell viper venous time (dRVVT) confirms heterogeneity among lupus anticoagulants. Blood Coagul Fibrinolysis 1:259-266, 1990.
9. Harris EN, Asherson RA, Hughes RV. Antiphospholipid antibodies—Autoantibodies with a difference. Annu Rev Med 39:261-271, 1988.
10. Sirridge MS, Shanron R. Laboratory Evaluation of Hemostasis and Thrombosis. Philadelphia: Lea & Febiger, 1983, pp 1-229.
11. Gaffney PJ. Distinction between fibrinogen and fibrin degradation products in plasma. Clin Chir Acta 65:109-115, 1975.
12. Mersky C, Johnson AJ, Lalezari P. Increase in fibrinogen and fibrin-related antigen in human serum due to in-vitro lysis of fibrin by thrombin. J Clin Invest 51:903-911, 1972.
13. Glueck CJ, Glueck HI, Tracy T, et al. Relationship between Lp(a), lipids, apolipoproteins, and fibrinolytic activity in 191 hyperlipidemic patients. Metabolism 42:236-246, 1993.
14. Brown BA. Hematology: Principles and Procedures. Philadelphia: Lea & Febiger, 1973, pp 184-185.
15. Donaldson MC, Weinberg DS, Belkin M, Whittemore AD, Mannick JA. Screening for hypercoagulable states in vascular surgical practice: A preliminary study. J Vasc Surg 11:825-831, 1990.
16. Nitecki S, Brenner B, Hoffman A, Lanir N, Schramek A, Torem S. Lower limb ischaemia in primary antiphospholipid syndrome. Eur J Vasc Surg 7:414-419, 1993.
17. Silver D. Heparin induced thrombocytopenia and thrombosis. Semin Vasc Surg 1:228-232, 1988.
18. Towne JB. Hypercoagulable states. Semin Vasc Surg 1:201-215, 1988.
19. Dahlack B. Physiologic anticoagulation: Resistance to activated protein C and venous thromboembolism. J Clin Invest 94:923-927, 1994.
20. Day HJ, Rao AK. Evaluation of platelet function. Semin Hematol 23:89-101, 1986.
21. Rodgers RPC, Levin J. A critical reappraisal of the bleeding time. Semin Thromb Hemost 1:1-20, 1990.
22. Fernandez F, Goudable C, Sie P, Ton-That H, Durand D, Suc JM. Low hematocrit and prolonged bleeding time in uraemic patients: Effect of red cell transfusions. Br J Haematol 59:139-148, 1985.

23. Remuzzi G, Livio M, Marchiaro G, Mecca G, de Gaitano G. Bleeding in renal failure: Altered platelet function in chronic uraemia only partially corrected by haemodialysis. Nephron 22:347-353, 1978.
24. Stuart MJ, Miller ML, Davey FR, Wolk JA. The post-aspirin bleeding time: A screening test for evaluating haemostatic disorders. Br J Haematol 43:649-659, 1979.
25. Saad EM, Kaplan S, El-Massry S, et al. Platelet aggregometry can accurately predict failure of externally-supported knitted Dacron femoropopliteal bypass grafts. J Vasc Surg 18:587-595, 1993.

67

The Effect of Smoking and Fibrinogen on Vein Graft Failure

DANIEL J. HIGMAN, F.R.C.S., ROBERT C.J. HICKS, F.R.C.S., JANET T. POWELL, M.D., Ph.D., and ROGER MALCOLM GREENHALGH, M.A., M.D., M.Chir., F.R.C.S.

In recent years vascular surgeons have become increasingly ambitious in their attempts to salvage ischemic limbs and to avoid major amputation. One area of treatment in which there has been a great deal of activity is in performing bypass surgery to increasingly distal arteries. Despite many technologic improvements in synthetic graft materials, it has become clear that the use of good quality autologous vein gives the best chance of long-term patency; it is perhaps not surprising that very great interest is now centered on the causes of vein graft failure and the factors associated with occlusion.

Poor patient selection and technical factors at the time of surgery probably account for most early graft occlusions during the first postoperative month. The annual 3% attrition rate of late graft occlusions after 2 or 3 years probably relates principally to the progression of underlying disease in the native arteries. Between these two time periods, a constant frustration for vascular surgeons is the continual occurrence of narrowing and occlusion in vein grafts that were apparently satisfactory at the original operation. Approximately 30% of vein grafts will develop perianastomotic intimal hyperplasia, localized stenoses, and strictures, that critically reduce the blood flow through the bypass and predispose to graft thrombosis. The importance of stenosis as a precursor to vein graft occlusion has been identified in many reports of graft surveillance programs. The poor outcome for limb salvage that follows graft occlusion has prompted much interest in the maintenance of graft patency, but although interventions such as percutaneous balloon angioplasty or patch angioplasty may produce encouraging secondary patency rates, there is currently no therapeutic measure available to inhibit the development of intimal hyperplasia and vein graft stenosis.[1] Such a measure is unlikely to emerge without a greater understanding of the vascular biology of vein grafts and the factors associated with failure. Most research has focused on the biology of the vascular smooth muscle cell.[1,2] We have been more concerned with how interactions at the blood vessel interface might predispose to graft failure.

THE MRC FEMOROPOPLITEAL BYPASS TRIAL AND VEIN GRAFT OCCLUSION

Much of our early work in this area is derived from the Medical Research Council–sponsored multicenter trial, which studied the effects of antiplatelet agents on the patency of femoropopliteal vein bypass grafts.[3] This was a randomized placebo-controlled trial in which patients either were allocated to receive aspirin and dipyridamole 2 days before bypass surgery and continuing indefinitely or to receive placebo tablets. The trial as a whole failed to show any beneficial effect of antiplatelet therapy on graft patency, although it did show that these drugs reduced the incidence of myocardial infarction and stroke in patients with cardiovascular disease. However, an important feature of the trial was the clinical and biochemical data that were recorded on patients with vein grafts. These data gave us important insights into other factors associated with femoropopliteal vein graft occlusion.

A subset of the original trial patients (n = 157) were prospectively studied in this way. In these 157 patients 159 infrainguinal vein grafts were performed for critical ischemia or disabling claudication.[4] In the first postoperative year, 44 of the vein grafts occluded. The single factor most closely associated with occlusion was the plasma

Supported by the British Heart Foundation and the A.F.G. Research Foundation.

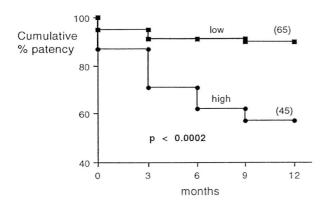

Fig. 1 Relation of patency of vein grafts and plasma fibrinogen concentration. Patients with concentrations lower than the median are represented by squares; patients with concentrations greater than the median are represented by circles. The numbers of patients with patent grafts are shown in parentheses.

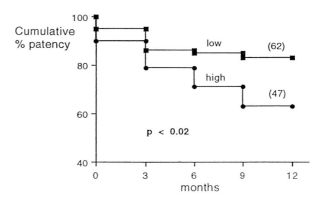

Fig. 2 Patency of femoropopliteal vein grafts in smokers (serum thiocyanate concentration >70 µmol/L; circles) and nonsmokers (serum thiocyanate concentration <70 µmol/L; squares). Numbers of patients with patent grafts are shown in parentheses.

concentration of fibrinogen; patients with occluded grafts had a median plasma fibrinogen concentration of 4.80 gm/L, compared with 3.90 gm/L in those patients with patent grafts ($p < .001$). Life-table analysis of graft patency at 12 months showed that patients with plasma fibrinogen levels lower than the median value had a patency of 90%, significantly higher than those with fibrinogen concentrations higher than the median value, with a patency of 57% ($p < .0002$) (Fig. 1). High concentrations of plasma fibrinogen appeared to be detrimental to the survival of vein grafts, providing an important insight into possible interactions between blood products and the vein graft wall.

Cigarette smoking is clearly the most important risk factor for atherosclerotic disease, and the majority of patients coming to bypass surgery will be current or former smokers. Smoking is also a potential cause of vein graft failure. The devoted smoker does not appear to be deterred by having undergone vascular reconstruction, and a large number of patients continue to smoke following surgery, despite firm advice to stop smoking. In the 157 patients with vein bypass grafts, the smoking markers carboxyhemoglobin and thiocyanate were prospectively measured throughout the follow-up period. Almost 45% of patients continued to smoke postoperatively despite strong advice to the contrary at every follow-up visit. Interestingly, less than half of these recalcitrant smokers admitted to their habit when questioned. This has been the problem with many studies in the past; smokers are reluctant to reveal their habit to vascular surgeons, and meaningful data on the effects of smoking should always take account of this fact and use objective smoking markers. One of the important features of this prospective study was the documentation of objective evidence of smoking among bypass patients.

The results showed conclusively that smoking has important effects on the outcome for patients with vein bypass grafts: smoking was clearly associated with an increased risk of graft occlusion. The smoking markers used for this study were carboxyhemoglobin (half-life about 5 hours) and thiocyanate (half-life 6 to 7 days). Results for the long half-life marker thiocyanate were the most revealing. The median plasma concentration of thiocyanate in patients with occluded grafts was 88 µmol/L, indicating a higher level of smoking than in those with patent grafts, who had a median thiocyanate level of 60 µmol/L ($p < .05$). Life-table analysis of vein graft patency showed that at 12 months' follow-up, 84% of nonsmokers had patent grafts, significantly more than the 63% of smokers with patent grafts ($p < .02$) (Fig. 2). The graft occlusion rate in smokers was double the occlusion rate in those who did not smoke or no longer smoked. This clear detrimental effect of smoking, coupled with the high prevalence of smokers in the bypass population, must give greater impetus to the efforts of vascular surgeons to persuade their patients to kick the smoking habit.

VEIN GRAFT STENOSIS

Graft occlusion is an end point with sinister implications for the ischemic limb. Best clinical practice now demands that the failing vein graft be identified with a view to preventing graft occlusion by timely intervention at an earlier stage. Accordingly, in 1992 a graft surveillance program was instituted in our unit. All vein grafts were examined throughout their length using color-coded Duplex scanning at intervals of 1 week, 1 month, and every 3 months in the first postoperative year, and all stenoses of 50% or greater were carefully recorded. At the 3- and 12-month visits, a blood sample was obtained for the estimation of smoking markers, lipids, and plasma fibrinogen. This program gave the opportunity to prospectively study the factors associated with the development of vein graft stenosis.

In our surveillance series we have reported the results of 79 consecutive vein grafts performed for critical ischemia (56 grafts), popliteal aneurysm (10 grafts), or disabling claudication, with a claudication distance of 50 meters or less (13 grafts).[5] At 1 month, 12 grafts had been excluded from the surveillance program because of early occlusion or death of the patient. Of the remaining 63 vein grafts, 20 (32%) developed stenoses of greater than 50% within the first 12 months. The only factor that was associated with the development of graft stenosis on univariate analysis was the plasma concentration of fibrinogen. For grafts with an above-median concentration of plasma fibrinogen (more than 4.4 gm/L), life-table analysis demonstrated that only 46% of grafts remained free of stenosis after 1 year, compared with 86% of those with below-median fibrinogen concentrations ($p = .009$) (Fig. 3).

In contrast to the situation with occluded grafts, smoking was not an independent risk factor for the development of vein graft stenoses. Multiple logistic regression was conducted to determine which factors were most closely associated with graft stenosis. A stepwise backward elimination procedure was used ($p = .2$ for terms to drop out of the model), and after removing the level of the distal anastomosis, sex, diabetes, preoperative smoking history, HDL cholesterol, and cholesterol as being not associated with stenosis, the remaining factors in the model were

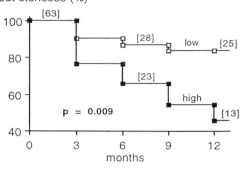

Fig. 3 The influence of fibrinogen on the development of vein graft stenoses. The cumulative graft survival, free of stenoses, is shown for patients with above-median fibrinogen concentration (closed squares) and for patients with below-median fibrinogen concentration (open squares). Eighty-six percent of patients with below-median fibrinogen concentrations had not developed stenoses by year 1, compared with 46% of grafts in patients with above-median concentrations. The numbers in parentheses give the number of grafts entering each time interval.

Table 1 Multivariate regression analysis for factors associated with the development of vein graft stenosis

Variable	Partial regression coefficient	p Value
Age (yr)	0.013	.085
Smoking at 3 mo (COHb%)	0.060	.237
Fibrinogen (gm/L)	0.151	.003
Ankle/brachial pressure index	0.640	.080

the age of the patient, the ankle/brachial pressure index at presentation, and the level of carboxyhemoglobin (i.e., continued smoking) at 3 months after surgery (Table 1).

These results suggest that smoking following vein graft surgery does influence the development of graft stenosis, but the association is not strong. It is well known that both smoking and advancing age increase the plasma concentration of fibrinogen, by approximately 5% to 10% of normal values. The association of smoking and advanced age with the development of vein graft stenosis may be explained in part by postulating that these factors exert their influence by increasing the plasma fibrinogen. Although this lends credence to the contention that to stop smoking is sensible advice for the patient with a bypass graft, circulating products of cigarette smoke may not have a direct influence on the development of intimal hyperplasia. The strong association between graft occlusion and smoking may be explained partly by the effect of smoking on fibrinogen levels but also by noting that smokers generally have a higher hematocrit level and plasma viscosity, and this increases the tendency for graft thrombosis to occur.

INTERACTION OF FIBRINOGEN WITH THE VESSEL WALL

This dominance of plasma fibrinogen as the factor most strongly associated with vein graft occlusion and stenosis provides an exciting new perspective on the biology of graft failure. Fibrinogen is the substrate in the coagulation cascade, and it might be assumed that high plasma concentrations of this protein would predispose to graft thrombosis by acting as a procoagulant. However, our more recent work suggests a more intriguing mechanism by which fibrinogen affects vein grafts, from a direct interaction of fibrinogen with the vessel wall. Until recently, fibrinogen has not been considered important in the pathogenesis of intimal hyperplasia, the principal cause of graft stenoses. There is accumulating experimental evidence to suggest mechanisms by which plasma fibrinogen influences cellular processes in the vessel wall. Fibrinogen cleavage products are mitogenic to the cells in the atherosclerotic lesion.[6] Of perhaps more relevance to the vein graft is the fact that fibrinogen binds to the adhesion molecule ICAM-1 on the venous endothelium. This interaction promotes leukocyte adhesion to the intima and cell signaling throughout the vessel wall. A recent clinical observation that fibrinogen is a potent risk factor for restenosis following coronary angioplasty[7] provides yet further evidence that fibrinogen directly promotes smooth muscle cell mitogenesis and intimal hyperplasia.

CONCLUSION

Clearly, much more needs to be known about the reasons that some vein grafts will go on working for years, whereas others stenose and occlude within a few months. Our work in this field has identified fibrinogen as one of the key factors involved in this process. Pharmacologic manipulation of plasma fibrinogen concentration or the modulation of its effects on the vein graft wall may well be the next major step toward the long-term preservation of graft patency. Similarly, lifestyle modification, stopping smoking, and exercising can help lower plasma fibrinogen concentrations and improve graft patency.

REFERENCES

1. Clowes AW. Intimal hyperplasia and graft failure. Cardiovasc Pathol 2(Suppl):S179-S186, 1993.
2. Davies MG, Hagen P-O. Pathobiology of intimal hyperplasia. Br J Surg 81:1254-1269, 1994.
3. McCollum CN, Kenchington G, Greenhalgh RM. Antiplatelet drugs in femoropopliteal vein bypasses: A mulicentre trial. J Vasc Surg 13:150-162, 1991.
4. Wiseman S, Kenchington G, Dain R, Marshall CE, McCollum CN, Greenhalgh RMG, Powell JT. Influence of smoking and plasma factors on patency of femoropopliteal vein grafts. BMJ 299:643-646, 1989.
5. Hicks RCJ, Ellis M, Mir-Hasseine R, Higman DJ, Nott D, Greenhalgh RM, Powell JT. The influence of fibrinogen concentration on the development of vein graft stenoses. Eur J Vasc Endovasc Surg 9:415-420, 1995.
6. Singh TM, Kadowaki MH, Glagov S, Zarins CK. Role of fibrinopeptide B in early atherosclerotic lesion formation. Am J Surg 160:156-159, 1990.
7. Montalescot G, Ankri A, Vicaut E, Drobinski G, Grosgogeat Y, Thomas D. Fibrinogen after coronary angioplasty as a risk factor for restenosis. Circulation 92:31-38, 1995.

SECTION VIII

Trauma and Complex Problems in Vascular Surgery

This section examines trauma and other complex problems in vascular surgery. Included are chapters on the optimal management of large- and medium-sized vein injuries, principles and techniques for managing carotid and vertebral artery trauma, surgical treatment of chronic mesenteric ischemia, and various methods for managing infected aortic and nonaortic prosthetic grafts. Additional chapters discuss techniques for first rib resection, management of upper extremity ischemia following angioaccess surgery, and techniques for dealing with vasculogenic impotence. The last three chapters are concerned with management of intractable venous ulcers, treatment of lymphatic complications following groin surgery, and treatment alternatives for deep venous thrombosis in pregnancy.

68

Update on Optimal Management of Trauma to Large- and Medium-Sized Veins

NORMAN M. RICH, M.D., MARK R. JACKSON, M.D., MAJ, MC, USA, and DAVID L. GILLESPIE, M.D., MAJ, MC, USA

Controversy continues concerning the appropriate management of injured veins, as reflected by the literature of the past 25 years.[1-50] Two textbooks, the first by Rich and Spencer[42] and the second by Hobson et al.,[17] provide additional details for further research. Civilian experience, as emphasized initially by Gaspar and Treiman[10] in 1960, has been elaborated over the past 15 years by Agarwal,[1] Aitken,[2] Barkun,[3] Bishara,[4] Blumoff,[5,6] Borman,[7] Brigham,[8] Gerlock,[11,12] Graham,[13] Hardin,[14] Hobson,[18,19] Jacobson,[21] Johnson,[22] Meyer,[25] Mullins,[26] Phifer,[27] Quast,[28] Richardson,[45] Sharma,[46] and Timberlake,[49] with their colleagues from many trauma centers in the United States and from South Africa (Aitken et al.[2]). Rich et al.,[29-41,43,44] Sullivan et al.,[47] and Wright et al.[50] provide additional details based on experience gained from the Vietnam Vascular Registry, established in 1966 at Walter Reed Army Medical Center. Specific associated research on effects of acute venous interruption carried out at Walter Reed Army Institute of Research are outlined by Hobson et al.,[15-17] Levin et al.,[23] Rich et al.,[33,42] and Swan et al.[48] Mattox et al.[24] reviewed the most extensive experience in managing civilian vascular injuries ever reported.

It is ironic to note that Dr. John B. Murphy recommended in 1897 that injured veins, like injured arteries, be repaired.[42] If one includes all medium- and large-caliber veins in a general description, it will only add to the confusion. It should be obvious that there is considerable difference in injury to the inferior or superior vena cava compared with the axillary or superficial femoral veins, with the latter two or more channels being duplicated more frequently. Recent controversy has centered on whether to ligate or repair large-caliber lower extremity veins. It has never been a question of whether the majority of patients can tolerate ligation of injured veins; rather, the challenge has been to determine which patients will not tolerate the ligation of medium and larger sized veins. Surgeons generally agree that the patient's overall condition must be considered first and that ligation may be necessary to save the life of a patient with multiple injuries. On the other hand, prevention of long-term disability, particularly from lower extremity swelling, should be considered with repair of major lower extremity veins when possible.

HISTORICAL NOTES

Schede and others identified successful efforts in repairing injured veins in the nineteenth century.[17,30,42] During the Balkan Wars before World War I, Soubbotitch noted that veins as well as arteries could be repaired successfully in managing arteriovenous fistulas and false aneurysms. Through World War II, there were a variety of conflicting recommendations regarding the management of injured veins and arteries. It is well recognized, however, that it was during the Korean Conflict that successful repair of injured arteries was first documented, at forward field hospitals, suggesting that this approach could prove acceptable for the repair of injured veins.[20] As with many wartime efforts that lead to advances in surgical procedures, the experience of approximately 600 well-trained American surgeons in Vietnam over an 8-year period (1965-1972) demonstrated that there should be an increased emphasis on the repair of major lower extremity veins, particularly the popliteal vein.[17,34,35,39-42,47]

The Vietnam consensus emphasizes that there were a number of patients who suffered from both acute venous hypertension, resulting

---

The views expressed in this article are those of the authors and do not reflect the official policy or position of the Department of the Army, Department of Defense, or the Uniformed Services University of the Health Sciences.

in the need for amputation in a number of patients, and chronic venous hypertension following acute interruption of large-caliber extremity veins. It was also realized that recanalization might be possible following early failure of an attempted venous repair. Particularly important was the refutation of previous concerns about the potential for increased incidence of thrombophlebitis and pulmonary embolism if venous repair was attempted. The clinical experience was verified in research at Walter Reed Army Institute of Research. Finally, long-term clinical follow-up added additional credibility to the desire to increase the effort to repair major extremity large-caliber veins, particularly the popliteal vein.

There have been an increasing number of reports from civilian medical centers in the United States and from around the world either confirming the experience of military surgeons in Vietnam or taking issue with the conclusions drawn from that experience. A number of reports have found that in civilian injuries for which injured veins were ligated, morbidity was not significant.[26,49] This is not surprising, considering that the wounds sustained by civilians, even from low-velocity handguns or knives, are typically less severe than the wounds of battle, with massive soft tissue destruction, interruption of lymphatics and venous collaterals, and associated fractures, all leading to increased morbidity with the ligation of major-caliber veins, particularly in the lower extremities.

It would be ideal to be able to determine which patients are at risk for complications. Phlebography and/or such examinations as ambulatory venous pressure could be of assistance; however, their use is frequently not practical because of the complexity and time involved. Because venous anatomy is inconsistent, it is vital to know the entire situation before determining success or failure of management. A knowledge of the numerous anatomic venous patterns that can exist underscores the importance of repairing one major-caliber lower extremity vein rather than repairing one of multiple conduits representing the venous return. There can be as many as one to five parallel superficial femoral veins in the deep femoral system, and the popliteal vein is known to be bifid on occasion. Gerlock et al.[11,12] have emphasized the importance of phlebography (venography); however, this approach has not been widely adopted. Those who are interested in evaluating and treating injured veins in the lower extremities recognize the value of repeated phlebograms to follow the changing developments. Color duplex scanning offers additional extremely valuable noninvasive evaluation of these patients.

Technique is extremely important in the repair of injured veins.[17,33,42] Recently Sharma et al.[46] documented the value of meticulous efforts in venous repair, leading to a higher degree of success than reported previously.

CONCLUSION

Although civilian casualties in general are distinct from the casualties generated on the battlefield, unfortunately, in the United States urban warfare is becoming more military in nature. As a result, the lessons learned on the battlefields from Korea and Vietnam to the Balkan peninsula are more relevant to the management of many civilian wounds. The evaluation of specific patients with either acute chronic venous insufficiency and/or chronic venous insufficiency remains a significant challenge. While phlebography provides the gold standard by mapping the venous anatomy, it is anticipated that advances such as color duplex scanning will help in evaluating these situations. Additional documentation and long-term follow-up will be required. Yet there is increasing evidence that there are patients with long-term disability from lower extremity swelling following ligation of medium- and large-caliber veins. The Vietnam Vascular Registry remains a repository of data that require additional follow-up evaluation. For a specific injured individual, the challenge continues to be determining whether repair of an injured major-caliber lower extremity vein will be of value to that patient.

REFERENCES

1. Agarwal N, Shah PM, Clauss RH, Reynolds DM, Stahl WM. Experience with 115 civilian venous injuries. J Trauma 22:827-832, 1982.
2. Aitken RJ, Matley PJ, Immelman EJ. Lower limb vein trauma: A long-term clinical and physiological assessment. Br J Surg 76:585-588, 1989.
3. Barkun JS, Terazza O, Daignault P, Chiu RC-J, Mulder DS. The fate of venous repair after shock and trauma. J Trauma 28:1322-1329, 1988.
4. Bishara RA, Schuler JJ, Lim LT, et al. Results of venous reconstruction after civilian vascular trauma. Arch Surg 121:607-611, 1986.
5. Blumoff RL, Proctor HJ, Johnson G Jr. Recanalization of a saphenous vein interposition venous graft. J Trauma 21:407-408, 1981.

6. Blumoff RL, Powell T, Johnson G Jr. Femoral venous trauma in a university referral center. J Trauma 22:703-705, 1982.
7. Borman KR, Jones GH, Snyder WH III. A decade of lower extremity venous trauma: Patency and outcome. Am J Surg 154:608-612, 1987.
8. Brigham RA, Eddleman WL, Clagett GP, Rich NM. Isolated venous injury produced by penetrating trauma to the lower extremity. J Trauma 23:255-257, 1983.
9. Danza R, Mauro L, Arias J, et al. Reconstruction of the femoro-popliteal vessels with a double graft (arterial and venous) in severe injury of the limb. J Cardiovasc Surg 11:60-64, 1970.
10. Gaspar MR, Treiman RL. The management of injuries to major veins. Am J Surg 100:171-175, 1960.
11. Gerlock AJ, Muhletaler CA. Venography of peripheral venous injuries. Radiology 133:77-80, 1979.
12. Gerlock AJ Jr, Thal ER, Snyder WH III. Venography in penetrating injuries of the extremities. Am J Roentgenol 126:1023-1027, 1976.
13. Graham JM, Mattox KL, Beall AC Jr. Portal venous system injuries. J Trauma 18:419-422, 1978.
14. Hardin WD Jr, Adinolfi MF, O'Connell RC, Kerstein MD. Management of traumatic peripheral vein injuries: Primary repair or vein ligation. Am J Surg 144:235-238, 1982.
15. Hobson RW II, Croom RD, Rich NM. Influence of heparin and low molecular weight dextran on the patency of autogenous vein grafts: Vein grafts in the venous system. Ann Surg 178:773-776, 1973.
16. Hobson RW II, Howard EW, Wright CB, Collins GJ, Rich NM. Hemodynamics of canine femoral venous ligation: Significance in combined arterial and venous injuries. Surgery 74:824-829, 1973.
17. Hobson RW II, Rich NM, Wright CB, eds. Venous Trauma; Pathophysiology, Diagnosis and Surgical Management. Mount Kisco: Futura, 1983.
18. Hobson RW, Yeager RA, Lynch TG, Lee BC, Jain K, Jamil Z, Padberg FT Jr. Femoral venous trauma: Techniques for surgical management and early results. Am J Surg 146:220-224, 1983.
19. Hobson RW, Lee BC, Lynch TG, Jain K, Yeager R, Jamil Z, Padberg FT Jr. Use of intermittent pneumatic compression of the calf in femoral venous reconstruction. Surg Gynecol Obstet 159:284-286, 1984.
20. Hughes CW. Arterial repair during the Korean War. Ann Surg 147:555-561, 1958.
21. Jacobson JH, Haimov J. Venous revascularization of the arm: Report of three cases. Surgery 81:599-604, 1977.
22. Johnson V, Eiseman B. Evaluation of arteriovenous shunts to maintain patency of venous autograft. Am J Surg 118:915-917, 1969.
23. Levin PM, Rich NM, Hutton JE Jr, Barker WF, Zeller JA. Role of arteriovenous shunts in venous reconstruction. Am J Surg 122:183-191, 1971.
24. Mattox KL, Feliciano DV, Burch J, Beall AC Jr, Jordan GL Jr, DeBakey ME. Five thousand seven hundred sixty cardiovascular injuries in 4459 patients: Epidemiologic evolution 1958 to 1987. Ann Surg 209:698-707, 1989.
25. Meyer JP, Walsh J, Schuler J, et al. The early fate of venous repair following civilian vascular trauma: A clinical hemodynamic and venographic assessment. Ann Surg 206:458-464, 1987.
26. Mullins RJ, Lucas CE, Ledgerwood AM. The natural history following venous ligation for civilian injuries. J Trauma 20:737-743, 1980.
27. Phifer TJ, Gerlock AJ, Rich NM, McDonald JC. Long-term patency of venous repairs demonstrated by venography. J Trauma 25:342-346, 1985.
28. Quast DC, Shirkey AL, Fitzgerald JB, Beall AC Jr, DeBakey ME. Surgical correction of injuries to the vena cava; An analysis of sixty-one cases. J Trauma 5:1-10, 1965.
29. Rich NM. Principles and indications for primary venous repair. Surgery 91:492-496, 1982.
30. Rich NM, Hobson RW II, Wright CB. Historical aspects of direct venous reconstruction. In Bergan JJ, Yao JST, eds. Symposium on Venous Problems in Honor of Geza de Takats. Chicago: Year Book, 1978.
31. Rich NM, Collins GJ Jr, Andersen CA, McDonald PT, Ricotta JJ. Venous trauma: Successful venous reconstruction remains an interesting challenge. Am J Surg 134:226-230, 1977.
32. Rich NM, Collins GJ, Andersen CA, McDonald PT. Autogenous venous interposition grafts in repair of major venous injuries. J Trauma 17:512-520, 1977.
33. Rich NM, Hobson RW II, Wright CB, Swan KG. Techniques of venous repair. In Swan KG, Hobson RW II, Reynolds DG, Rich NM, Wright CB, eds. Symposium on Venous Surgery in the Lower Extremities. St Louis: Warren H Green Publishers, 1975, pp 243-256.
34. Rich NM, Hobson RW II, Wright CB, Fedde CW. Repair of lower extremity venous trauma: A more aggressive approach required. J Trauma 14:639-652, 1974.
35. Rich NM, Baugh JH, Hughes CW. Acute arterial injuries in Vietnam: 1,000 cases. J Trauma 10:359-369, 1970.
36. Rich NM, Hughes CW. Vietnam vascular registry: A preliminary report. Surgery 65:218-226, 1969.
37. Rich NM, Sullivan WG. Clinical recanalization of an autogenous vein graft in the popliteal vein. J Trauma 12:919-920, 1972.
38. Rich NM, Hobson RW II. Historical background of repair of venous injuries. In Witkin E, et al, eds. Venous Diseases, Medical and Surgical Management. The Hague, The Netherlands: Mouton, 1974.
39. Rich NM, Hobson RW II, Wright CB, Fedde CW. Repair of lower extremity venous trauma: A more aggressive approach required. J Trauma 14:639-652, 1974.
40. Rich NM, Jarstfer BS, Geer TM. Popliteal artery repair failure: Causes and possible prevention. J Cardiovasc Surg 15:340-351, 1974.
41. Rich NM, Hobson RW II, Collins GJ Jr, Anderson CA. The effect of acute popliteal venous interruption. Ann Surg 183:365-368, 1976.
42. Rich NM, Spencer FC. Vascular Trauma. Philadelphia: WB Saunders, 1978.
43. Rich NM. Management of venous trauma. Surg Clin North Am 68:809-821, 1988.
44. Rich NM. Venous injuries. In Sabiston DC Jr, ed. Textbook of Surgery, 13th ed. Philadelphia: WB Saunders, 1986, pp 2009-2018.
45. Richardson JB Jr, Jurkovich GJ, Walker GT, Nenstiel R, Bone EG. A temporary arteriovenous shunt (Scribner) in the management of traumatic venous injuries of the lower extremity. J Trauma 26:503-509, 1986.

46. Sharma PVP, Shah PM, Vinzona AT, Pallan TM, Clauss RH, Stahl WM. Meticulously restored lumens of injured veins remain patent. Presented at the Fourth Annual Meeting of the Eastern Vascular Society. Boston: May 10-13, 1990.
47. Sullivan WG, Thorton FG, Baker LH, LaPlante ES, Cohen A. Early influence of popliteal vein repair in the treatment of popliteal vessel injuries. Am J Surg 122: 528-531, 1971.
48. Swan KG, Hobson RW, Reynolds DG, Rich NM, Wright CB, eds. Venous Surgery in the Lower Extremities. St. Louis: Warren H Green Publishers, 1975.
49. Timberlake GA, O'Connell RC, Kerstein MD. Venous injuries: To repair or ligate, the dilemma. J Vasc Surg 4:533-538, 1986.
50. Wright CB, Hobson RW II, Swan KG, Rich NM. Extremity venous ligation: Clinical and hemodynamic correlation. Am Surg 41:203-208, 1975.

69

Current Principles for Managing Carotid and Vertebral Artery Trauma

MALCOLM O. PERRY, M.D.

The highest incidence of vascular injuries in the neck is seen in urban areas where violence is endemic; penetrating trauma resulting from knives and bullets is the usual cause. Steering wheel injuries, deceleration forces, falls, and blows to the neck occasionally cause vascular wounds. Because of the frequency of multiple wounds, a careful assessment is required. This is especially true of wounds of the brachiocephalic vessels because not only is hemorrhage and airway compromise a threat, but there also may be neurologic problems.

MECHANISMS OF INJURY

Most penetrating injuries in the neck are caused by stabbing or by bullets traveling at a low velocity, and the damage is confined to the wound tract.[1] Knife wounds usually produce punctures, lacerations, and occasionally transections of the vessel, but the damage from missiles is extensive and complete vessel transection is more likely. High-velocity missiles traveling at speeds of more than 1500 feet per second can damage vessels remote from the wound tract because of the concussive effect. Secondary missiles consisting of splinters of bone or fragments of the bullet can injure other structures remote from the entry site. These destructive effects may not be suspected from initial inspection of the skin where there may be only a small entrance wound. Close-range shotgun wounds also often cause a great deal more damage to the interior structures than is apparent from superficial inspection.

Motor vehicle accidents and industrial mishaps are the primary causes of blunt trauma to the neck, but an increase in injuries from assaults is being seen. The hyperextension injury of the internal carotid artery results from extension and rotation of the head and the internal carotid artery at the base of the skull is stretched over the body of C2 and the transverse process of C3, producing multiple intimal and medial tears (Fig. 1). Avulsion of the carotid artery as it enters the carotid foramen may occur, but more often the stretch injury results in thrombosis, perhaps with embolization into the head. There can be a protracted time between the injury and the appearance of the neurologic deficit.[2]

Special problems are often encountered in these patients because there may be neurologic damage and there also may be wounds of the pharynx, esophagus, trachea, and major nerves.[3,4] Large injuries of the trachea are usually obvious but penetration of the oropharynx may be more difficult to detect. Patients who have combined injuries of the major vessels and the brachial plexus often present a difficult

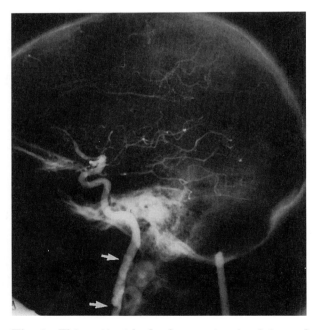

Fig. 1 This patient had a hyperextension injury of the internal carotid artery resulting in multiple injuries to the arterial wall (arrows). The artery was replaced with a saphenous vein graft.

diagnostic problem; this is particularly true if the patient has associated head injuries and altered consciousness because of closed head trauma.

DIAGNOSIS

In the evaluation of penetrating trauma to the neck it is helpful to divide the neck into three zones as described by Monson et al.[5] Zone 1 extends inferiorly from 1 cm above the manubrium to include the thoracic outlet. Zone 2 extends from zone 1 to the angle of the mandible and zone 3 from the angle of the mandible to the base of the skull. Vascular injuries in zone 2 often can be approached directly for definitive repair, but injuries in zones 1 and 3 may require special incisions for proper exposure. Penetrating injuries that pierce the platysma muscle over the anterior triangles of the neck and the root of the neck are more likely to result in major vascular wounds. In contrast, patients who have sustained blunt trauma may have an occult arterial injury without superficial evidence in the form of bruises, cuts, or lacerations. The detection of associated injuries of the sympathetic chain or major nerves may alert the surgeon to the possibility of other pathology.

In the evaluation of patients with carotid artery trauma, it is helpful to divide them into three groups for purposes of evaluation (Table 1). Group 1, which is the largest group, includes those patients who have no neurologic deficit. Group 2 comprises those patients with a mild neurologic deficit and group 3 contains patients with a severe neurologic deficit that often includes spastic hemiplegia and alterations in consciousness. The eventual outcome in these patients is largely determined by the severity and degree of the neurologic deficit prior to treatment.[3]

A careful neurologic examination is essential in the assessment of these patients. A thorough baseline neurologic examination should include evaluation of the recurrent laryngeal nerves as well as the other major nerves in the neck.

ADJUNCTIVE DIAGNOSTIC METHODS

Plain radiographs may not expose the injury, but the presence of air in the tissues or distortions of normal anatomy may assist in the detection of other wounds. Collections of air, fluid, or blood are usually evidence of an underlying wound. An upright x-ray film of the chest may reveal a mediastinal injury and perhaps an associated wound of major vessels in the thoracic

Table 1 Carotid trauma

Group	Neurologic deficits	No.
1	None	58
2	Mild	12
3	Severe	15

outlet. A mediastinal shadow that is wider than 8 cm in the second interspace suggests bleeding in the mediastinum, and although this is usually of venous origin it alerts the surgeon. Distortion of the aortic shadow, obscuring of the aortic knob, and deviation of an endotracheal or nasogastric tube also suggest the possibility of injury of the great vessels.

In stable patients ultrasound examination may help in the detection of vascular wounds. Although large hematomas in the neck interfere with ultrasonography, these studies may expose a false aneurysm or an arterial or venous injury. Normal findings do not rule out an arterial wound.[6]

Most patients who have had blunt trauma will have a CT scan of the head (or perhaps an MRI scan) to evaluate closed head injuries. These studies may also be of help in examining the cervical spine and the spinal cord. Arteriography continues to be the most useful test in the evaluation of these patients, and some authorities suggest that any patient with penetrating or blunt trauma of the neck should have a four-vessel arteriogram with intracranial radiographs.[7] There is no consensus regarding this opinion, and other trauma surgeons suggest that selective arteriography is satisfactory. Arteriograms are obtained mainly for one of three reasons: (1) to detect an injury not otherwise discernable by clinical methods, (2) to exclude the need for an exploratory operation in a patient who has no other indications for surgery, or (3) to plan an operation where special maneuvers may be required such as exposure of vessels in the thoracic outlet or at the base of the skull.

Patients who have penetrating trauma thought to involve vessels in zone 2, but who have no neurologic deficits, are often operated on without arteriography. Patients who have a neurologic deficit and those who have injuries in zones 1 and 3 may be benefitted by preoperative arteriography (Fig. 2). If the patients are stable these studies can be obtained in the arteriogra-

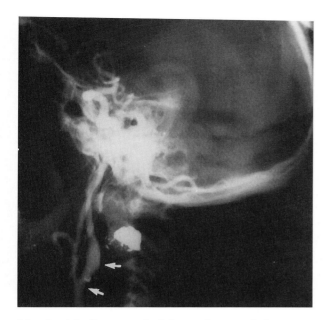

Fig. 2 A bullet wound of the neck caused these two injuries to the carotid artery (arrows). The patient was asymptomatic. At operation three false aneurysms containing clot were repaired with interrupted sutures.

phy suite, but if the patients are unstable they should be taken to the operating room and if further diagnostic studies are needed they can be performed there.

INITIAL TREATMENT

During resuscitation attention to the airway and control of bleeding are the first priorities, and it is usually obvious what is necessary. A more dangerous situation can exist if the patient has achieved a degree of cardiopulmonary stability via internal compensatory mechanisms, and then when these adjustments deteriorate hemodynamic collapse may be sudden.

Once the airway is secure and control of external bleeding has been obtained, vital signs are assessed, an overall evaluation is carried out, and treatment priorities are set. After emergency procedures such as closed thoracostomy or stabilization of cervical spine injuries are completed, appropriate catheters and intravenous lines are inserted.

Arterial lines and Swan-Ganz catheters are helpful in managing these patients if they are hemodynamically unstable or if they have known cardiovascular disease. A radial artery catheter is inserted for monitoring of blood pressure after a normal Allen test. Insertion of a central line and a Swan-Ganz catheter can be performed through the subclavian vein if there are no injuries on that side of the neck or chest, but it is better to use a peripheral vein rather than direct subclavian puncture if there is an injury in that area. A difficult vein puncture may produce an additional vascular injury and complicate care of the patient. Most patients with penetrating trauma to the neck do not require a nasogastric tube, but if other injuries dictate nasogastric decompression the tube should be inserted with care; dislodgement of a clot in the neck may cause fresh bleeding. In patients with cervical spine injuries, manipulations attending nasogastric intubation may cause further damage to the spinal cord. If there is penetrating trauma to the chest and a hemopneumothorax, thoracostomy tubes should be inserted prior to beginning pressure-assisted ventilation.

SELECTION OF PATIENTS

The results of several studies support surgical repair of all carotid artery injuries in patients who have no neurologic deficit or have only a mild neurologic deficit.[3,4,7] All of the patients in groups 1 and 2 should undergo repair of isolated carotid artery injuries. This decision is easily reached when the arterial injury is bleeding actively but may be more difficult when there is complete carotid artery occlusion and no neurologic symptoms are present. In such patients technical problems encountered during surgery could produce injury, although this has been a rare occurrence in the reported experience. Careful neurologic and arterial studies are required before an operation is undertaken in these patients. It is the author's practice to repair all carotid artery injuries in patients who have no neurologic deficit or who have a neurologic deficit but have continued prograde flow in the carotid artery. In patients who have complete occlusion of the internal carotid artery as a result of blunt trauma and who have no neurologic deficit, or have occlusion and a profound neurologic deficit with altered consciousness, operative intervention is probably not indicated.

It is the author's practice to explore all penetrating wounds that pierce the platysma muscle and enter the anterior triangles of the neck. Although biplane arteriography in these patients may offer valuable evidence regarding the presence or absence of an arterial injury, it is not infallible. Moreover, those tests that are used to evaluate the aerodigestive tract have been shown to have a small but definite incidence of false negative results.[8,9] They cannot be depended on in every instance to rule out injury to these structures, and definitive repair of the injuries in these patients is recommended. Patients who have penetrating injuries in other areas of the neck, which on careful examination can be determined not to have threatened major vascular structures, can be treated nonoperatively.

OPERATIVE MANAGEMENT

The carotid arteries are approached through the standard incision made along the anterior border of the sternomastoid muscle. Proximal control of the common carotid artery is obtained before the area of suspected injury is exposed. Bleeding from a laceration or a puncture of the artery usually can be controlled with gentle finger pressure while the artery proximal and distal to the injury is encircled with a soft vascular tape. An injury of the external carotid artery is controlled with vascular clamps and is repaired or ligated, depending on the status of the other arteries and its role as a collateral. Unless there is evidence that the external carotid artery is a major cerebral arterial collateral, it is usually neither grafted nor shunted but is repaired with simple sutures.

More often the common and internal carotid arteries are injured—the left slightly more frequently then the right. Injuries to the carotid artery in zone 2 can usually be repaired simply with sutures or with resection and an end-to-end anastomosis. Once bleeding is controlled, backflow from the internal carotid artery is assessed and if it is brisk and pulsatile that is evidence of adequate cerebral perfusion. If there is any question, measurements of carotid artery back pressure may be obtained, and if these pressures are greater than 70 mm Hg that is acceptable.[10] If the back pressure is below 70 mm Hg or if the backflow from the internal carotid artery is scanty and shunts are selected, a simple inlying tube is usually chosen. Most surgeons administer systemic heparin when shunts are in place and anticoagulants are not contraindicated, although it would appear to be equally important to heparinize the patient if the distal carotid artery is filled with a stagnant column of blood. Most studies of carotid artery trauma do not

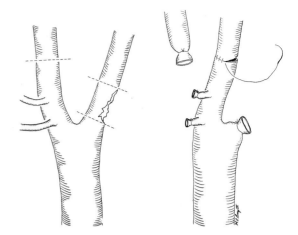

Fig. 3 If the external carotid artery is not a major collateral vessel, it can be transposed to repair wounds of the proximal internal carotid artery.

document the need for shunting or heparinization during these operations.

If the damage to the internal carotid artery is such that direct repair cannot be obtained, one can substitute the external for the internal carotid artery (Fig. 3). In other patients the surgeon may choose to use an autogenous graft taken from the saphenous vein in the groin to reestablish vascular continuity. If in such a patient an inlying shunt is chosen because of scanty backflow or low back pressures in the internal carotid artery, it may be inserted as shown in Fig. 4.

Penetrating injuries of the internal carotid artery at the base of the skull may be difficult to expose, but resection of the digastric muscle and excision of the styloid process usually enable the surgeon to see the artery up to the entrance into the carotid foramen. In some patients, if this exposure is not satisfactory, anterior subluxation of the mandible may be needed to gain adequate exposure.[11] These maneuvers require preoperative placement of dental wires and appliances to ensure adequate subluxation without damage. Some trauma surgeons alternatively elect to perform a vertical osteotomy of the mandibular ramus to facilitate this exposure. These procedures require consultation and assistance from oral surgeons and are best arranged preoperatively.

Bleeding from the root of the neck or staining of the carotid sheath as it enters the neck are

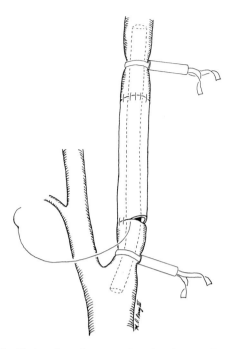

Fig. 4 Extensive damage to the internal carotid artery can be repaired with an interposition vein graft. If a temporary inline shunt is required, this is a useful technique.

indications that proximal injuries may be present and adequate control of these vessels is best obtained by extension of the neck incision into a median sternotomy. If the preoperative evaluation suggests an injury in zone 1, at the root of the neck, the initial incision should include a median sternotomy. Once proximal control of the great vessels is obtained in the mediastinum, the danger of exsanguination is averted and a controlled repair may be made. Injuries of the common carotid artery in the root of the neck rarely require a shunt, and repair of these large vessels can be achieved with simple suture techniques or resection and anastomosis. If grafts are required, the vessels are large and a plastic prosthesis may be needed; most trauma surgeons choose polytetrafluoroethylene. During repair it is necessary to debride only that portion of the artery that appears injured on inspection with the naked eye. It is important to secure a smooth intimal surface, particularly in the internal carotid artery, and careful placement of monofilament sutures is required.

In patients with penetrating trauma there may be concomitant injuries of the trachea or the esophagus, and repair and drainage of these wounds will be required. If drains are used, it is advisable that they be routed away from the repaired artery and all fascial layers closed between the wounds. Early removal of the drain is important to prevent exposure to bacterial contamination. Carotid artery ligation may be needed in a very small group of patients: those with complete internal carotid artery occlusion caused by blunt trauma and severe neurologic deficits including alterations in consciousness.[4,12] Revascularization of a carotid artery injured by blunt trauma near the base of the skull may not be possible and complete removal of all clots is essential to avoid postoperative thromboembolism. Completion arteriography in these patients is an important part of management to ensure that all clots have been removed and the distal carotid system is free of obstruction. This information will document the adequacy of the repair and show the status of the intracranial circulation. The latter information may be of particular value if a postoperative neurologic deficit appears. Intraoperative duplex scanning may also be helpful to assess the repair and the distal extracranial internal carotid artery.

Injuries of the jugular vein are common with penetrating trauma to the carotid artery and associated structures, but it is unusual for anything other than simple suture repair of these vessels to be undertaken. They are rarely grafted.

INJURIES TO THE VERTEBRAL ARTERY

Although in the past it was believed that vertebral artery injuries were rare, most patients did not undergo four-vessel studies and the actual incidence is unknown. More recent data suggest that injuries to the vertebral artery occur with greater frequency than was previously suspected but are often asymptomatic. It is not unusual for one vertebral artery to be dominant, but in the absence of four-vessel arteriograms this information would not be available. The circle of Willis is intact as depicted in anatomy books in less than 50% of patients. One of the common anomalies is a missing posterior communicating artery or one of the vertebral arteries can end in a posterior inferior cerebellar artery. The vertebral artery enters the bony canal at the C6 level and emerges again at C2. It is relatively protected from trauma while in the bony canal, although gunshot wounds that hit the spine can produce serious injuries to the vertebral artery and its associated veins. In most patients injuries to the vertebral artery are treated by ligation when outside the bony canal and by combinations of ligation, suturing, and packing when within the canal. Symptomatic injuries of a dominant vertebral artery are repaired, and in a few instances autogenous veins have been employed to restore continuity. These operations are extensive and require a careful arteriographic evaluation before they are undertaken. Few have been performed. There is little support in the literature for repair because ligation has been used most often. Nevertheless, it is advisable when such injuries are suspected to obtain a careful preoperative survey and to plan the repair according to the cerebral vascular architecture. In many cases the collateral circulation is such that simple ligation may be acceptable and extensive repairs may not be required.

POSTOPERATIVE CARE

The long-term results of repair of carotid artery injuries are generally good, and if the patient is admitted without a preoperative neurologic deficit, recovery is without incident in most cases (Table 2). Although false aneurysms, arteriovenous fistulas, and bleeding may complicate any vascular wound, they are uncommon in the carotid system.

Postoperatively the patients are carefully monitored for neurologic and vascular complications on an hourly basis for at least 6 hours and then every 4 hours during the first day. If a new neurologic deficit develops, it is usually the result of a technical problem at the repair site and the patient is returned immediately to the operating room for exploration. This is likely to be successful if blood flow can be restored before a cerebral infarction occurs. If minor neurologic events emerge, and there is no evidence of internal carotid artery occlusion by noninvasive studies and clinical evaluation, repeat arteriograms are recommended to evaluate the cerebral circulation. A distal embolus is then treated in the appropriate manner, usually with anticoagulation. These events are rare, and most of these patients can be expected to have an uncomplicated convalescence if the initial repair is successful (Table 3).

Table 2 Carotid trauma

Group	No.	Mortality (%)
1	0	0
2	1	8.3
3	5	33

Table 3 Collected review of repair vs. ligation of carotid artery for injuries in patients without preoperative neurologic deficit*

Results	Repaired	Ligated
No neurologic deficit	153	6
Transient deficit	6	0
Permanent deficit	2	2
Death	0	1
TOTAL	161	9
Favorable results	99%	67%

*Modified from Liekweg WG, Greenfield LJ. Management of penetrating carotid arterial injury. Ann Surg 188:587-592, 1978.

REFERENCES

1. Perry MO. Management of Acute Vascular Injuries. Baltimore: Williams & Wilkins, 1981, pp 67-81.
2. Perry MO, Snyder WH, Thal ER. Carotid artery injuries caused by blunt trauma. Ann Surg 192:74-77, 1980.
3. Thal ER, Snyder WH, Hays RJ, Perry MO. Management of carotid artery injuries. Surgery 76:955-962, 1974.
4. Liekweg WG, Greenfield LJ. Management of penetrating carotid arterial injury. Ann Surg 188:587-592, 1978.
5. Monson DO, Saletta JD, Freeark RJ. Carotid vertebral trauma. J Trauma 9:987-999, 1969.
6. Bynoe RP, Miles WS, Bell RM, et al. Noninvasive diagnosis of vascular trauma by duplex ultrasonography. J Vasc Surg 14:346-352, 1991.
7. Fry WJ, Fry RE. Management of carotid artery injury. In Bergan JJ, Yao JST, eds. Vascular Surgical Emergencies. Orlando: Grune & Stratton, 1987, pp 153-162.
8. Roon AJ, Christensen N. Evaluation and treatment of penetrating cervical injuries. J Trauma 19:391-397, 1979.
9. Bishara RA, Pasch AR, Douglas DD, et al. The necessity of mandatory exploration of penetrating zone II neck injuries. Surgery 100:655-660, 1986.
10. Ehrenfeld EK, Stoney RJ, Wylie EJ. Relation of carotid stump pressure to safety of carotid artery ligation. Surgery 93:299-305, 1983.
11. Fisher DF, Clagett GP, Parker JI, et al. Mandibular subluxation for high carotid exposures. J Vasc Surg 1:727-731, 1984.
12. Ledgerwood AM, Mullins RJ, Lucas CE. Primary repair vs ligation for carotid artery injuries. Arch Surg 115:488-496, 1980.

70

Surgical Treatment of Chronic Mesenteric Ischemia

DONALD E. PATTERSON, M.D., KEITH D. CALLIGARO, M.D., MATTHEW J. DOUGHERTY, M.D., and DOMINIC A. DeLAURENTIS, M.D.

Chronic mesenteric ischemia is relatively rare but familiar to all vascular surgeons. Occlusion of the mesenteric arteries was first described by Chiene[1] more than a century ago. The relationship between abdominal pain and chronic mesenteric ischemia was reported by Schnitzler[2] in 1901. This syndrome was first successfully treated by endarterectomy, as reported by Shaw and Maynard[3] in 1958. Since that time, much has been written to clarify the disease process and treatment alternatives. Revascularization techniques and results are also now well documented in the literature. We will review the pathophysiology of mesenteric ischemia and its clinical presentation, diagnosis, and treatment.

CAUSE AND DIAGNOSIS

Stenosis or occlusion of the visceral arteries is primarily caused by atherosclerosis.[4] Fibromuscular dysplasia and external compression on the celiac axis by the arcuate ligament of the diaphragm are less common causes of arterial insufficiency in the mesenteric circulation. In general, chronic mesenteric ischemia presents clinically only when there is compromise of at least two of the three major visceral vessels.[5,6] In this setting, collateral visceral perfusion maintains intestinal viability but cannot meet the need for augmented perfusion that is required for digestion.

The term "abdominal angina" has been applied to the symptom complex associated with chronic mesenteric ischemia.[7] Patients present with a dull or gnawing abdominal pain located in the periumbilical and epigastric region. The pain usually begins 15 to 30 minutes after consumption of a meal and lasts for 1 to 4 hours. With repeated episodes of eating followed by pain, the patient develops a "food fear," since even the smallest of meals can lead to the onset of symptoms. This begins a cycle that leads to weight loss, inanition, and severe malnutrition. Patients can develop an alteration in bowel activity consisting of diarrhea or constipation.[8] Malabsorption has been reported but only rarely is the cause of weight loss. Because many patients presenting with mesenteric infarction report a history of these symptoms, it is likely that bowel infarction represents the natural history of this condition.

The presenting symptom complex of chronic intestinal ischemia usually generates an extensive gastrointestinal evaluation. Patients often undergo CT imaging of the abdomen, upper and lower gastrointestinal endoscopy, and other studies before the mesenteric circulation is considered. The interval between symptom onset and the confirmatory diagnostic aortography averages 17 months.[5,6]

Cachexia and findings of atherosclerotic occlusive disease elsewhere are often noted on physical examination. An epigastric bruit is often noted. Although newer technologies such as magnetic resonance angiography and spiral CT scan are being explored, the "gold standard" for diagnosis of mesenteric arterial disease is the biplanar aortogram. In addition to detailing the level and severity of the disease, the collateral circulation can be visualized.

Anatomic location of occlusive disease has varied among published reports. Murray and Stoney[7] noted that both the origin of the celiac and the superior mesenteric arteries were involved in 94% of patients. In a report by Hollier et al.,[9] 77% of patients had involvement of two or three visceral arteries, whereas 23% had isolated celiac or superior mesenteric artery (SMA) disease associated with symptoms. Calderon et al.[10] noted that the majority of symptomatic patients had at least two-vessel disease. In Taylor and Porter's series[11] of 48 patients,

---

Supported by a grant from the John F. Connelly Foundation.

all had stenosis or occlusion of the SMA, 77% had celiac artery disease, and 60% had inferior mesenteric artery occlusion. Only 8% had isolated SMA disease.

Atherosclerotic involvement of the renal arteries can be seen in approximately a third of patients with mesenteric occlusive disease. Infrarenal aortic aneurysmal or occlusive disease was present in approximately one fourth of patients in a large series by Cunningham et al.[12]

Symptomatic patients with multivessel visceral artery disease should undergo revascularization. We will categorize interventions as (1) endarterectomy techniques, (2) bypass techniques, and (3) endovascular techniques.

ENDARTERECTOMY

In the first report of operative intervention for chronic mesenteric ischemia, Shaw and Maynard[3] described endarterectomy through a superior mesenteric arteriotomy. In the two cases presented, little technical detail is given to the exact repair and closure of the arteriotomy. Transaortic endarterectomy was later advanced by Rob[13] and Rapp et al.,[14] and is especially suitable for atherosclerotic visceral artery disease as the lesions tend to occur at the ostia of the vessels. Exposure of the visceral vessels for transaortic endarterectomy can be accomplished via a thoracoretroperitoneal approach[14,15] or by a transabdominal approach using medial visceral rotation.[12] Using the latter technique, a lateral dissection plane is created between the stomach, spleen, pancreas, and left colon while the left kidney remains in its anatomic location. The abdominal viscera are displaced medially and upward. The entire abdominal aorta can then be exposed to facilitate surgery at the celiac level. After complete control of the abdominal aorta and lumbar arteries within the region, a "trapdoor" arteriotomy is made to include the orifices of both the SMA and celiac arteries as required.[12,16] An en bloc endarterectomy is performed, removing the aortic plaque with its extensions into the visceral orifices. This procedure can be performed in concert with removal of disease from the distal abdominal aorta. Sleeve aortic endarterectomy and renal artery transaortic endarterectomy can also be performed if so indicated. Following the endarterectomy, the aortotomy is closed with running monofilament sutures. Concomitant infrarenal aortic replacement can also be performed. Occlusive disease extending well beyond the ostium may be difficult to treat in this fashion, and adjunctive bypass or patch angioplasty may be necessary. Transmural calcification of the visceral aorta also favors alternative techniques.

MESENTERIC BYPASS

Visceral arterial bypass procedures have been described wherein the graft originates from either the supraceliac or infrarenal abdominal aorta. Classic articles by Rob[13] and Morris et al.[17] describe revascularization of the mesenteric circulation using the infrarenal abdominal aorta. Advantages of this technique include (1) ease of construction of the bypass, (2) familiarity with the regional anatomy by most surgeons, (3) avoidance of supraceliac aortic clamping, and (4) proximity during other intra-abdominal procedures such as aortic aneurysm repair or bowel resection.

Retrograde bypass from the infrarenal aorta is performed by anastomosing the proximal graft to the infrarenal abdominal aorta in an end-to-side fashion.[6,11] Saphenous vein or prosthetic material can be used. Grafts can be placed in the SMA, celiac, or hepatic artery in an end-to-side or end-to-end manner. Kinking of the bypass is a major concern with retrograde reconstructions, particularly of the SMA, because displacement of the bowel for anastomosis makes predicting length and orientation of the graft difficult. Placing long prosthetic grafts in a wide loop to avoid this tendency is advocated by Taylor and Porter.[11] Grafts to the celiac artery are usually tunneled in the retropancreatic space. Retrograde bypass should be avoided when the infrarenal aorta is severely diseased or encased in scar tissue and there is no indication for aortic replacement.

Other authors have advocated supraceliac aortovisceral bypass, since this allows the placement of the graft in a more anatomically favorable position, decreasing the likelihood of the graft's kinking.[18] The supraceliac aorta is also more likely to be free of atheromatous disease, permitting a technically easier proximal anastomosis. A disadvantage may be potentially higher morbidity of aortic clamping at this level.[6,11] However, we and others have not found this to be the case.[18,19] The crus of the diaphragm is divided to expose the anterior aspect of the aorta. A partially occluding clamp can be used; blood pressure must be carefully controlled with vasodilators. Single-limb or bifurcated prosthetic grafts are used. For celiac revascularization, an end-to-end anastomosis to the celiac trunk or an end-to-side anastomosis to the hepatic artery is employed. Grafting to the SMA may require tunneling in the retropancreatic plane. However, if there is a short proximal lesion of the SMA, the cephalad border of the pancreas can be retracted inferiorly and the bypass to the SMA performed cephalad to the pancreas.

Mortality varies between 4.9% and 30% in published series, but in recent reports from major centers, averages have been under 10%.* Several authors have reviewed their experience and attempted to correlate the extent of revascularization with survival, graft patency, and recurrence of symptoms. Improved relief of symptoms was seen when revascularization was carried beyond single-vessel reconstruction.

PERCUTANEOUS TRANSLUMINAL ANGIOPLASTY

Recently, interest has been increasing for the use of percutaneous transluminal angioplasty (PTA) for chronic visceral ischemia. Less invasive techniques are attractive for these generally elderly and malnourished patients.[24] The ostial location of atherosclerotic visceral artery disease and its association with aortic plaque make achieving a good technical result difficult. The published literature includes only small series with limited follow-up. Initial technical success has been reported as high as 80% for a balloon dilatation procedure for the celiac and SMA distribution.[25] Primary patency at 24 months has ranged from 40% to 100%. Recurrent symptoms have developed in up to 45% of patients. Complications of PTA occur in 12% to 16% of patients and include arterial rupture and arterial wall dissection.

CONCLUSION

Chronic mesenteric ischemia secondary to atherosclerotic disease of the celiac and mesenteric arteries should be treated surgically to prevent the debilitating spiral of weight loss, malnutrition, inanition, and bowel infarction. Endarterectomy and bypass procedures remain the mainstay of surgical reconstruction, with long-term successful results. Complete revascularization should be performed to prevent recurrence of symptoms. Data on the long-term success of PTA are lacking, and this procedure should be reserved for patients who are not candidates for surgery. Techniques for correction of visceral artery stenosis by this approach continue to be refined.

REFERENCES

1. Chiene J. Complete obliteration of celiac and mesenteric arteries. J Anat Physiol 3:65, 1869.
2. Schnitzler F. Zur Symptomatik des Darmarterien-Verschlusses. Wien Med Wochenschr 11/12:506-509, 1901.
3. Shaw R, Maynard E. Acute and chronic thrombosis of the mesenteric arteries associated with malabsorption. New Engl J Med 258:874-878, 1958.
4. Derrick J, Pollard H, Moore R. The pattern of arteriosclerotic narrowing of the celiac and superior mesenteric arteries. Ann Surg 149:684-689, 1959.
5. Stoney R, Cunningham C, Ehrenfeld W. Chronic visceral ischemia: A surgical condition. In Veith F, Hobson R, Williams R, Wilson S, eds. Vascular Surgery Principals and Practice, 2nd ed. New York: Mc-Graw-Hill, 1994, pp 781-793.
6. Taylor L, Porter J. Treatment of chronic visceral ischemia. In Rutherford R, ed. Vascular Surgery, 4th ed. Philadelphia: WB Saunders, 1995, pp 1301-1311.
7. Murray S, Stoney R. Chronic visceral ischemia. Cardiovasc Surg 2:176-179, 1994.
8. Morris G, Crawford E, Cooley D, DeBakey M. Revascularization of the celiac and superior mesenteric arteries. Arch Surg 84:113-125, 1962.
9. Hollier L, Bernatz P, Pairolero P, Payne W, Osmundson P. Surgical management of chronic intestinal ischemia: A reappraisal. Surgery 90:940-946, 1981.
10. Calderon M, Reul G, Gregoric I, Jacobs M, Ducan J, Ott D, Livesay J, Cooley D. Long-term results of the surgical management of symptomatic chronic intestinal ischemia. J Cardiovasc Surg 33:723-728, 1992.
11. Taylor L, Porter J. Treatment of chronic intestinal ischemia. Semin Vasc Surg 3:186-199, 1990.
12. Cunningham C, Reilly L, Rapp J, Schneider P, Stoney R. Chronic visceral ischemia: Three decades of progress. Ann Surg 214:276-288, 1991.
13. Rob C. Surgical diseases of the celiac and mesenteric arteries. Arch Surg 93:21-32, 1966.
14. Rapp J, Reilly L, Qvarfordt P, Goldstone J, Ehrenfeld W, Stoney R. Durability of endarterectomy and antegrade grafts in the treatment of chronic visceral ischemia. J Vasc Surg 3:799-806, 1986.
15. Stoney R, Wylie E. Recognition of surgical management of visceral ischemic syndromes. Ann Surg 164:714-722, 1969.
16. Stoney R, Ehrenfeld W, Wylie E. Revascularization methods in chronic visceral ischemia caused by atherosclerosis. Ann Surg 186:468-476, 1977.
17. Morris G, Crawford E, Cooley D, DeBakey M. Revascularization of the celiac and superior mesenteric arteries. Arch Surg 84:113-125, 1962.

---

*References 9, 10, 12, 16, 17, 19-23.

18. Hermreck A, Thomas J, Iliopoulos J, Pierce G. Role of supraceliac aortic bypass in visceral artery reconstruction. Am J Surg 162:611-614, 1991.
19. Beebe H, MacFarlane S, Raker E. Supraceliac aortomesenteric bypass for intestinal ischemia. J Vasc Surg 5:749-754, 1987.
20. Rheudasil J, Stewart M, Schellack J, Smith R, Salam A, Perdue G. Surgical treatment of chronic mesenteric arterial insufficiency. J Vasc Surg 8:495-500, 1988.
21. Crawford E, Morris G, Myhre H, Roehm J. Celiac axis, superior mesenteric artery, and inferior mesenteric artery occlusion; Surgical considerations. Surgery 82:856-866, 1977.
22. McAfee M, Cherry K, Naessens J, Pairolero P, Hallet J, Gloviczki P, Bower T. Influence of complete revascularization on chronic mesenteric ischemia. Am J Surg 164:220-224, 1992.
23. Harwood T, Brooks D, Flynn T, Seeger J. Multiple organ dysfunction after mesenteric artery revascularization. J Vasc Surg 18:459-469, 1993.
24. Golden D, Ring E, McLean G, Freiman D. Percutaneous transluminal angioplasty in the treatment of abdominal angina. AJR 139:247-249, 1982.
25. Matsumoto A, Tegtmeyer C, Fitzcharles E, Selby J, Tribble C, Angle J, Kron I. Percutaneous transluminal angioplasty of visceral arterial stenosis: Results and long-term clinical follow-up. J Vasc Intervent Radiol 6:165-174, 1995.

71

Management of Aortic Graft Infection By Graft Excision and Extra-Anatomic Revascularization: Long-Term Results With the Standard Treatment

DAVID C. BREWSTER, M.D.

Aortic graft infection remains the most feared and difficult to manage complication of aortic surgery. Although the incidence of aortic graft infection is low, it has remained relatively constant (0.5% to 3.0%) despite improvements in surgical techniques, graft materials, and systemic antibiotics.[1] The incidence of infection is lowest for intracavitary (tube, aortoiliac) grafts, and several-fold higher for aortofemoral grafts that involve groin incisions.

GOALS OF THERAPY

Irrespective of the treatment strategy selected, the common goals of all forms of management include the following: (1) eradicate infection, (2) maintain adequate extremity circulation, and (3) avoid procrastination and delay, which can result in sequelae such as systemic sepsis, anastomotic disruption, and erosion into adjacent organs.

ACCEPTED PRINCIPLES OF MANAGEMENT

All forms of treatment acknowledge certain basic principles as an integral part of successful management of aortic graft infection.
1. Need for organism-specific antibiotics, based on cultures of blood, perigraft fluid or tissue, or the graft material itself
2. Need for adequate debridement of infected or devitalized tissues in the area of graft infection
3. Use of monofilament sutures to repair involved vessels
4. Recognition of the importance of the nutritional and immunologic status of the patient

TREATMENT OPTIONS

Although the goals of therapy are widely accepted, considerable controversy exists as to how best to achieve them. A wide variety of strategies have evolved and a voluminous amount of literature generated. Treatment options may be broadly classified into groups as listed below and shown in Fig. 1.
1. Graft excision alone, no revascularization
2. Graft excision (complete or partial) and extra-anatomic revascularization
3. Graft excision (complete or partial) and in situ graft replacement
4. Graft preservation and localized wound management

It is clear that the major differences among the various management strategies centers on several fundamental questions. First, is graft excision necessary? If so, must the entire prosthesis be removed or only the obviously infected portion? Second, if the infected graft is removed, is revascularization required and by what method (extra-anatomic, in situ, or endovascular)? What is the best new conduit (autogenous tissue, new prosthetic, or allograft)? Finally, what is the best staging of excision and revascularization (preliminary, simultaneous, or delayed revascularization)?

TRADITIONAL TREATMENT

It is generally accepted that standard or conventional treatment of aortic graft infection involves removal of the entire prosthesis, oversewing of the aortic stump, and lower extremity revascularization by extra-anatomic (ex situ) bypass. The fundamental tenets of this management scheme are that the prosthetic graft is a foreign body and nidus for infection that cannot be reliably eradicated without removing the graft. In addition, it is thought that excision of only part of the prosthesis will likely lead to an unacceptable incidence of persistent or recurrent infection in the remaining portion of the graft. To minimize the possibility of reinfection of a new

437

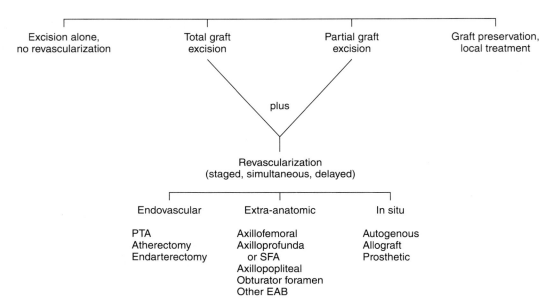

Fig. 1 Treatment options for infected aortic grafts. SFA = superficial femoral artery.

conduit placed to maintain lower extremity circulation, a blood supply should be restored by new grafts from a noninfected inflow artery to a noninfected outflow vessel via a remote route through clean, noninfected tissue planes.

Although some authors have previously recommended that revascularization be performed on a selective basis after removal of the infected graft, the adequacy of lower extremity perfusion after graft removal is difficult to predict preoperatively or assess objectively in the immediate postoperative period, unless the infected graft is already occluded. Numerous series have documented better results if revascularization is performed when patent infected grafts are removed.[1-4] Therefore, a policy of routine early revascularization as part of an optimal management plan seems advisable.

Although not firmly established, available evidence also suggests a more favorable outcome (reduced amputation and mortality rates) if the extra-anatomic bypass (EAB) is performed prior to removal of the infected graft if clinical circumstances allow. Therefore, unless emergent operation for active anastomotic bleeding or gastrointestinal hemorrhage is required, and if the diagnosis of graft infection is reasonably well established, EAB is performed prior to removal of the infected graft, either as the first step in a simultaneous combined procedure or by an interval of 1 to 6 days if a staged approach is preferred. The rationale for preliminary EAB, which appears valid, is to avoid the deleterious effects of superimposing the metabolic consequences of prolonged leg ischemia on the already substantial blood loss and stresses of aortic graft resection if this is removed first. In addition, the presence of the functioning EAB minimizes the hemodynamic effects of aortic clamping for graft removal and makes heparinization unnecessary during this portion of the procedure. With appropriate intravenous antibiotic treatment, there is no evidence of increased risk of EAB infection with implantation prior to removal of the infected graft.

KEY FEATURES OF THE "MODERN" STANDARD APPROACH

Initial EAB typically utilizes the axillary artery for inflow. Axillo-bifemoral grafts are employed if the groins are uninvolved with infection. If there is groin involvement, axillo-superficial femoral or axillo-profunda bypass is used depending on the anatomic pattern of disease present, or axillopopliteal bypasses may be inserted if required. Recent improved results of axillofemoral grafts employing externally supported 8 mm polytetrafluoroethylene (PTFE) grafts suggest that this is the best choice of conduit for EAB under these circumstances. EAB incisions must be in clean, uninfected areas and must be carefully protected by adhesive

Table 1 Recent (1989-1994) series of treatment of aortic graft infection by graft excision and EAB

Study	No. of cases	Operative mortality (%)	Early amputation (%)	Stump blowout (%)	EAB reinfection (%)	1-year survival (%)
Schmitt et al. (1989)[7]	20	15	5	6	5	75
Yeager et al. (1990)[8]	22	14	10	4	22	77
Quiñones-Baldrich et al. (1991)[9]	45	24	11	0	17	65
Ricotta et al. (1991)[10]	18	17	11	0	0	85
Bacourt et al. (1992)[11]	98	24	10	8	7	70
Bunt (1993)[12]	22	9	14	0	5	—
Lehnert et al. (1993)[13]	21	10	0	0	5	80
Sharp et al. (1994)[14]	20	5	0	0	5	90
Cumulative results	266	14.8	7.6	2.3	8.3	77.4

barrier drapes following closure prior to removal of the infected prosthesis.

Following EAB, the surgeon may proceed immediately to graft removal or wait 1 to 6 days. A transperitoneal approach for graft excision provides the most flexibility for dissection of both limbs and allows omental pedicle coverage of the aortic stump. Perigraft dissection is best done within the old graft capsule. Temporary suprarenal aortic clamping is frequently advisable to maximize the available length of infrarenal aorta and allow proper debridement and secure closure of the aortic stump. Following takedown of the proximal anastomosis and ligation of the aorta, the clamp can be transferred to a position just below the renal arteries and renal perfusion restored.

Management of the aortic stump is paramount and the following steps should be taken: debridement back to healthy tissue, two-layer closure (a proximal row of 3 or 4 adjacent mattress sutures and distal over-and-over running sutures to the stump itself), coverage with omentum, debridement of the graft bed and perigraft tissues as necessary, and placement of drains in areas where there is significant contamination.

Graft limbs should be freed as distally as possible, taking care to avoid injury to the ureters. Distal graft limbs are then divided and oversewn, and the abdomen is closed.

Attention is then turned toward the groin muscles, which are reopened and the graft and native vessels controlled. Following takedown of the graft anastomosis, the arteriotomy sites are closed primarily, or with venous or autogenous tissue (endarterectomized proximal segment of superficial femoral artery if chronically occluded). Use of patches are quite helpful if the intent is to preserve retrograde plevic blood flow from the profunda. Ligation of the femoral artery may be advisable, however, if heavy local contamination or sepsis is present.

Removal of the distal detached graft limb is the final step of the procedure. This is usually easily accomplished, as it has been previously divided proximally and is now detached from the femoral artery. Usually a bit of dissection along the old graft limb just under the inguinal ligament allows it to be withdrawn through the groin incision.

RESULTS OF MODERN STANDARD TREATMENT

Historically, traditional management of infected aortic grafts has resulted in high perioperative mortality (25% to 75%) and morbidity (15% to 40% amputation) rates. Critics also emphasize the risk of aortic stump dehiscence, poor long-term patency of EAB used for revascularization, and the risk of reinfection of the EAB. Much of the data that influenced the anticipated poor results of traditional therapy were drawn from initial series reporting results of treatment of graft infection in the early literature. As shown in Table 1, more recent results of surgical management based on the previously outlined principles are much improved. Pooled data from series detailing results of standard treatment of aortic graft infection within the past 5 years demonstrate a reduction of the perioperative mortality rate to approximately 15%, with the amputation rate and the incidence of infection of the new EAB both less than 10%.[7-14] Recognition of the important concepts and techniques necessary to acheive secure closure of the aortic stump has made stump blowout quite infrequent (2.3%) in current practice. One-year survival has also improved to an acceptable 77%. Long-term patency of EAB, although not specifically discussed in many of these reports, has also been documented to be substantially improved in several other recent series of axillofemoral bypasses in noninfected patients, possibly related to the use of externally supported conduits.[15,16] It is also important to recognize that mortality rates will vary from one series to another depending on the frequency of aortoenteric fistulas (AEF). For instance, in the multicenter retrospective report of Bacourt et al.[11] from France, nearly 50% of patients underwent urgent graft excision and EAB for AEF, no doubt explaining in large part the higher mortality rate in that series. Such difficult clinical problems are not present in many series of alternative methods purporting "better" results. In addition, the report of Quiñones-Baldrich et al.,[9] which also noted a 24% mortality rate, describes experience with patients treated over a long period (1970 to 1988), which may not truly be an accurate reflection of contemporary practice and results.

Such overall improvement in results of modern standard therapy are in large part attributable to advances in anesthesia and perioperative supportive care in the intensive care unit following these major procedures in critically ill patients. In part, however, they reflect evolution and refinements of ingenious approaches, which facilitate revascularization while avoiding contaminated areas,[17,18] as well as improved diagnostic capabilities, which allow for earlier diagnosis and better planning of elective treatment in most cases. Indeed, these current results are those to which the results of proposed alternative strategies must be compared.

ALTERNATIVE STRATEGIES

The impetus for the development of a variety of alternative approaches to treatment of aortic graft infection by innovative and experienced surgeons was clearly the perceived poor outcome long attributed to standard therapy. All alternative strategies share the goal of seeking an easier and more expedient solution to the problem of graft infection, which is potentially safer for the patient and less challenging and demanding for the surgeon. However, all alternatives share a potential deficiency—the higher risk of persistent or recurrent infection. Indeed, a review of the literature on all alternative methods suggests that although perioperative morbidity and mortality may occasionally be lessened by such approaches, in many instances differences in early outcome are not significant when compared to current results of conventional therapy. Most important, the incidence of failure to successfully eradicate infection when alternative strategies are employed is clearly much higher than with standard treatment. Therefore the risks, technical difficulties, and costs of the subsequent reoperations that are required when alternative methods are unsuccessful must also be considered, not merely the morbidity and mortality of the primary intervention for graft infection.

Partial graft excision offers the advantage of less extensive surgery, but requires very accurate evaluation of the extent of infection by various imaging modalities or operative exploration.[1,19,20] Despite a probably reduced perioperative mortality risk, recurrent or persistent graft infection has been noted in many series. In the 1984 report of Reilly et al.,[2] only 33% of patients with apparent localized graft infection treated with partial graft excision were cured of infection. The remaining 67% either died of persistent sepsis (33%) or required subsequent removal of the remainder of the graft (34%). In a review of the literature since 1991, Bunt[12] noted a failure rate of 44% for partial excision methods. Ricotta et al.[10] reported a 25% incidence of reinfection and reoperation for partial graft excision. Our own experience showed a similar 30% incidence; in contrast, no patients with total graft excision in our series had any evidence of recurrent infection or required reoperation for this problem.

Similarly, possible management utilizing in situ graft replacements has been proposed to simplify treatment, reduce amputation rates because of improved patency with such in-line reconstructions, and obviate the dangers of aortic stump blowout.[21,22] Many of these reports, however, involve small or anecdotal series with only short-term follow-up. The long-term efficacy of such therapies remains unproved. Some series, such as that of Walker et al.,[21] still had a 22% mortality (60% if frank retroperitoneal purulence was present) and a 17% incidence of anastomotic disruption at the new aortograft anastomosis, which is in many ways akin to stump blowout. Most series of in situ prosthetic graft replacements acknowledge the poor results with this method when extensive graft infection or gross retroperitoneal sepsis is present and recommend its use only in selected situations of limited graft involvement and low virulence infections.[1,19,22-26] Use of antibiotic-impregnated grafts for in situ replacement remains an appealing theory but is still experimental at present, because no such grafts are currently available.[27] Use of autogenous tissue for in situ replacement is notable for the difficulty and extensive additional surgery that is often needed to obtain satisfactory conduits.[2,28] Use of allografts is likely to be limited by the degenerative changes common in such homograft tissue.[29]

If used for replacement of the entire original graft, a major drawback of in situ graft replacement, in my opinion, is the devastating consequences of recurrent infection involving the new aortic prosthesis. Obtaining an adequate length of intact aorta for secure stump closure during the first operation for an infected aortic graft is difficult enough. Reoperation for infection of a new anastomosis is sure to be more difficult, if not impossible. It is almost axiomatic that the surgeon frequently has only one chance at secure closure of the aortic stump. In instances of infection involving the body and/or proximal anastomosis of an aortic graft, this one opportunity is best seized for secure stump closure rather than implantation of another prosthesis.

The growing interest in possible graft preservation based on aggressive local wound care and use of possible muscle flaps has a failure rate ranging from 20% to 40% in many series.[12,30,31] The prolonged hospitalization, perhaps in an ICU setting if close observation of an anastomotic area is necessary, required for such methods offsets much of the possible cost savings. Finally, although such attempts at graft preservation may succeed, all series still report mortality and morbidity secondary to complications such as persistent infection or anastomotic rupture. It should also be recalled that no patients selected for graft preservation in these series had AEF or other more extensive manifestations of graft infections known to increase risk. Therefore, in many instances, these methods cannot be directly compared to traditional management, since conventional graft excision and EAB are often employed for more extensive problems.

CURRENT RECOMMENDATIONS

It is evident that there is no single "best" treatment for aortic graft infection. Each case must be evaluated individually. Factors to be considered are the nature (virulence) of the organism, extent of infection, anatomy of the infected graft and native arteries involved, and condition of the patient. Alternative strategies may be considered under certain carefully selected circumstances such as infections of limited extent caused by a low-virulence organism in a patient with no signs of systemic sepsis.[1,4] Most often these requirements may be met by patients who present with late, low-grade infections involving only one groin of an aortobifemoral graft. If the clinical picture is consistent with biofilm infection (*Staphylococcus epidermidis*) and the remainder of the graft seems well incorporated and uninvolved, then partial graft excision, in situ replacement, local wound measures, or various combinations of all of these alternative approaches may be considered. In most other circumstances suggestive of more extensive graft involvement, traditional treatment appears to be the best choice.

It is important to stress that very specific criteria must be present to warrant deviation from the well-established principles of traditional treatment. The current improved results of such management are indeed the standard to which the long-term efficacy of various new approaches must be compared.

REFERENCES

1. Bandyk DF. Aortic graft infection. Semin Vasc Surg 3:122-132, 1990.
2. Reilly LM, Altman H, Lusby RJ, et al. Late results following surgical management of vascular graft infection. J Vasc Surg 1:36-44, 1984.
3. O'Hara PJ, Hertzer NM, Beven EG, Krajewski LP. Surgical management of infected abdominal aortic grafts: Review of a 25-year experience. J Vasc Surg 3:725-731, 1986.
4. Calligaro KD, Veith FJ. Diagnosis and management of infected prosthetic aortic grafts. Surgery 110:805-813, 1991.
5. Reilly LM, Stoney RJ, Goldstone J, Ehrenfeld WK. Improved management of aortic graft infection: The influence of operation sequence and staging. J Vasc Surg 5:421-431, 1987.
6. Trout HH, Kozloff L, Giordano JM. Priority of revascularization in patients with graft enteric fistulas, infected arteries or infected arterial prostheses. Ann Surg 199:669-683, 1984.
7. Schmitt DD, Seabrook GR, Bandyk DF, Towne JB. Graft excision and extra-anatomic revascularization: The treatment of choice for the septic aortic prosthesis. J Cardiovasc Surg 31:327-332, 1990.
8. Yeager RA, Moneta GL, Taylor LM, et al. Improving survival and limb salvage in patients with aortic graft infection. Am J Surg 159:466-469, 1990.
9. Quiñones-Baldrich WJ, Hernandez JJ, Moore WS. Long-term results following surgical management of aortic graft infection. Arch Surg 126:507-511, 1991.

10. Ricotta JJ, Faggioli GL, Stella A, et al. Total excision and extra-anatomic bypass for aortic graft infection. Am J Surg 162:145-149, 1991.
11. Bacourt F, Koskas F, and the French University Association for Research in Surgery. Axillobifemoral bypass and aortic exclusion for vascular septic lesions: A multicenter retrospective study of 98 cases. Ann Vasc Surg 6:119-126, 1992.
12. Bunt TJ. Vascular graft infections: A personal experience. Cardiovasc Surg 1:489-493, 1993.
13. Lehnert T, Gruber HP, Maeder N, Allenberg JR. Management of primary aortic graft infection by extra-anatomic bypass reconstruction. Eur J Vasc Surg 7:301-307, 1993.
14. Sharp WJ, Hoballah JJ, Mohan CR, et al. The management of the infected aortic prosthesis: A current decade of experience. J Vasc Surg 19:844-850, 1994.
15. Harris EJ, Taylor LM, McConnell DB, et al. Clinical results of axillobifemoral bypass using externally supported polytetrafluoroethylene. J Vasc Surg 12:416-421, 1990.
16. El-Massry S, Saad E, Sauvage LR, et al. Axillofemoral bypass with externally supported, knitted Dacron grafts: A follow-up through twelve years. J Vasc Surg 17:107-115, 1993.
17. Nunez AA, Veith FJ, Collier P, et al. Direct approaches to the distal portions of the deep femoral artery for limb salvage bypasses. J Vasc Surg 8:576-581, 1988.
18. Veith FJ, Ascer E, Gupta SK, Wengerter KR. Lateral approaches to the popliteal artery. J Vasc Surg 6:119-123, 1987.
19. Bandyk DF, Bergamini TM, Kinney EV, et al. In situ replacement of vascular prostheses infected by bacterial biofilm. J Vasc Surg 13:575-583, 1991.
20. Miller JH. Partial replacement of an infected arterial graft by a new prosthetic polytetrafluoroethylene segment: A new therapeutic option. J Vasc Surg 17:546-558, 1993.
21. Walker WE, Cooley DA, Duncan JM, et al. The management of aortoduodenal fistula by in situ replacement of the infected abdominal aortic graft. Ann Surg 205:727-732, 1987.
22. Robinson JA, Johansen K. Aortic sepsis: Is there a role for in situ graft reconstruction? J Vasc Surg 13:677-684, 1991.
23. Bandyk DF, Berni GA, Thiele BL, Towne JB. Aortofemoral graft infection due to Staphylococcus epidermidis. Arch Surg 119:102-108, 1984.
24. Towne JB, Seabrook GR, Bandyk D, et al. In situ replacement of arterial prosthesis infected by bacterial biofilms: Long-term follow-up. J Vasc Surg 19:226-235, 1994.
25. Jacobs MJHM, Reul GJ, Gregoric I, Cooley DA. In-situ replacement and extra-anatomic bypass for the treatment of infected abdominal aortic grafts. Eur J Vasc Surg 5:83-86, 1991.
26. Fichelle JM, Tabet G, Cormier P, et al. Infected infrarenal aortic aneurysms: When is in situ reconstruction safe? J Vasc Surg 17:635-645, 1993.
27. Colburn MD, Moore WS, Chrapil M, et al. Use of an antibiotic-bonded graft for in situ reconstruction after prosthetic graft infections. J Vasc Surg 16:651-660, 1992.
28. Clagett GP, Bowers BL, Lopez-Viego MA, et al. Creation of a neo-aortoiliac system from lower extremity deep and superficial veins. Ann Surg 218:239-249, 1993.
29. Kieffer E, Bahini A, Koskas F, et al. In situ allograft replacement of infected infrarenal aortic prosthetic grafts: Results in forty-three patients. J Vasc Surg 17:349-356, 1993.
30. Perler BA, Vander Kolk CA, Manson PM, Williams GM. Rotational muscle flaps to treat localized prosthetic graft infection: Long-term follow-up. J Vasc Surg 18:358-365, 1993.
31. Calligaro KD, Veith FJ, Schwartz ML, et al. Selective preservation of infected prosthetic arterial grafts: Analysis of a 20-year experience with 120 extra-cavitary-infected grafts. Ann Surg 220:461-471, 1994.

72

Treatment of Infected Aortic Prostheses Using Deep and Superficial Lower Extremity Vein Grafts for In Situ Replacement

G. PATRICK CLAGETT, M.D.

Treatment of aortoiliac prosthetic infections by in situ replacement with a new prosthesis has met with limited success. Although the approach remains an option in high-risk patients who have limited infections caused by low virulence organisms and no evidence of widespread contamination, it is a less than ideal solution because of the potential for reinfection, the possible involvement of the proximal aortic anastomoses with life-threatening consequences, and the probable need for lifelong antibiotic therapy. In situ replacement with autogenous grafts fashioned from endarterectomized arterial segments and saphenous veins has been eminently successful in eradicating infection, as well as resisting reinfection[1-3]; however, this approach has been plagued with unsatisfactory patency of these conduits. In situ allograft replacement for infected aortic prostheses has been championed as a satisfactory alternative approach [4,5]; however, use of allografts is limited by the degenerative changes common in such homograft tissue.

The most important tenets in treating extensive aortic prosthetic infection include excision of all infected prosthetic material and restoration of adequate pelvic and lower extremity arterial circulation. The operative strategies available to achieve these and the contemporary mortality and amputation rates are listed in Table 1. Currently, the most widely favored operative approach is extra-anatomic bypass through uninfected tissues with removal of the aortic prosthesis. In data pooled from major contemporary series, the overall mortality rate with this approach is 19% (95% confidence interval [CI], 15% to 24%), and the amputation rate is 14% (95% CI, 8% to 19%).[6-12,16,18-21] Most experts prefer staging these procedures, with extra-anatomic bypass preceding prosthesis removal by a 2- to 3-day interval. However, critical analysis of the data (see Table 1) demonstrates little difference in outcome between a staged or simultaneous operative approach.

A limitation to extra-anatomic bypass and removal of the aortic prosthesis is the potential for infection of the new prosthesis and aortic stump blowout. In data pooled from major series reported since 1980, the rate of infection of the extra-anatomic bypass is 16% (95% CI, 10% to 21%) and the incidence of fatal aortic stump blowout is 8% (95% CI, 5% to 12%).[6-8,17,18-20,22,23] These problems can also occur with allograft in situ replacement, and reinfection of homografts and fatal homograft rupture have been reported.

One of the most disappointing features of extra-anatomic bypass is the high rate of acute occlusion. This often occurs in patients with extensive vascular disease and complex extra-anatomic bypasses such as axillo–unilateral popliteal or profunda bypasses. Thrombosis of these reconstructions limited by poor outflow is usually sudden, catastrophic, and leads to amputation in a large number of cases. In a recently reported series of patients with extra-anatomic bypasses placed for aortic prosthetic infection, the primary patency rate was 43% at 3 years and approximately one third of all survivors required major amputation.[8]

Dissatisfaction with extra-anatomic prosthetic bypasses stimulated the development of an in situ autologous reconstruction using major lower extremity veins. Building on the experience of others who used greater saphenous veins,[1-3,17] an approach was developed using the superficial femoropopliteal veins or deep veins to reconstruct the aortoiliac femoral system.[24] For simplicity, it is termed a neoaortoiliac system (NAIS).

443

Table 1 Pooled data from series of infected aortic prostheses reported since 1980

Operations	References	Mortality			Amputation		
		No. of patients	Incidence (%)	(95% CI)	No. of patients	Incidence (%)	95% CI
Excise prosthesis, no revascularization	6-11	18/47	38.3	(24.4-52.3)	18/38	47.4	31.5-63.3
In situ prosthetic replacement	12-15	7/29	24.1	(8.4-39.7)	—	—	—
Autogenous reconstruction	2, 3, 7, 16, 17	11/41	26.8	(13.2-40.4)	8/41	19.5	7.4-31.6
Extra-anatomic bypass, excise prosthesis (any sequence, with or without delay)	6-12, 16, 18-22	53/276	19.2	(14.6-23.8)	20/147	13.6	8.1-19.1
Excise prosthesis first, followed by extra anatomic bypass	7, 8, 9, 12, 23	22/85	25.9	(16.6-35.2)	10/40	25.0	11.6-38.4
Extra-anatomic bypass first, followed by excision of prosthesis (with or without delay)	7, 11, 12, 18-21	39/183	21.3	(15.4-27.2)	10/90	11.1	4.6-17.6
Extra-anatomic bypass first, delayed excision of prosthesis	7, 11, 18, 19	8/45	17.8	(6.6-29.0)	4/34	11.8	1.0-22.6
Extra-anatomic bypass first, no delay in excision of prosthesis	7, 12, 18, 21	29/132	22.0	(14.9-29.1)	5/50	10.0	1.7-18.3

CI = confidence interval.

OPERATIVE DETAILS

Large venous autografts are important for successful NAIS reconstruction. It is important to assess preoperatively the size of the greater saphenous and deep veins. Experience shows that only very large saphenous veins, at least 8 mm in distended diameter, perform satisfactorily for this approach. Smaller veins are prone to develop focal stenoses and diffuse neointimal hyperplasia, which require multiple revisions and replacement procedures. I currently favor the use of deep veins in most instances and avoid using greater saphenous veins. It is also important to image the superficial femoropopliteal veins with duplex ultrasonography before performing the operation. I have noted occasional anomalies as well as areas of occlusion and recanalization in the deep veins that preclude their successful use. The anomaly encountered most frequently (in approximately 5% of patients) is a dominant profunda system that communicates directly with the distal popliteal vein. In these circumstances the superficial femoropopliteal vein is usually small and incomplete. Shulman et al.[25] reported finding a dominant profunda venous system in approximately 7% of patients undergoing femoropopliteal bypass with deep vein grafts. Fortunately this anomaly is most often unilateral and a reconstruction can be planned using the normal deep vein from one extremity and a segment of greater saphenous vein from the other. It is important to preserve the greater saphenous vein in the extremity from which the deep vein is harvested. Limb edema can occur if both veins are harvested from the same extremity.

The operation begins with vein harvest, and every effort is made to ensure that this remains a sterile procedure. Infected femoral wounds are excluded from the field by secure placement of adherent iodine-impregnated plastic drapes over grossly infected wounds, which are dressed with dry gauze sponges to absorb contaminated fluids during the operation. A two-team approach is preferred with one team harvesting veins while the other removes the infected aortic prostheses.

In harvesting deep vein autografts, the lateral border of the sartorius muscle is mobilized from the upper thigh to the knee joint. The sartorius muscle is freed along its lateral border and reflected medially and posteriorly to preserve its blood supply, which enters the muscle belly from the inferomedial aspect. Hunter's canal is exposed and care is taken to preserve the major collateral branches of the superficial femoral and popliteal arteries, the saphenous nerve, and the ipsilateral greater saphenous vein. Saphenous neuralgia will occur if the saphenous nerve is injured. This complication is vexing to patients, although it is usually temporary, lasting several weeks to months. The adductor canal is opened by incising the tendinous portion of the adductor magnus muscle, and multiple branches of the superficial femoropopliteal vein are carefully ligated and divided; large branches are doubly ligated or suture ligated. Secure ligation of these branches cannot be overemphasized. They are prone to displacement as the large-caliber conduits are passed through the restricted space of the tunnels fashioned in the retroperitoneum to the femoral sites. The most tedious portion of the dissection occurs in the adductor canal region where the vein has multiple large branches and is in close apposition to the artery and the aponeurosis of the adductor magnus.

A critically important feature in preventing excessive venous hypertension is the careful preservation of the junction of the profunda femoris vein with the common femoral vein. The entrance of the profunda femoris vein into the common femoral vein is identified, and the proximal superficial vein is transected and oversewn flush with this junction. The popliteal vein is mobilized distally until a length adequate for NAIS reconstruction is acquired. This often requires mobilization of the vein to the knee joint or just below it.

Vein grafts are distended with chilled whole blood or a cold solution consisting of Ringer's lactate (1 L), heparin (5000 U), albumin (25 gm), and papaverine (60 mg). Because the vein is largest in diameter proximally, the valves are fractured by retrograde passage of a Mills-Leather valvulotome so that the large-caliber end can be anastomosed comfortably to the aortic stump. There are usually only three or four major valves in the long deep vein autograft. Valves within 10 to 15 cm of either the proximal or distal end can be easily excised after exposing them by everting the graft. Vein grafts are stored in solutions maintained at a temperature of 4° C until they are required for NAIS reconstruction. Vein harvest incisions are irrigated copiously with antibiotic solutions and closed completely.

All prosthetic material is excised, and the aorta and periaortic tissues are liberally debrided to achieve a clean proximal anastomotic site for the deep vein autograft. Aortic debridement can be facilitated by suprarenal aortic control either by cross-clamping at the diaphragmatic level or with intraluminal balloon control. The proximal anastomotic technique favored most involves simply suturing the deep vein autograft end to end to the debrided aorta (Fig. 1). Standard continuous polypropylene (4-0) suture technique is used, taking care to make slightly more advancement on the aorta than the venous autograft because of the greater circumference of the aorta. To date, I have encountered three patients with very large proximal aortas, two with dilatation and the other with frank aneurysmal change. In these situations the deep veins were joined and sewn to the aneurysmal aorta.

Infected femoral wounds are opened and debrided, and all prosthetic material is removed from below. The retroperitoneal tunnels are irrigated with antibiotic solutions and mechanically debrided by pulling gauze sponges through them. Venous grafts are brought through the old tunnels and anastomosed directly to the debrided femoral vessels. The venous autografts are brought through the old tunnels in an undistended state, avoiding twisting and kinking. Creation of new tunnels is dangerous because of limited space and retroperitoneal inflammation and scarring. I frequently dilate the old, fibrotic tunnels by simple finger insertion or passage of a large-caliber graft passer. This dilatation is important because portions of the deep vein graft have a larger diameter than the tunnel.

Examples of NAIS reconstructions are illustrated in Fig. 2. The most satisfactory experience has been with a simple deep vein autograft anastomosed to the terminal aorta and to a

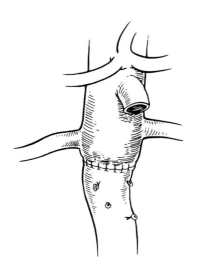

Fig. 1 Proximal aortic end-to-end anastomosis with a deep vein autograft. The diameter of the deep vein autograft is usually only slightly smaller than that of the aorta, which allows for a comfortable anastomosis with standard suture techniques.

Fig. 2 Schematic representation of NAIS reconstructions. **A,** Aorto–unilateral femoral bypass with a deep vein autograft and femorofemoral bypass with another deep vein graft or greater saphenous vein graft. **B,** Conjoined greater saphenous veins anastomosed end to end to the aorta. **C,** Conjoined greater saphenous veins sewn end to side to the anterior aorta following oversewing of the aortic stump. **D,** Aorto–left femoral bypass with deep vein autograft and right femoral limb (deep vein autograft or greater saphenous vein graft) anastomosed end to side. **E,** Replacement of unilateral infected aortobifemoral bypass limb with deep vein or saphenous vein autograft. **F,** This patient originally had greater saphenous vein graft replacement of an infected right aortobifemoral bypass limb and experienced an infected left femoral false aneurysm 4 years later. The remainder of the prosthesis was replaced by deep vein autografts that were conjoined proximally to accommodate anastomosis to an aneurysmal aorta. **G,** Aortoiliac replacement fashioned from deep vein autografts. **H,** The right common iliac artery is anastomosed end to side to an aorto–left iliac bypass constructed from a deep vein autograft. **I,** This patient had recurrent aortobifemoral bypass occlusions secondary to intimal hyperplasia at distal anastomosis to profunda femoral arteries. Both limbs were replaced by greater saphenous vein autografts. (From Clagett GP, Bowers BL, Lopez-Viego MA, Rossi MB, Valentine RJ, Myers SI, Chervu A. Creation of a neo-aortoiliac system from lower extremity deep and superficial veins. Ann Surg 218:239-249, 1993.)

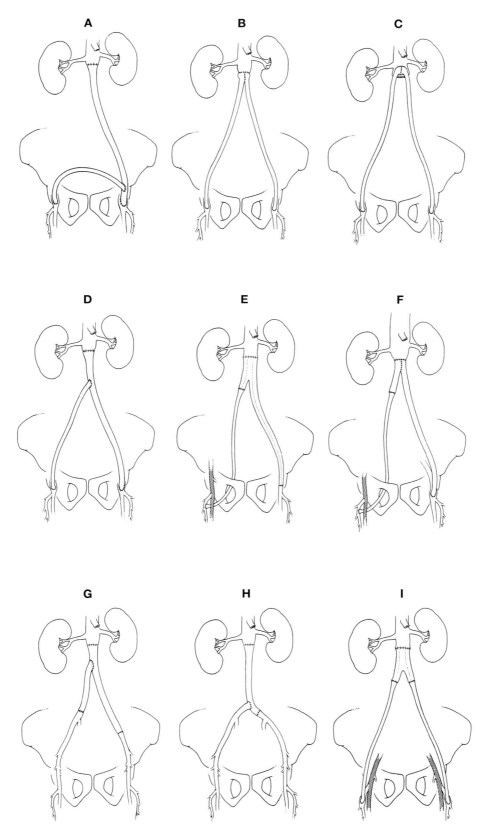

Fig. 2 For legend see opposite page.

femoral or iliac artery. A second deep vein autograft is anastomosed end to side to the autograft in place and then passed through a retroperitoneal tunnel to the contralateral femoral vessel. Distal anastomoses have been fashioned to the common femoral artery, the profunda femoris artery, and the superficial femoral artery with relatively equal frequency. At the completion of NAIS reconstruction, the debrided subcutaneum of the femoral wounds is closed over the venous autografts and the skin left open. It has not been necessary to cover the venous autografts with muscle flaps. Drainage is rarely employed and antibiotics are discontinued within 5 to 7 days after the operation. These patients are particularly prone to deep venous thrombosis caused by stasis in the residual distal popliteal vein. An important adjunct to prevent this complication is intermittent pneumatic compression combined with low-dose heparin prophylaxis.

UNIVERSITY OF TEXAS SOUTHWESTERN MEDICAL CENTER EXPERIENCE

The Center's early experience with the NAIS reconstruction has been reported,[24] and an update will now be provided. Thirty-four patients have undergone NAIS reconstruction at the University of Texas Southwestern Medical Center. Twenty-six patients underwent NAIS reconstruction because of aortic prosthetic infection (26 infected aortobifemoral bypasses, two aortoenteric fistulas, and one aortoenteric erosion). Eight patients had the operation because of complex aortic problems. These included patients who had contraindications to standard prosthetic reconstruction because of ongoing regional infections (e.g., advanced peroneal, scrotal, and pubic hydradenitis suppurativa or gastrointestinal fistulas) that could not be cleared in a timely fashion. These patients also had failed attempts at interventional radiologic approaches to achieve revascularization. Other patients in the category of complex aortic problems included those with multiple recurrent prosthetic aortobifemoral bypass thromboses from exuberant anastomotic neointimal hyperplasia or severely restricted outflow that would not support prosthetic reconstruction. My experience with this latter group of patients suggests that severely restricted outflow along with exceedingly small aortoiliac vessels leads to an unacceptable rate of occlusion with a standard aortobifemoral prostheses.[26]

Among the patients with infected prostheses, 19 had paninfected aortobifemoral bypasses or aortoiliac prostheses with pus surrounding the body and limbs of the prostheses, and seven patients had a single aortobifemoral bypass limb involvement. The majority of these patients had infected knitted Dacron prostheses, most of which were placed for occlusive disease. However, three patients had expanded polytetrafluoroethylene aortic graft (ePTFE) limb replacements that subsequently became infected. The mean (±SD) interval between the original aortic operation and the diagnosis of prosthetic infection was 68 ± 54 months (range, 4 to 192 months), and the modes of presentation included femoral abscesses, chronic draining groin sinuses, infected femoral anastomotic aneurysms, fever, anemia, and gastrointestinal bleeding. Almost all patients complained of malaise and chronic fatigue. Risk factors for prosthetic infection included multiple femoral reoperations after initial aortic procedure (mean, 3 ± 2; range, 0 to 10), usually for anastomotic aneurysms, limb thromboses, or wound complications. Other risk factors seen in individual patients included renal failure requiring dialysis, immunosuppressive therapy with cyclophosphamide for an autoimmune disorder, and multiple chronically infected cutaneous squamous cell carcinoma lesions.

More conservative local procedures had failed in at least one half of the patients in this series. These included removal of a single aortobifemoral bypass limb with extra-anatomic bypass (obturator bypass, axillofemoral superficial femoral bypass, and axillopopliteal bypass), continuous irrigation with antibiotic solutions coupled with multiple debridements, muscle flap coverage, and debridement with in situ replacement with ePTFE. All of these patients were treated with prolonged oral or parenteral antibiotics and the femoral wounds had healed before signs of recurrent, more extensive infection developed. Organisms cultured from excised prosthetic material or pus surrounding prostheses and number of patients are listed below.

Staphylococcus epidermidis (10)
S. aureus (5)
Pseudomonas aeruginosa (2)
Escherichia coli (1)
β-hemolytic streptococcus (1)
Enterobacter aerogenes (1)

Bacteroides bivius (1)
Proteus mirabilis (1)
Serratia marcescens (1)
Propionibacterium acnes (1)
Candida albicans (1)

Consistent with most contemporary reports, gram-positive organisms, especially *S. epidermidis*, predominated; however, there were also gram-negative infections that included *P. aeruginosa, E. coli,* and *P. mirabilis.*

Veins harvested for NAIS reconstruction included bilateral saphenous veins (seven patients), deep veins and greater saphenous veins from opposite limbs (three patients), bilateral deep veins (12 patients), and unilateral deep veins (12 patients). The mean operative time was 6.5 ± 1.8 hours (range, 4.5 to 10 hours) and intraoperative blood transfusion requirement was 4 ± 4 units (range, 0 to 9 units). When two teams were used, operative time was less than 5 hours. Supraceliac aortic control was required in five patients.

None of the patients died during surgery. However, three patients died at prolonged intervals (more than 30 days after operation) from peritonitis, sepsis, and multisystem organ dysfunction. Interestingly, all of these patients presented with aortoenteric fistula or erosion. There were two acute amputations in survivors for an overall procedure-related mortality and amputation rate of 9% and 6%, respectively. Other major morbidity included gastrointestinal complications with peritonitis in four patients. In these cases, the ability of the deep veins to resist infection was demonstrated. Peritonitis developed in these patients from a perforated duodenal diverticulum with septic pancreatitis, ischemic small bowel necrosis, acute cholecystitis, and gangrene of the gallbladder. Three of these patients had diffuse peritonitis and the deep vein autografts were bathed in polymicrobial pus (*E. aerogenes, P. maltophilia,* and *C. albicans*). The vein grafts were inspected during exploratory surgery on multiple occasions, and the NAIS vein grafts and anastomoses were found to be intact and uninfected. Deep venous thrombosis occurred in two patients, and one patient sustained a major pulmonary embolism. The site of deep venous thrombosis was on the side of the deep vein harvest in both cases.

The mean follow-up time has been 32 ± 23 months (range; 2 to 90 months). There have been four deaths related to cardiac disease and none directly attributable to the NAIS reconstruction. One patient required amputation because of progression of distal disease.

The difference in behavior between the greater saphenous vein and deep vein autograft as noted on long-term follow-up was interesting. Three patients with greater saphenous vein NAIS developed total occlusion within 1 year following surgery, which resulted from progressive, diffuse, neointimal hyperplasia documented by angiography and biopsy at reexploration. One of these patients underwent secondary prosthetic extra-anatomic bypass, and the remaining two patients have noncritical lower extremity ischemia with severe claudication and desire no further intervention. Four patients developed focal stenoses in the greater saphenous vein autografts and three required reoperation with patch angioplasty or femoral crossover limb replacement. Small greater saphenous veins were particularly prone to failure (Fig. 3, *A*). In contrast, large saphenous veins had sustained patency. Discrete stenoses were likely to develop at areas of kinking and at valve sites. Aortic anastomoses with greater saphenous vein were also problem prone (Fig. 3, *B*). All failures were apparent within the first year after operation and were manifested by falling ankle pressure indices, changes on duplex surveillance (decrease in luminal caliber and focal areas of jet-flow velocity), and onset of intermittent claudication. Despite the high failure rate of greater saphenous veins, no amputations have been required. In contrast, all NAIS reconstructions from larger caliber deep vein autografts have remained patent and free of stenoses (Fig. 4). The overall failure rate (defined as occlusion or stenosis requiring reintervention) of greater saphenous vein NAIS reconstruction was 64% compared to 0% for deep vein NAIS reconstruction ($p = .01$).

Because of the tendency of greater saphenous vein grafts used for NAIS reconstruction to develop focal stenoses as well as diffuse intimal hyperplasia, it is important to monitor these vein grafts with frequent duplex ultrasound examinations and clinical assessment, especially in the first year after placement. Focal stenoses are corrected by timely reintervention. Despite this limitation, occlusion following greater saphenous vein NAIS reconstruction is more gradual than the sudden thrombotic occlusion experienced by patients with extra-anatomic bypasses who frequently present with profound, irrevers-

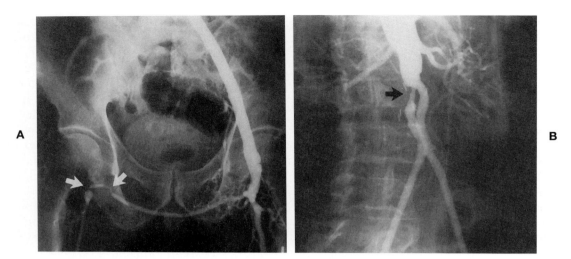

Fig. 3 A, Focal stenoses (arrows) developing in a small greater saphenous vein femoral crossover bypass at sites of kinks and angulation. The aorto–left femoral deep vein autograft is widely patent. This patient experienced progressive right lower extremity intermittent claudication and underwent prosthetic femoral crossover bypass. **B,** Focal stenoses (arrow) developing at site of kinking in proximal aortic anastomosis of conjoined greater saphenous vein autografts. This patient had progressive right leg intermittent claudication, falling ankle pressure indices, and elevated flow velocities on duplex ultrasound at the site of stenosis. (From Clagett GP, Bowers BL, Lopez-Viego MA, Rossi MB, Valentine RJ, Myers SI, Chervu A. Creation of a neo-aortoiliac system from lower extremity deep and superficial veins. Ann Surg 218:239-249, 1993.)

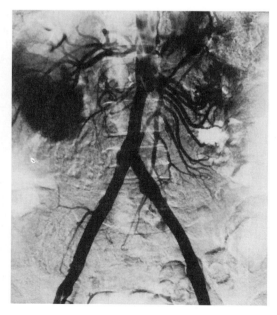

Fig. 4 NAIS reconstruction similar to that shown schematically in Fig. 2, *D,* with wide patency of both limbs fashioned from deep vein autografts.

ible limb ischemia. The slowly progressive occlusion in patients with greater saphenous vein NAIS reconstructions has allowed for early detection, reintervention, and in some cases, development of collateral circulation.

I currently favor deep vein autografts for NAIS reconstructions and rarely use greater saphenous veins unless they are large (≥ 8 mm in diameter). I have not observed focal or diffuse intimal hyperplasia in deep vein autografts. The superficial femoropopliteal vein has a diameter of 1.0 to 1.5 cm, which allows end-to-end anastomosis to a normal-caliber aorta with relative ease. Another advantage of the deep vein autografts is that minor kinks and areas of intimal hyperplasia at valve sites do not produce hemodynamic disturbances to the degree produced by similar-size defects in small-caliber greater saphenous vein grafts. A potential problem with the deep vein autograft is the development of mural thrombosis. This has been reported with the use of deep vein autografts greater than 1.2 cm in diameter for femoropopliteal bypass. Failure resulted from mural thromboembolism. I have not observed this and predict that it will not occur because of the better size match between the aortoiliac femoral system and the deep vein autografts. Aneurysmal dilatation of deep vein grafts is also a serious concern. I have not observed this condition, but continue to monitor all patients with serial duplex ultrasonography, CT, and in some cases repeat angiography.

Of the 27 patients (39 limbs) who had unilateral or bilateral deep vein harvest, only four (15%) have had significant chronic limb edema requiring use of compression stockings. These patients either had ipsilateral venous thrombosis with presumed valvular injury or prior harvest of the ipsilateral greater saphenous vein, usually for a prior distal bypass. The absence of significant limb edema has been gratifying. This has also been the experience of Shulman et al.,[27] who pioneered the use of the deep vein autograft for femoropopliteal reconstructions. Schanzer et al.[28] reported mild calf enlargement along with a pattern on strain-gauge plethysmography indicative of venous outflow obstruction in most patients who had deep vein harvest for femoropopliteal bypass. Despite this, clinically significant edema requiring use of compression stockings was rare and there was no functional disability. This is in agreement with the findings of Masuda et al.,[29] who studied the long-term hemodynamic and clinical outcomes in patients who had ligation of the superficial femoral vein. These investigators concluded that there was no correlation between physiologic obstruction of this vein and the presence or absence of limb edema. They further observed that obstruction is well tolerated when the profunda femoris and ipsilateral greater saphenous veins are intact. Although Schulman et al.[27] did not find significant edema in limbs from which both greater saphenous and deep veins were removed, I caution against this. I also believe that preservation of the profunda femoris vein is critical in preserving sufficient venous collateral flow to prevent excessive venous hypertension.

CONCLUSION

Venous autografts resist infection when used for NAIS reconstructions. Small greater saphenous veins are prone to failure as a result of the development of focal stenoses and intimal hyperplasia. In contrast, deep veins perform well, anastomose comfortably with the proximal aorta, and have sustained patency. Furthermore, deep vein harvest is well tolerated with no functional disability and minimal problems with limb edema as long as the profunda and common femoral veins remain intact and the ipsilateral greater saphenous vein is preserved. NAIS reconstruction can be a successful option in patients with aortic prosthetic infections and other complex aortic problems.

REFERENCES

1. Ehrenfeld WK, Wilbur BG, Olcott CN, Stoney RJ. Autogenous tissue reconstruction in the management of infected prosthetic grafts. Surgery 85:82-92, 1979.
2. Quiñones-Baldrich WJ, Gelabert HA. Autogenous tissue reconstruction in the management of aortoiliofemoral graft infection. Ann Vasc Surg 4:223-228, 1990.
3. Lorentzen JE, Nielsen OM. Aortobifemoral bypass with autogenous saphenous vein in treatment of paninfected aortic bifurcation graft. J Vasc Surg 3:666-668, 1986.
4. Bahnini A, Ruotolo C, Koskas F, Kieffer E. In situ fresh allograft replacement of an infected aortic prosthetic graft: Eighteen months' follow-up. J Vasc Surg 14:98-102, 1991.
5. Snyder SO, Wheeler JR, Gregory RT, Gayle RG, Zirkle PK. Freshly harvested cadaveric venous hemografts as arterial conduits in infected fields. Surgery 101:283-291, 1987.
6. Ricotta JJ, Faggioli GL, Stella A, Curl GR, Peer R, Upson J, D'Addato M, Anain J, Gutierrez I. Total excision and extra-anatomic bypass for aortic graft infection. Am J Surg 162:145-149, 1991.
7. Reilly LM, Stoney RJ, Goldstone J, Ehrenfeld WK. Improved management of aortic graft infection: The influence of operation sequence and staging. J Vasc Surg 5:421-431, 1987.
8. Quiñones-Baldrich WJ, Hernandez JJ, Moore WS. Long-term results following surgical management of aortic graft infection. Arch Surg 126:507-511, 1991.
9. Schellack J, Stewart MT, Smith RB, Perdue GD, Salam A. Infected aortobifemoral prosthesis—A dreaded complication. Am Surg 54:137-141, 1988.
10. Lorentzen JE, Nielsen OM, Arendrup H, Kimose HH, Bille S, Andersen J, Jensen CH, Jacobsen F, Roder OC. Vascular graft infection: An analysis of sixty-two graft infections in 2411 consecutively implanted synthetic vascular grafts. Surgery 98:81-86, 1985.
11. Casali RE, Tucker WE, Thompson BW, Read RC. Infected prosthetic grafts. Arch Surg 115:577-580, 1980.
12. Yeager RA, Moneta GL, Taylor LM, Harris EJ Jr, McConnell DB, Porter JM. Improving survival and limb salvage in patients with aortic graft infection. Am J Surg 159:466-469, 1990.
13. Robinson JA, Johansen K. Aortic sepsis: Is there a role for in situ graft reconstruction? J Vasc Surg 13:677-684, 1991.
14. Walker WE, Cooley DA, Duncan JM, Hallman GL Jr, Ott DA, Reul GJ. The management of aortoduodenal fistula by in situ replacement of the infected abdominal aortic graft. Ann Surg 205:727-732, 1987.

15. O'Mara CS, Williams GM, Ernst CB. Secondary aortoenteric fistula, a 20 year experience. Am J Surg 142:203-209, 1981.
16. Yeager RA, McConnell DB, Sasaki TM, Vetto RM. Aortic and peripheral prosthetic graft infection: Differential management and causes of mortality. Am J Surg 150:36-43, 1985.
17. Seeger JM, Wheeler JR, Gregory RT, Snyder SO, Gayle RG. Autogenous graft replacement of infected prosthetic grafts in the femoral position. Surgery 93:39-45, 1983.
18. Bacourt F, Koskas F, French University Association for Research in Surgery. Axillobifemoral bypass and aortic exclusion for vascular septic lesions: A multicenter retrospective study of 98 cases. Ann Vasc Surg 6:119-126, 1992.
19. O'Hara PJ, Hertzer NR, Beven EG, Krajewski LP. Surgical management of infected abdominal aortic grafts: Review of a 25-year experience. J Vasc Surg 3:725-731, 1986.
20. Trout HH, Kozloff L, Giordano JM. Priority of revascularization in patients with graft enteric fistulas, infected arteries, or infected arterial prostheses. Ann Surg 6:669-682, 1984.
21. Olah A, Vogt M, Laske A, Carrell T, Bauer E, Turina M. Axillo-femoral bypass and simultaneous removal of the aortofemoral vascular infection site: Is the procedure safe? Eur J Vasc Surg 6:252-254, 1992.
22. Schmitt DD, Seabrook GR, Bandyk DF, Towne JB. Graft excision and extra-anatomic revascularization: The treatment of choice for the septic aortic prosthesis. J Cardiovasc Surg 31:327-332, 1990.
23. Turnipseed WD, Berkoff HA, Detmer DE, Acher CW, Belzer FO. Arterial graft infections. Delayed vs. immediate vascular reconstruction. Arch Surg 118:410-414, 1983.
24. Clagett GP, Bowers BL, Lopez-Viego MA, Rossi MB, Valentine RJ, Myers SI, Chervu A. Creation of a neo-aortoiliac system from lower extremity deep and superficial veins. Ann Surg 218:239-249, 1993.
25. Schulman ML, Schulman LG, Lledo-Perez AM. Unusual autogenous vein grafts. Vasc Surg 26:257-264, 1992.
26. Valentine RJ, Hansen ME, Myers SI, Chervu A, Clagett GP. The influence of sex and aortic size on late patency following aortofemoral revascularization in young adults. J Vasc Surg 21:296-306, 1995.
27. Schulman ML, Badhey MR, Yatco R. Superficial femoral-popliteal veins and reversed saphenous veins as primary femoropopliteal bypass grafts: A randomized comparative study. J Vasc Surg 6:1-10, 1987.
28. Schanzer H, Chiang K, Mabrouk M, Peirce EC. Use of lower extremity deep veins as arterial substitutes: Functional status of the donor leg. J Vasc Surg 14:624-627, 1991.
29. Masuda EM, Kistner RL, Ferris EB III. Long-term effects of superficial femoral vein ligation: Thirteen-year follow-up. J Vasc Surg 16:741-749, 1992.

73

Long-Term Follow-Up of More Than 100 Infected Extracavitary Arterial Prosthetic Grafts

KEITH D. CALLIGARO, M.D., FRANK J. VEITH, M.D., MICHAEL L. SCHWARTZ, M.D., JAMIE GOLDSMITH, R.N., MATTHEW J. DOUGHERTY, M.D., and DOMINIC A. DeLAURENTIS, M.D.

Routine graft excision has been the traditional method used to treat infected peripheral prosthetic arterial grafts, but it has been associated with high mortality (9% to 36%) and limb loss (27% to 79%) rates.[1-5] This method has been proposed as a means to prevent anastomotic hemorrhage and systemic sepsis.[6-8] At Montefiore Medical Center, Veith[9] and Samson et al.[10] were among the first to suggest that selective graft preservation may be an improved method of treating these complications. At Pennsylvania Hospital a similar strategy has been used, and we have noted better results compared to routine graft excision.[11] This chapter details an updated series of more than 100 infected extracavitary prosthetic arterial grafts treated at both medical centers over the past 20 years.

METHODS

Since the early 1970s we have treated more than 100 infected prosthetic grafts anastomosed to an extracavitary artery at Montefiore Medical Center in New York and Pennsylvania Hospital in Philadelphia (Table 1). Patients ranged in age from 34 to 91 years (mean, 66 years). There were 63 men and 57 women. The infected graft was polytetrafluoroethylene (PTFE) in 95 cases and Dacron in 25 (Table 2). Fourteen infections involved the femoral anastomosis of aortofemoral grafts (see Table 2). The infection involved the anastomosis in 109 cases and was confined to the body of the graft in 11 cases. The bypasses were

Supported by grants from the John F. Connelly Foundation, the United States Public Health Service (HL 02990-01), the James Hilton Manning and Emma Austin Manning Foundation, the Anna S. Brown Trust, and the New York Institute for Vascular Studies.

Table 1 Site of infection involving 120 extracavitary prosthetic arterial grafts

Site of infection	No.
Anastomotic infections	
Femoral artery*	85
Tibial artery	13
Popliteal artery	10
Axillary artery	1
TOTAL	109
Infection confined to the body of the graft	
Thigh	5
Flank	2
Chest	1
Knee	1
Calf	1
Ankle	1
TOTAL	11

*Femoral = common, superficial, or deep femoral arteries in the groin in all cases.

Table 2 Type of infected extracavitary prosthetic arterial graft*

	No.	PTFE	Dacron
Femoropopliteal	50	44	6
Femorotibial	32	32	0
Aortofemoral†	14	0	14
Femorofemoral crossover	10	10	0
Femoral interposition	8	4	4
Axillofemoral	6	5	1
TOTAL	120	95	25

*Femoral = common, superficial, or deep femoral arteries.
†Patients who presented with aortofemoral graft infections were included in this series only if the infection was confined to the groin based on clinical, CT scan, sinogram, arteriographic, and initial operative findings.

performed for limb salvage in 101 cases, for disabling claudication in 11 cases, and for noninfected aneurysms or pseudoaneurysms in eight cases. Follow-up averaged 3 years (range, 1 month to 20 years).

Complete graft preservation was attempted in 51 cases when the following criteria existed: (1) the anastomosis was intact, (2) the graft was patent, and (3) the patient was not septic.

If patients presented with a disrupted anastomosis (20 cases) or sepsis (6 cases), they were treated by graft excision. The entire graft was removed in septic patients to eradicate any potential source of continuing infection. In patients who presented with a disrupted anastomosis, the infected segment of graft was excised. The remainder of the graft was left intact only if it was found to be well incorporated and uninvolved with the infection, based on results of preoperative radiologic studies, intraoperative Gram stain, and operative exploration. This strategy proved especially useful when a patient presented with a disrupted distal anastomosis of an aortobifemoral graft. If there was no evidence of infection involving the proximal part of the graft, only the infected distal limb was excised. Through a separate flank incision, the proximal uninvolved limb of the graft was divided and oversewn or used as inflow for revascularization of the threatened limb via an uninfected route.[9,12]

Patients who had infected thrombosed grafts and intact anastomoses (43 cases) were treated by subtotal graft excision except for a 2 to 3 mm remnant in the wound to maintain patency of the underlying artery (partial graft preservation). This strategy proved particularly useful for infections involving an occluded graft in the groin where patency of the deep femoral artery was essential for limb salvage.[13] Subtotal graft excision to treat occluded infected grafts often obviated the need for additional revascularization procedures. This technique allowed simple oversewing of the most proximal or distal cuff of the graft without having to dissect out arteries in wounds with extensive scarring. A clamp could be placed across the graft immediately above or below the intact anastomosis after thrombus was extracted. The remainder of the occluded graft could then be excised and the cuff of graft on the artery oversewn leaving a graft remnant as a patch.

Appropriate intravenous antibiotics were administered through a central venous catheter for at least 6 weeks based on aerobic and anaerobic cultures that were obtained from the infected wounds. When revascularization was necessary to salvage a threatened extremity after total or subtotal graft excision, we preferred tunneling a new graft through uninfected, usually lateral, routes. Since most of the infections involved prosthetic grafts in the groin, proximal inflow sites included the axillary and iliac arteries and the infrarenal or thoracic aorta.[9,12,14] The new graft was tunneled lateral to the groin wound to a patent outflow artery such as the distal deep or superficial femoral or popliteal arteries.[15,16] In a stable patient the infected wound was isolated with adhesive dressings, and the secondary bypass was performed prior to graft excision.

A critical adjunct to achieve successful wound healing included wound excision or aggressive operative debridement of all infected tissue in the wound including exudate on the graft or artery. Debridement was repeated under anesthesia in the operating room as often as necessary to ensure a healing wound. Patients were observed in a special care unit where 1% povidone-iodine or antibiotic-soaked dressing changes were performed three times a day.[17] This protocol was carried out until healthy granulation tissue covered the anastomosis. Wound healing by secondary intention was attempted in conjunction with complete graft preservation in 42 cases; in nine other cases a muscle flap was used (3 sartorius, 2 gracilis, 2 rectus abdominis, 1 semimembranous, and 1 soleus).[18]

RESULTS

Management of 120 infected extracavitary prosthetic grafts using the preceding protocol resulted in a hospital mortality rate of 12% (14/120) (Table 3). Death was attributed to sepsis in seven patients (4 treated by total graft excision, 3 by complete graft preservation), myocardial infarction in four patients (2 treated by partial graft preservation, 2 by complete graft preservation), pneumonia in one patient (treated by complete graft preservation), stroke in one patient, and recurrent hemorrhage in one patient (both treated by initial total graft excision). Surprisingly, patients who presented with oc-

Table 3 Results of treatment of 120 infected extracavitary prosthetic arterial grafts

	Hospital mortality rate	Amputation rate*	Wound healing rate†
Graft excision for bleeding (20) or sepsis (6)	23% (6/26)	15% (3/20)	95% (19/20)
Partial graft salvage for occluded grafts	5% (2/43)	22% (9/41)	85% (35/41)
Total graft preservation‡	12% (6/51)	4% (2/45)	71% (32/45)
p value§	NS	<.05	<.05
TOTAL	12% (14/120)	13% (14/106)	81% (86/106)

*Amputation rate in survivors.
†Wound healing rate in survivors after long-term follow-up (mean, 3 years; range, 1 month to 20 years).
‡Patients who presented with patent grafts, intact anastomoses and were not septic (51) were treated by attempted complete graft preservation.
§p values relate to statistically significant differences in results between any of the three treatment groups. No statistically significant differences in mortality rates existed between any one treatment group compared to either of the other two treatment groups, but there were significant differences in amputation and wound healing rates between one treatment group compared to either of the other two.

cluded grafts had the lowest mortality rate (5%; 2/43). Not surprisingly, mortality rates were highest for patients who presented with bleeding or sepsis (23%; 6/26). The mortality rate for patients treated by complete graft preservation was 12%.

Major amputations (8 above-knee, 6 below-knee) were required in 13% (14/106) of the surviving patients (see Table 3). Amputation rates were significantly higher in patients who presented with occluded grafts and underwent attempted partial graft salvage (22%; 9/41) compared to patients who had sepsis or bleeding (15%; 3/20) or were treated by attempted complete graft preservation (4%; 2/45) (p <.05). Revascularization procedures were not attempted in any of the 14 patients who lost a limb because the threatened extremity was not considered salvageable, the critical medical condition precluded a prolonged operative procedure, or the lack of an adequate outflow artery precluded a distal bypass.

Thirty-two of 45 grafts in the survivors initially treated by complete graft preservation remained healed after long-term follow-up. Two patients had hemorrhaging at the original infected site 3 and 12 months, respectively, after they were first seen. Eleven other patients developed nonhealing wounds or recurrent infection after 2 weeks to 38 months of follow-up and required total graft excision. None of the 32 patients successfully treated by complete graft preservation required a secondary revascularization procedure. Among the 13 patients in whom this approach failed, six required a secondary bypass, five did not require further revascularization procedures to maintain a viable limb, and two underwent above-knee amputations.

Nineteen of 20 grafts in surviving patients who were treated initially by total graft excision for sepsis or a disrupted anastomosis remained healed during the period of long-term follow-up. Four years after complete graft excision, one patient had a delayed arterial hemorrhage, which required further arterial interruption and an above-knee amputation. All 20 patients had initially been treated by oversewing or ligation of the involved artery. Of the 20 surviving patients who had sepsis or a disrupted anastomosis and who were treated by graft excision, 11 maintained viable limbs without revascularization, six required a secondary bypass, and three required amputation.

Thirty-five of 41 occluded grafts in survivors treated by subtotal graft excision with oversewing of a 2 to 3 mm graft remnant remained healed after long-term follow-up. Three wounds did not heal after 2 to 4 weeks of aggressive local wound care and required excision of the residual prosthetic patch and ligation or oversewing of the artery. Three other patients had delayed anastomotic bleeding at the site of the prosthetic patch after 1 week, 8 months, and 34 months of follow-up, and all were treated by excision of the residual prosthetic patch and ligation or division and oversewing of the ends of the artery. Of the 41 surviving patients who initially presented with occluded grafts, 19 did not require a secondary revascularization procedure because adequate collateral circulation was maintained, 13 required a secondary bypass, and nine others

Table 4 Bacteriology of 120 infected extracavitary prosthetic arterial grafts

Bacteria	No.
Gram-positive bacteria	
Staphylococcus (69)	
aureus	40
epidermidis	29
Streptococcus (33)	
faecalis	23
viridans	6
Group D nonenterococcus	4
Diphtheroides	5
Corynebacterium	4
Clostridium	1
Gram-negative bacteria	
Pseudomonas aeruginosa	25
Proteus mirabilis	12
Escherichia coli	10
Serratia marcescens	6
Bacteroides (6)	
fragilis	5
cloaca	1
Morganella morganii	4
Enterobacter	4
Acinetobacter	3
Klebsiella	1
Salmonella	1
Acinetobacter	1

underwent major amputations during their hospital stay.

Of the surviving 106 patients, long-term wound healing was successfully accomplished in 86 patients (81%) (see Table 3). Total excision of the graft resulted in higher rates of wound healing (95%; 19/20) than partial graft preservation (85%; 35/41) or attempted complete graft preservation (71%; 32/45) ($p <.05$).

Gram-positive bacteria only were cultured from 55 wounds, gram-negative bacteria only from 28 wounds, and both types of bacteria from 37 wounds (Table 4). *Staphylococcus aureus* was the most common gram-positive organism cultured and *Pseudomonas aeruginosa* was the most common gram-negative organism cultured. This expanded updated series confirms our previous finding that successful graft preservation was as likely when gram-negative bacteria were cultured from the wound as when gram-positive bacteria were cultured with the exception of *Pseudomonas*.[19]

DISCUSSION

The 12% mortality rate in our current series is similar to the most favorable results of other reported series of infected peripheral grafts (9% to 36%).[1-6,20] However, our amputation rate represents an overall improvement compared to most other series.[1-6] We believe that our low amputation rate is primarily due to three factors: (1) attempted complete graft preservation had been successfully achieved in about three fourths of surviving patients (32/45), (2) patency of the underlying artery and important collateral vessels was maintained by leaving an oversewn prosthetic graft cuff on the artery when subtotal graft excision was necessary to treat occluded infected grafts, and (3) an aggressive approach to limb salvage was used by carrying out extra-anatomic bypass in clean fields throughout this 20-year period when a secondary revascularization was required after infected graft excision or occlusion.[13,21]

Complete graft preservation under certain conditions, even when the graft-artery anastomosis is involved in the infectious process, represents the most important new aspect of our management scheme. By preserving the arterial supply to the threatened limb, successful graft preservation often obviates the need to perform complex secondary bypasses. The highest amputation rates among surviving patients were found in those who required subtotal or total graft excision for occluded grafts (22%) or for sepsis and bleeding (15%), respectively (see Table 3). In comparison, the amputation rate was only 4% for patients who could be treated by attempted complete graft preservation.

Many of our patients with infected occluded prosthetic grafts did not require secondary revascularization procedures to achieve limb salvage because we chose to oversew a small cuff of prosthetic graft on the underlying artery after excision of the thrombosed remainder of the graft. This technique maintained the patency of the artery and often allowed adequate perfusion of the threatened extremity through important collateral vessels. We have demonstrated that the majority of wounds treated in this manner remained healed after long-term follow-up. Oversewing of a small graft patch is most applicable for infected occluded prosthetic grafts in the groin to maintain the patency of the deep femoral artery.[13] Others have proposed placing an autologous tissue patch (vein or endarterectomized segment of occluded superficial femoral artery) on the involved arteriotomy or using in situ autologous conduits following prosthetic graft excision.[20,22-24]

A key to successful graft preservation was aggressive wound debridement. Excision of all infected tissue in the wound and all exudate or fibrin on the exposed graft must initially be performed in the operating room. Even when the anastomosis was involved in the infectious process, as in the majority of grafts in this series, complete graft preservation could usually be accomplished. The vast majority of our patients were successfully managed with repeated operative wound debridement and antibiotic or Betadine-soaked dressing changes until the wounds healed by delayed secondary intention. Advancement of a muscle flap onto an exposed, infected graft has been reported to be an important adjunct to achieve successful graft preservation.[18,25] We believe that placement of a muscle flap is not essential to achieve a high rate of success in graft preservation. However, we have recently been using this technique more frequently because it may shorten the hospital stay. In our experience, however, this should only be done when healthy granulation tissue is present and the wound has minimal evidence of residual infection.[18]

Bandyk et al.[26] have achieved good results by replacing an infected prosthetic graft with a new PTFE graft when coagulase-negative *S. epidermidis* is the only organism cultured from the wound. We continue to propose that these cases are more easily managed by graft preservation of the original infected graft, if the other criteria for complete graft preservation exist.

We found similar rates of successful graft preservation whether gram-negative or gram-positive bacteria were cultured from the wound, with one notable exception.[19] *Pseudomonas* was the only bacteria identified that correlated with a low rate of successful graft preservation. *Pseudomonas* was cultured in 25 wounds in the current series, but complete graft preservation was attempted in only 10 patients who fulfilled our previously mentioned criteria. A successful outcome was achieved in only 40% of these cases (4 patients). *P. aeruginosa* is relatively resistant to antibiotics, has a high adaptability to a wide variety of physical conditions, and produces elastase and alkaline protease, which lead to arterial wall disruption by inhibiting phagocytosis and degrading elastin, collagen, and fibrin.[27] These considerations may explain the poor results of attempted graft preservation when *Pseudomonas* is cultured, and for these reasons we generally favor graft excision in these cases unless no other alternative for revascularization exists.

Complete graft preservation was attempted in less than half (51 cases) of the infected grafts because the other patients had contraindications to graft preservation such as a disrupted anastomosis, sepsis, or an occluded graft. Patients with infected grafts who present with hemorrhage, pseudoaneurysm, or systemic sepsis represent extremely virulent manifestations of infection. We believe that this virulence is related more to individual host-bacterial interaction than to the identities of the causative organisms, per se. In the present series almost one quarter of the patients who had one of these virulent manifestations died despite immediate graft excision. Although there have been occasional reports of successful graft preservation in the setting of anastomotic disruption,[25] we believe the safest method for preventing recurrent hemorrhage in these cases is graft excision.[7,9] Similarly, patients with infected extracavitary prosthetic grafts who present with severe systemic sepsis are best managed by immediate total graft excision.[7-9] To rid these critically ill patients of infection as quickly as possible, all infected prosthetic material must be removed. In addition, an occluded graft mandates at least subtotal graft excision, since organized thrombus in the graft cannot be sterilized and will continue to be a focus of infection.[6]

Secondary revascularization procedures were generally accomplished by performing a new bypass tunneled laterally through sterile fields to avoid the infected wound. This approach has proved to be simpler than and as effective as obturator bypass.[8,28] Often it is necessary to tunnel the graft lateral to the anterior superior iliac spine if the groin wound extends far laterally. For groin infections involving a femorodistal graft, we have preferentially used the thoracic aorta or the abdominal aorta or the iliac artery approached through a retroperitoneal incision as proximal inflow sources. We also have used the axillary artery in poor-risk patients or when the aortoiliac system is diseased. Preoperative arteriography of the aortic arch, aortoiliac system, and outflow tract is recommended, if possible, before all secondary bypasses.[9,29]

Although our management scheme continues to evolve, we believe our current strategy for treating extracavitary prosthetic graft infections results in improved amputation rates without sacrificing patient survival. Selective graft preservation can be effective in many patients but is especially applicable in patients with multiple risk factors who cannot tolerate complete graft excision and an associated revascularization procedure.

REFERENCES

1. Veith FJ, Hartsuck JM, Crane C. Management of aortoiliac reconstruction complicated by sepsis and hemorrhage. N Engl J Med 270:1389-1392, 1964.
2. Liekweg WG, Greenfield LJ. Vascular prosthetic infections: Collected experience and results of treatment. Surgery 81:335-342, 1977.
3. Lorentzen JE, Nielsen OM, Arendrup H, et al. Vascular graft infection: An analysis of sixty-two graft infections in 2411 consecutively implanted synthetic vascular grafts. Surgery 98:81-86, 1985.
4. Kikta MJ, Goodson SF, Bishara RA, Meyer JP, Schuler JJ, Flanigan DP. Mortality and limb loss with infected infrainguinal bypass grafts. J Vasc Surg 5:566-571, 1987.
5. Yeager RA, McConnell DB, Sasaki TM, Vetto RM. Aortic and peripheral prosthetic graft infection: Differential management and causes of mortality. Am J Surg 150:36-43, 1985.
6. Szilagyi DE, Smith RF, Elliott JP, Vrandecic MP. Infection in arterial reconstruction with synthetic grafts. Ann Surg 16:321-333, 1972.
7. Bunt TJ. Synthetic vascular graft infections. I. Graft infections. Surgery 6:733-746, 1983.
8. Shaw RS, Baue AE. Management of sepsis complicating arterial reconstructive surgery. Surgery 53:75-79, 1963.
9. Veith FJ. Surgery of the infected aortic graft. In Bergan JJ, Yao JST, eds. Surgery of the Aorta and Its Body Branches. New York: Grune & Stratton, 1979, pp 521-533.
10. Samson RH, Veith FJ, Janko GS, Gupta SK, Scher LA. A modified classification and approach to the management of infections involving peripheral arterial prosthetic grafts. J Vasc Surg 8:147-153, 1988.
11. Calligaro KD, Westcott CJ, Buckley M, Savarese RP, DeLaurentis DA. Infrainguinal anastomotic arterial graft infections treated by selective graft preservation. Ann Surg 216:74-79, 1992.
12. Calligaro KD, Veith FJ. Diagnosis and management of infected prosthetic aortic grafts. Surgery 110:805-813, 1991.
13. Calligaro KD, Veith FJ, Gupta SK, et al. A modified method for management of prosthetic graft infections involving an anastomosis to the common femoral artery. J Vasc Surg 11:485-492, 1990.
14. DeLaurentis DA. The descending thoracic aorta in reoperative surgery. In Bergan JJ, Yao JST, eds. Reoperative Arterial Surgery. Orlando: Grune & Stratton, 1986, pp 195-203.
15. Veith FJ, Ascer E, Gupta SK, Wengerter KR. Lateral approach to the popliteal artery. J Vasc Surg 6:119-123, 1987.
16. Nunez AA, Veith FJ, Collier P, Ascer E, White Flores S, Gupta SK. Direct approaches to the distal portions of the deep femoral artery for limb salvage bypasses. J Vasc Surg 8:576-581, 1988.
17. Lineaweaver W, Howard R, Soucy D, et al. Topical antimicrobial toxicity. Arch Surg 120:267-270, 1985.
18. Calligaro KD, Veith FJ, Sales CM, Dougherty MJ, Savarese RP, DeLaurentis DA. Comparison of muscle flaps and delayed secondary intention wound healing for infected lower extremity arterial grafts. Ann Vasc Surg 8:31-37, 1994.
19. Calligaro KD, Veith FJ, Schwartz ML, Savarese RP, DeLaurentis DA. Are gram-negative bacteria a contraindication to selective preservation of infected prosthetic arterial grafts? J Vasc Surg 16:337-346, 1992.
20. Ehrenfeld WK, Wilbur BG, Olcott CN, Stoney RJ. Autogenous tissue reconstruction in the management of infected prosthetic grafts. Surgery 85:82-92, 1979.
21. Veith FJ, Gupta SK, Samson RH, et al. Progress in limb salvage by reconstructive arterial surgery combined with new or improved adjunctive procedures. Ann Surg 194:386-401, 1981.
22. Kieffer E, Bahnini A, Koskas F, Ruotolo C, Le Blevec D, Plissonnier D. In situ allograft replacement of infected infrarenal aortic prosthetic grafts: Results in forty-three patients. J Vasc Surg 17:349-356, 1993.
23. Seeger JM, Wheeler JR, Gregory RT, Snyder SO, Gayle RG. Autogenous graft replacement of infected prosthetic grafts in the femoral position. Surgery 93:39-45, 1983.
24. Clagett GP, Bowers BL, Lopez-Viego MA, et al. Creation of a new aortoiliac system from lower extremity deep and superficial veins. Ann Surg 218:239-249, 1993.
25. Perler BA, Vander Kolk CA, Dufresene CR, et al. Can infected prosthetic grafts be salvaged with rotational muscle flaps? Surgery 110:30-34, 1991.
26. Bandyk DF, Bergamini TM, Kinney EV, Seabrook GR, Towne JR. In situ replacement of vascular prostheses infected by bacterial biofilms. J Vasc Surg 13:575-583, 1991.
27. Pollack M. Pseudomonas aeruginosa. In Mandell GL, ed. Principles and Practice of Infectious Disease. 3rd ed. New York: Churchill-Livingstone, 1990, pp 1673-1691.
28. Guida PM, Moore WS. Obturator bypass technique. Surg Gynecol Obstet 128:1307-1316, 1969.
29. Calligaro KD, Ascer E, Veith FJ, et al. Unsuspected inflow disease in candidates for axillofemoral bypass operations: A prospective study. J Vasc Surg 11:823-827, 1990.

74

Transaxillary First Rib Resection With Extrapleural T2 Ganglion Thoracic Sympathectomy

DAVID B. ROOS, M.D.

For patients who have intolerable pain, paresthesias, and weakness of the upper extremities from thoracic outlet syndrome and in whom a reasonable attempt at conservative management has failed to control these symptoms through mild stretching exercises of the neck and shoulder muscles and medication for muscle relaxation and pain control, surgical decompression of the affected nerves of the brachial plexus may still offer substantial relief. If the symptoms seem to affect the lower nerves of the brachial plexus, C8 and T1, causing pain from the back of the neck and scapular area and down the arm from the posterior axilla through the inner arm, elbow, and T1 area of the forearm to the ring and small fingers, decompression of the lower nerves is the treatment of choice. This is best accomplished by transaxillary first rib resection, which provides the clearest and safest exposure and access to the thoracic outlet from below without having to operate down through the large subclavian vessels and brachial plexus to remove the bony floor of the outlet and skeletal attachments of the anterior and middle scalene muscles. The anomalous fibromuscular bands that are always found in such patients are best seen and eliminated from below.

If the patient has typical symptoms of causalgia, with burning pain and skin hypersensitivity (allodynia and hyperpathia) of the arm and hand, a selective T2 extrapleural thoracic sympathectomy can readily be performed at the time of transaxillary first rib resection, often resulting in dramatic relief. Reflex sympathetic dystrophy (RSD) with a hand that is ice-cold, discolored, somewhat swollen and painful, and often sweaty commonly responds to the same procedure. It is now considered that brachial plexus compression and irritation of thoracic outlet syndrome (TOS) may be the driving force for the RSD symptoms, and that outlet decompression combined with a sympathectomy will offer a much greater chance of favorable response than sympathectomy alone, such as with the thoracoscope or transthoracic technique.

If the patient has symptoms predominantly from *upper* plexus, C5, C6, and C7 nerves, compression and irritation with severe pain in the anterolateral aspect of the neck spreading from the clavicle up through the brachial plexus to the mandible and ear, sometimes even into the face, and down into the upper chest, then across the trapezius ridge into the outer arm and down the radial distribution, removal of the anterior scalene muscle offers the best chance of relief. In every case with these symptoms, anomalies of the anterior scalene muscle will be found with unusual muscle fiber attachments to the perineurium of the upper nerves of the plexus, usually a sheet of abnormal scalene muscle tissue covering the middle and lower trunks of the plexus, and sometimes even anomalies of the brachial plexus itself, with the C5 nerve lying on the *anterior* surface of the anterior scalene muscle immediately lateral to the phrenic nerve. Dividing this muscle (scalenotomy) usually offers no relief because the muscle will predictably reattach by a heavy pseudotendon of fibrocartilaginous tissue that shortens and tightens the remaining part of the anterior scalene muscle even more than it originally was, thus increasing the compression and tugging effect on the nerves of the brachial plexus. Complete removal of the anterior scalene muscle with replacement by prescalene fat to cover the bare nerves of the plexus offers the best chance of relief of the distressing upper plexus symptoms.

Thus it is of utmost importance for the physician, and especially the surgeon responsible for choosing and performing the operation for TOS, to determine which nerves of the plexus are especially involved, since the surgical techniques differ for the upper nerves, C5-7, compared with the lower nerves, C8 and T1. The operation should be chosen specifically to match the patient's symptom pattern rather than "shotgunning" the symptoms by decompressing both the upper and lower nerves in every case, because many patients will not require combined anterior scalenectomy and rib resection. The scar tissue recurrence rate is many times greater for the neck surgery than for the transaxillary rib resection. Therefore I think we should avoid scalenectomies whenever possible, unless there are compelling indications for decompressing the upper nerves of the plexus to minimize the risk of the patient's later developing severe scar tissue entrapment of these nerves. This would require further high-risk neurolytic surgery, when the patient might not have needed the neck procedure in the first place if he or she had only lower plexus symptoms—the most common presentation—which is best managed through the transaxillary approach.

A few points of special importance should be emphasized. The patient should be in the straight lateral decubitus position rather than in a supine position, then tilted slightly back toward the surgeon so he or she can operate from the axilla directly downward through the axillary tunnel to the thoracic outlet. The transverse incision is located in the axillomammary crease, demonstrated by compressing the shoulder joint and breast together (Fig. 1). It should lie in the *lower* axilla over the third rib and not be placed in the midaxilla or apex to avoid operating through extensive axillary fat that lies precariously close to the axillary vessels and brachial plexus.

The anterior scalene muscle should be finger-dissected from surrounding areolar tissue to isolate it from the subclavian artery and vein, then hooked with a right-angle hemostat to protect the major vessels from injury as the muscle is divided at its insertion on the first rib. The tendon of the subclavian muscle is cleared from surrounding fat anterior to the subclavian vein and divided to provide greater access to the anterior end of the first rib for it to be resected with the rib shears and rongeurs up to the costocartilage and to help decompress the vein. The attachments of the middle scalene and intercostal muscles between the first and second ribs are then taken down with raspatories (periosteal elevators) being careful to leave the periosteum intact on the rib to reduce scar tissue formation from retained periosteal tissue in the bed of the resected rib.

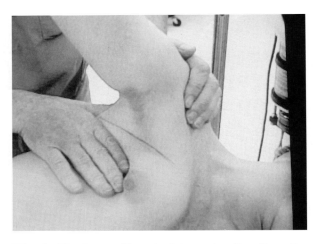

Fig. 1 The low axillary incision extending from the latissimus dorsi to the pectoralis major muscle edges is shown by compressing the shoulder joint and the breast toward each other after the patient has been turned in the lateral decubitus position.

The small nerve shield retractor is quite beneficial in protecting the T1 nerve and the lower trunk of the brachial plexus as the rib is resected posteriorly with the right-angle rib shears and shortened with rongeurs nearly to the transverse process of the T1 vertebra. The rib must be resected this short to prevent a long posterior stump of first rib from impinging against the T1 nerve and lower trunk of the plexus, with a high risk of scar fixation of these nerves to the stump causing severe recurrent lower plexus symptoms. After the first rib is removed, the entire thoracic outlet exposure expands considerably. The surgeon should examine the area carefully for the anomalous fibromuscular bands that these patients always seem to have in the region of the plexus and subclavian vessels (Fig. 2). These bands should be carefully separated from the T1 nerve, artery, and vein, then put on stretch with a long forceps or hemostat and fully resected so they cannot reattach and cause compression or scarring later. Merely removing the rib and closing the incision is now not considered an adequate operation without looking for and excising all fibromuscular structures in the outlet, which can be accomplished much more thoroughly and safely through the axillary approach than through the neck approach.

In the past 2 years I have been sealing the posterior stump of rib with bone wax, then

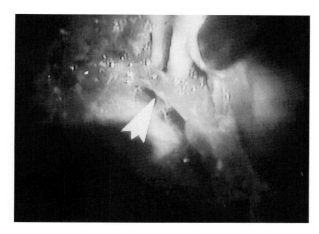

Fig. 2 This surgical photograph through the right axilla shows a typical type VII taut fibromuscular band from the middle scalene muscle passing under the T1 nerve and subclavian artery (arrow), and attaching to the costocartilage in front of the vein. This tough, anomalous band is intact after complete removal of the first rib and must be separated from the nerve and vessels, then totally resected to permit complete decompression of the neurovascular structures in the outlet.

covering the stump with the middle scalene muscle by drawing down the lower divided end and suturing it to fibromuscular tissue under the neck and stump of the first rib with absorbable suture. This interposes normal scalene muscle between the stump and T1 nerve without pressure on the nerve that was so prominent when the abnormally large middle scalene muscle was stretched far out to the middle third of the first rib, causing an unusual pressure point against the T1 nerve and lower trunk of the plexus. When I reoperate for scar tissue recurrence of lower plexus symptoms, I always find especially hard scar tissue that developed from the posterior stump of rib that attaches to the T1 nerve. By isolating the stump behind the reattached middle scalene muscle, the chance of such scar forming from the stump grasping the T1 nerve will be reduced.

If the patient needs a thoracic sympathectomy for associated causalgic burning pain or RSD of the arm and hand, the sympathectomy can be readily performed after the first rib resection. The mediastinal parietal pleura is carefully stripped down by finger dissection as far as the third or fourth rib. The sympathetic chain is located beneath the areolar tissue of the mediastinum as it passes obliquely in a posterior direction from the stellate ganglion, just below always between the subclavian artery and T1 nerve of the plexus. The top edge of the second rib can easily be felt with long scissors and the sympathetic chain freed from enveloping areolar tissue crossing the second rib. The chain is divided at the top edge of the second rib, just below the lower tip of the stellate ganglion. The chain is elevated as rami communicantes are severed down to the top edge of the third rib, where the chain is divided again to remove the second thoracic ganglion. This is the ganglion that provides most of the sympathetic innervation to the upper extremity, mainly through the T1 nerve and ulnar nerve of the arm, so more extensive resection of the chain is usually not required. The stellate ganglion is left completely undisturbed, which greatly reduces the incidence of Horner's syndrome and aberrant sweating. The T2 ganglionectomy usually relieves the causalgic burning pain and severe vasospasm of RSD that causes the ice-cold, clammy, discolored, somewhat swollen, and painful hand.

A suction catheter is placed over the apex of the lung to the mediastinum, brought out over the second rib and through the lateral chest wall, then is attached to the suction device to provide constant suction drainage from the outlet and base of the neck postoperatively. If the pleura has been torn, the same tube is threaded through the hole in the pleura and down the mediastinum a short distance, brought out the axilla, over the second rib, and attached to the suction device to provide constant suction drainage from the pleural cavity as well. Insertion of a standard argyle chest tube through an intercostal space is unnecessary, carries a risk of lacerating the visceral pleura if adhesions are present, and causes much more pain.

The shoulder is lowered and the subcutaneous tissue and skin are closed in two layers with absorbable suture, using a subcuticular closure for the skin. I use collodion to seal the incision and drain site, then apply a small gauze dressing. The drain is left overnight to remove blood and serum and to monitor postoperative bleeding. After the drain is removed, the patient is allowed to shower, usually on the second postoperative day, and advised to wash the axilla with soap and water. Deodorants and powder may then be used as desired.

A quiet convalescence is imperative for the best chance of favorable results from surgery.

Physical therapy should be strictly avoided, because some therapists do not understand the type of surgery that has been performed and tend to press these patients into a vigorous exercise program to correct the weakness of the arm and hand. This is unnecessary and merely stimulates the pain and muscle spasms the surgery is trying to relieve. The only "therapy" required is a power squeeze of the hand to improve strength and relieve any swelling and to elevate the extremity in the abducted position to 180 degrees twice a day to avoid a stiff shoulder joint. Patients should not return to heavy, strenuous jobs in most cases, such as heavy construction work or even floor nursing, because of the high risk of reinjury with a great chance of causing severe recurrent symptoms. Therefore some patients have to change their employment or career to protect the favorable results that may accrue from the surgical decompression of the outlet for TOS and the sympathectomy for RSD.

Careful selection of patients, meticulous technique, good assistance, appropriate instruments, and clear exposure with bright illumination result in a safe operation, rare complications, and results the patients are pleased with in 85% to 90% of cases that were unresponsive to all conservative measures available.

75

Pathogenesis and Management of Upper Extremity Ischemia Following Angioaccess Surgery

HARRY SCHANZER, M.D., MILAN SKLADANY, M.D., RICHARD J. KNIGHT, M.D., ELIZABETH B. HARRINGTON, M.D., MARTIN HARRINGTON, M.D., and MOSHE HAIMOV, M.D.

Upper extremity ischemia related to the presence of an arteriovenous fistula (AVF) or bridge AVF (BAVF) constructed for hemodialysis is a relatively infrequent but potentially devastating complication. Distal steal, induced by the fistula, is the underlying pathophysiologic mechanism. Correction of this problem has been attempted using different surgical techniques such as ligation of the AVF or BAVF, narrowing of the angioaccess, elongation of the bridge, and ligation of the artery distal to the fistula plus bypass. The purpose of this chapter is to review our experience with this pathologic entity and, based on our findings, discuss the clinical aspects of this condition, its pathogenesis, and the results of different therapeutic approaches.

PATIENTS AND METHODS
Study Population

Over a 7-year period (1987 to 1994), 34 patients with end-stage renal failure requiring hemodialysis developed severe ischemia in the extremity carrying the angioaccess. Twenty-two of these patients were women (64.7%) and 28 had diabetes (82.4%). The mean age was 60.1 ± 15.7 years. Twenty-nine patients had a polytetrafluoroethylene (PTFE) brachioaxillary BAVF, four patients had a radiocephalic AVF, and one patient had a brachiocephalic AVF. Thirty patients had severe ischemia with threatened loss of function and tissue in the hand. Gangrenous changes had already occurred in seven of these patients. The remaining four patients had pain in the affected extremity during dialysis or exercise. In 27 patients symptoms developed immediately after construction of the access. The remaining seven patients had late onset of ischemia (range, 5 months to 5 years).

Diagnosis of Steal

The clinical diagnosis of steal was confirmed by forearm Doppler pressure measurements and/or forearm and digital pulse wave pneumoplethysmographic recordings with and without manual compression of the fistula. An increase in pressure or improvement in the pulse wave after compression confirmed the presence of a hemodynamic steal.

Indications for Surgery

A corrective procedure was performed when proved hemodynamic steal coexisted with any of the following clinical conditions: (1) severe ischemic symptoms early after construction of the angioaccess (rest pain, severe numbness, paralysis, cyanosis of digits), (2) persistence of mild symptoms for more than 1 month after the angioaccess operation, or (3) presence of new limb-threatening symptoms in a patient with no previous symptoms.

Corrective Techniques

Several different surgical corrective techniques were used throughout this study. These included simple ligation of the access in seven patients, banding of the access in four, and ligation of the artery distal to the takeoff of the AVF or BAVF plus bypass in 23 (after AVF in four and after BAVF in 19).

The choice of procedure depended on the surgeon's preference and the particular clinical situation (i.e., ligation was often used in patients with ischemia of the access-bearing extremity and no further need for hemodialysis). In the ligation procedure, a simple monofilament tie was placed on the arterial end of the bridge graft. In the banding procedure, narrowing of the outflow of the BAVF was achieved by applying tangential staples or sutures to the graft close to the arterial anastomosis. The technique of arterial ligation-bypass has been previously described in detail.[1] Briefly it involves ligating the artery distal to the inflow of the AVF/BAVF and establishing an arterial bypass from a point

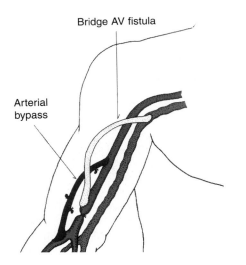

Fig. 1 Schematic representation of the distal arterial ligation-bypass procedure. (From Schanzer H, Skladany M, Haimov M. Treatment of angioaccess-induced ischemia by revascularization. J Vasc Surg 16:861-866, 1992.)

5 cm proximal to the AVF/BAVF inflow to a point just distal to the ligation (Fig. 1). The ligature abolishes the reversal of flow in the distal artery, and the bypass re-establishes normal arterial flow to the distal extremity. Materials used for bypass included saphenous vein in 12 patients, basilic arm vein in one patient, and PTFE in 10 patients.

Evaluation of Function

Patency of the arterial bypass was estimated by palpation of distal pulses and confirmed by Doppler arterial pressure measurements. Function of the access was assessed by palpation of a thrill and auscultation of a bruit. Patency rates were calculated using life-table analysis.

RESULTS
Ligation Procedure

In all seven patients, this procedure was used to relieve severe symptoms of arm ischemia that had begun immediately after construction of the access. Six of these patients had complete resolution of symptoms after the procedure, but in one patient pain persisted, despite good arm and hand perfusion, because of residual ischemic neuropathy.

Banding Procedure

Four patients underwent banding of the BAVF. Indications for this procedure included rest pain in three patients and hand claudication in one. All of these patients had thrombosis of their grafts within 1 day, 1 month, 2 months, and 3 months of the banding procedure.

Arterial Ligation-Bypass Procedure

All 23 patients treated by this technique showed immediate signs of improvement after surgery. One patient with advanced gangrenous changes in the upper extremity at the time of the corrective procedure (2 months after the original access surgery) required amputation of the forearm 13 months later. Three patients had partial improvement with some residual ischemic neuropathic symptoms. The remaining 19 patients had complete resolution of the ischemia and healing of the gangrenous lesions. Among the five patients with AVFs that required revascularization, two bypasses thrombosed at 17 and 23 months, respectively, and two remained patent at 8 and 24 months of follow-up. BAVF patency was 73% at 1 year and 45.5% at 2 years (Fig. 2). Bypass patency was 95.6% at 1 and 2 years (Fig. 3). Only one PTFE bypass failed at 2 months.

DISCUSSION

Ischemia of the upper extremity following construction of an AVF or BAVF occurs in approximately 10% of cases. Usually it is mild, its only manifestations being coldness, some numbness, and pain during dialysis. In most cases the problem is self-correcting and the symptoms are completely reversed within approximately 1 month.[1] More severe ischemia requiring treatment has been reported in approximately 1% of patients with AVFs (most commonly when the fistula is performed at the elbow level using the brachial artery as the inflow source) and in approximately 2.7% to 4.3% of patients with BAVFs.[2-6]

The majority of patients who are affected by this condition have diabetes and/or severe obstructive disease of the arteries distal to the brachial artery. Symptoms of severe ischemia can occur immediately after construction of the arteriovenous connection or later after surgery. In our experience, severe ischemia requiring surgical correction became apparent very early after construction of the fistula in more than three fourths of the patients. In the remaining fourth the ischemia occurred between 5 months and 5 years after access surgery.

Much has been written about the importance of careful preoperative evaluation of the circula-

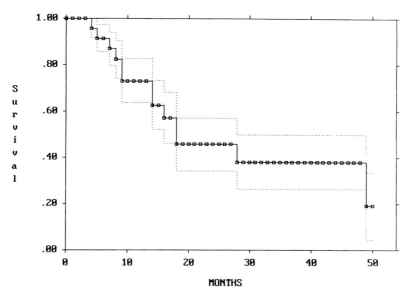

Fig. 2 Life-table curve of BAVF in patients with ischemic steal treated with the arterial ligation-bypass procedure. (From Schanzer H, Skladany M, Haimov M. Treatment of angioaccess-induced ischemia by revascularization. J Vasc Surg 16:861-866, 1992.)

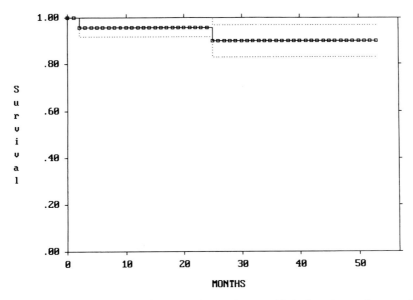

Fig. 3 Life-table curve of arterial bypasses in patients with ischemic steal treated with the arterial ligation-bypass procedure. (From Schanzer H, Skladany M, Haimov M. Treatment of angioaccess-induced ischemia by revascularization. J Vasc Surg 16:861-866, 1992.)

tory status and the collateral potential of the limb as a means of predicting and preventing ischemia.[1] In our experience, however, even the most thorough physical examination cannot accurately predict which arms are at risk. It is, therefore, of the utmost importance to be able to recognize in a timely manner the existence of ischemia and if it is severe, to initiate immediate treatment.

The pathophysiologic basis of these ischemic complications has been discussed in detail by Barnes.[7] The lower pressure system present at the outflow side of the arteriovenous connection induces reversal of flow in the portion of the artery distal to the fistula. This alteration in the direction of flow has been labeled "steal,"[8] and when it is of sufficient magnitude and cannot be compensated by collateral flow, it will result in ischemic manifestations. This is particularly likely to occur in diabetic individuals, who may have diffuse arterial occlusive disease. Hemodynamic studies performed by us, which directly measure the direction and amount of blood flow in the different components of the fistula, have demonstrated that steal occurs in 73% of AVFs and 91% of BAVFs.[9]

If the ischemic manifestations are severe and threaten the viability of the limb, surgical treatment is required. Several techniques have been used for this purpose. The simplest and most direct means of treating ischemic steal is ligation of the outflow of the fistula. This will instantaneously reverse the steal and improve distal perfusion. The obvious drawback of this technique is that the angioaccess is lost.

Another widely used procedure is the so-called banding technique, which involves producing a stenosis in the outflow portion of the AVF/BAVF close to the anastomosis. Many variations of the banding technique, all intended to produce a narrowing and consequent reduction in flow, have been reported.[10-14]

Manufacturers are producing grafts designed to prevent steal phenomena. These grafts are tapered and the narrowest portion is intended to be anastomosed to the artery. The rationale for this design is grounded in the concept that by increasing the resistance to the outflow of the fistula, steal will be prevented.

The practical problems associated with banding techniques or the use of tapered grafts stem from difficulties in establishing the precise degree of stenosis required for elimination of the steal while still allowing sufficient flow to sustain patency of the outflow fistula. In our experience thrombosis of the access is common, even if the amount of narrowing is determined by means of careful hemodynamic measurements (direct flow measurements or digital plethysmography). The explanation for this is discouraging because of the fact that at the level of "critical stenosis" that results from the banding procedure, a minimal further reduction in fistula flow, produced, for example, by mild hypotension, can induce thrombosis of the graft.

Another technique that has been used is elongation of the BAVF.[15] The purpose of this procedure is also to increase peripheral resistance of the fistula outflow, but it is associated with the same difficulties as banding.

A recently described technique,[16] offered as a solution to the problem of early steal after brachial artery to axillary vein BAVF, is the use of a branch of the axillary artery for inflow and the brachial vein for outflow. The explanation proposed for the success of this technique is that the reduced amount of flow delivered by the axillary branch prevents ischemic steal. Under similar circumstances, we have used the axillary artery itself as the inflow source with comparable results. Our explanation for the success of this technique is that the axillary artery is very rich in collateral circulation and this overcomes the steal.

With regard to the technique of distal arterial ligation and bypass, which we described in 1988,[1] we believe it offers the most rational and effective approach for correction of the hemodynamic disturbances produced by the presence of an AVF/BAVF. Ligation of the artery distal to the AVF/BAVF by itself will eliminate reversal of flow. Intraoperative pressure measurements have demonstrated that this maneuver improves (but does not normalize) pressure in the distal artery.[1] The addition of the arterial bypass provides the distal vascular bed with normal perfusion pressure and flow. This results in an immediate reversal of the ischemic condition. Our results show that these theoretical expectations occur in clinical situations. The 23 extremities treated by this approach showed a dramatic improvement in subjective as well as objective ischemic manifestations immediately after surgery. Because of advanced irreversible ischemic damage at the time of the corrective bypass surgery, one extremity was eventually lost and three patients continued to complain of mild symptoms of neuropathy. The remaining 19 patients had complete reversal of ischemia, even with healing of advanced gangrenous lesions. This was accomplished without affecting the durability of the angioaccess.

CONCLUSION

To achieve a complete reversal of ischemic symptoms, prompt diagnosis and treatment are required. A delay in treatment may result in nonreversible ischemic manifestations. Ligation is an effective method for achieving reversal of steal but it results in loss of the access. Although banding is theoretically an appealing procedure, its practical application is unsatisfactory. Often the result is thrombosis of the access or nonresolution of the symptoms. The technique of distal arterial ligation plus bypass produces immediate resolution of ischemia without affecting the function and longevity of the angioaccess. In our view it is the procedure of choice for correction of AVF/BAVF-induced ischemic steal.

REFERENCES

1. Schanzer H, Schwartz M, Harrington E, Haimov M. Treatment of ischemia due to "steal" by arteriovenous fistula with distal artery ligation and revascularization. J Vasc Surg 7:770-773, 1988.
2. Duncan H, Ferguson L, Faris I. Incidence of the radial steal syndrome in patients with Brescia fistula for hemodialysis: Its clinical significance. J Vasc Surg 4:144-147, 1986.
3. Haimov M, Burrows L, Schanzer H, Neff M, Baez A, Kwun K, Slifkin R. Experience with arterial substitutes in the construction of vascular access for hemodialysis. J Cardiovasc Surg 21:149-154, 1980.
4. Porter JA, Sharp WV, Walsh EJ. Complications of vascular access in a dialysis population. Curr Surg 42:298-300, 1985.
5. Zibari GB, Rohr MS, Landreneau MD, Bridges RM, DeVault GA, Petty FH, Costley KJ, Brown ST, McDonald JC. Complications from permanent hemodialysis vascular access. Surgery 104:681-685, 1988.
6. Winsett OE, Wolma FJ. Complications of vascular access for hemodialysis. South Med J 78:513-517, 1985.
7. Barnes RW. Hemodynamics for the vascular surgeon. Arch Surg 115:216-223, 1980.
8. Bussell JA, Abbott JA, Lim RC. A radial steal syndrome with arteriovenous fistula for hemodialysis. Ann Intern Med 75:387-394, 1971.
9. Kwun KB, Schanzer H, Finkler N, Haimov M, Burrows L. Hemodynamic evaluation of angioaccess procedures for hemodialysis. Vasc Surg 13:170-177, 1979.
10. Corry RJ, Natvarlal PP, West JC. Surgical management of complications of vascular access for hemodialysis. Surg Gynecol Obstet 51:49-54, 1980.
11. Drasler WJ, Wilson GJ, Jenson ML, Klement P, George SA, Protonotarios EL, Dutcher RG, Possis ZC. Venturi grafts for hemodialysis access. ASAIO Trans 36:M753-M760, 1990.
12. Khalil IM, Livingston DH. The management of steal syndrome occurring after access for dialysis. J Vasc Surg 7:572-573, 1988.
13. Mattson WJ. Recognition and treatment of vascular steal secondary to hemodialysis prostheses. Am J Surg 154:198-201, 1987.
14. West JC, Bertsch DJ, Peterson SL, Gannon MP, Norkus G, Latsha RP, Kelly SE. Arterial insufficiency in hemodialysis access procedures: Correction by "banding" technique. Transplant Proc 23:1838-1840, 1991.
15. West JC, Evans RD, Kelly SE, et al. Arterial insufficiency in hemodialysis access procedures: Reconstruction by an interposition polytetrafluoroethylene graft conduit. Am J Surg 153:300-301, 1987.
16. Jendrisak MD, Anderson CB. Vascular access in patients with arterial insufficiency. Ann Surg 212:187-193, 1990.

76

Techniques and Results of Vascular Surgery for Impotence: Large and Small Vessel Options

RALPH G. DePALMA, M.D.

Interest in vasculogenic impotence began with Leriche's 1923 observation[1] that aortoiliac atherosclerosis related to erectile failure resulting from inadequacy of cavernosal perfusion.[2] Because aortic operations themselves often caused postoperative impotence,[3] in the 1970s techniques were developed to minimize this complication.[4] The use of vascular surgical procedures to revascularize cavernous bodies[5,6] became a subject of increasing interest in the late 1970s.

In 1982 stimulation of erection by intracorporal injection of the vasoactive agents papaverine[7] and phentolamine[8] changed this emphasis. Not only did the use of intracavernous injection (ICI) lead to effective methods for better delineation of erectile physiology, but ICI also developed as an important diagnostic and effective therapeutic tool. Although the original vasoactive substances remain valuable for certain applications, because of the risks of priapism and legal issues in the United States, prostaglandin E_1 is currently preferred for ICI.[9]

Modern research emphases shifted from methods to increase arterial inflow or diminish venous outflow toward detailed study of the cavernosal smooth muscle itself. Notable advances include delineation of the roles of nitric oxide[10] and oxygen tension[11] on erectile function. Current diagnosis and therapy rely on noninvasive studies of blood as well as the effects of therapy with vasoactive drugs in planning initial treatment. The majority of men respond to medical therapy; however, a subset of men—approximately 6% to 7% of those who present with impotence—exhibit well-defined arterial or venous abnormalities. These men ultimately become candidates for vascular intervention. Depending on cause, approximately 70% of these men respond favorably to appropriate vascular surgical interventions.[12]

Impotence is a symptom, not a disease. Table 1 classifies causes of vasculogenic impotence. Although vasculogenic abnormalities are common, erectile failure is also caused by endocrine, metabolic, neurologic, and psychogenic factors. Any of these can coexist with vasculogenic impotence, or even in a sense be etiologic, inasmuch as erectile failure is a vascular dysfunction. Some form of arterial inflow abnormality is associated with impotence in 45% of men screened by noninvasive methods.[12,13] Most of these patients respond to nonoperative treatment; cavernosal leakage syndrome, however, may be more refractory to medical therapy.

In understanding the pathogenesis of penile erectile dysfunction, the clinician must understand two interrelated hemodynamic processes responsible for normal erectile function: an adequate arterial flow increase and closure or marked reduction of venous outflow. Both pro-

Table 1 Causes of vasculogenic impotence

Arterial	
Large vessel	Aortoiliac occlusion
Small vessel	Internal iliac anterior division, pudendal and penile arteries
Cavernosal factors	
Arteriolar	Functional or helicine artery abnormality
Fibrosis	Postpriapic, drug injection, aging
La Peyronie	Deformity, cavernosal leakage
Smooth muscle	Diabetes, hormonal lack, blood pressure medication
Venous	
Acquired	Tunic albuginea abnormalities: patterns include dorsal vein, crural, and spongiosum leaks
Congenital	Cavernous spongiosum leak existing since childhood
Mixed	Leakage with inadequate arterial inflow of any cause

cesses depend on relaxation of the cavernosal smooth muscle, which in turn depends on intact neural mechanisms as well as the physiology of the smooth muscle endothelial complex itself. To achieve normal erectile function, an adequate supply of oxygenated arterial flow is needed. Relaxation of the subalbugineal smooth muscle conditions closure of cavernosal outflow and the normal smooth muscle function that is also needed for a normal erection. The hemodynamics of the erectile process have been recently reviewed.[13] During normal erection, intracavernous pressure increases from approximately 15 mm Hg in the flaccid state to 80 to 90 mm Hg in the erect state. Higher and even suprasystolic pressures are generated by perineal muscle contraction.

CLINICAL PRESENTATION

Gradual erectile failure in the absence of traumatic life events and in the presence of symptomatic lower extremity vascular disease suggests large-vessel arteriogenic impotence. In these men both the intensity and duration of risk factors predisposing to atherosclerosis, such as cigarette smoking, hypertension, diabetes, and hyperlipidemia, contribute to arteriogenic impotence. Aortoiliac aneurysms or ulcerative disease can cause embolic pudendal or penile artery occlusion. A recent observation is that even small aortoiliac aneurysms, particularly at the bifurcation of the distal common iliac artery,[12] can relate to abrupt onset of impotence as documented by penile Doppler and plethysmographic studies.

In a recent summary on experience with occult aortoiliac disease,[14] men with arteriogenic impotence resulting from aortoiliac disease averaged 64 years of age. During the same period, impotent men with small-vessel penile or pudendal disease or venous leakage averaged 42 to 47 years of age. In these categories of men, risk factors for atherosclerosis were much less frequent. In some cases of diffuse penile arterial disease, particularly in men in their third or fourth decades, risk factors were virtually absent. Many men with diabetes and hypertension who are receiving medication present with impotence but have no abnormalities of penile arterial perfusion. These patients are not candidates for vascular reconstruction. In patients with diabetes, neuropathy is an important factor and can be documented by testing of the appropriate somatic pathways. The immediate onset of impotence following rectal, urologic, or vascular surgery is a critical historical point that also suggests neurovascular testing. Finally, drug or alcohol use may correlate with the onset of impotence, and patients may improve when these are discontinued (e.g., use of nasal inhalants or change in antihypertensive medication).

When femoral pulsations are absent or an aneurysm is present, atherosclerosis involves the aortoiliac segments and the proximal segments of the internal iliac artery. These findings suggest large-vessel arteriogenic impotence and may be indications for intervention, not for impotence, per se, but also taking into account accompanying lower extremity ischemia or occult aneurysms. In screening more than 1000 men,[14] approximately one in 100 was found to have an aortoiliac aneurysm, almost always less than 5 cm in diameter, that was previously undetected.

Examination and invasive testing for smallvessel disease, venous leakage, and cavernosal dysfunction are complex. Before invasive tests are done, I recommend that penile brachial indices (PBI) and pulse volume recordings be obtained.[15,16] A PBI of about 0.75 suggests that no major occlusion exists between the aorta and the distal measurement point on the penis, whereas a PBI of less than 0.6 suggests major vascular occlusion. Abnormal plethysmographic findings can occur with either, but with normal indices, flat plethysmographic recordings appear to be associated with small-vessel or cavernosal disease. A sequence of neurovascular testing[15] is useful, because neurologic disorders also contribute to erectile failure. Approximately 28% of impotent men exhibit some type of neurologic disorder, elicited by testing of pudendal, lumbar, and somatosensory evoked potentials and measurements of bulbocavernosus reflux time.[17-19] Abnormalities in these somatic pathways usually contraindicate vascular reconstruction for impotence. Obtaining these tests is also useful in selecting the initial dosage of prostaglandin for ICI during the first office visit. This expedites timely assessment of the erectile process using direct observation.

PATIENT SELECTION FOR SURGICAL INTERVENTION

From January 1983 to March 1994, 1145 men (average age, 55.5 years) were screened using PBI and penile plethysmography.[14] These men presented with a complaint of impotence. Four hundred eighty-four exhibited some form of abnormal penile arterial flow, with 77 exhibiting aortoiliac disease. The remainder had probable involvement in the distal penile or pudendal arteries or abnormalities within the corporeal bodies themselves.

Men with normal arterial flow and an inability to respond to medical treatment or to ICI of vasoactive agents using prostaglandin E_1, up to 40 µg were investigated for venous leakage using dynamic infusion cavernosometry and cavernosography.[20] Men selected for selective pudendal arteriography similarly failed to respond to ICI or medical treatment. The cause of cavernous leakage can often be remote from the structure of the cavernous bodies. Important underlying pathologic states in venous leakage can relate to undiagnosed arterial disease with subsequent failure of smooth muscle relaxation. For example, among men screened for venous leakage on the basis of noninvasive neurovascular testing and employing dynamic cavernosometry and cavernosography for suspected venous leakage, we found that 23% have unsuspected arterial lesions demonstrated by selective pudendal arteriography.[21] This has led to the recommendation that both pudendal arteriography and dynamic infusion cavernosometry and cavernosography are needed before considering venous interruption or any type of microvascular reconstruction.

DUPLEX SCANNING AND NOCTURNAL PENILE TUMESCENCE

Color-flow duplex scanning can be used to examine penile arteries at intervals after ICI or ICI combined with visual sexual stimulation (VSS).[22,23] Values for normal middle-aged men after ICI using prostaglandin E_1 and VSS have been suggested to be a 70% increase in deep cavernosal artery diameter and systolic peak blood flow velocities above 30 cm/sec. Duplex scanning might also suggest venous leakage in the presence of high diastolic cavernosal artery flow. Here the data are less secure, and ultimately the duplex scan is used to select for arteriography or dynamic infusion cavernosometry and cavernosography. If an aneurysm is suspected, an appropriate probe can be used at this time to examine the abdomen. In contrast to Doppler measurement of PBI and plethysmography, duplex scanning is time intensive and requires a physician's presence. Patients must be observed in the clinic to ensure subsidence of the induced erection. A recent report underlined the diagnostic difficulties of duplex scanning in evaluating the corporeal veno-occlusive mechanism.[24] False positive results were noted in 22% of patients when compared with results of nocturnal penile tumescence (NPT) studies.

NPT is a useful study, particularly when psychogenic impotence is likely and in cases with medicolegal problems. NPT is done optimally in a sleep laboratory setting using 3 nights of monitoring[25] and measurement of erectile rigidity during maximum tumescence. Normal penile rigidity is determined at 400 to 500 g of buckling pressure. Although NPT testing is time consuming and expensive, a normal sleep erection virtually rules out organic erectile dysfunction. Such men are not candidates for further interventions.

INVASIVE TESTING

Dynamic Infusion Cavernosometry and Cavernosography. This evaluation provides a measure of venous afflux and localizes sites of cavernosal leakage. Flow to maintain erection (FME) is a valid measure if complete muscular relaxation has been obtained to produce a linear pressure flow relationship, as recently described.[26] ICI in this setting requires much larger doses and sometimes reinjection. We consider FME in excess of 40 ml/min to be abnormal.

ARTERIOGRAPHY

To detect pudendal or penile arterial occlusion and to determine candidacy for microvascular interventions, selective arteriographic studies are needed. Conventional aortoiliac studies to demonstrate large-vessel disease should be used first when PBI or lower extremity pulses are abnormal. Highly selective internal iliac arteriography using nonionic contrast media and ICI to produce partial penile tumescence (not full erection) are needed to display pudendal and penile vascular anatomy. As mentioned previously, both dynamic infusion cavernosometry and cavernosography and selective arteriography are both required in potential candidates for microvascular reconstructions or venous ablation.

PATTERNS OF VASCULAR INVOLVEMENT

As a result of noninvasive and invasive testing of men with impotence, four subsets of patterns can be recognized:

Aortoiliac disease
Pudendal or penile artery segmental obstructions
Diffuse distal penile artery disease
Cavernosal leakage, acquired or congenital

Aortoiliac disease is usually caused by atherosclerosis, although fibromuscular hyperplasia has been seen.[27] In men with the sole complaint of impotence, aortoiliac involvement can be aneurysmal or occlusive; in the latter instance claudication is often minimal or overlooked by inactive patients. Ankle/brachial indices in these cases are usually 0.6 or less, as are penile brachial indices.

TREATMENT OF VASCULOGENIC IMPOTENCE

Revascularization of penile vessels or venous interruption should offer ideal options in men failing to respond to ICI or a trial of vacuum constrictor services (VCD). Presently penile revascularization is being reappraised.[28,29] Skepticism exists because reported results range from 33% to 100% success rates, with scanty life-table data to support these claims.[30] No uniform methods of postoperative surveillance have been agreed on, and the true success rates of these procedures are currently unknown. This situation is similar to the early era of coronary revascularization. Penile artery bypass, deep dorsal vein arterialization, and venous interruption are evolving procedures; however, with accurate preoperative evaluation they appear to be useful for carefully selected patients. Techniques of aortoiliac surgery that perfuse the internal iliac arteries and spare autonomic nerves are less controversial and more effective. In a recent analysis of 10 years' experience, 23 among 1145 men screened for impotence ultimately underwent aortoiliac procedures for aneurysms or occlusive disease.[12,14] These procedures, with comparison of these results to penile interventions, have been described in detail.[14]

Each of four subsets of impotent men with differing patterns of vascular pathology requires a specific approach. These include a variety of interventions for macrovascular aortoiliac disease, microvascular reconstruction of pudendal or penile artery local occlusions, deep dorsal arterialization for diffuse penile obstructive disease, and correction of cavernosal leakage based on elevated FME and visualization of leakage sites. As mentioned, approximately one man of 100 impotent men exhibits an aneurysm; these aneurysms may be small. Although atheroembolism with abrupt onset of impotence can be discerned in some cases, treatment does not always reverse this process. In addition, a discrete incidence of aneurysmal disease in men in their sixth or seventh decades is not unexpected; some of these aneurysms may be coincidental.

Microvascular bypass to the dorsal penile artery uses the inferior epigastric artery[31]; the best responders are young men with isolated pudendal artery involvement or those lesions that are caused by trauma.[32] Diffuse penile arterial disease not suitable for bypass or mixed arterial and venous impotence has been treated using deep dorsal vein arterialization.[31,33,34] This procedure has the disadvantage of the potential for glans hyperemia, with ulceration as an early or late complication. Additionally, the physiologic mechanism by which this procedure improves erectile function is puzzling. The direction of arterial flow appears to be mainly into the spongiosum as we have seen[35] and as documented by others using MRI.[36] Similar to my experience, in recent follow-ups approximately half to a third of these patients report spontaneous function,[37,38] whereas 70% achieve erections with ICI, which had been previously ineffective.[12]

Venous interruption efficacy clearly correlates with correction of abnormally elevated FME from 80 ml/min or more to postoperative values of 40 ml/min or less. If this reduction is not obtained, there is failure to achieve an erection either spontaneously or with ICI. Although immediate postoperative function rates are high after venous ligation, a falloff in function over the ensuing 36 months occurs regularly. Again, 70% of men function overall with ICI following venous interruption. Studies using postoperative dynamic infusion cavernosometry and cavernosography have shown the development of sequential leakage from other sources, which accounts for this falloff in function.[39] Thus as complete an interruption as possible is a desirable goal of the initial procedure. Anatomic factors favoring success, in my experience, are dominant leakage from the deep dorsal vein[40]; diffuse cavernous spongiosum leakage offers a poor prognosis.

TECHNICAL APPROACHES AND RESULTS

Group I: *Aortoiliac Disease.* Of 23 men with aortoiliac disease, we repaired aneurysms in 11 men using inlay grafts with nerve-sparing techniques and with anastomoses at the junction of the internal and external iliac arteries.[27] Three of these were probably due to emboli from small aneurysms with debris in the distal common iliac arteries. When return of erectile function did occur, this event was correlated with improved PBI and penile plethysmography.

In 12 men with occlusive disease, with ankle/brachial indices of <0.6, a variety of reconstructive techniques were used, including femorofemoral bypass, transluminal angioplasty of common or external iliac arteries, and internal iliac endarterectomy. All exhibited improved penile and extremity indices. Two did not regain erectile function; this outcome was associated with continued need for drug use (lithium and propranolol) postoperatively.

In analyzing results with follow-ups ranging from 33 to 48 months, 60% of men in this group reported spontaneous erectile function, 15% responded to ICI or VCD, and 25% remained impotent. The average age of 64 years for this group, as compared with the average age of groups II through IV (42 years) was significantly different ($p < .001$). Despite the older age of men with aortoiliac disease, the frequency of spontaneous erectile postoperative function was more favorable as compared with groups II through IV ($p < .05$ by chi-square).

Group II: *Dorsal Penile Artery Bypass.* This procedure was performed in 12 men using the inferior epigastric artery as a donor source and microvascular anastomoses to the dorsal penile artery with 10-0 nylon.[35] The most favorable candidates were previously potent men with pelvic trauma and those younger than 60 years. End-to-end anastomoses using the bifid inferior epigastric artery into both proximal and distal segments of a divided dorsal penile artery have been most recently favored. At follow-ups ranging from 14 to 72 months, 27% of men reported spontaneous erections. In these cases Doppler signals were audible over the grafts. When ICI was added, 72% reported function that had not been present preoperatively.

Group III: *Deep Dorsal Vein Arterialization.* We performed deep dorsal vein arterialization in 12 men. This operation was selected when penile arterial disease was diffuse and when no suitable anastomotic site in the dorsal arteries could be located. Postoperative arteriography demonstrated prograde venous flow into the spongiosium. In all cases the inferior epigastric artery appeared to be suitable and was used for anastomosis to the deep dorsal vein. Two cases of glans hyperemia with ulceration required secondary intervention; this was the only significant morbidity associated with these procedures. Overall at follow-up of 18 to 19 months, 33% of these men had spontaneous erections; 47% responded to ICI.

Group IV: *Venous Interruption.* Techniques have been previously described using dorsal vein interruption, resection,[40] and coil embolization.[27] Venous interruption was utilized in 27 men. At follow-ups ranging from 20 to 70 months, 33% function spontaneously and 44% use ICI. The importance of an accurate diagnosis to rule out arterial insufficiency,[21] a complete initial operation, and the favorable anatomic pattern of dorsal vein leakage are all factors in successful outcome.

CONCLUSION

Overall, 6% to 7% of men with four distinct forms of vasculogenic impotence appear to be candidates for vascular interventions. The results of this type of surgery will probably improve with better selection criteria, surgical techniques, and more critical follow-up methods. For the general vascular surgeon, men with aortoiliac disease are an important albeit small subset of those with impotence. A careful workup for small aneurysms or ulcerated aortic lesions is indicated in this group of men. Dilatation of the common or external iliac artery appears to be worthwhile. Although not described in this experience, dilatation of the internal iliac artery or its branches has not been successful in cases I have seen. Among men failing medical treatment for impotence, approximately 70% overall will function after vascular surgical interventions, including men who will find ICI effective postoperatively. For the general vascular surgeon it is important to underscore the efficacy of aortoiliac procedures, as compared with the more specialized microvascular penile reconstructions and venous interruptions. This appears to be a consistent trend despite the more advanced age of men with aortoiliac disease.

REFERENCES

1. Leriche R. Des oblitérations artérielle hautes (oblitération de la termination de l'aorte) comme cause insufficances circulatoire des membres inferiurs [abst]. Bull Mem Soc Chir 49:1404, 1923.
2. Leriche R, Morel A. The syndrome of thrombotic obliteration of the aortic bifurcation. Ann Surg 127:193-206, 1948.
3. May AG, Rob CB, DeWeese JA. Changes in sexual function following operation on the abdominal aorta. Surgery 65:41-47, 1969.
4. DePalma RG, Levine SB, Feldman S. Preservation of erectile function after aortoiliac reconstruction. Arch Surg 113:902-958, 1978.
5. DePalma RG, Kedia K, Persky L. Surgical options in the correction of vasculogenic impotence. Vasc Surg 14:92-102, 1980.
6. Michal V, Kramar L, Pospichal J, Hejel L. Gefasschirurgia erektiver Impotenz. Sexual Medicine Sondertruck 5:15-20, 1976.
7. Virag R. Intravenous injections of papaverine for erectile failure. Lancet 2:938, 1982.
8. Brindley GS. Pilot experiments on the actions of drugs injected into the corpus cavernosum penis. Br J Pharmacol 87:495-500, 1986.
9. Waldhauser M, Schramek P. Efficiency and side effects of prostaglandin in treatment of erectile dysfunction. J Urol 140:525-527, 1988.
10. Rajfer J, Aronson WF, Bush PA, Dorey FJ, Ignarro LF. Nitric oxide as a mediator of the corpus cavernosum in response to nonadrenergic noncholinergic neurotransmission. N Engl J Med 329:90-94, 1992.
11. Azadzoi KM, Negra A, Siroky MB. Effects of cavernosal hypoxia and oxygenation on penile erection. Int J Impot Res 6(Suppl I):D4, 1994.
12. DePalma RG, Olding M, Yu GW, et al. Vascular interventions for impotence: Lessons learned. J Vasc Surg 21:576-585, 1995
13. DePalma RG. Mechanisms of vasculogenic impotence. In White RA, Hollier LA, eds. Vascular Surgery: Basic Science and Clinical Correlations. Philadelphia: JB Lippincott, 1994, pp 359-368.
14. DePalma RG, Massarin E. Occult aortoiliac disease in men with primary complaint of erectile dysfunction. Int J Impot Res 6(Suppl I):A10, 1994.
15. DePalma RG, Emsellem HA, Edwards CA, et al. A screening sequence for vasculogenic impotence. J Vasc Surg 5:228-236, 1987.
16. DePalma RG, Michal V. Point of view; Deja vu again: Advantages and limitations of methods for assessing penile arterial flow. Urology 36:199-200, 1990.
17. Emsellem HA, Bergsrud DW, DePalma RG, Edwards CM. Pudendal evoked potentials in the evaluation of impotence [abst]. J Clin Neurophysiol 5:359, 1988.
18. Opsomer RJ, Guerit FM, Wese FX, Van Cough PJ. Pudendal cortical somatosensory evoked potentials. J Urol 135:1216-1218, 1986.
19. Fisher-Santos BL, de Dues Viera AL, dos Santos ES. Bulbocavernosus reflex and evoked potentials in evidentally normal males. Int J Impot Res 6(Suppl I):A12, 1994.
20. DePalma RG, Schwab FJ, Emsellem HA, et al. Noninvasive assessment of impotence. Surg Clin North Am 70:119, 1990.
21. DePalma RG, Dalton CM, Gomez CA, et al. Predictive value of a screening sequence for venogenic impotence. Int J Impot Res 4:143-148, 1992.
22. Lewis RW, King BF. Dynamic color Doppler sonography in the evaluation of penile erectile disorders. Int J Impot Res 6(Suppl I):A30, 1994.
23. Lue TF, Hricak H, Marich KW, Tanagho EA. Vasculogenic impotence evaluated by high-resolution ultrasonography and pulsed Doppler spectrum. Radiology 155:777-781, 1985.
24. Mansour MOA. Anxiety mediated impotence misdiagnosed as venogenic impotence by color duplex scanning: A comparison with nocturnal tumescence monitoring. Int J Impot Res 6(Suppl I):A36, 1994.
25. Ware JC, Kryger MH, Roth T, Dement WC, eds. Principles and Practice of Sleep Medicine. Philadelphia: WB Saunders, 1989, pp 689-695.
26. Udelson D, Hatzichristou DG, DeTejada IS, et al. A new methodology of pharmacocavernosometry which enables hemodynamic analysis under conditions of known corporal smooth muscle relaxation. Int J Impot Res 6(Suppl I):A17, 1994.
27. DePalma RG, Edwards CM, Schwab FJ, Steinberg DL. Modern management of impotence associated with aortic surgery. In Bergan JJ, Yao JST, eds. Arterial Surgery: New Diagnostic and Operative Techniques. Orlando: Grune & Stratton, 1988, pp 337-348.
28. Furlow WF. Vascular surgery in the treatment of impotence. Int J Impot Res 6(Suppl I):A58, 1994.
29. Sohn M. Is there an indication for invasive diagnostic workup and vascular surgery in patients with erectile dysfunction? Int J Impot Res 6(Suppl I):A58, 1994.
30. Sharlip I. A critical evaluation of short- and long-term results of penile revascularization. Int J Impot Res 6(Suppl I):A59, 1994.
31. DePalma RG, Olding MJ. Surgery for vasculogenic impotence. In Greenhalgh RM, ed. Vascular and Endovascular Surgical Techniques, 3rd ed. London: WB Saunders, 1994, pp 239-244.
32. Krane RG, Goldstein I, DeTejada IS. Impotence. N Engl J Med 321:1648-1659, 1989.
33. DePalma RG. Surgery for sexual impotence. In Jamieson CW, Yao JST, eds. Rob and Smith's Operative Surgery, 5th ed. London: Chapman and Hall, 1994, pp 292-297.
34. Furlow WL, Knoll LD, Benson RC. Deep dorsal vein applications in the Furlow-Fischer modification in 156 patients with vasculogenic impotence [abst]. Int J Impot Res 4:187, 1992.
35. DePalma RG, Olding MF. Surgery for vasculogenic impotence. In Greenhalgh RM, ed. Vascular Surgical Techniques: An Atlas. London: WB Saunders, 1989, pp 167-172.
36. Sohn MH, Sikora RR, Bolundorf KK, et al. Objective follow-up after penile revascularization [abst]. Int J Impot Res 4:73, 1992.

37. Schramek P, Engelmann U, Kaufmann F. Microsurgical arterialization in treatment of vasculogenic impotence. J Urol 147:1028-1032, 1992.
38. Cookson MS, Phillips DL, Huff ME, Fitch WP III. Analysis of microsurgical penile revascularization by etiology of impotence. J Urol 149:1308, 1993.
39. Yu GW, Schwab FJ, Melograna FS, DePalma RG, Miller HC, Richoft AL. Preoperative and postoperative dynamic cavernosometry and cavernosography: Objective assessment of venous ligation for impotence. J Urol 147:618-622, 1992.
40. DePalma RG, Schwab FJ, Druy EM, Miller HC, Emsellem HA, Edwards CM, Bergrud D. Experience in diagnosis and treatment of impotence caused by cavernosal leak syndrome. J Vasc Surg 2:117-121, 1989.

77

Management of Venous Ulceration: The Relative Role of Radical Excision for Intractable Ulcers

BEN U. MARSAN, M.D., and JOHN J. RICOTTA, M.D.

It is estimated that 0.5% to 1% of the population in the United States is affected by venous stasis ulceration.[1] As such, this is one of the most common problems encountered in vascular surgery. The cost of treating patients with these chronic ulcers is staggering. Projected annual figures range from $775 million to $1 billion.[2] Morbidity can cause diminished working capacity and job loss, resulting in changes in patient's lifestyle. This chapter reviews the current understanding of chronic venous insufficiency (CVI) and the pathophysiology underlying venous ulceration. Topics discussed include nonoperative medical management and the various surgical approaches to CVI in the treatment of venous ulceration. The principles and rationale behind radical ulcer excision and early split-thickness skin grafting are presented along with results in patients treated at our institution. In addition, the advantages and disadvantages of skin grafting and free flaps are discussed.

PATHOPHYSIOLOGY OF CHRONIC VENOUS INSUFFICIENCY AND ULCERATION

In the lower extremities, venous blood flows through the superficial and deep systems interconnected by the perforator veins. Under gravitational forces, venous foot vein pressure normally ranges from 90 to 100 mm Hg. During calf muscle exercise, the pressure drops to 30 mm Hg.[3] Competent valves maintain a unidirectional venous blood flow from the superficial system to the deep system and from the periphery toward the heart. These venous valves and the muscle pump action play a critical role in preventing chronic venous hypertension. Injury to the valves can lead to chronic venous reflux with stasis, venous hypertension, and ulceration. Venous ulceration is most common in the perimalleolar (gaiter) area corresponding to the site of maximally elevated venous pressure. Venous insufficiency may be primary or the result of venous thrombosis. It is estimated that in approximately 40% to 50% of limbs with CVI the condition is due to primary valvular incompetence. Usually the valves are floppy and elongated because of the degeneration of elastic tissue.[4,5] This primary incompetence may result from disease of the valve segments or dilatation of the vein itself with stretching of valve cusps. Venous thrombosis will result in development of collateral circulation, which lacks valves. Thrombosed segments can themselves recanalize but again with loss of valvular function. Therefore venous thrombosis will lead to reflux from both recanalization and newly developed incompetent collateral vessels.[6] In approximately 5% of patients, venous outflow obstruction may be the cause of chronic venous hypertension, usually as a result of intraluminal thrombosis or extraluminal compression. Venous abnormalities may develop in the superficial, deep, or perforating veins. In 20% to 30% of cases, only superficial incompetence is present but in the majority, two or more systems are involved.[3,4,6] Regardless of the cause of venous hypertension, 20% of patients with venous hypertension will develop venous stasis ulcers. The time between the onset of hypertension and ulceration is usually years. Theories concerning venous ulceration are numerous. Two theories have been advanced to explain the etiology of venous ulceration associated with venous hypertension.[5,7-9] Capillary elongation and dilatation are the first signs of venous hypertension. Increased venous pressure causes local changes in the microcirculation increasing capillary permeability. Locally, lymph flow and the concentration of fibrinogen in the lymph are increased. This results in the deposition of fibrin and fibrinogen in the interstitial and perivascular spaces. Microscopically, this perivascular fibrin deposition is believed to decrease diffusion and create local hypoxia. Although this may play some role in venous ulceration, it is not thought to be sufficient to completely explain the process. In addition to fibrin deposition, macrophages and lymphocytes[7,9] are sequestered and trapped in areas of venous hypertension. These cells become activated and release superoxide radicals and proteolytic enzymes leading to local tissue damage. Tissue hypoxia and malnutrition follow producing further skin changes and subcutaneous tissue injury resulting in fibrosis. Ultimately, local skin death and necrosis results leading to ulceration. Furthermore, these ulcers can easily become secondarily infected causing more extensive damage. Thus current efforts to treat and prevent venous ulceration are based on relieving local venous hypertension and reversing the local changes that inhibit wound healing.[5,7-11]

PHYSIOLOGIC BASIS FOR TREATMENT OF CHRONIC VENOUS INSUFFICIENCY

Nonoperative medical management has focused on compression therapy to reduce local venous hypertension with or without pharmacologic topical agents to treat the venous ulcers. Unna's boot has been the standard bandage used. Recently developed medical treatments have combined compression therapy with topical dressings such as hydrocolloid, platelet-derived growth factors, or arginine-glycine-aspartic acid analogs (RGD). Some of these have shown an increased ability to heal large ulcers but only when combined with compression.[12]

Operative approaches directly address venous hypertension by removal or ligation of incompetent veins or repair of incompetent valves. Ligation of incompetent perforating veins can isolate a competent superficial system from an incompetent deep one. Patients with isolated superficial venous insufficiency are effectively treated by removal of incompetent superficial veins, relying on competent deep veins to provide adequate venous outflow. Venous reconstructive procedures are aimed at either bypassing obstructed venous segments or replacing incompetent valves. Indications for reconstructive surgery are restricted and long-term results often depend on continued compression therapy.

The treatment of venous ulceration, once established, is directed at relief of local venous hypertension. This may be achieved by the use of elevation and compression dressings. Surgically,

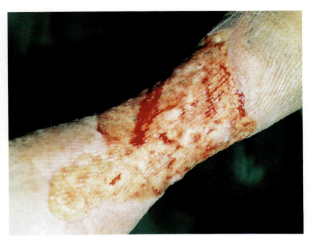

Fig. 1 Large left extremity chronic circumferential (260 cm^2) draining ulcer. Despite adequate conservative treatment (note compression markings), the ulcer did not heal and became infected. This patient had two large ulcers and underwent bilateral radical excision with immediate skin grafting.

local venous hypertension can be corrected by removal of incompetent superficial veins or ligation of incompetent perforating veins. Valvular reconstruction or venous bypass can be used in selected cases when obstruction or insufficiency is the cause of hypertension. All these approaches share the common feature of local relief of venous hypertension in the area of the ulcer. The ulcer is then left to heal by secondary intention. In cases when the ulcerated area is smaller or moderate in size, this is a highly effective approach. However, in patients with extensive venous ulcerations (Fig. 1), the preceding measures are less likely to be successful. The large ulcers are often a source of low-grade sepsis and usually resist reepithelialization by secondary intention. Furthermore, they represent a considerable morbidity as a source of pain and drainage for the patient. The preferred method for management of large ulcers at our institution is complete excision of the venous ulcer with early skin grafting. Postoperatively the venous hypertension is managed with compression stockings.[13-16]

COMPRESSION AND PHARMACOTHERAPY OF VENOUS ULCERS

Several topical, oral, and intravenous agents have been developed to treat venous ulceration with mixed results. These products can be separated into those that address the local nutritive defects, deficient fibrinolysis, and white blood cell sequestration. The main disadvantage of these products is that they fail to address the underlying pathophysiology of the venous ulceration. To be effective they must be combined with long-term compression therapy.

Adequate hygiene, good local wound care, elevation, and compression stockings can achieve a 90% healing rate for venous stasis ulcers. However, this requires multiple dressing changes, visits by a nurse, and occasionally hospitalization. The treatment characteristically requires 3 to 6 months. In 1896 the German dermatologist Unna[17] developed the paste gauze boot. This treatment has been used for decades in the management of CVI and venous ulceration. The paste gauze is impregnated with zinc oxide, calamine lotion, and glycerin. Unna's boot provides both topical and compression therapy. In a recent prospective trial comparing Unna's boot with the hydroactive dressing DuoDERM (HD), patients treated with Unna's boot had a much higher rate of ulcer healing and fewer complications.[18] The authors concluded that the main difference between these two treatment regimens was the compression provided by Unna's boot. Unna's boot is an effective form of therapy but requires prolonged dressing care, patient compliance, and continuous support from health care professionals. It is not easily applied to patients with infected or draining ulcers. However, it is often the treatment of choice for uncomplicated small venous ulcers.

Platelet-derived wound healing growth factors have been used as stimulants to macrophages and fibroblasts with the intent of accelerating wound healing. These proteins have been proved to be potent mitogens for mesenchymal cells and chemoattractants to neutrophils and monocytes. However, in a prospective randomized trial, platelet-derived wound healing growth factors failed to provide an additional benefit in ulcer healing compared to placebo.[19]

In the early 1970s, cryopreservation of keratinocytes and epithelial cells became feasible. These cells can be grown in layers and applied for temporary wound coverage. Release of growth factors promotes migration and stimulation of the recipient keratinocytes. In a recent multicenter trial, 17 patients with 25 chronic venous ulcers averaging 21.5 cm^2 were treated by this method. A total of 106 grafts were used. Only 15 ulcers healed completely. The greatest disadvantage with this treatment is that the underlying ulcer and involved skin are left in place. The ulcer is only cleaned and covered with successive grafts. In addition, there is great difficulty in maintaining these grafts over the long term.[20,21]

Ketanserin, a potent 5-hydroxytryptamine (serotonin) receptor antagonist, has been used to promote ulcer healing. Serotonin has been shown to produce several undesirable effects resulting in increased lymphocyte adherence, impaired red blood cell deformability, and platelet aggregation and degranulation. In the microcirculation these side effects promote an increase in blood viscosity resulting in further local tissue ischemia. In 1991 a double-blind, placebo-controlled clinical trial with 2% Ketanserin ointment was conducted.[22] The study involved 299 patients with decubitus, venous stasis, diabetic, and arterial ulcers. One hundred thirty-four patients had venous stasis ulcers, and 70 patients were randomized to the treatment group. Unlike the positive response reported with decubitus, diabetic, or arterial ulcers, the healing rate for venous ulcers did not differ from that of the placebo control group.

Two drugs initially thought to show great promise for treatment of venous ulcers in small series have been ineffective in randomized trials.[23-26] Stanozolol, an androgenic steroid that enhances fibrinolytic activity, has been used in several clinical trials. The drug is given by mouth and the fibrinolytic activity of the blood is measured each month during the treatment. Earlier reports showed encouraging results.[25] To further evaluate this drug, a trial was performed in a controlled crossover fashion in 23 patients. One group of patients received 5 mg twice daily with placebo; both groups used elastic compression stockings. Improvement was noted with both treatments but the difference was not statistically significant. A more recent study failed to demonstrate a clinical benefit.[23,27] In addition, as with other steroids, adverse effects can be expected.[24] In the early 1970s, significant interest in the flavonoids of the rutoside group (O, B-hydroxyethyl rutoside) was exhibited as clinical studies reported relief of symptoms in patients with CVI. The effect was attributed to a decrease in the capillary filtration rate reducing localized lower extremity edema. In 1981, 28 patients with venous stasis ulcers were involved in a double-blind trial with oral O, B-hydroxyethyl rutoside. The results did not

Table 1 Classification for chronic venous insufficiency

Class	Clinical		Anatomic location	Origin
	Current symptoms	Prior		
0	Asymptomatic	Same	0 Unknown	0 Unknown
1	Mild	Same	1 Superficial veins	1 Congenital
2	Moderate	Same	2 Perforators	2 Postthrombotic
3	Severe (ulceration)	Same	3 Deep—calf	
			4 Deep—thigh	
			5 Deep—iliofemoral	
			6 Deep—caval	
			7 Combination of 2-5 (any)	

From Subcommittee on Reporting Standards in Venous Disease, Ad Hoc Committee on Reporting Standards, Society for Vascular Surgery/North American Chapter, International Society for Cardiovascular Surgery. Reporting standards in venous disease. J Vasc Surg 8:172-178, 1988.

show a significant improvement in venous symptoms or ulcer healing rates between the two groups.[26]

Several drugs have shown some ability to accelerate the healing of venous ulcers. Pentoxifylline, a hemorrheologic agent that reduces blood viscosity and increases red blood cell deformity, also increases fibrinolytic activity, decreases the release of superoxide free radicals, and abrogates the inflammatory response from neutrophils. In a recent multicenter study, patients treated with Trental demonstrated a statistically significant increase in venous ulcer healing compared to control subjects.[28-30]

Prostaglandin E_1 and prostaglandin I_2 are potent vasodilators that also reduce the white blood cell inflammatory response and inhibit platelet aggregation. Patients with venous ulcers who were involved in a prospective, double-blind, placebo-controlled study using intravenous prostaglandin E_1 showed significant improvement in ulcer healing compared to controls.[31,32]

SURGICAL THERAPY

Surgery should be considered when medical therapy has failed or when there is an isolated remediable cause of venous hypertension. Surgical therapy is directed at relieving local venous hypertension in the area of ulceration. Usually patients with stage II or stage III venous insufficiency are candidates for surgical intervention (Table 1).[33] Proper patient selection is crucial to surgical success. The site or sites of venous abnormalities (i.e., superficial, deep, or perforating veins) need to be accurately defined. Best results are achieved when local physiology is returned to normal.

Ligation and stripping of the saphenous system is the procedure of choice in patients with venous ulcers secondary to isolated superficial venous insufficiency. In these cases it can reliably relieve venous hypertension and results in a low venous ulcer recurrence rate. Patients can be selected by a combination of duplex ultrasonography and plethysmography. This approach is best used for patients with small or healed ulcers with mild skin changes. If the venous ulcer is large or lipodermatosclerosis is severe, an incision may be required through the ulcer itself and may involve closure of diseased skin. This can sometimes be obviated by stripping only the proximal saphenous vein to the knee. However, in large ulcers there is still the problem of the primary wound.

Venous ulceration from perforator incompetence responds well to subfascial ligation of incompetent perforator veins with or without saphenectomy. These procedures are reserved for severe stage II and stage III CVI and resulting ulceration. In a recent review of the literature on surgery for incompetent perforator veins, the ulcer healing rates averaged 71% in 680 limbs. The procedure can be performed through a medial vertical[34] or posterior incision[35,36] and more recently an endoscopic approach has been described.[37] Wound infection (13% to 19%) and skin necrosis (2.7%) are the major complications reported.[38] Again this procedure yields the best results in patients with moderate lipodermatosclerosis and medium-sized ulcers.

The main objective of venous reconstruction is to restore the normal physiology of the venous system. In practice this is rarely possible because of the multifocal nature of most venous disease.

Currently, reconstructive options include internal or external valvuloplasty with or without a Dacron sleeve,[39] Dacron sleeve in situ,[39,40] axillary valve transfer,[41] and Kistner segment transfer.[42] These procedures work best in patients with primary valve incompetence. Although venous reconstruction has produced satisfactory early hemodynamic improvement in postphlebitic patients, long-term results have been mixed. Valve reconstruction for patients with postphlebitic syndrome with ulceration has not been shown to be superior to elevation and compression. Reported ulcer healing rates for the various procedures range from 60% to 88% within the first 12 months to 33% to 63% at 24 months.[39]

DIRECT TREATMENT OF ULCERS

A variety of local therapies directed at closure of the dermal defect itself have been evaluated. These approaches have generally been considered for very large or indolent ulcers that have not responded to compression therapy. They have commonly been employed in patients who are not suitable for venous excision alone. Occasionally debridement and grafting are used as primary therapy, usually with poor results. In its simplest form the ulcer is treated with dressings or debridement to achieve a granulating base, and a split-thickness skin graft or pinch grafts are applied. Although early results are acceptable, the late recurrence rate is high. This is because the grafted skin is covering an unstable base and the underlying venous physiology remains unchanged.[43,44]

A somewhat more aggressive approach in the treatment of venous ulceration is layered shaving followed by partial skin grafting. The goal of this procedure is complete removal of all infected tissue and diseased microcirculation. Immediate grafting is performed to cover the ulcerated area. The surgical method involves shaving the infected and granulated tissue with a skin graft knife. Approximately three to four passes are required to completely clean the surrounding skin and ulcer bed. Once the ulcer is completely clean, a partial skin graft is placed without sutures but overlapping the surrounding skin. In a recent study, layered shaving and grafting was performed in 32 patients with 58 ulcers averaging 66.5 cm^2. Using this method, more than 90% healing was achieved.[45] However, no patient follow-up or ulcer recurrence rates were reported. We have had no experience with this technique. The major disadvantages of this procedure are the base of the ulcer is left intact and is only covered by the skin graft and, most important, ligation of the perforators is not performed. Proponents argue that ligation of the perforators is not necessary for the leg ulcers to heal. However, it is well documented that an increase in ambulatory venous pressure is closely correlated with perforator and deep valvular incompetence.[46] In addition, patients with ambulatory venous pressure greater than 80 mm Hg have a 73% incidence of leg ulceration.[47] In treating large venous ulcers, we believe it is necessary to treat the ulcer and the underlying venous hypertension.

Free flaps have recently been proposed to treat resistant venous ulcers. This type of grafting entails excision of the lipodermatosclerotic tissue bed and reconstruction with a free flap containing normal tissue microcirculation. The theory behind this procedure is that the autotransplanted tissue contains multiple competent venous valves, thus potentially eliminating the local tissue effects of CVI. In a recent retrospective study, six young patients had eight free flaps placed after complete ulcer excision.[48] The scapular region was the main site for the donor flap. One arterial and two venous vascular microanastamoses were performed in an end-to-side fashion. All flaps remained healed after 7 years. Skin biopsies taken at 2 and 7 years showed no signs of lipodermatosclerosis. The major disadvantages of this procedure are the need for a donor site for the free flap, intravenous heparinization, and a microsurgical anastomosis.[45] In addition, postoperative compression stockings were used in all of the patients, and although the free flap postoperative venous refill time measured by photoplethysmography improved significantly, the underlying CVI pathophysiology was not corrected.

We believe that radical excision with skin grafting presents several advantages over other local methods for treatment of large venous ulcers. The difference between this surgical approach and the less extensive procedures is that complete excision of the ulcer and ligation of incompetent veins (including perforators) are performed. The dermatosclerotic process and the infection are removed in one setting. This approach includes all involved skin and subcutaneous tissue down to and including the muscular fascia. Ligation of the perforating veins is done to reduce the increased local venous hypertension.

Immediate skin grafting is performed, and CVI is managed with elastic compression stockings. Compared to free flap transfer, this approach is much less complex. It is more readily applied to our patients, many of whom are elderly, obese, and sedentary. All of these patients have large indolent ulcers with superinfection and extensive lipodermatosclerosis. The patients selected for this procedure have documented deep venous insufficiency and have failed conservative medical treatment. Patients may need to be admitted to the hospital for 1 to 2 days of elevation, antibiotics, and topical treatment. The patients are scheduled for surgery once the peripheral edema and cellulitis show significant improvement. Blood loss occasionally may be significant and all patients are crossed-matched preoperatively. To minimize blood loss, a lower extremity tourniquet may be used in rare instances.

The surgery is usually performed under spinal anesthesia. To completely excise the ulcer, an incision is made in healthy skin and extended deeply through the subcutaneous tissues down to the fascia. The lipodermatosclerotic ulcerated tissue is carefully resected down to and including the muscular fascia. Care is taken not to damage the tendons. The saphenous vein and perforators are ligated as they are encountered. Once the complete ulcer had been excised, pulsatile irrigation is performed. The wound is covered immediately with a partial skin graft in a 1.5:1 meshed ratio nonexpanded (Figs. 2 to 6). Postoperatively the patients are treated with topical Sulfamylon and kept on absolute bed rest for 10 to 14 days. Elderly patients may require a posterior splint to protect the skin graft. When ambulation is begun, venous hypertension is first controlled with Unna's boots and then by graduated compression stockings.

Since 1988, 13 patients with 18 large intractable ulcers have been treated in this manner. Patients ranged in age from 34 to 85 years (mean, 63 years), and average duration of ulceration was 106 ± 7 months (range, 6 to 216 months) prior to surgery. Mean ulcer size at the time of excision was 177 ± 35 cm^2 (median, 130 cm^2). Four patients had bilateral ulceration. One patient had squamous cell carcinoma in bilateral chronic ulcers that had been present for more than 15 years. Twelve patients had gross venous insufficiency on duplex evaluation, and one had extensive occlusive disease. Circumferential excision was required in seven ulcers.

Sixteen ulcers (89%) have remained healed over a mean follow-up period of 29 ± 7 months (median, 24 months). Two patients developed new ulcerations in a different location from the original grafted site. Foot edema has been a

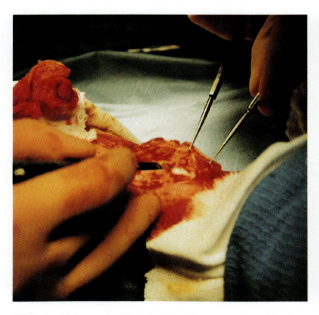

Fig. 2 Using a knife, the lipodermatosclerotic ulcer tissue is resected including the muscular fascia.

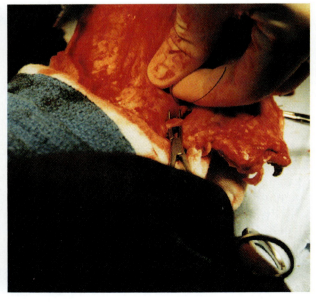

Fig. 3 Large perforators and greater saphenous vein are ligated as the ulcer bed is resected. Photograph shows a large perforator.

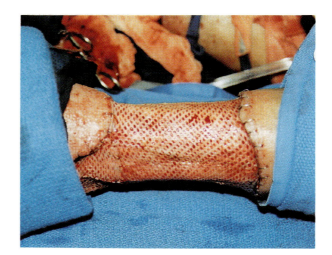

Fig. 4 Application of partial skin graft, 1.5:1 meshed ratio.

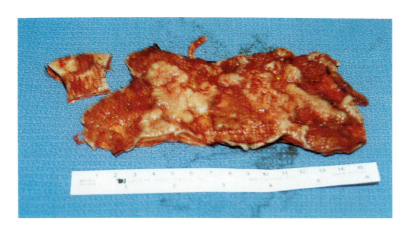

Fig. 5 Resected specimen showing complete excision of the lipodermatosclerotic ulcer tissue.

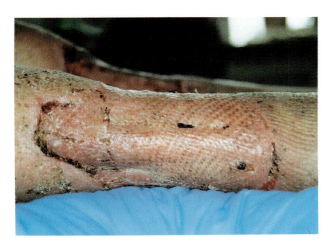

Fig. 6 Skin graft 14 days postoperatively.

transient problem in patients with circumferential excision but has been managed successfully with a sequential compression pump followed by compression stockings. It is important to note, that all patients except one had documented venous insufficiency on venous duplex and impedance plethysmography. That patient had extensive deep vein obliteration with resulting venous obstruction and has continued to be troubled by recurrent ulceration in both legs and bilateral osteomyelitis.

Radical excision and early grafting with compression therapy provides a successful approach to chronic draining venous ulceration. This approach avoids the need for extensive venous reconstruction if ligation of the perforator veins is performed. Free flap transfer is not necessary. In our series, radical excision of the ulcer with partial split-thickness grafting has been shown to be durable with low ulcer recurrence rates. It is particularly interesting to note that although two patients developed recurrent ulcers, they did so in an area distinct from their initial resection. This further emphasizes the durability of skin grafting when accompanied by venous ligation. Radical excision and early grafting should be considered as an alternative to long-term topical treatment in patients with indolent venous ulceration.

REFERENCES

1. Immelman EJ, Jeffery PC. The postphlebitic syndrome: Pathophysiology, prevention and management. Clin Chest Med 5:537-550, 1984.
2. Phillips TJ, Jeffrey SD. Leg ulcers. J Am Acad Dermatol 25:965-987, 1991.
3. Pollack AA, Wood EH. Venous pressure in the saphenous vein at the ankle in man during exercise. J Appl Physiol 1:649-662, 1949.
4. O'Donnell TF. Chronic venous insufficiency: An overview of epidemiology, classification and anatomic considerations. Semin Vasc Surg 1:60-65, 1988.
5. Browse NL. The pathogenesis of venous ulceration: A hypothesis. J Vasc Surg 7:468-472, 1988.
6. Sumner DS. Pathophysiology of CVI. Semin Vasc Surg 1:66-72, 1988.
7. Thomas PRS, Nash GB, Dormandy JS. White cell accumulation in the dependent legs of patients with venous hypertension: A possible mechanism for trophic changes in the skin. Br Med J 296:1693-1695, 1988.
8. Coleridge Smith PD, Thomas P, Scurr JH, Dormandy JS. Causes of venous ulceration: A new hypothesis. Br Med J 296:1726-1727, 1988.
9. Wilkinson LS, Bunker C, Edwards JCW, Scurr JH, Smith PDC. Leukocytes: Their role in the pathogenesis of skin damage in venous disease. J Vasc Surg 17:669-675, 1993.
10. Ersek RA, Jones MH, Tilak SP, Howard JM. Studies of the peripheral lymphatics following femoral vein occlusion in the dog. Surgery 57:269-274, 1965.
11. Ganchi RH, Irizarry E, Nackman GB, Halpern VJ, Mulcare RJ, Tilson MD. Analysis of the connective tissue matrix and proteolytic activity of primary varicose veins. J Vasc Surg 18:814-820, 1993.
12. Cheatle TR, Scurr JH, Coleridge Smith PD. Drug treatment of chronic venous insufficiency and venous ulceration: A review. J R Soc Med 84:354-358, 1991.
13. Wilson NM, Rutt DL, Browse NL. Repair and replacement of deep vein valves in the treatment of venous insufficiency. Br J Surg 78:388-394, 1991.
14. Masuda EM, Kistner RL. Long-term results of venous valve reconstruction: A four-to twenty-one–year follow-up. J Vasc Surg 19:391-403, 1994.
15. Cheatle TR, Perrin M. Venous valve repair: Early results in fifty-two cases. J Vasc Surg 19:404-413, 1994.
16. Welch HJ, McLaughlin RL, O'Donnell TF Jr. Femoral vein valvuloplasty: Intraoperative angioscopic evaluation and hemodynamic improvement. J Vasc Surg 16:694-700, 1992.
17. Unna PG. Ueber paraplaste eine neue form medikamentoser pflaster. Wien Med Wochenschr 43:1854-1856, 1896.
18. Kikta JM, Schuler JJ, Meyer JP, Durham JR, Elrup-Jorgensen J, Scwarcz HT, Flanigan DP. A prospective, randomized trial of Unna's boots versus hydroactive dressing in the treatment of venous stasis ulcers. J Vasc Surg 7:478-486, 1988.
19. Krupski CW, Reilly LM, Perez S, Moss MK, Cromble Holme PA, Rapp HJ. A prospective randomized trial of autologous platelet-derived wound healing factor for treatment of chronic nonhealing wounds: A preliminary report. J Vasc Surg 14:526-536, 1991.
20. Deluca M, Albanese E, Cancedda R, Viecova A, Faggione A, Zambruno G, Gianetti A. Treatment of leg ulcers with cryopreserved allogeneic cultured epithelium. Arch Dermatol 128:633-638, 1992.
21. Brysk MM, Rainer SS, Pupo R, Bell T, Rajaman S. Grafting of leg ulcers with undifferentiated keratinocytes. J Am Acad Dermatol 25:238-244, 1991.
22. Rooman RP, Janssen H. Ketanserin promotes wound healing: Clinical and preclinical results. In Borbul A. Clinical and Experimental Approaches to Dermal and Epidermal Repair: Normal and Chronic Wounds. New York: Wiley-Liss, Inc, 1991, pp 115-128.
23. McMullin GM, Walker GT, Coleridge Smith PD, Surr JH. The efficacy of fibrinolytic enhancement with stanozolol in the treatment of venous insufficiency. Aust NZ J Surg 61:306, 1991.
24. Does stanozolol prevent venous ulceration? Drug Ther Bull 23:91-92, 1985.
25. Browse NL, Jarret PEM, Morland M, Burnand K. Treatment of liposclerosis of the leg by fibrinolytic enhancement: A preliminary report. Br Med J 2:434-435, 1977.
26. Mann RJ. A double blind trial of oral O,B-hydroxyl ethyl rutoside for stasis leg ulcers. Br J Clin Pract 35:79-81, 1981.
27. Burnand K, Clemenson G, Morland M, Jarret PEM, Browse NL. Venous lipodermatosclerosis: Treatment by fibrinolytic enhancement and elastic compression. Br Med J 280:7-11, 1980.

28. Weitgasser H. The use of pentoxifylline (Trental 400) in the treatment of leg ulcers: The results of a double blind trial. Pharmatherapeutica 3(Suppl):143-151, 1983.
29. Sullivan GW, Carper HT, Novick WJ, Mandell GL. Inhibition of the inflammatory action of interleukin-1 and tumor necrosis factor (alpha) on neutrophil function by pentoxifylline. Infect Immunol 56:1722-1729, 1988.
30. Angelides NS, Weil von Derahe CA. Effects of oral pentoxifylline therapy on venous lower extremity ulcers due to deep venous incompetence. Angiology 40:752-763, 1989.
31. Moneta LG, Nehler MR, Chitwood RW, Porter JM. The natural history, pathophysiology and nonoperative treatment of chronic venous insufficiency. In Rutherford RB, ed. Vascular Surgery, 4th ed. Philadelphia: WB Saunders, 1995, pp 1837-1850.
32. Rudofsky G. Intravenous PGE_1 in the treatment of venous ulcers. A double-blind, placebo-controlled trial. Vasa 28(Suppl):39-43, 1989.
33. Subcommittee on Reporting Standards in Venous Disease, Ad Hoc Committee on Reporting Standards, Society for Vascular Surgery/North American Chapter, International Society for Cardiovascular Surgery. Reporting standards in venous disease. J Vasc Surg 8:172-181, 1988.
34. Linton RR. John Homan's impact on diseases of the veins of the lower extremity, with special reference to deep thrombophlebitis and the post-thrombotic syndrome with ulceration. Surgery 81:1-11, 1977.
35. Dodd H. The diagnosis and ligation of incompetent perforating veins. Ann R Coll Surg Engl 34:186-196, 1964.
36. Lim RC, Blaisdell FW, Subrin J, et al. Subfascial ligation of perforating veins in recurrent stasis ulceration. Am J Surg 119:246-249, 1970.
37. Gloviczki P, Merrell SW, Bower TC. Femoral vein valve repair under direct vision without venotomy: A modified technique with use of angioscopy. J Vasc Surg 14:645-648, 1991.
38. Coleman EJ, Bouchier-Hayes D. Surgery in the treatment of varicose veins. Semin Vasc Surg 1:92-100, 1988.
39. Raju S, Fredericks R. Valve reconstruction procedures for nonobstructive venous insufficiency: Rationale, techniques, and results in 107 procedures with two- to eight-year follow up. J Vasc Surg 7:301-310, 1988.
40. Raju S. Multiple-valve reconstruction for venous insufficiency: Indications, optimal technique, and results. In Veith FJ, ed. Current Critical Problems in Vascular Surgery, 4th ed. St. Louis: Quality Medical Publishing, 1992, pp 122-125.
41. Taheri SA, Lazar L, Elias S, et al. Surgical treatment of postphlebitic syndrome with vein valve transplant. Am J Surg 144:221-224, 1982.
42. Kistner R. Surgical technique of external venous valve repair. Proceedings of the Straub Pacific Health Foundation 55:15-16, 1990.
43. Mol AEM, Manning PB, Van Eendenburg JP, Westerhof W, Mekles JR, Vanginkel JWC. Grafting of venous leg ulcers. J Am Acad Dermatol 24:77-82, 1991.
44. Davies DM, Wood MK. Use of split skin grafting in the treatment of chronic leg ulcers. Ann R Coll Surg Engl 77:222-223, 1995.
45. Quaba AA, McDowall RAW, Hackett MEJ. Layered shaving of venous leg ulcers. Br J Plast Surg 40:68-72, 1987.
46. Nicolaides AN, Zukowski AJ. The value of dynamic venous pressure measurements. World J Surg 10:919-924, 1986.
47. Nicolaides AN, Summer DS. Investigation of Patients With Deep Vein Thrombosis and Chronic Venous Insufficiency. Los Angeles: Med-Orion, 1991, p 30.
48. Dunn MR, Fudem MG, Walton LR, Anderson AF, Malhadra R. Free flap valvular transplantation for refractory venous ulceration. J Vasc Surg 19:525-531, 1994.

78

Treatment of Lymphatic Complications: A Comparison of Conservative Therapy and Lymphazurin-Assisted Early Ligation Techniques

HARRY SCHANZER, M.D., MARK A. SCHWARTZ, M.D., MILAN SKLADANY, M.D., MOSHE HAIMOV, M.D., and JEFFREY S. STEIN, M.D.

BACKGROUND

Lymphatic leakage, especially at the groin level, is a well-known complication following vascular procedures. It has been estimated that this complication occurs in approximately 1.8% of all arterial reconstructive procedures.[1] The femoral triangle remains the most common location. Various arterial and venous reconstructive procedures have been found to precede the development of lymphatic complications.[1,2] Lymphatic leaks have also been reported following various intra-abdominal and intrathoracic procedures.[2] The pathogenesis and management of this clinical problem remain unclear. The initial event in development of lymphatic leakage is thought to be the transection of lymphatic channels during dissection. The reason for the persistence of leakage may be related to elevated lymphatic pressures, altered wound healing, the presence of foreign material, or coexistent infection. This may account for an increased incidence of lymphatic complications in cases involving insertion of prosthetic material or in extensive dissections or in patients who have undergone multiple groin procedures.[3,4] Clinically, this abnormality is manifested either as a lymphocutaneous fistula or a lymphocele.

Since the first description of lymphatic leakage following a vascular procedure, many different treatments have been proposed. Nonoperative treatments have commonly included bed rest, leg elevation, compressive dressings, and prophylactic antibiotic therapy. Lymphoceles have also been managed by multiple aspirations, sclerotherapy, radiation therapy, and cyst wall excision.[5,6] Attempts to control lymphatic fistulas have included lymphovenous anastomosis, wound marsupialization, and instillation of thrombotic agents.[7,8] All of these modalities have resulted in varying degrees of success, but they have been hampered by the need for prolonged therapy, risk of graft infection, and frequent recurrences.

An aggressive approach, consisting of wound exploration and ligation of the leaking lymphatic vessels, was first described by Kwaan et al.[1] in 1979. They used Evans blue dye (0.5% aqueous solution) to assist in localizing transected lymphatics. The dye was injected subdermally in the first interdigital web space ½ to 1 hour before exploration. Problems with this dye, related to its high affinity for protein binding, consisted of the prolonged time necessary to travel through the lymphatics and its tendency to diffusely stain the surrounding tissues when in the groin, making identification of the leaking point difficult. Kwaan et al. concluded that early exploration significantly shortened the hospital stay and decreased the incidence of wound infections when compared with standard nonoperative protocols.

A variation of this method was reported by Weaver and Yellin[9] in 1991. They used isosulphan blue dye (Lymphazurin, Hirsch Industries, Richmond, Va.), which, in contrast to Evans blue dye, travels rapidly through lymphatics, is water soluble, and does not stain surrounding tissues.[10,11] They reported success with this approach in six patients with groin lymphorrhea following lower extremity revascularization and in two cases of lymphoceles following renal allotransplantation. No complications or recurrences occurred in their series.

OUR EXPERIENCE

Since 1991, we at Mount Sinai Medical Center have been treating lymphatic leaks either with a conservative approach (bed rest, leg elevation, prophylactic antibiotics, compressive dressings, and intermittent aspiration) or an aggressive surgical approach consisting on early wound exploration and selective lymphatic ligation, assisted by Isosulphan blue. Seventeen lymphatic complications were identified over a 3-year period. Seven patients (41%) were treated solely by nonoperative means. Ten patients (59%) were treated initially by nonoperative means, followed by operative ligation assisted by dye injection. In the operative group, six patients had lymphoceles and four had lymphatic fistulas. In the nonoperative group, four patients had lymphoceles and three had lymphatic fistulas. The type of complication (lymphocele vs. lymphorrhea) did not differ significantly in the two groups.

Various operative procedures led to the development of lymphatic complications. In the operative group the initial procedure was infrainguinal bypass in three patients, transfemoral angioplasty in two, lymph node dissection in two, repair of pseudoaneurysm in two, and aortobifemoral bypass in one patient. In the conservative group the initial procedure was infrainguinal bypass in four patients, femoral valvuloplasty in two, and aortobifemoral bypass in one patient.

Both patient populations had similar clinical and demographic characteristics. The mean age of patients in the operative group was 63 ± 19.42 years (range, 35 to 88 years), and in the nonoperative group was 61 ± 16.22 years (range, 38 to 82 years). The operative group consisted of five men and five women vs. four men and three women in the nonoperative group.

Lymphoceles were diagnosed by the presence of a subcutaneous fluid collection, which on aspiration showed clear fluid with no infection or hematoma. Lymphatic fistulas were diagnosed by the presence of clear fluid draining from the wound margins. In the operative group there were six lymphoceles and four lymphorrheas; in the conservative group there were four lymphoceles and three lymphorrheas.

Initially all patients underwent a trial of nonoperative therapy including bed rest, leg elevation, compressive dressings, and prophylactic antibiotic administration. Lymphoceles were additionally treated with aspiration therapy. Unsatisfactory results, such as prolongation of hospital stay, overall length of treatment, and high complication rate, prompted us to look for an alternative, more aggressive therapeutic modality. Since March 1992, all patients with lymphatic complications that failed to resolve after 2 to 3 weeks of conservative management have been treated surgically. Operative procedure included ligation of the leaking lymphatic following the technique described by Weaver and Yellin.[9] The patients received general anesthesia, and 2 ml of 1% isosulphan blue solution was injected subdermally in divided doses into the dorsal aspect of the first and second interdigital web space of the ipsilateral foot. Following injection, the patient was placed in the Trendelenburg position. The groin wound was prepared in the standard sterile fashion. Fifteen minutes later the incision was opened widely and the wound thoroughly explored. The leaking lymphatic channels were identified by the presence of the blue dye appearing from the area of transection. Lymphatic vessel ligation was then accomplished by placing interrupted absorbable sutures. The cavity was then irrigated with gentamicin-bacitracin solution. A closed-suction drain was placed and the wound closed with interrupted absorbable sutures and skin clips.

The results of this experience can be summarized as follows: all wounds in these 17 patients were initially deemed noninfected on clinical grounds. Five wounds subsequently developed infections (cellulitis, purulent drainage, and/or positive cultures). Cultures yielded *Staphylococcus aureus* in four patients and *Pseudomonas* in one. All infections developed in lymphoceles that had been treated by multiple aspirations. One patient was subsequently treated by operative ligation and the remaining four were treated by nonoperative methods. Two cases of wound infection occurred in patients who had undergone bypass procedures; neither was associated with prosthetic material, and no instance of disruption or loss of bypass grafting was found.

The mean hospital stay in the nonoperative group was 19 days (range, 14 to 42 days), compared with 2.4 days (range, 1 to 4 days) in the operative group. In addition, in the nonoperative group there was significant coexistent morbidity. The total duration of therapy, which included outpatient treatment, was substantially longer in the nonoperative group (74 days) when compared with those patients who underwent operative ligation (18 days). It must be emphasized, however, that the majority of days required for treatment in the operative group included the preoperative period of conservative therapy.

One patient treated with operative ligation

augmented by dye injection developed an immediate recurrence. This patient had been managed by lymphatic ligation in addition to complete excision of the lymphatic capsule. This operative strategy differed from subsequent operations in that in the remaining patients the capsule was left intact after lymphatic ligation. The recurrence was managed by reexploration. A new, different transected lymphatic vessel was found and ligated. This patient responded favorably to treatment, and no recurrence was noted after a follow-up of 2 years.

In all cases of dye-assisted ligation there was clear and precise identification of the transected lymphatic vessels. No complications occurred in the operative group. As mentioned previously, five cases of wound infection developed in the group subjected to multiple aspirations. All aspirations were performed using sterile technique with small-gauge needles.

The average follow-up period in the operative group was 2.1 years. All seven patients treated in the nonoperative group eventually resolved, with an average follow-up of 1.3 years.

CONCLUSION

Lymphatic complications following vascular surgery remain a relatively rare occurrence. Although some patients respond to a short course of conservative treatment, the majority require prolonged therapy and possibly multiple attempts at aspiration therapy, which may jeopardize underlying vascular grafts. The present study confirms Weaver and Yellin's results and demonstrates the superiority of this approach compared with conservative treatment. In our experience, the use of isosulphan blue allows a rapid and accurate identification of all transected lymphatics. No reported cases of ulceration, local tissue reaction, or postoperative edema existed. As previously stated, we did have one recurrence following dye-assisted ligation. This occurred in our first operative case involving a lymphocele. We believe this patient had a recurrence because of the extensive dissection required to remove the lymphatic capsule, exposing adjacent lymphatics to injury. In support of this, we noted that an area of dye extravasation was found in a different location from the previous ligature.

Our current practice is to avoid dissection around the capsule to prevent further injury to adjacent lymphatics. Our results show that early operative ligation, assisted by dye injection, may also lead to a shorter hospital stay and fewer wound complications, compared with standard conservative therapy. In our view, this is the preferred treatment for groin lymphatic fistulas and lymphoceles.

REFERENCES

1. Kwaan JHM, Berstein JM, Connolly JE. Management of lymph fistula in the groin after arterial reconstruction. Arch Surg 114:1416-1418, 1979.
2. Croft RJ. Lymphatic fistula: A complication of arterial surgery [letter]. BMJ 2:205, 1978.
3. Wolfe JHN. Treatment of lymphedema. In Rutherford RB, ed. Vascular Surgery, 3rd ed. Philadelphia: WB Saunders, 1989, pp 1668-1678.
4. Johnston KW. Nonvascular complications of vascular surgery. In Rutherford RB, ed. Vascular Surgery, 3rd ed. Philadelphia: WB Saunders, 1989, pp 536-540.
5. Van Sonnenburg E, Wittich G, Casula G, et al. Lymphoceles: Characteristics and percutaneous management. Radiology 161:593-596, 1986.
6. Pope AJ, Ormiston MC, Bogod DG. Sclerotherapy in the treatment of a recurrent lymphocele. Postgrad Med J 58:573-574, 1982.
7. Judd ES, Nix JT. Spontaneous and traumatic lymph fistulas: Data on 40 cases. Surg Clin North Am 29:1035-1047, 1949.
8. Smellie GD, Wallace JR. Lymph fistulas and lymphocysts after peripheral vascular surgery. J R Coll Surg Edinb 26:78-81, 1981.
9. Weaver FA, Yellin AE. Management of postoperative lymphatic leaks by use of isosulphan blue [letter]. J Vasc Surg 14:566-567, 1991.
10. Kinmouth JB. Lymphangiography in clinical surgery and particularly in the treatment of lymphoedema. Ann R Coll Surg Engl 15:300-315, 1954.
11. Hirsch JI, Banks WI Jr, Sullivan JS, et al. Noninterference of isosulphan blue on estrogen-receptor activity. Radiology 171:109-110, 1989.

79

Treatment Alternatives for Deep Venous Thrombosis in Pregnancy: Anticoagulation vs. Vena Caval Filtration Devices

ALI F. ABURAHMA, M.D.

Deep venous thrombosis (DVT) of the lower extremities in pregnancy is an infrequent complication. However, if appropriate treatment is not instituted, significant maternal and/or fetal morbidity and mortality can occur.

INCIDENCE AND PATHOPHYSIOLOGY

The incidence of antepartum DVT has been reported to be no greater than 0.36% of deliveries[1] and postpartum DVT is three to five times more common. DVT is three to 16 times more common in women who deliver by cesarean section than in those who have vaginal deliveries. Acute iliofemoral venous thrombosis is six times more frequent in pregnant women than nonpregnant women.[1] Approximately one in 2000 pregnancies is complicated by a pulmonary embolus, which remains an important cause of maternal mortality, second only to abortion. Of particular importance, pulmonary embolism occurs in 15% to 24% of patients with untreated DVT, resulting in a 12% to 15% mortality rate. With appropriate therapy the incidence of pulmonary embolism is reduced to 4.5%, with an overall mortality rate of 0.7%.

Virchow's triad, specifically stasis, hypercoagulability, and vessel wall injury, continues to form the basis of venous thrombosis. Each element of this triad is present at some time during pregnancy. In general, there is no firm evidence that vascular injury plays a role in causing venous thrombosis during pregnancy. However, significant vascular damage can occur at delivery. An increase in venous capacitance produces stasis. In the early part of the second trimester, the femoral venous pressure rises and continues to do so until term, when it falls rapidly after delivery. This increase in venous pressure appears to be secondary to mechanical obstruction. Pregnancy has been described as an acquired hypercoaguable state. Underlying the changes in the element of the hemostatic system is a low-grade, chronic, disseminated intravascular coagulation within the placental bed and deposition of fibrin in the spiral arteries, which gradually replaces the internal elastic lamina and smooth muscles. The levels of coagulation factors I, V, VII, VIII, IX, X, and XII increase during pregnancy. Fibrinogen undergoes the most marked increase with the total circulating amount almost doubling in preparation for the formation of a hemostatic endometrial fibrin mesh when the placenta separates. Platelet count remains in the normal range. In addition, plasma fibrinolytic activity is decreased, perhaps secondary to an increase in fibrinolysis inhibitors (e.g., inhibitors of urokinase), which may return to normal within an hour of delivery of the placenta. The net effect is an increased potential for thrombosis because of increased levels of clotting factors and decreased fibrinolysis. This change is most marked at term and immediate puerperium and helps to control blood loss after placental separation. A deficiency of antithrombin III, protein C, and protein S levels has also been implicated in the development of DVT during pregnancy.[2]

DIAGNOSIS

Approximately one half of patients with clinical symptoms and signs of DVT have been proved not to have thrombosis after objective testing. The most common symptoms and signs are pain, tenderness, swelling, Homan's sign, change in limb color, and a palpable cord. When venous thrombosis is accompanied by massive swelling, discoloration, pain, and fever (phlegmasia cerulea dolens, "the blue leg," and phlegmasia alba dolens, "the white leg"), a diagnosis can be confidently based on the physical examination. Because therapy entails significant risk, treatment of thromboembolic disease should never be initiated solely on the basis of a clinical diagnosis. The diagnosis must be objectively confirmed prior to the initiation of treatment.

Several diagnostic tests, including venography and noninvasive testing, have been used to diagnose venous thrombus. Visualization of a well-defined filling defect on more than one radiologic view during venography is required. Suggested signs include abrupt termination, absence of opacification, or diversion of flow. False positive study results may occur because of poor technique, leg muscle contraction, or a pathologic condition such as external compression. Unfortunately, the pelvic veins and deep femoral veins cannot be evaluated adequately so large nonobstructive thrombi in the common femoral vein can be missed. Since the clinical findings associated with DVT are common in pregnancy, the clinician may be reluctant to use ascending venography because the fetus may be unnecessarily exposed to ionizing radiation and the use of pelvic shielding may invalidate the results. Because of the time, expense, and potential risks involved with venography, a number of noninvasive tests have been developed that may be used for evaluation.

Noninvasive Testing

The most commonly used noninvasive tests include Doppler ultrasound, impedance plethysmography (IPG), and standard and color duplex ultrasound. Although the physiologic noninvasive tests are usually reliable, their accuracy may be affected by physiologic alterations associated with pregnancy. Recently, standard and color duplex ultrasound has been used more frequently and has practically replaced most, if not all, physiologic testing.

Doppler Ultrasound. This test detects popliteal, femoral, and iliac thrombosis. Thrombi that completely occlude proximal veins cause an absence of blood flow sound. Those not large enough to obstruct blood flow may escape detection. Doppler ultrasonography is relatively insensitive for small, proximal, and partially occluding thrombi. The patient is normally examined in the supine position. However, in the third trimester, 25% of patients may demonstrate obstructed flow in this position. Therefore the patient's position during Doppler ultrasound examination must be noted to avoid an incorrect diagnosis.

Plethysmography. These techniques, including impedance (IPG), strain-gauge (SPG), and phleborheography (PRG), have all been used to estimate the extent to which venous occlusion interferes with venous drainage. Although the instrumentation varies, the physiologic basis of these tests remains the same. IPG is the most popular of all these tests. Its principle is based on the observation that changes in the blood volume are reflected by changes in electrical resistance. Sensitivity and specificity are high for proximal thrombosis but low for distal thrombosis. In comparison with venography, the sensitivity and specificity of IPG for detecting proximal venous thrombosis is 90%. However, for calf vein thrombosis alone, the sensitivity is poor and less accurate than Doppler ultrasound for detecting thrombi. It must be remembered that venous thrombosis confined to the soleal plexus, the profunda femoris, or the hypogastric veins will not be detected by these simple noninvasive tests.

Duplex Ultrasonography. Compression ultrasonography or color duplex imaging has been shown to have an accuracy of over 90% for the diagnosis of venous thrombi located within the femoral and popliteal venous segments.[3] The imaging protocol consists of using distention of the common femoral vein in response to a Valsalva maneuver to exclude obstructing thrombus in the iliac veins. The remainder of the femoropopliteal venous system is surveyed with color-flow Doppler imaging with flow augmentation in the femoral and popliteal veins to exclude nonobstructing thrombosis. Compression ultrasonography is also performed along the course of the femoral and popliteal veins with a transducer held transverse to the vein. A normal vein has a spontaneous phasic-augmented signal. DVT is diagnosed when a venous segment is noncompressible and does not show any flow signal.

TREATMENT

The choice of therapy is not well defined and has been widely debated.[1,2,4-9] Orally administered warfarin passes through the placenta to the fetus and may cause frequent fetal complications and/or death. Heparin, in contrast, does not cross the placental barrier and is considered a more effective therapy for DVT.[2] However, long-term venous administration during pregnancy may be impractical and increases the risk of osteoporosis, alopecia, and neurologic complications.[4] The rationale of heparin therapy is to prevent further thrombosis and pulmonary embolization and possibly to minimize the effect of postthrombotic changes in the lower extremity. A review of published reports on pregnancies in which heparin was administered demonstrates conflicting results. Some show significant fetal and maternal morbidity and mortality,[6] whereas other conclude that heparin can be safely used.[7] It has also been reported that 36% to 90% of patients have chronic venous insufficiency after receiving conventional anticoagulation.[10]

In a comprehensive review of heparin therapy for treatment of DVT in pregnancy, Hall et al.[6] noted that only two thirds of pregnancies in women treated with heparin during gestation resulted in normal births. Moreover, this figure did not differ from those treated with warfarin. The heparin-associated abnormalities included stillbirths, spontaneous abortions, and a high incidence of prematurity. This report has been criticized by Weiner,[1] who noted that in this study pregnancy loss in patients taking warfarin was usually related to placental abruption, fetal anomalies, or fetal/neonatal intracranial hemorrhage—each related to warfarin. In contrast, pregnancy loss in patients taking heparin was predominantly secondary to preterm delivery. A recent review of 22 children of mothers who took warfarin during pregnancy revealed no significant difference compared to controls. This suggests that the incidence of significant abnormalities may be lower than previously reported.[11] However, the alarming report by Hall et al.[6] cannot be ignored.

Once the diagnosis of DVT has been confirmed, a sufficient quantity of heparin should be administered to prolong the partial thromboplastin time (PTT) to 1.5- to 2-fold over the baseline. Heparin may be administered either subcutaneously or by continuous infusion with similar results.[8] Using the intravenous route, a loading dose of 110 U/kg is given, followed by a continuous infusion of heparin (initially 1000 U/hr). The PTT should be monitored every 2 hours and adjustments made in the infusion rate until a stable prolongation time has been achieved. The subcutaneous route requires a loading dose of 150 U/kg given intravenously, followed by 20,000 units of heparin every 12 hours. The PTT is monitored at midintervals until the plasma heparin level achieved with subcutaneous injection is stable. Although there is no difference in efficacy between 8- and 12-hour dose intervals, the 8-hour interval may be preferred when the volume of heparin injected exceeds 1 ml. The duration of intravenous heparin infusion is quite variable but should be continued for a minimum of 2 days with DVT and 5 days with pulmonary embolism, depending on the severity of the disease. Historically, the goal was to continue intravenous heparin until active thrombosis had stopped, thrombi were firmly attached to the vessel wall, and organization had begun. Although many authors recommended intravenous heparin therapy for 7 to 10 days, adequate therapeutic response may be achieved by the use of subcutaneous heparin.[8] The period of continuous intravenous infusion is followed by therapeutic subcutaneous injection for the duration of the pregnancy. Postpartum thromboembolism should be treated with therapeutic anticoagulation for a minimum of 6 weeks for DVT and 3 months for pulmonary embolism.

It is recommended that the platelet count be checked prior to beginning heparin and every 2 to 3 days thereafter to detect developing thrombocytopenia. The patient should be instructed not to inject heparin once regular uterine contractions have begun. If delivery appears likely within 12 hours of the last heparin injection, an episiotomy should be avoided. Uterine hemostasis is unaffected by heparin.

Generally there are three basic choices to be made regarding peripartum management. One approach is to continue therapeutic heparinization, which is recommended for high-risk patients such as those with recent pulmonary embolism, iliofemoral thrombosis, or heart valve prosthesis. As a more uniform low therapeutic heparin level is desired, the patient may be switched from subcutaneous injection to continuous intravenous infusion, aiming for a heparin level of 0.1 to 0.2 U/ml or a low therapeutic PTT (1.5 of normal). Except for episiotomy hematomas, patients who have vaginal deliveries have similar blood losses regardless of whether they are therapeutically anticoagulated. However, patients who are receiving therapeutic heparin and have cesarean sections have a significantly greater blood loss than usual. The second approach is to reduce the subcutaneous dose of heparin to 5000 units every 12 hours. This is suggested for patients with recent thromboembolism. The third approach is to discontinue intravenous heparin administration 4 hours before delivery. However, if the dose is being given subcutaneously, the last injection should be given 6 hours prior to delivery. If the PTT is more than 60 seconds in the second stage, protamine sulfate reversal may be considered to minimize bleeding from lacerations. The effect of heparin is quickly reversed with 1 mg of protamine for every 100 units of heparin. Larger doses should be avoided since excess protamine may act as an antithrombin.

The postpartum period is associated with the greatest risk of thromboembolism. As soon after delivery as feasible, the patient should receive a subcutaneous injection since it takes 2 to 4 hours before a therapeutic plasma level of heparin can be obtained. Heparin should be initiated no more than 6 hours after labor. Heparin (5000 units subcutaneously every 12 hours) should be continued for 6 to 8 weeks postpartum. Warfarin can be initiated after 4 to 7 days of heparin for nonlactating women and the dose should be adjusted to keep the prothrombin time (PT) to 15 to 20 seconds. A progestational contraceptive should be considered for the anticoagulated ovulating woman to reduce the risk of hemorrhagic corpus luteum and menorrhagia. Postpartum suppression of lactation with estrogen is associated with a much higher incidence of thromboembolism and is contraindicated. Many physicians recommend either calf or thigh high compression stockings for prophylaxis.

ALTERNATIVE TREATMENTS

The role of anticoagulation in the treatment of DVT in general is to prevent pulmonary embolism and to minimize the long-term sequelae characterized by the postphlebitic syndrome. Heparin anticoagulation has been somewhat effective in achieving the former but ineffective in preventing valvular damage and, as a consequence, avoiding the postphlebitic syndrome. Comerota[10] summarized the findings reported in 13 studies that compared the benefits of heparin sodium with those of thrombolytic therapy, as judged by pretreatment and posttreatment phlebography. Of 227 patients who underwent heparin therapy, significant lysis of thrombi occurred in the legs in only 6% of patients and partial lysis in an additional 12% of patients. The remaining 82% of patients showed no improvement and there was an actual extension of the degree of thrombosis as visualized in the pretreatment phlebogram. In addition, bleeding from heparin probably occurs in approximately 5% to 10% of patients, but may affect as many as one third of patients.[2] Based on these concerns and the fact that two pregnant patients in our medical center in 1 year had major complications while taking heparin (one with significant retroperitoneal bleeding and one with pulmonary embolus), other alternatives of therapy were explored.

Vena Caval Filters

To achieve the goal of DVT therapy, the prevention of pulmonary embolism and the long-term sequelae, we began a protocol of inserting a Greenfield filter for the prevention of pulmonary embolism in patients with iliofemoral DVT who were at high risk for this complication. In addition, a lower dose of heparin (dose-adjusted for a PTT of 1.5 of the control) was used to prevent further thrombotic processes and as prophylaxis for DVT during the course of pregnancy. The introduction of the percutaneous Greenfield filter has made the procedure less invasive and more attractive. Fluoroscopy is required briefly when the filter is placed. It has been estimated that 2 minutes of fluoroscopy to the abdomen exposes the area to 0.5 rads of irradiation. None of our patients has required more than 2 minutes of fluoroscopy.

The indications for vena caval interruption in the treatment of DVT during pregnancy are similar to the indications in a nonpregnant state. Another potential indication, primarily for prevention of pulmonary embolism, could be in pregnant patients with iliofemoral DVT in the third trimester, combined with lower-dose heparin, to prevent further venous thrombosis.

Other alternative therapies for iliofemoral venous thrombosis during pregnancy include thrombectomy and temporary arteriovenous fistula combined with heparin therapy as proposed by Mogensen et al.,[9] who reported favorable results.

Thromboembolic Prophylaxis

Patients at high risk for thromboembolic disease in pregnancy should be considered for anticoagulant prophylaxis during pregnancy, including patients with a past history of DVT or pulmonary embolism during or prior to pregnancy or operative delivery; patients with preeclampsia or eclampsia; patients with concurrent malignant disease; patients with an artificial heart valve; patients who are older; patients with higher parity; obese patients; and patients who have primary hypercoagulable disorders such as an antithrombin III, protein S, or protein C deficiency. A patient with a thromboembolic event during an earlier pregnancy may receive prophylaxis throughout a later pregnancy. If thromboembolism is not associated with pregnancy, opinions vary as to the need for prophylaxis during pregnancy, but it is agreed that prophylaxis is important during the puerperium. A protocol for prophylaxis in pregnancy has not yet been clearly established, but low-dose heparin administration is reasonable, with close clinical follow-up essential. Uteroplacental coagulation and platelet activity increase as the pregnancy progresses, leading to progressive neutralization of heparin. Doses must, therefore, be increased from 5000 units to 7500 units and possibly 10,000 units every 12 hours in the third trimester. A dose of 8000 units is suggested for the puerperal period.

CLINICAL EXPERIENCE

Of 25,907 deliveries during a 6-year period (1987 to 1993) at our medical center, 22 patients were diagnosed as having DVT of the lower extremity with or without a pulmonary embolism during their pregnancy.

The clinical diagnosis of DVT was confirmed in each case by duplex ultrasound and/or phlebography. Two treatment protocols were used for treatment of DVT in pregnancy during this period. Conventional therapy consisted of continuous full-dose intravenous heparin for 7 to 10 days (5000 to 10,000 units intravenous bolus, the dosage adjusted by an activated partial thromboplastin time [APTT] of 1.5 to 2.5 of the control), followed by an adjusted dose of subcutaneous heparin every 8 to 12 hours in a dose that maintained the midinterval APTT at 1.5 to 2 times the control until delivery, followed by 5000 units of subcutaneous heparin every 12 hours until 6 to 8 weeks after delivery. Nonconventional therapy was used for patients with iliofemoral DVT. Patients were treated with lower-dose subcutaneous heparin for 7 to 10 days with Greenfield filter insertion (5000 to 10,000 units intravenous bolus, then 5000 to 10,000 units every 8 to 12 hours subcutaneously with the dosage adjusted for an APTT of 1.5 of the control), followed by 5000 units of subcutaneous heparin every 12 hours until 6 to 8 weeks after delivery. Four patients who received conventional therapy and two who had nonconventional therapy, who were not lactating, were maintained on 5 mg warfarin (Coumadin) daily for 6 to 8 weeks after delivery instead of subcutaneous heparin.

In both groups, subcutaneous heparin was discontinued when active labor commenced and reinstituted as soon as possible following delivery. All patients were kept in bed with their legs elevated until the acute swelling was resolved. Prescription support stockings were used during ambulation.

All patients, except three, were examined in the vascular laboratory for evidence of leg swelling or other symptoms and signs of chronic venous insufficiency. They also had a late (more than 6 months) color venous duplex ultrasound of the lower extremity to verify DVT resolution. Patients with filters had an x-ray film of the abdomen to check the level of their filters.

RESULTS

The mean age of patients in this series was 24 years (range, 17 to 39 years). Follow-up ranged from 6 to 90 months (mean, 42.4 months). The clinical diagnosis of DVT was confirmed in each case by duplex ultrasound (18 patients) and/or phlebography (four patients). Seventeen cases were diagnosed in the third trimester, four in the second trimester, and one in the first trimester. Fifteen of the 22 cases were in the left lower extremity. The venous thrombosis was located in the iliofemoral vein in 13 patients, the femoral in six patients, the femoropopliteal in two patients, and the popliteal in one patient. Fifteen patients had their protein C, protein S, and antithrombin III levels estimated and 13 patients had lupus anticoagulant studies. Three patients had a protein C deficiency and two patients had a protein S deficiency.

Thirteen patients received conventional therapy. Two of these were given full-dose heparin for 24 hours and, because of complications (one bleeding and one pulmonary embolism), were converted to a lower-dose heparin regimen. Eleven patients received nonconventional therapy. Both groups were comparable regarding age and risk factors for DVT.

Ten patients who received nonconventional therapy had Greenfield filters inserted, including one for pulmonary embolism, one for bleeding complications that occurred during full-dose intravenous continuous heparin regimen for 24 hours (after filter insertion, heparin was switched to a subcutaneous low-dose regimen), two for free-floating iliofemoral DVT, and six to prevent pulmonary embolism in patients with iliofemoral DVT. The filters were inserted through the right internal jugular vein by cutdown in four patients (stainless steel filters) and percutaneously (titanium filters) in six patients.

Immediate and Late Outcomes. In the patients who received conventional therapy, there were three immediate major complications: two pulmonary embolisms, one of which was fatal, and one case of significant retroperitoneal bleeding that necessitated a blood transfusion (3 of 13 patients [23%]). There were no immediate major complications or complications related to the insertion of the Greenfield filters or misplacement of the filters in the patients who received nonconventional therapy (0 of 11; Fisher's exact two-tailed test, $p = .14$). There was no fetal morbidity or mortality in either group.

In long-term follow-up, three (38%) of eight patients who received conventional therapy had significant leg swelling with partial resolution of DVT in one and venous occlusion in two demonstrated by duplex ultrasound. This is in contrast to three (27%) of 11 patients in those who received nonconventional therapy. Two patients had partial resolution and one suffered a venous occlusion (Fisher's exact two-tailed test, $p = .506$). Three patients who received conventional therapy did not have long-term follow-up. There was one death secondary to massive pulmonary embolism after delivery and two patients refused to participate in follow-up care.

CONCLUSION

In our series, patients who received low-dose subcutaneous heparin and had a Greenfield filter inserted tended to do better than those who received full-dose continuous intravenous heparin treatment. However, since the number of patients in this study was small, further verification is needed.

Based on our previous clinical experience, we conclude that the use of heparin during pregnancy demands an individualized, well-planned regimen with careful control. Generally accepted treatments include (1) conventional full-dose heparin anticoagulation before delivery, withdrawal of heparin during delivery, and reinstatement after delivery; and (2) heparin before and after delivery with insertion of an inferior vena caval filter prepartum to prevent pulmonary embolism in patients with iliofemoral DVT with onset less than 30 days before labor begins.

REFERENCES

1. Weiner CP. Diagnosis and management of thromboembolic disease during pregnancy. Clin Obstet Gynecol 28:107-118, 1985.
2. Rutherford SE, Phelan JP. Thromboembolic disease in pregnancy. Clin Perinatol 13:719-739, 1986.
3. Polak JF, Wilkinson DL. Ultrasonographic diagnosis of symptomatic deep venous thrombosis in pregnancy. Am J Obstet Gynecol 165:625-629, 1991.
4. Hull RD, Raskob GE, Pineo GF, et al. Subcutaneous low-molecular-weight heparin compared with continuous intravenous heparin in the treatment of proximal-vein thrombosis. N Engl J Med 326:975-982, 1992.
5. Teodorescu V, Schanzer H. Management of thrombophlebitis in the prepartum period. J Cardiovasc Surg 33:448-450, 1992.
6. Hall JG, Pauli RM, Wilson KM. Maternal and fetal sequelae of anticoagulation during pregnancy. Am J Med 68:122-140, 1980.
7. Rosenfeld JC, Estrada FP, Orr RM. Management of deep venous thrombosis in the pregnant female. J Cardiovasc Surg 31:678-682, 1990.
8. Hommes DW, Bura A, Mazzolai L, et al. Subcutaneous heparin compared with continuous intravenous heparin administration in the initial treatment of deep vein thrombosis. Ann Intern Med 116:279-284, 1992.
9. Mogensen K, Skibsted L, Wadt J, et al. Thrombectomy of acute iliofemoral venous thrombosis during pregnancy. Surg Gynecol Obstet 169:50-54, 1989.
10. Comerota AJ. Thrombolytic Therapy. New York: Grune & Stratton, 1988, pp 76-77.
11. Chang MKB, Harvey D, DeSwiet M. Follow-up study of children whose mothers were treated with warfarin during pregnancy. Br J Obstet Gynaecol 91:70-73, 1984.

SECTION IX

Venous Disease Update

This section offers differing views on venous valve repair techniques. It also details the importance of the plantar venous plexus and methods for improving venous flow that involve applying sequential venous compression devices to the foot. Finally, there are chapters in this section that deal with updates on the use of stents and lytic agents for large vein occlusive disease and treatment of pulmonary embolism.

80

Valve Repair Techniques for Chronic Venous Insufficiency: When, How, and By Whom Should They Be Performed?

THOMAS F. O'DONNELL, Jr., M.D., and AGUSTIN A. RODRIGUEZ, M.D.

Recent advances in deep venous reconstructive surgery have been associated with excellent long-term results in selected patients.[1] This report will review the indications, diagnostic evaluation, surgical techniques, and results of surgical treatment for deep valvular incompetence.

INDICATIONS

Patients with recurrent venous ulcers who have failed standard nonsurgical therapy consisting of elastic compression and local wound care are considered candidates for vascular reconstruction of the deep venous system. In our experience, most patients have had an ulcer for a mean of 6 or 7 years and have experienced three to four recurrences.[2] Younger patients and those with active lifestyles may be offered surgery following a shorter duration of their venous ulcers. Rarely, selected individuals with advanced stage II disease who are deemed "pre-ulcer" may undergo surgery. Deep venous reconstructive surgery is not offered for the initial episode of venous ulceration, without first attempting optimal medical management.

DIAGNOSTIC EVALUATION

Duplex scans enable both anatomic and physiologic assessment of the deep and superficial venous systems. Because our institution is a referral center, only approximately 15% of our patients with venous ulcers have superficial venous system involvement alone,[3] but this incidence rises to 40% to 50% in community-based practices. Duplex scanning (B mode) characterizes the morphologic status, whereas spectral analysis allows for functional assessment of the deep venous system. Typical recanalization changes suggest postthrombotic destruction of valves, whereas visualization of valve leaflets makes primary valvular incompetence (PVI) more likely.[4] Measurement of duplex-derived valve closure times at the superficial femoral and popliteal vein levels provides objective information regarding valvular dysfunction.[5] A recent prospective study using descending phlebography as the "gold standard" showed that there was good correlation between a combined popliteal and superficial femoral vein valve closure time of more than 4 seconds and Kistner's grade III/IV venous reflux by descending phlebography.[6] Patients with reflux solely to the superficial femoral vein (SFV) level are usually not deemed candidates for deep venous reconstruction.

Ascending phlebography is used to rule out venous obstruction, especially proximal in the iliofemoral segment, and to demonstrate both the presence and sites of incompetent communicating veins and perforators. In addition, recanalization changes suggesting postthrombotic syndrome (PTS) or the presence of valve structures may be helpful in selecting the type of procedure. Descending phlebography is carried out to confirm the level of valvular incompetence.[4]

Air plethysmographic measurements of the venous filling index, ejection fraction, and residual volume fraction provide functional information regarding the degree of hemodynamic impairment and should be regarded as complementary to the duplex scan. The venous filling index, a measure of reflux, is usually increased to 9 to 10 ml/sec or greater, whereas the residual volume fraction, a reflection of ambulatory venous pressure,[7,8] is usually elevated in excess of 50%.[9] In patients with documented deep venous thrombosis, a hypercoagulable screen is performed to eliminate patients with a circulating lupus anticoagulant or antithrombin III deficiency. Duplex assessment of perforating vein competence permits concomitant treatment of incompetent perforating veins and is important for complete resolution of the pathophysiologic impairment.[10]

SURGICAL TECHNIQUE

The type of deep venous reconstruction is dictated by the underlying pathologic findings (Table 1). Proximal venous outflow obstruction of a physiologic significance, as determined by the arm/foot method of Raju and Fredericks,[11] should be corrected first. Perforator vein incompetence should be corrected prior to or concomitant with deep venous reconstruction. The pathology of valvular incompetence dictates the surgical approach, and in general a direct approach is used for PVI and an indirect approach is used for postthrombotic valvular dysfunction.

PRIMARY VALVULAR INCOMPETENCE

Patients with PVI require some form of *direct* valve repair. Initially this was accomplished by means of an open valve repair through a transverse venotomy.[12,13] However, we now prefer a closed, angioscopically guided repair (Fig. 1).[14] The first valve located in the proximal SFV is generally repaired with interrupted 7-0 monofilament mattress sutures (Fig. 2). Angioscopic repair has the following advantages: (1) it can be performed more rapidly because there is no need for a venotomy, (2) it is less traumatic to the vein, and (3) it provides a more accurate physiologic intraoperative evaluation of the valve repair—competence is easily demonstrated in the operating room. The angioscope is introduced via a side branch as shown, and a two-team approach is employed. One surgeon places the sutures to "reef-up" the valve cusps, while another observes their placement.[14]

POSTTHROMBOTIC VALVULAR DYSFUNCTION

Transposition of the profunda femoris vein or the greater saphenous vein valve[15] (Fig. 3) and *transplantation* of a valve-bearing segment from the axillary vein[16] (Fig. 4) are the two preferred surgical alternatives to this problem. Because of

Table 1 Surgical options in the management of chronic venous insufficiency

Valvular Reflux
Primary venous insufficiency
Valvuloplasty
  Open
  Closed (angioscopic)
External venous support
  Diameter reduction of vein by interrupted sutures
  Psathakis external sling
  Dacron "cuff"
Postthrombotic syndrome
  Valve autotransplantation
  Vein segment transposition

Venous Outflow Obstruction
Iliac vein obstruction
  Autogenous femorofemoral crossover graft
  Prosthetic femorofemoral crossover graft
Femoral vein obstruction
  Autogenous saphenopopliteal bypass
  Prosthetic saphenopopliteal bypass

Superficial Venous Insufficiency
Ligation and stripping
  Greater saphenous and/or tributaries
  Lesser saphenous and/or tributaries
  Interruption of perforating veins

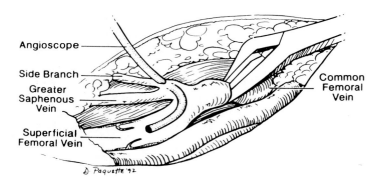

Fig. 1 Angioscopically guided valvuloplasty. The angioscope is being introduced via a side branch of the greater saphenous vein. This allows for closed placement of sutures under direct visualization. (From Welch HJ, McLaughlin RL, O'Donnell TF Jr. Femoral vein valvuloplasty: Intraoperative angioscopic evaluation and hemodynamic improvement. J Vasc Surg 16:694-700, 1992.)

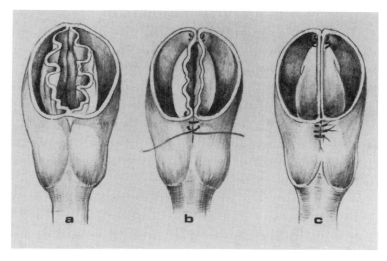

Fig. 2 Artist's rendering of the direct valvuloplasty technique. **A,** Incompetent valve with redundant, floppy cusps. **B,** Following placement of interrupted sutures at each commissure, the valve is rendered competent. **C,** Final result.

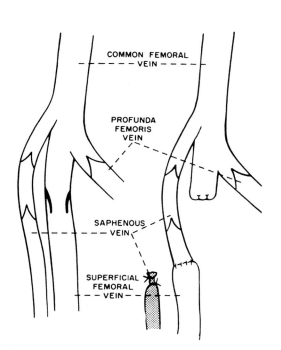

Fig. 3 Technique of femoral vein transposition to the greater saphenous vein. Advantage is taken of a competent vein valve at the saphenofemoral junction to prevent proximal reflux in the SFV. (From Queral LA, Whitehouse WM, Flinn WR, et al. Surgical correction of chronic deep venous insufficiency by valvular transposition. Surgery 87:690, 1980.)

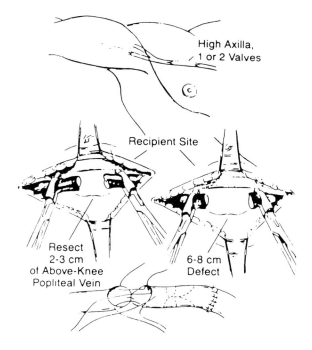

Fig. 4 Axillary-to-popliteal vein-valve transplant. A 5 to 7 cm segment of brachial vein is harvested through a longitudinal incision parallel to the neurovascular bundle to bridge a 2 to 3 cm segment of resected diseased popliteal vein. The distal followed by the proximal anastomosis is fashioned using interrupted monofilament 7-0 suture. (From O'Donnell TF, Mackey WC, Shepard AD, Callow AD. Clinical, hemodynamic and anatomic follow-up of direct venous reconstruction. Arch Surg 122:474-482, 1987.)

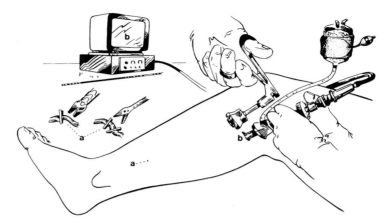

Fig. 5 Typical setup for laparoscopic interruption of communicating veins. The laparoscope is introduced through a small incision (b), away from the "underprivileged tissue" overlying the incompetent perforators (a), which are double clipped and divided. (From O'Donnell TF Jr. Surgical management of incompetent communicating veins. In Bergan JJ, Kistner RL, eds. Atlas of Venous Surgery. Philadelphia: WB Saunders, 1992, pp 111-124.)

the critical role of the popliteal vein in modulating the hemodynamic function of the calf muscle venous pump, we prefer this site for transplantation.[2] In addition, the larger axillary vein segment is used because it affords a better size match, which might prevent later incompetence secondary to venous dilatation. The above-knee popliteal vein is isolated and the axillary vein valve segment is interposed end to end with interrupted monofilament sutures (Fig. 4).

Postoperative care for all deep venous reconstructions entails maintenance of intermittent pneumatic compression boots until the patient becomes ambulatory to promote increased venous flow, thereby mitigating stasis at the operative site, conversion of perioperative heparin to Coumadin (for a period of at least 6 months), and custom-fitted elastic compression stockings to control edema.[4] With the use of selective subfascial vein ligation sites by our own laparoscopic approach (Fig. 5), hospitalization time is reduced.[10]

RESULTS
Primary Valvular Incompetence

The long-term follow-up report of Matsuda and Kistner[17] has documented the efficacy of deep venous reconstruction for PVI. Fifty-one limbs (57% of which had venous ulceration) were followed for periods of up to 10 years, with 60% of patients showing significant clinical improvement. Maintenance of valve competence correlated with long-term results, so that 86% of patients with normal limbs had excellent function according to duplex scans. Ulcers recurred within 4 years in the majority (12 of 15) of cases.

Raju and Fredericks[13] reported their experience with 107 venous valve reconstructions followed over a period of 2 to 8 years. Most patients in this series had PVI and 71% had stasis ulceration. These patients underwent direct open valvular repair as well as ligation of the saphenofemoral junction. Sixty-nine percent of patients exhibited clinical healing of ulcers and/or marked symptomatic improvement.

Cheatle and Perrin studied 52 limbs in which valvuloplasty of the SFV was performed for recurrent ulceration or severe stasis. Most patients (94%) underwent simultaneous ligation of perforating veins. Eighty-five percent of patients were free of ulcers at 1-year follow-up and 68% had normalization of their venous refill time.

Eriksson and Almgren[19] reported on 22 limbs with PVI in which valvuloplasty plus peforator ligation was performed; follow-up in these cases ranged from 6 to 84 months. Fifty-three percent of limbs showed improvement at 84 months' follow-up. Doppler examination revealed competent valves in all patients at 6 months' follow-up, and the seven late clinical failures all had phlebographically documented incompetence of their repaired valves. This group was the first to call attention to the importance of profunda femoris vein competence in these patients. Only those patients with documented preoperative competence of the profunda femoris vein showed

Table 2 Results of surgical therapy for chronic venous insufficiency

Series	No. of limbs (preop)	% Ulcers*	% Ulcer healing Short†	% Ulcer healing Long†
Valvuloplasty				
Matsuda and Kistner[17]	51	57	?	57
Raju and Fredericks[13]	107	78	85	63
Cheatle and Perrin[18]	52	40	?	?
Eriksson and Almgren[19]	22	?	64	62
Sottiurai[20]	20	100	?	80
Simkin et al.[21]	7	100	?	50
O'Donnell et al.[2]	9	100	100	100
Venous Transposition				
Ferris and Kistner[24]	14	?	80	?
Johnson et al.[25]	12	33	100	67
O'Donnell et al.[2]	9	100	100	78
Vein Valve Transplant				
Taheri et al.[26]	43	40	?	94
Raju and Fredericks[11]	24	80	79	42
Bry et al.[23]	15	100	100	62
External Venous Support				
Psathakis[27]	44	23	100	100

*Refers to percentage of limbs that had chronic ulceration as the indication for surgery.
†Short and long refer to percentage of ulcers healed over the short (<18 months) and long term (>48 months).

improvement in physiologic parameters (ambulatory venous pressure and venous refill time) postoperatively.

Sottiurai[20] described a novel approach that combined transverse and vertical venotomy to attain better exposure for valvular exposure and reported his results with 20 limbs so treated. All patients in this series had recurrent ulcers and were followed up for a mean of 37 months. Eighty percent of these patients showed healing of their ulcers.

Simkin et al.[21] reported their experience with seven patients, three of whom underwent Kistner valvuloplasty and four of whom underwent intraluminal femoral and popliteal valvuloplasty. This latter technique involves placement of multiple U-shaped monofilament sutures to reduce the caliber of the vein. Fifty percent of the patients in this small group were ulcer free after an unspecified follow-up interval.

Our group has recently reported results of SFV valvuloplasty in nine limbs with recurrent venous ulcers. In addition to valvuloplasty, five patients required subfascial ligation of perforating veins, and three underwent superficial stripping and ligation. The last five valvuloplasties were evaluated intraoperatively by means of an angioscope and in the last two an angioscopically guided closed technique was used.[14] Mean follow-up was 20 months and all patients showed healing of their ulcers. Duplex quantitation of valve closure time and air plethysmography–derived venous filling index almost normalized following angioscopically guided repair.

These results (Table 2) show that valvuloplasty for reflux in patients with PVI and stage III disease is associated with healing of ulcers as well as hemodynamic improvement, provided patients have a competent profunda femoris vein. Patients with incompetent perforating veins should have these addressed before or at the time of valvuloplasty. Furthermore, angioscopic evaluation of vein valve repair appears to improve hemodynamic and functional results.

Postthrombotic Valvular Incompetence

The results with treatment of this form of valve incompetence are less durable than those obtained with primary valvular reconstruction,[22,23] which arises from the greater potential for recurrent thrombosis in the former. In addition, preexisting venous changes associated with concomitant obstruction and diminished compliance may adversely affect the results. Venous valve transplantation is indicated in the setting of deep venous insufficiency secondary to PTS.

Patients who also have an element of proximal venous outflow obstruction may be candidates for staged repair, with correction of the venous outflow being done first.

Chronic deep venous involvement usually presents with recanalization changes on B-mode imaging, and valvular incompetence secondary to PTS is characterized by either absent or markedly thickened valves. Motionless, scarred valves that fail to coapt are seen on B-mode scan.

We prefer to interpose a valve-bearing segment of axillary vein at the popliteal vein level

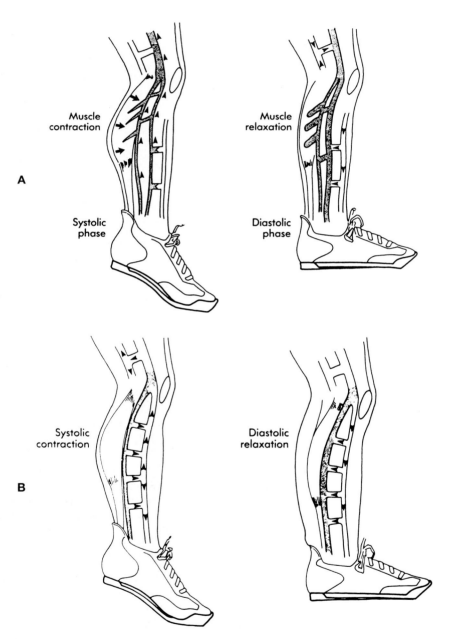

Fig. 6 The direction of venous flow following activation of the calf muscle pump in the normal limb **(A)** is from superficial to deep during the systolic phase, without reflux during the diastolic phase, in sharp contrast to that found in the limb with chronic venous insufficiency **(B),** where blood flows into the superficial system during systole and there is a significant amount of reflux in diastole. The importance of the popliteal vein valve lies in its ability to act as a "gatekeeper" to the calf muscle pump mechanism.

(see Fig. 4) to take advantage of the "gatekeeper" function of the popliteal valve in the calf muscle pump mechanism (Fig. 6, *A* and *B*). Both proximal and distal anastomoses are constructed using interrupted 7-0 monofilament sutures. If there is incompetence of the communicating veins, these are divided prior to or concomitant with the vein valve transplant procedure.

CONCLUSION

We have reported our experience with 15 patients who underwent popliteal vein valve transplant and were followed up for a mean of 5 years.[23] All patients achieved healing of their ulcers, and the mean ulcer-free interval was 4 years. Table 2 summarizes the results in the largest reported series. Although patency and long-term results are quite variable, 70% of patients do enjoy good clinical results.

Venous surgery is technically demanding and as unforgiving as arterial surgery, maybe more so. Wilson et al.[28] have accurately pointed out that "optimum surgical treatment of venous insufficiency requires the correction of all abnormalities including the perforating veins." The accurate preoperative evaluation and careful selection of patients (segregating PVI vs. PTS), followed by meticulous surgery by someone experienced in the technique, and taking advantage of angioscopy to eliminate the need for venotomy should result in improved outcome.

REFERENCES

1. Kistner RL. Valve repair and segment transposition in primary valvular insufficiency. In Bergan JJ, Yao JST, eds. Venous Disorders. Philadelphia: WB Saunders, 1991, pp 261-272.
2. O'Donnell TF, Mackey WC, Shepard AD, Callow AD. Clinical, hemodynamic and anatomic follow-up of direct venous reconstruction. Arch Surg 122:474-482, 1987.
3. McEnroe CS, O'Donnell TF, Mackey WC. Correlation of clinical findings with venous hemodynamics in 386 patients with chronic venous insufficiency. Am J Surg 156:142-152, 1988.
4. O'Donnell TF. The surgical management of deep venous valvular incompetence. In Rutherford RB, ed. Vascular Surgery, 3rd ed. Philadelphia: WB Saunders, 1989, pp 1612-1626.
5. van Bemmelen PS, Beach K, Bedford G, Strandness DE. The mechanism of venous valve closure. Arch Surg 125:617-619, 1990.
6. Welch HJ, Faliakou EC, McLaughlin RL, et al. Comparison of descending phlebography with quantitative photoplethysmography, air plethysmography, and duplex quantitative valve closure time in assessing deep venous reflux. J Vasc Surg 16:13-20, 1992.
7. Christopoulos DG, Nicolaides AN, Szendro G, et al. Air plethysmography and the effect of elastic compression on venous hemodynamics of the leg. J Vasc Surg 5:148-159, 1987.
8. Nicolaides AN, Hussein MK, Szendro G, et al. The relation of venous ulceration with ambulatory venous pressure measurements. J Vasc Surg 17:414-419, 1993.
9. Welkie JF, Comerota AJ, Katz ML, et al. Hemodynamic deterioration in chronic venous disease. J Vasc Surg 16:733-740, 1992.
10. O'Donnell TF Jr. Surgical management of incompetent communicating veins. In Bergan JJ, Kistner RL, eds. Atlas of Venous Surgery. Philadelphia: WB Saunders, 1992, pp 111-124.
11. Raju S, Fredericks R. Venous obstruction: An analysis of 137 cases with hemodynamic, venographic and clinical correlations. J Vasc Surg 14:305-313, 1991.
12. Kistner RL. Surgical repair of the incompetent femoral vein valve. Arch Surg 110:1336-1342, 1975.
13. Raju S, Fredericks R. Valve reconstruction procedures for nonobstructive venous insufficiency: Rationale, techniques, and results in 107 procedures with two to eight year follow-up. J Vasc Surg 7:301-310, 1988.
14. Welch HJ, McLaughlin RL, O'Donnell TF Jr. Femoral vein valvuloplasty: Intraoperative angioscopic evaluation and hemodynamic improvement. J Vasc Surg 16:694-700, 1992.
15. Kistner R, Sparkuhl MD. Surgery in acute and chronic venous disease. Surgery 85:31-41, 1979.
16. Taheri SA, Pendergast DR, Lazar E. Vein valve transplantation. Am J Surg 150:201-202, 1985.
17. Matsuda EM, Kistner RL. Long-term results of venous valve reconstruction: A four- to twenty-one–year follow-up. J Vasc Surg 19:391-403, 1994.
18. Cheatle TR, Perrin M. Surgical options in the post-thrombotic syndrome. Phlebology 8:50-57, 1993.
19. Eriksson JI, Almgren B. Surgical reconstruction of incompetent deep vein valves. Uppsala J Med Sci 93:139-143, 1988.
20. Sottiurai VS. Surgical correction of recurrent venous ulcer. J Cardiovasc Surg 32:104-109, 1991.
21. Simkin R, Estebam JC, Bulloj R. Bypass veno-venosos y valvuloplastias en el tratamiento quirurgico del sindrome post-trombotico. Angiologia 1:30-34, 1988.
22. Nash T. Long-term results of vein valve transplants placed in the popliteal vein for intractable postphlebitis venous ulcers and pre-ulcer skin changes. J Cardiovasc Surg 29:712-716, 1988.
23. Bry JDL, Muto PM, O'Donnell TF Jr, Isaacson L. The clinical and hemodynamic results after axillary-to-popliteal vein valve transplantation. J Vasc Surg 21:110-119, 1995.
24. Ferris EB, Kistner RL. Femoral vein reconstruction in the management of chronic venous insufficiency. Arch Surg 117:1571-1579, 1982.
25. Johnson ND, Queral LA, Flinn WR, et al. Late objective assessment of venous valve surgery. Arch Surg 116:1461-1468, 1981.
26. Taheri SA, Lazar E, Elias SM, et al. Vein valve transplantation. Surgery 91:28-33, 1982.
27. Psathakis ND. The substitute "valve" operation by technique II in patients with post-thrombotic syndrome. Surgery 95:542-548, 1984.
28. Wilson NM, Rutt DL, Browse NL. Repair and replacement of deep vein valves in the treatment of venous insufficiency. Br J Surg 78:388-394, 1991.

81

Optimal Technique for Venous Valve Repair: Which Patients Should Have the Procedure?

SESHADRI RAJU, M.D.

Technical options for venous valve reconstruction have expanded beyond the original internal technique described by Kistner[1] for "primary" reflux. A variety of new techniques are now available, many of them applicable to postthrombotic reflux as well. It is now possible to choose a technique that is optimal for an individual case and pathologic condition.

Internal valvuloplasty is a reliable, proven technique that yields a long-term cure rate of 50% to 60% for stasis ulcers.[2] The results are extraordinarily durable, with minimal decay beyond 3 years after surgery. It is, however, the most demanding among technical choices currently available and is time-consuming. For these reasons it is not expedient for use when multiple valve reconstructions are indicated. It is generally not possible to repair valves in small-caliber veins by the internal technique. In our hands the use of internal valvuloplasty is restricted to the superficial femoral vein. The first superficial femoral vein valve is located immediately distal to the profunda orifice and is invariably present unless destroyed by postthrombotic changes. The second superficial femoral vein valve is located 1 to 2 inches distal to the first; it is a good standby if for some reason the first valve cannot be repaired. In approximately 16% of cases, a superficial femoral vein valve that is initially refluxive is seen to become competent by the strip test as the vein goes into mild venospasm after surgical manipulation.[3] This phenomenon is seen more commonly in smaller caliber veins, in as many as 50% of crural veins below the knee, and in approximately 40% of profunda femoral explorations. When such a situation is encountered, it has been our practice to apply a prosthetic jacket of either Dacron or ringed polytetrafluoroethylene to fit the valve station in its slightly contracted position to maintain valve competency in the postoperative state. This technique is relatively simple and rapid and does not require a venotomy. The results are durable and comparable to those obtained with internal valvuloplasty. It is an optimal and often usable technique with small-caliber veins. Used as outlined, there is a negligible incidence (<5%) of hemodynamic stenosis from the application of the prosthetic jacket. Other authors have extended the principle underlying the technique by tightening the jacket (or external prosthetic device) to stenose the valve station to the point at which overt reflux ceases.[4] We have not applied the prosthetic sleeve technique in this manner to correct refluxive valves that remain overtly incompetent even after the onset of surgically induced venospasm, for fear of producing iatrogenic stenosis. Until recently our choice for correction of such overtly refluxive valves has been application of the external repair technique described by Kistner.[5] This repair method closes the commissural valve angle, which is often wide (>11%) in the presence of overt reflux, uncorrected by mild venospasm; a venotomy is not required and the technique is rapid and applicable to small-caliber veins. Precise identification of valve attachment lines by careful adventitial dissection is essential for carrying out the procedure. This technique, however, has been superseded by the transcommissural technique described by Gloviczki et al.,[6] who used it under angioscopic control (Fig. 1). The external technique closes the commissural valve angle by partial-thickness intramural sutures traversing the venous wall along the valve attachment lines; the transcommissural technique employs externally applied full-thickness sutures that traverse the venous lumen and the valve leaflets near their base where they are attached to the venous wall. This results not only in the closure of the commissural angle but also in the tightening of the valve cusps. The latter crucial step, absent in the external technique, is in our opinion a desirable element in achieving a complete and durable repair. In performing this repair, it is not necessary to use the angioscope for the actual placement of the transcommissural sutures. Rather,

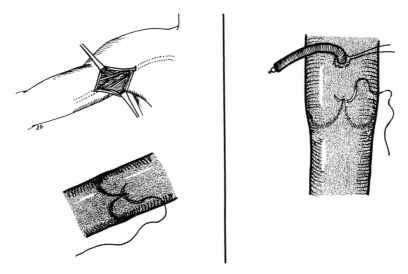

Fig. 1 Transcommissural repair under angioscopic control. Use of the angioscope is optional. The transcommissural technique is our choice for repair of an incompetent axillary vein valve in situ before transfer.

the use of an angioscope is optional for assessment of valve abnormalities, confirmation of a good repair *after* the placement of sutures, and checking for restoration of valve competence with angioscopic irrigation. The transcommissural technique is also our first choice for "bench" repair of incompetent axillary valves before transfer (Fig. 1). It is more consistently successful than the external valvuloplasty technique in restoring competency to a leaky axillary valve before transfer. The transcommissural repair can be performed as rapidly as the external valvuloplasty and can be used in small-caliber veins as well. "Redo" valve reconstruction procedures may be required when a valve repair fails after time. This is an infrequent occurrence (<5% incidence); however, recurrence of ulcers after initially successful valve reconstruction is often due to the appearance of reflux in venous segments not previously addressed or missed. In the rare instance when a redo procedure is required, general principles well established in reoperative vascular surgery should be followed. It is preferable to approach a new valve station in the axial vein unmolested by previous surgery, thus avoiding the old surgical incision. If not previously exposed during the initial surgery, the second superficial femoral vein valve may be approached by extending the old surgical incision distally (Fig. 2). A valve is commonly present

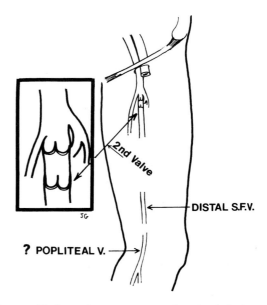

Fig. 2 Redo valve reconstruction is infrequently required. After previous proximal femoral valve reconstruction, repeat valve reconstruction may be performed on the second superficial femoral vein valve or the distal superficial femoral vein valve at the adductor hiatus. The popliteal vein valve is less satisfactory (see text).

in the superficial femoral vein at the adductor hiatus; this is our preference for a redo procedure in the event of failure of the initial repair at the groin level. The popliteal vein has a thick adventitia and valve stations are difficult to identify.

"PRIMARY" VALVE REFLUX

Approximately 55% of patients currently undergoing valve reconstruction in our center fall under this category. Worldwide experience[7] with single valve reconstruction in this pathologic entity indicates that 60% to 80% successful results can be expected short term (1 to 2 years) and approximately 50%, long term (>5 years). It is open to question whether these results can be further improved by performing multiple valve reconstructions, abolishing additional segments of venous reflux, in this entity. Multisegment, multilevel reflux is typically present. Ambulatory venous pressure recovery times are significantly improved in multiple valve reconstructions compared to single valve repairs (54% vs. 25% improvement, respectively).[8]

POSTTHROMBOTIC REFLUX

Indications for multiple valve reconstructions in postthrombotic reflux are more clear. Collateral reflux is a prominent feature of postthrombotic syndrome. Refluxive collateral vessels may be axioaxial or tributary axial (e.g., profunda-popliteal). In extreme cases in which the axial vein has failed to recanalize satisfactorily, an axial tributary feeding the collateral vessel may enlarge dramatically (axial transformation), functioning as the major outflow (and reflux) conduit. Even when the axial vein has become satisfactorily recanalized, the collaterals once formed persist without regressing. Significant collateral reflux is probably present in most cases of postthrombotic syndrome. Thrombotic destruction of axial vein valves resulting in reflux after recanalization may also be present. Various derangements of the calf venous pump, such as capacitance and compliance reduction due to the organizing thrombus, add further complexity to the hemodynamic abnormalities present in the postphlebitic limb. Although little can be done to correct calf venous pump abnormalities, the collateral and axial reflux that may be present in a symptomatic limb can be corrected. Axillary vein transfer, an inferior technical choice in primary reflux, is by default the mainstay of treatment in postthrombotic syndrome. A seemingly simple technique on the surface, axillary vein transfer in practice has proved to be technically demanding and prone to failure from even minor technical imperfections. The axillary vein valve apparatus appears to be architecturally different from those in the lower limb, with shorter valve cusps, shallower sinuses, and a wider commissural valve angle. Malcoaptation and reflux are easily produced with even minor torsional defects or suboptimal tension. Competent in the axillary position, axillary vein valves were mildly incompetent after their insertion into the femoral position in 16% of cases in our experience. Late dilatation and recurrent reflux may occur after successful insertion because of compliance mismatch. A fitted prosthetic sleeve may prevent this late failure. When executing an axillary vein transfer, it is our practice to complete the upper suture line first. We then monitor the valve for reflux through the open lower end with the proximal clamp off, while adjusting the graft for proper tension and torsional orientation and completing the distal suture line. When a suitable axillary vein valve is unavailable or unusable, a *de novo valve reconstruction* may be performed fashioning new valve cusps from a segment of saphenous or axillary vein (Fig. 3). The luminal surface of the inserted valve cusps does not have an intimal covering. In a limited experience of seven cases (mean follow-up, 1 year), there have been no instances of thrombosis despite the presence of a thrombogenic surface on the newly created valve cusps. Therapeutic anticoagulation was used. Functional benefit was evident in five of seven patients with rapid healing of stasis ulceration.

In 75% of limbs with advanced postthrombotic syndrome (PTS grades IV to VI), reparable valves were absent at groin level and axillary vein transfer or de novo valve reconstruction was required. In a surprising 87% of patients with less severe postthrombotic changes (PTS grade II or III), the first superficial femoral vein valve was spared, allowing repair by an open or closed valve reconstruction technique described earlier. The presence of such a redundant valve is an enigma and raises many questions that remain unanswered. Did the thrombotic process result from a "primary" redundant valve or did the

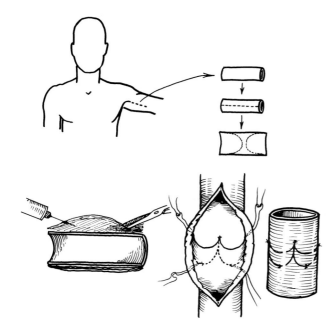

Fig. 3 In a de novo valve reconstruction, a segment of axillary vein is harvested and the adventitia is thinned out with the aid of intramural saline injection. U-shaped cusps are fashioned from an intima-like thinned-out wall and sewn in place within the host vein. The technique is facilitated by initial placement of three anchoring sutures with the knots tied outside. The horizontal mattress running suture connects the three anchors.

thrombotic process in some way render a previously competent valve refluxive? Postthrombotic reflux is generally ascribed to valve destruction and not to reflux through retained redundant valve cusps as we encountered in our experience. That the uppermost femoral valve was spared by the thrombotic process in and of itself is not surprising because venous thrombosis in the lower limb is overwhelmingly distal. The consistent presence of reflux in such a spared valve is surprising. This suggests that it may be the result rather than the cause of the thrombotic process itself. Angioscopic inspection of the postthrombotic valve reveals redundant valve cusps similar to those seen in primary valve reflux; the cusps are somewhat smaller and seated within the fibrosed venous lumen. The venous wall at the valve station has a noticeable lack of compliance under angioscopic irrigation, and postthrombotic wall changes are clearly evident in the lumen and on external inspection. We speculate that the valve redundancy resulting in reflux is secondary to these restrictive wall changes associated with postthrombotic fibrosis and luminal contraction (Fig. 4). Such wall changes may extend proximally beyond the level of actual thrombosis. The series of duplex studies of Killewich et al.[9] following venous thrombosis is supportive of such a hypothesis. These authors

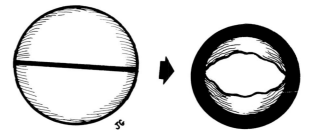

Fig. 4 Proposed explanation for the invariable presence of reflux in the femoral valve when spared in a postthrombotic limb. Restrictive wall changes may result in secondary valve redundancy similar in appearance to primary valve reflux.

reported development of reflux in valves of proximal venous segments not directly involved by the distal venous thrombus.

COMBINED OBSTRUCTION/REFLUX

It is now apparent that combined obstruction/reflux is the most common morphologic outcome of deep venous thrombus. Obstruction is compensated to a varying degree in most patients, however. Most sequelae, especially stasis ulceration, are believed to be the result of a hemodynamically significant reflux element and not the

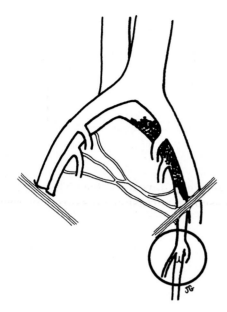

Fig. 5 Valve reconstruction below an occluded vein remains surprisingly patent and functional (see text for details).

obstruction itself. We have observed patients whose conditions evolved gradually over a period of years from an obstructive picture with leg swelling and pain to one of stasis ulceration as they develop reflux as demonstrated by serial duplex examination. The proper therapeutic approach to patients with combined obstruction/reflux is undetermined. The femoral valve was reconstructed *below* an occluded iliac vein (Fig. 5) in 11 patients with stasis ulceration. All 11 reconstructions have remained patent below the obstructed iliac vein for a mean follow-up period of 4 years. Stasis ulcers have recurred in two of 11 patients. These results are similar to those obtained in patients with primary reflux with an open iliac vein.

REFERENCES

1. Kistner RL. Surgical repair of venous valve. Straub Clin Proc 34:41-43, 1968.
2. Masuda EM, Kistner RL. Long-term results of venous valve reconstruction: A four- to twenty-one–year follow-up. J Vasc Surg 19:391-403, 1994.
3. Raju S. Technical options in venous valve reconstruction (submitted for publication).
4. Jessup G, Lane RJ. Repair of incompetent venous valves: A new technique. J Vasc Surg 8:369-373, 1988.
5. Kistner RL. Surgical technique: External venous valve repair. Straub Found Proc 55:15-16, 1990.
6. Gloviczki P, Merrell SW, Bower TC. Femoral vein valve repair under direct vision without venotomy: A modified technique with use of angioscopy. J Vasc Surg 14:645-648, 1991.
7. O'Donnell TF, Rodriguez AA. Angioscopic valvuloplasty. In Raju S, Villavicencio JL, eds. Surgical Management of Venous Disease. Baltimore: Williams & Wilkins (in press).
8. Raju S, Fredericks R, Neglen P. Venous function after venous valve reconstruction (submitted for publication).
9. Killewich LA, Bedford GR, Beach KW, Strandness DE Jr. Spontaneous lysis of deep venous thrombi: Rate and outcome. J Vasc Surg 9:89-97, 1989.

82

The Plantar Venous Plexus and Applications of A-V Impulse System Technology

JOHN V. WHITE, M.D., and JOSEPH I. ZARGE, M.D.

Although anatomically distinct, the arterial and venous circulations of the lower extremity are inextricably linked. Each component plays a vital but dependent role in tissue perfusion and any alteration in that role is readily evident in the function of the microvasculature. Arterial blood is transported from the heart to the periphery by vessels that continually increase in number and decrease in diameter until ultimately the capillary bed is reached. With each successive division of the arterial tree, blood becomes slightly more diluted until a hematocrit level of approximately 30% is reached within the microcirculation.[1] This increase in liquid content enhances the diffusion of oxygen and nutrients from the capillaries into the tissues. As the fluid component of blood leaves the lumen to bathe the pericapillary tissues, hemoconcentration occurs and the hematocrit level and colloid oncotic pressure begin to rise. Toward the venous end of the capillary bed, pressure and oncotic gradients favor the movement of fluid from the tissues into the microvasculature, enhancing the removal of metabolic waste products. Residual tissue fluid is taken up and transported to the heart by the lymphatic system.

Since flow across the capillary bed is primarily determined by the pressure gradient established by arterial inflow and venous outflow, higher arterial inflow pressures and lower venous outflow pressures favor capillary blood flow. Arterial inflow pressures are increased by elevating mean arterial blood pressure, whereas venous outflow pressures can be reduced by venous pump mechanisms. In the setting of a constant venous outflow pressure, flow through the microcirculation is proportional to arterial inflow pressure. Conversely, in the setting of a fixed arterial inflow pressure, tissue perfusion is inversely proportional to venous outflow pressure. These principles dictate that either a substantial reduction of arterial inflow pressures or an escalation of venous outflow pressures will lead to a decrease in capillary blood flow. This reduction in microvascular perfusion pressure can result in tissue hypoxia and death, such as that seen in deep venous thrombosis, phlegmasia cerulea dolens, and arterial insufficiency. In each of these disorders, capillary pressure gradients are significantly altered, resulting at times in severe tissue edema and ischemia.

An understanding of the mechanisms by which venous outflow of the lower extremity is maintained is critical, then, not only for the prevention of venous disease but also for the preservation of adequate and appropriate tissue perfusion.

BASIC MECHANISMS OF VENOUS FLOW

The traditional understanding of venous outflow is based on the concept of the calf muscle pump.[2] In the late 1960s, Ludbrook[3,4] studied the impact of muscular compression on flow within the intramuscular venules and its effect on proximal venous flow, demonstrating that compression of the gastrocnemius and soleal muscles causes the forceful ejection of blood from the venules, which increases flow through the popliteal vein. On relaxation of the muscles, blood is drawn into the venules from the periphery. This action reduces the pressure within the regional venous system to less than half that of the static standing venous pressure.

The mechanism by which blood is ejected from the more distal leg and foot veins is less clear. It was previously believed that the calf muscles compressed the veins in a bellowslike fashion. On relaxation of the muscles, blood was presumably drawn from the periphery and subcutaneous veins into the deep venous system. There are, however, many fundamental problems with this concept. In an ambulating adult venous pressure within the tibial veins frequently exceeds 100 mm Hg.[5] Compartment pressures rarely exceed 60 mm Hg, so it would not be possible for

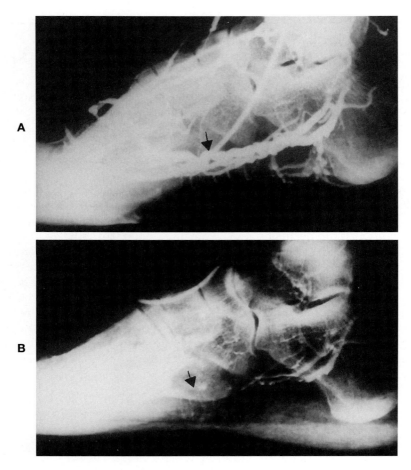

Fig. 1 The appearance of the plantar venous plexus. **A,** Plexus full (arrow). When the foot is relaxed and in a dependent position, the plantar venous plexus, which spans the plantar surface of the foot under the arch, fills. **B,** Plexus empty (arrow). On weight bearing, the veins are stretched slightly and empty rapidly upward.

the muscle to pump blood from the interstitium into the veins.[6] Thus it is unlikely that the calf muscles are the principal or sole mechanism by which the tibial and pedal veins empty.

Recent investigations have documented the presence of a plantar venous reservoir that may also play a significant role in venous outflow of the leg.[7-9] Using videophlebography, Gardner and Fox[7] injected contrast medium into a vein of the forefoot and studied the pattern of upward flow. In doing so, they were able to identify a pool of dye remaining within the foot that was unaffected by ankle dorsiflexion or plantar flexion (Fig. 1, A). This reservoir is composed of the venae comitantes of the lateral plantar artery veins, located between the superficial and deep intrinsic muscles of the foot. As weight is placed simultaneously on the heel and metatarsal heads, these veins become stretched and forcefully compressed, ejecting blood into the deep venous system of the calf (Fig. 1, B). This physiologic foot pump is capable of generating local venous pressures of over 100 mm Hg, suggesting it can propel blood upward even in an upright individual.[10] The synchronized upward displacement of blood into the calf may be required for appropriate function of the calf muscle pump. Based on this information, a mechanical device, the A-V Impulse System (The Kendall Co., Mansfield, Mass.), has been developed for the enhancement of the plantar venous foot pump.

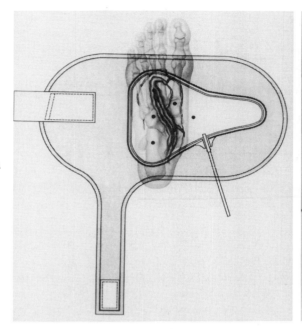 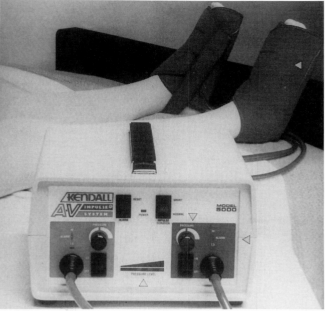

Fig. 2 Schematic representation of the ImPad foot cover and the A-V Impulse System. **A,** The air bladder within the foot cover is sufficiently sized to span the length and breadth of the plantar venous plexus on the sole of the foot. The foot covers containing the air bladders are connected to an air impulse generator by small flexible air hoses. **B,** The controller is capable of regulating the amount of pressure delivered to the air bladders in the sole of the foot.

THE A-V IMPULSE SYSTEM FOOT PUMP

The A-V Impulse System was developed to simulate the impact of weight bearing on the plantar venous plexus in a nonambulatory patient. The system consists of a foot cover, or boot, containing an air bladder (ImPad foot cover, The Kendall Co.) that, when appropriately applied, spans the area on the sole of the foot that overlies the plantar venous reservoir (Fig. 2). The air bladder is inflated within 0.4 second to a pressure of 50 to 200 mm Hg by an air impulse generated by a controller and transmitted by a flexible hose. Inflation pressure can be adjusted on the controller. The rigid sole of the foot cover beneath the inflation pad contains and directs the air impulse and ImPad inflation toward the sole of the foot. The controller rapidly inflates the ImPad to flatten and stretch the plantar arch, mimicking the natural effects of weight bearing. A 3-second impulse is then applied to the sole of the foot approximately every 20 seconds, allowing time for the plantar venous plexus to refill. Inflation pressure is precisely maintained by the controller's feedback mechanism, a unit that contains alarms which sound automatically if inflation pressure is too high or too low for effective use.

The impact of the A-V Impulse System device on venous outflow from the lower extremity has been assessed in the vascular laboratory. Both Doppler ultrasound and color-flow duplex imaging have demonstrated a 250% increase in mean blood flow velocity through the popliteal vein, which is transmitted to the common femoral vein.[11] These results suggest that augmentation of the plantar venous pump can enhance venous outflow and reduce venous pressure within the lower extremity.

APPLICATIONS OF THE A-V IMPULSE SYSTEM FOOT PUMP

By enhancing venous outflow and reducing venous pressure, the A-V Impulse System can reduce the risk of deep venous thrombosis, decrease posttraumatic lower extremity edema, and improve flow across the capillary bed resulting in increased tissue perfusion.

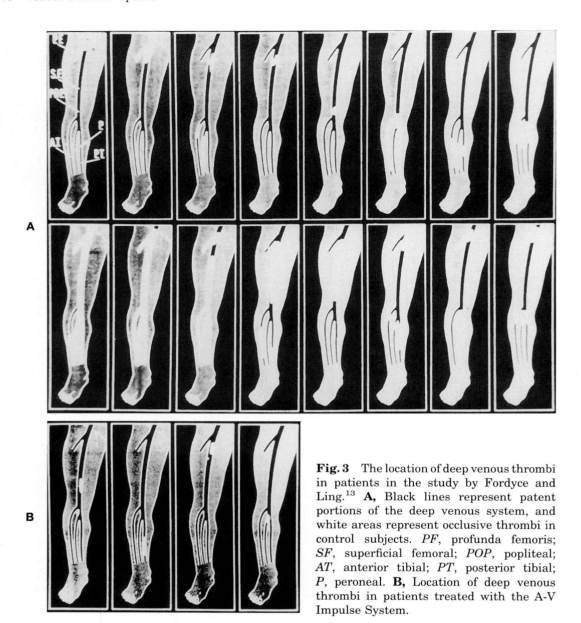

Fig. 3 The location of deep venous thrombi in patients in the study by Fordyce and Ling.[13] **A,** Black lines represent patent portions of the deep venous system, and white areas represent occlusive thrombi in control subjects. *PF*, profunda femoris; *SF*, superficial femoral; *POP*, popliteal; *AT*, anterior tibial; *PT*, posterior tibial; *P*, peroneal. **B,** Location of deep venous thrombi in patients treated with the A-V Impulse System.

Numerous studies have documented the effectiveness of the system for the prevention of deep venous thrombosis after joint surgery. Wilson et al.[12] evaluated the A-V Impulse System in a prospective randomized trial of 60 patients undergoing total knee replacement. The incidence of major deep venous thrombosis was reduced from 59.4% in the untreated group to 17.8% in those using the foot pump. These observations were expanded by Fordyce and Ling,[13] who assessed the system for deep venous thrombosis prophylaxis in patients undergoing total hip arthroplasty. Thrombi were noted in 16 of 40 (40%) of untreated patients but in only two of 39 (5%) of patients who used the A-V Impulse System (Fig. 3). In a study of 74 patients undergoing total hip replacement, Bradley et al.[14] added the foot pump to a prophylactic regimen of 5000 U of heparin administered subcutaneously every 12 hours and 400 mg of hydroxychloroquine sulphate, also given every 12 hours. There was an overall incidence of deep venous thrombosis of 27.3% in the 44 patients for when the pump was not prescribed and 6.6% in

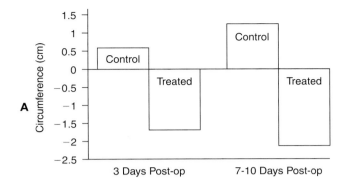

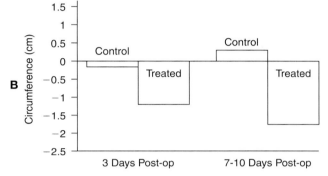

Fig. 4 Mean reduction in swelling in calf and thigh of treated vs. control group. Use of the A-V Impulse System in patients sustaining lower extremity trauma, after leg surgery or traumatic leg injury, resulted in significantly reduced swelling in both the thigh **(A)** and the calf **(B)**. (From Stranks SJ, McKenzie NA, Grover ML, Fail T. The A-V Impulse System reduces deep-vein thrombosis and swelling after hemiarthroplasty for hip fracture. J Bone Joint Surg [Br] 74B:775-778, 1992.)

30 patients who had the pump added to their prophylactic regimen. Santori et al.[15] compared 65 hip replacement patients who used the A-V Impulse System with 67 patients treated with calcium-heparin alone. The incidence of deep venous thrombosis in the two groups was 13.4% and 35.4%, respectively, and in the heparin group there was one fatal pulmonary embolism.

These studies confirm that the mechanical activation of the plantar venous foot pump is effective for the enhancement of venous outflow of the lower extremity in nonambulatory patients.

The A-V Impulse System is also capable of reducing leg swelling after soft tissue injury. Gardner et al.[16] noted that maintenance of the plantar foot pump function was an effective method for reducing posttraumatic swelling. In 11 patients with severe tibial fractures, the authors noted a rapid reduction in both swelling and compartment pressures in more than half of the study patients. Similar results were noted by Myerson and Henderson[17] studying patients with acute swelling after major elective or posttraumatic surgery of the foot or ankle. In a prospective, randomized, controlled trial, Stranks et al.[18] evaluated the impact of the A-V Impulse System on thigh and calf swelling in 82 patients undergoing hip arthroplasty after hip fracture. They noted a significant ($p < .001$) reduction in both thigh and calf swelling in patients treated with the device compared with control subjects (Fig. 4).

THE A-V IMPULSE SYSTEM AND POSTREVASCULARIZATION EDEMA

Because of the ability of the system to reduce posttraumatic injury, we have undertaken a study to determine its effects on postrevascularization edema. Postrevascularization edema is multifactorial. It is recognized that it occurs in more than 50% of patients undergoing peripheral revascularization and results in wound complications in a significant number of these cases.[19] Altered capillary perfusion pressures, increased capillary leakage, and altered lymphatic function have all been implicated as causes.[20-22] The A-V Impulse System is capable of increasing capillary flow by augmenting venous outflow, which may result in a reduction of fluid extravasation from the capillary bed and a decrease in postrevascularization edema.

To evaluate this benefit of the system, a protocol was established in which patients were treated either with compression bandaging or the A-V Impulse System pumping of the foot of the operative leg, beginning in the recovery room and continuing for 7 days. Patients undergoing distal vascular reconstruction for limb salvage were randomized to the control or pump group at the time of surgery. The ability of the system to augment femoral and popliteal venous velocity was evaluated preoperatively and on postoperative day 7. Calf and ankle circumferences were measured daily, beginning immediately preoperatively and continuing until postoperative day 7. The preoperative calf and ankle circumferences of the operative leg were taken as baseline values. Wound complications were also recorded.

As demonstrated in volunteers, there was a significant increase in venous velocities within both the common femoral and popliteal veins despite the presence of significant lower extremity ischemia (Fig. 5). Preliminary results in 10 patients demonstrated a significant benefit of intermittent pneumatic compression of the plantar venous plexus by the A-V Impulse System after lower extremity revascularization. Over the 7-day period of observation, control subjects demonstrated a progressive increase in calf circumference that was greatly reduced in patients who used the device (Fig. 6). This increase in calf circumference occurred despite early limited ambulation in the postoperative period. Control subjects also demonstrated progressive ankle edema, which was very prominent on postoperative day 1 and peaked on postoperative day 5 (Fig. 7). There was then a reduction of ankle edema that may have correlated to the onset of ambulation. The system markedly reduced ankle edema during the first 5 postoperative days.

The relationship between the A-V Impulse System and postrevascularization edema was well demonstrated in one patient (Fig. 8) in whom edema in the immediate postoperative period was well controlled by the system. On postoperative day 2, the patient underwent a second toe amputation unrelated to the use of the foot pump. Because of this, the device was not used for 24 hours. On postoperative day 3, before the system was again placed, the patient demonstrated significant ankle edema. This ankle edema resolved with resumption of the use of this device. In this small series there were no wound complications in the immediate postoperative period in patients treated with the system; however, wound complications occurred in three of five patients in the control group (Fig. 9).

Perhaps most interesting is the use of the A-V Impulse System to enhance capillary blood flow in patients with arterial occlusive disease. Previous studies of the effects of intermittent sequential pneumatic compression on the lower extremity have demonstrated that in addition to augmenting venous flow, PGI_2 production and plasmin activity are increased and venous pressure and thrombin activity are reduced.[23,24] It is also recognized that patients with severe chronic distal ischemia may experience fibrin deposition within the distal arterial tree. Morgan et al.[25] recently studied the impact of intermittent pneumatic compression of the plantar venous plexus on arterial inflow in the setting of significant arterial occlusive disease and distal ischemia. They studied 10 control subjects and 10 subjects with peripheral vascular disease and a mean ankle/brachial index of 0.62. Assessing arterial flow by noninvasive means, the investigators demonstrated a mean increase in popliteal artery flow of 93% over resting flow in control subjects. They also demonstrated a mean popliteal artery flow increase of 84% over resting flow in patients with peripheral vascular disease.

Based on these interesting results, we have undertaken a study to determine whether augmentation of venous outflow can result in enhanced arterial inflow in patients with severe peripheral arterial occlusive disease. Although this study has only recently been undertaken and just four selected patients have been treated, it appears as though the A-V Impulse System may be of benefit in patients with severe distal

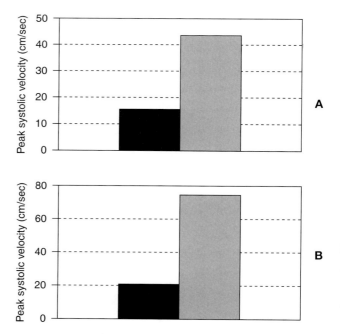

Fig. 5 The impact of the A-V Impulse System on common femoral and popliteal vein velocities in patients with lower extremity ischemia. Baseline flow (black) in the common femoral vein **(A)** and the popliteal vein **(B)** was significantly augmented by the system (gray) despite significant peripheral ischemia.

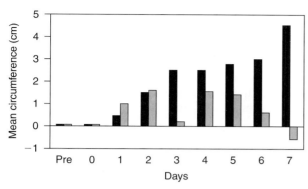

Fig. 6 Postrevascularization calf edema after femorotibial bypass. Control subjects demonstrated a progressive and significant increase in calf circumference (black bars), which was greatly reduced by the A-V Impulse System (gray bars). Note that by day 7, there is not only a reduction in postrevascularization edema, but also a decrease in baseline calf circumference suggesting resolution of the perioperative dependent edema.

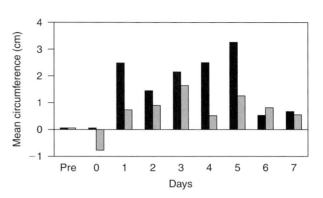

Fig. 7 Postrevascularization ankle edema after femorotibial bypass. There was immediate onset of ankle edema and an increase in ankle circumference in all control subjects (black bars). Ankle edema began to resolve spontaneously by postoperative day 6. Ankle edema during the first 5 postoperative days was significantly reduced by the application of the A-V Impulse System (gray bars).

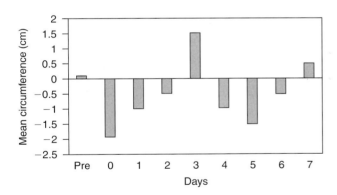

Fig. 8 Interruption of the A-V Impulse System in postrevascularization ankle edema. This profile of postoperative ankle circumference in a patient who had undergone a femorodistal posterior tibial in situ bypass demonstrates that the reduction in postoperative edema achieved with the system is dependent on continuous use of the device. On postoperative day 2 the device was removed and the patient was taken to the operating room for amputation. The device was replaced on postoperative day 3 after measurement of ankle circumference.

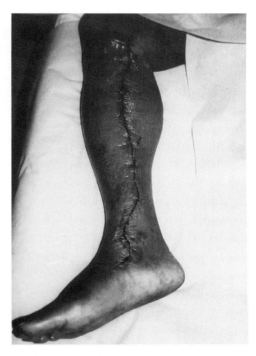

Fig. 9 Postrevascularization edema in a patient undergoing a femoral–dorsalis pedis in situ bypass. Note blackening of the wound edges and early signs of peri-incisional skin sloughing. This patient eventually required skin grafting for wound closure.

ischemia and unreconstructable vascular disease.

The following case illustrates the results we have seen. A 44-year-old blind diabetic woman presented with severe right leg ischemia. As expected, noninvasive studies revealed falsely elevated pressures throughout. Angiography demonstrated a 5 cm occlusion of the left superficial femoral artery with reconstitution of the above-knee popliteal artery and discontinuous runoff to the foot by peroneal and anterior tibial arteries (Fig. 10). The posterior tibial artery was occluded at the level of the ankle, and no dorsalis pedis pulse was identified. Because the patient was deemed unsuitable for very distal arterial reconstruction, she underwent balloon angioplasty of the superficial femoral arterial lesion with an excellent technical result. However, she continued to have severe rest pain of the left foot with no change in

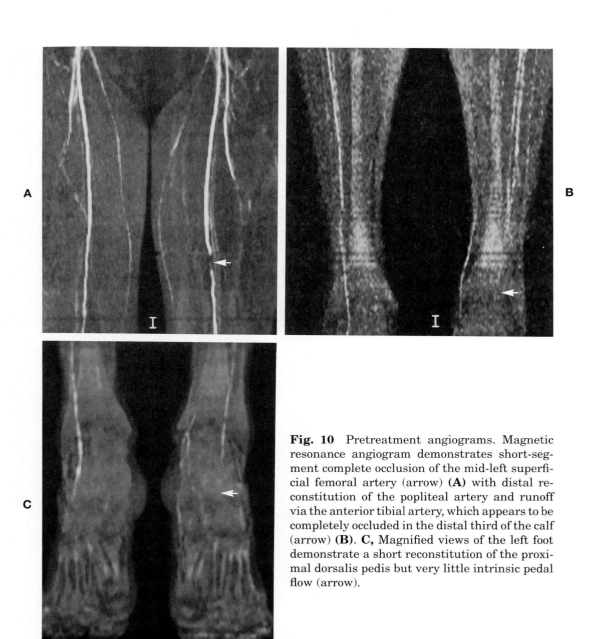

Fig. 10 Pretreatment angiograms. Magnetic resonance angiogram demonstrates short-segment complete occlusion of the mid-left superficial femoral artery (arrow) **(A)** with distal reconstitution of the popliteal artery and runoff via the anterior tibial artery, which appears to be completely occluded in the distal third of the calf (arrow) **(B)**. **C,** Magnified views of the left foot demonstrate a short reconstitution of the proximal dorsalis pedis but very little intrinsic pedal flow (arrow).

her manifestations of severe left foot ischemia. Therefore the patient was placed in a 15-degree reverse Trendelenburg position, and the A-V Impulse System was used to decrease peripheral venous pressures in the hopes of augmenting arterial inflow. After 3 days of intermittent use of the pump, the patient's foot warmed significantly and 2 days later, she had a palpable dorsalis pedis pulse. Repeat angiography demonstrated continuous flow by the superficial femoral and popliteal arteries through the anterior tibial artery into the dorsalis pedis, with reconstitution of the pedal arch (Fig. 11).

It is likely that enhancement of venous outflow and a reduction of distal venous pressures permitted both increased arterial inflow and activation of the regional lytic system, resulting in peripheral thrombolysis. The patient's necrotic toe lesions completely resolved.

CONCLUSION

The plantar venous plexus appears to play a critical role in venous outflow from the lower extremity. Compression of this vascular plexus rapidly ejects blood from the foot and initiates flow through the tibial veins. This flow is augmented by the calf muscle pump of the soleus and gastrocnemius muscle groups. A reduction of venous pressures and augmentation of venous flow have numerous benefits that may significantly extend the vascular surgeon's ability to treat patients with peripheral arterial and venous disease. By reducing pressures and augmenting local thrombolytic pathways, posttraumatic and postrevascularization edema can be reduced and arterial inflow augmented. Further investigation is certainly warranted to more clearly define the role of this technology in the future of vascular therapy.

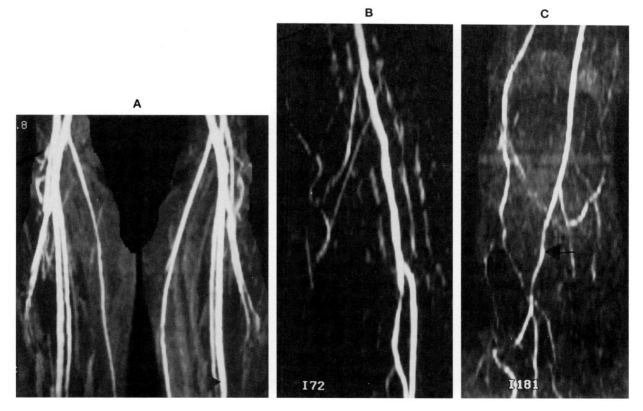

Fig. 11 Posttreatment magnetic resonance angiogram. **A,** Excellent results were achieved after balloon angioplasty of the left superficial femoral artery. **B,** Reconstitution of the distal superficial femoral artery and popliteal artery with runoff via the anterior tibial artery. **C,** Flow through the anterior tibial artery was continuous to the ankle, and magnified views of the foot showed a completely patent dorsalis pedis as well as an increased number of pedal vessels.

REFERENCES

1. Intaglietta M. Microcirculatory effects of hemodilution: Background and analysis. In Tuma RF, White JV, Messmer K, eds. The Role of Hemodilution in Optimal Patient Care. San Francisco: W. Zuckschwerdt Verlag, 1989, pp 21-41.
2. Sumner DS. Hemodynamics and pathophysiology of venous disease. In Rutherford RB, ed. Vascular Surgery, 3rd ed. Philadelphia: WB Saunders, 1989, pp 1483-1504.
3. Ludbrook J. The musculovenous pumps of the human lower limb. Am Heart J 71:635, 1966.
4. Ludbrook J. Aspects of Venous Function in the Lower Limbs. Springfield, Ill.: Charles C Thomas, 1966.
5. Husni EA, Ximenes JOC, Goyette EM. Elastic support of the lower limbs in hospital patients: A critical study. JAMA 214:1456, 1970.
6. Alimi YS, Barthelemy P, Juhan C. Venous pump of the calf: A study of venous and muscular pressures. J Vasc Surg 20:728-735, 1994.
7. Gardner AMN, Fox RH. The venous pump of the human foot: Preliminary report. Bristol Med Chir J 98:109-112, 1983.
8. Koslow AR, DeWeese JA. Anatomical and mechanical aspects of a plantar venous plexus. Presented at the Jobst Symposium on Current Issues in Venous Disease, Chicago, 1988.
9. Gardner AMN, Fox RH. The venous footpump: Influence on tissue perfusion and prevention of venous thrombosis. Ann Rheum Dis 51:1173-1178, 1992.
10. Gardner AMN, Fox RH. The Return of Blood to the Heart, 2nd ed. London: John Libbey, 1993.
11. Laverick MD, McGivern RC, Crone MD, Mollan RAB. A comparison of the effects of electrical calf muscle stimulation and the venous foot pump on venous blood flow in the lower leg. Phlebology 5:285-290, 1990.
12. Wilson NV, Das SK, Kakkar VV, Maurice HD, Smibert JG, Thomas EM, Nixon JE. Thrombo-embolic prophylaxis in total knee replacement. J Bone Joint Surg [Br] 74B:50-52, 1992.
13. Fordyce MJF, Ling RSM. A venous foot pump reduces thrombosis after total hip replacement. J Bone Joint Surg [Br] 74B:45-49, 1992.
14. Bradley JG, Krugener GH, Jager HJ. The effectiveness of intermittent plantar venous compression in prevention of deep venous thrombosis after total hip arthroplasty. J Arthroplasty 8:57-61, 1993.
15. Santori FS, Vitullo A, Stopponi M, Santori N, Ghera S. Prophylaxis against DVT in total hip replacement: Comparison of heparin and foot impulse pump. J Bone Joint Surg 76:579-583, 1994.
16. Gardner AMN, Fox RH, MacEachern AG, Lawrence C, Bunker TD, Ling RSM. Reduction of post-traumatic swelling and compartment pressure by impulse compression of the foot. J Bone Joint Surg [Br] 72B:810-815, 1990.
17. Myerson MS, Henderson MR. Clinical applications of a pneumatic intermittent impulse compression device after trauma and major surgery to the foot and ankle. Foot Ankle 14:198-202, 1993.
18. Stranks SJ, McKenzie NA, Grover ML, Fail T. The A-V Impulse System reduces deep-vein thrombosis and swelling after hemiarthroplasty for hip fracture. J Bone Joint Surg [Br] 74B:775-778, 1992.
19. Schwartz ME, Harrington EB, Schanzer H. Wound complications after in situ bypass. J Vasc Surg 7:802-807, 1988.
20. Porter JM, Lindell TD, Lakin PC. Leg edema following femoropopliteal autogenous vein bypass. Arch Surg 105:883-888, 1972.
21. Schubart PJ, Porter JM. Leg edema following femorodistal bypass. In Bergan JJ, Yao JST, eds. Reoperative Arterial Surgery. Orlando: Grune and Stratton, 1986, pp 311-330.
22. AbuRahma AF, Woodruff BA, Lucente FC. Edema after femoropopliteal bypass surgery: Lymphatic and venous theories of causation. J Vasc Surg 11:461-467, 1990.
23. Guyton DP, Khayat A, Husni EA, Schreiber H. Elevated levels of 6-keto-prostaglandin-$F_{1\alpha}$ from a lower extremity during external pneumatic compression. Surg Gynecol Obstet 166:338-342, 1988.
24. Weitz J, Michelsen J, Gold K, Owen J, Carpenter D. Effect of intermittent pneumatic calf compression on postoperative thrombin and plasmin activity. Thromb Haemost 56:198-201, 1986.
25. Morgan RH, Carolan G, Psaila JV, Gardner AMN, Fox RH, Woodcock JP. Arterial flow enhancement by impulse compression. Vasc Surg 25:8-16, 1991.

83

Aggressive Interventional Treatment for Acute Iliofemoral Venous Thrombosis: Are Surgical Thrombectomy and Regional Catheter-Directed Urokinase Beneficial?

ANTHONY J. COMEROTA, M.D.

Patients with iliofemoral deep venous thrombosis (DVT) that fits the description of phlegmasia cerulea dolens often have a high risk of pulmonary emboli, have significant acute extremity morbidity, and are likely to have severe, chronic posthrombotic sequelae.[1,2] Although traditional teaching indicates that bed rest, leg elevation, and anticoagulation therapy are adequate for rapid and uneventful recovery, this is not the case in patients with an occlusive thrombus in the iliofemoral venous system. When treating patients with acute iliofemoral venous thrombosis, the intuitive desire is to eliminate the thrombus and restore unobstructed venous drainage from the involved leg. This was the theory behind initial attempts at venous thrombectomy. Although the preliminary reports were encouraging,[3,4] the long-term results failed to sustain the initial optimism. Operative morbidity was an issue and problems included pulmonary emboli, significant blood loss necessitating transfusion, and prolonged hospitalization frequently associated with operative mortality.[5] Although more recent reports indicate substantially improved outcomes,[6,7] venous thrombectomy has not been accepted as a reasonable treatment for these patients in the United States.

Thrombolytic therapy is an alternative with the potential to restore patency to the occluded iliofemoral venous system with the use of drugs. Although patients with infrainguinal DVT have a reasonably good chance of experiencing clot lysis if treated with intravenous infusions of thrombolytic agents, recanalization is frequently not attained in patients with iliofemoral venous thrombosis treated with systemic fibrinolysis.[8,9] The failure of these patients to respond to systemic lytic therapy is understandable. The iliofemoral clot is packed into the iliofemoral venous segment and has little, if any, exposure to flowing blood. Since blood carries the plasminogen activator, only a slight amount of activator ever reaches the thrombus. These patients therefore require delivery of the plasminogen activator by a method other than that used in patients with infrainguinal DVT. I believe that thrombolytic therapy can be successful if the drug reaches the clot. Therefore I recommend direct intraclot infusion for patients with iliofemoral venous thrombosis. Ipsilateral intra-arterial infusion with systemic doses of plasminogen activators has been used in patients with severe phlegmasia cerulea dolens with impending gangrene. Whether this is more advantageous than direct intraclot infusion remains to be established, although it is my impression that infrainguinal thrombus can be lysed with this technique. However, the iliofemoral thrombus persists, necessitating direct methods of therapy (intraclot infusion or thrombectomy).

The rationale for aggressive therapy is that iliofemoral DVT is associated with severe acute and chronic morbidity. The acute symptoms are easily recognized on presentation. Long-term morbidity is the rule with iliofemoral venous thrombosis. Contemporary studies evaluating venous function following thrombosis indicate that the severity of the postthrombotic sequelae is related to the magnitude of the acute thrombosis.[10] The pathophysiology of postthrombotic syndrome is ambulatory venous hypertension, and the pathologic components leading to ambulatory venous hypertension are valvular incompetence and luminal obstruction. The most severe manifestations of postthrombotic syn-

---

Supported in part by National Institutes of Health grant K07HL02658-01.

drome occur in patients who have both obstruction and valvular incompetence.[11] Recent studies have demonstrated that valvular function can be preserved after physiologic lysis of DVT, especially when lysis occurs over a relatively short period.[12,13] Better preservation of long-term valvular function would thus be expected with therapeutic fibrinolysis, if lysis were successful. This has been demonstrated in three prospective randomized series.[14-16] Postthrombotic sequelae following thrombolytic therapy typically occur if treatment has failed or thrombosis has recurred, not if lysis has been successful and vessels remain patent. Similarly, when patients with iliofemoral venous thrombosis undergo surgery, the best results are achieved if patency is restored to the iliofemoral venous system.[6] We instituted a strategy of aggressive regional therapy using contemporary venous thrombectomy technique or catheter-directed lysis. Our initial experience was favorable and indicates that our approach is substantially better than standard anticoagulation therapy.[17]

MATERIAL AND METHODS

Between May 1988 and May 1994, 14 patients were admitted with occlusive iliofemoral venous thrombosis. Ages ranged from 20 to 60 years (mean, 40 years). The average duration of leg symptoms was 4 to 5 days (range, 2 to 10 days) with an average of 4.2 days (range, 2 to 8 days) for patients who had surgery and 4.6 days (range, 2 to 10 days) for those treated with catheter-directed thrombolysis. The diagnosis was established in all patients by means of venous duplex imaging and iliofemoral phlebography. Venous duplex imaging was used to evaluate the infrainguinal deep venous system. Iliofemoral phlebography was selectively performed to assess the proximal extent of thrombus; however, routine contralateral iliocavagraphy was used to evaluate the contralateral iliofemoral system and vena cava. Although four patients were known to have had a recent pulmonary embolism, the remainder had no symptoms of pulmonary embolism. Although eight patients underwent ventilation/perfusion scanning before treatment, routine posttreatment ventilation/perfusion scanning was not performed. Patients who had a pulmonary embolism during the present thrombotic episode had a vena caval filter inserted. If the patient had large, irregular, and nonocclusive vena caval clots, a vena caval filter was also inserted. We

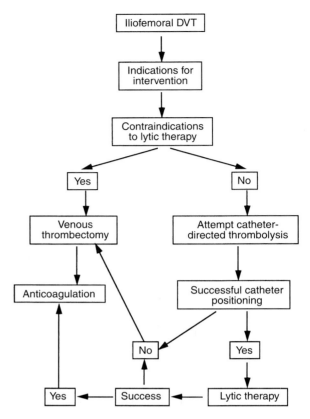

Fig. 1 Algorithm for treatment of iliofemoral venous thrombosis.

have not routinely placed caval filters preoperatively or before catheter-directed thrombolysis if the thrombus is limited to the iliofemoral venous system. However, six of the patients had caval filters in place at the time of treatment. Three patients had occlusive vena caval thrombosis extending above a previously placed filter, and three patients had a caval filter inserted as part of the current therapy.

In patients who had no contraindication to thrombolytic therapy, catheter-directed thrombolysis was attempted. Patients in whom the catheter-directed approach failed and those with an absolute contraindication to thrombolytic therapy or multiple relative contraindications underwent venous thrombectomy and construction of an arteriovenous fistula (AVF) under general anesthesia (Fig. 1). A cross-pubic venous bypass was constructed if unobstructed ipsilateral iliofemoral venous patency could not be restored.

The cause of acute venous thrombosis was established in all patients. Postoperative and/or posttraumatic thrombosis occurred in eight pa-

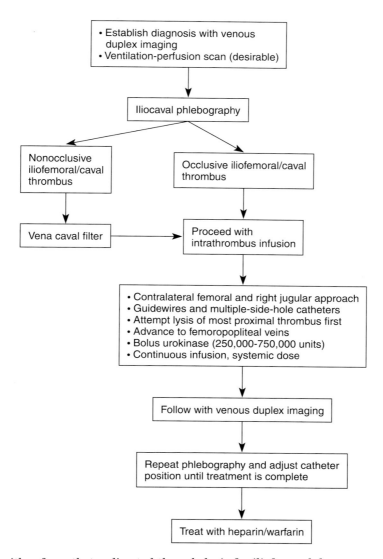

Fig. 2 Algorithm for catheter-directed thrombolysis for iliofemoral deep venous thrombosis.

tients, malignancy was found in four, and an underlying hypercoagulable state was found in two patients. Follow-up was 8 to 72 months (mean, 29 months). Two patients were lost to follow-up after 11 and 36 months, and two patients died of metastatic cancer 2 weeks and 8 months, respectively, after therapy.

CATHETER-DIRECTED THROMBOSIS

The technique of catheter-directed thrombolysis for iliofemoral DVT is summarized in Fig. 2. Direct infusion is achieved by placing a catheter from the contralateral femoral vein or the right jugular vein, or both. Alternately, an ipsilateral femoral vein catheter can be used at the discretion of the surgeon. Use of the contralateral femoral vein or the jugular vein allows placement of a vena caval filter, if indicated, before the infusion is begun. Although I do not routinely insert vena caval filters before catheter-directed lytic therapy, they were inserted in three patients (two had a pulmonary embolism and one had a large, nonocclusive caval thrombus). The indications for caval filtration in this setting are evolving. If a venous thrombectomy is subsequently required, a caval filter imposes technical limitations that can compromise operative results.

Once a guidewire is appropriately positioned in the thrombus, catheters with multiple side holes are advanced into the thrombus to ensure maximal delivery of the lytic agent to the fibrin-bound plasminogen. Systemic doses of plasminogen activators are used. I administer urokinase as a 250,000- to 500,000-unit bolus followed by a continuous infusion of 250,000 units/hr. In three patients, bolus doses (10 mg) of recombinant tissue plasminogen activator (rt-PA) followed by urokinase infusion (250,000 U/hr) were used to take advantage of potential synergistic fibrinolysis.[9-11] Venous duplex imaging is used to track the lysis of the infrainguinal clot and visualize as much of the iliac venous system as possible. Phlebography is performed through the infusion catheters and repeated at 12- to 24-hour intervals. Therapy is continued until maximal lysis is achieved. Routine coagulation studies are performed before treatment. During treatment, prothrombin times, partial thromboplastin times, fibrinogen levels, and fibrin(ogen) split product measurements are monitored at 12-hour intervals. If the fibrinogen level falls below 100 mg/dl, the lytic agent is stopped for 6 to 12 hours and additional heparin is given. Lytic infusion is resumed when the fibrinogen level rises above 100 mg/dl. After completion of the lytic infusion, patients continue to receive heparin and, later, oral anticoagulants. If the infusion catheters cannot be appropriately positioned within the iliac vein thrombus, a venous thrombectomy is performed.

VENOUS THROMBECTOMY

Although a venous thrombectomy can be performed with the patient under local anesthesia, general anesthesia is preferred. Because most patients are receiving heparin and continue to receive anticoagulants after the operation, regional (spinal or epidural) anesthesia is contraindicated. I prefer to use general endotracheal anesthesia with application of at least 10 cm of positive end-expiratory pressure. Patients have 2 units of blood cross-matched, and autotransfusion devices are used routinely to minimize transfusion requirements.

A vertical inguinal incision is made over the femoral vessels, and the common femoral, superficial femoral, deep femoral, and saphenous veins are mobilized and controlled. Heparin (100 U/kg or more) is administered to achieve systemic anticoagulation. A transverse or slightly oblique venotomy is made in the distal common femoral vein just proximal to the saphenofemoral junction. The proximal thrombus is removed with passage of an 8 or 10 Fr venous thrombectomy catheter. Balloon catheter occlusion of the vena cava from the contralateral femoral vein is not attempted before thrombectomy because the likelihood of pulmonary embolism is low.[18,19] Positive end-expiratory pressure is applied during the thrombectomy, further minimizing the possibility of pulmonary embolism. Patients who are awake can perform the Valsalva maneuver. If the patient has a vena caval filter in place, fluoroscopy is used to guide the passage of the thrombectomy catheter, and liquid contrast medium is used to inflate the balloon.

The proximal venous segment is always assessed by completion phlebography, which is carried out by injection of 25 to 30 ml of contrast material through the common femoral venotomy. In light of the inflow occlusion, this technique generally provides good visualization of the entire iliac venous system. An alternative method is to use direct venoscopy with an angioscope as reported by Loeprecht.[20] I have not had success with venous angioscopy because of an inability to adequately clear the lumen of blood draining from collateral veins.

If patency cannot be restored to the proximal venous segment or if it is found to be extrinsically compressed, a cross-pubic venous bypass is performed with an 8 to 10 mm externally supported polytetrafluoroethylene (PTFE) graft.[17,21] A 3 to 4 mm AVF is created approximately 4 to 6 cm distal to the origin of the superficial femoral artery. Alternatively, a simple cross-pubic venous bypass can be performed with bilateral end-to-side anastomoses and the AVF constructed with the saphenous vein or a large proximal branch anastomosed to the superficial femoral artery.

After proximal thrombectomy, the distal thrombus is removed. As much clot as possible is extracted by the extrusion technique either by stroking along the course of the distal veins or by wrapping a tight Esmarch bandage proximally from the foot. Attempts are then made to pass a Fogarty venous thrombectomy catheter distally, although its passage is usually prohibited by venous valves. Others have reported exploration of the posterior tibial vein into which a catheter is introduced and advanced to the common femoral vein. A thrombectomy catheter is attached and guided distally, and a thrombectomy of the entire leg can then be performed.[18] I have used this technique only once, and it may represent an improvement over what can be achieved by compression/extrusion alone; however, the endothelial damage created by balloon catheters is always a concern. Venography can be performed through the distal point of access to assess the adequacy of thrombectomy.

An AVF is constructed with a large proximal branch of the greater saphenous vein or the proximal greater saphenous vein itself if a branch is not available. In most patients the proximal greater saphenous vein usually requires thrombectomy to restore patency prior to AVF; therefore one does not sacrifice it for the AVF. Because the saphenous vein enters the deep venous system below the iliofemoral venous occlusion, its contribution to collateral venous drainage is not a consideration. However, if only the proximal segment is thrombosed, every effort is made to preserve the vein by performing a proximal thrombectomy and creating an AVF to a branch, if available. A small piece of 4 mm PTFE graft is placed around the vein before anastomosis with the superficial femoral artery. This ensures that the arteriovenous communication will not enlarge to create a vascular steal. The superficial femoral artery is mobilized 4 to 6 cm distal to its origin, and an end-to-side anastomosis, no greater than 4 mm in diameter, is performed. A double loop of Prolene suture is passed around the vein segment (PTFE graft) and the ends are joined with a silver or titanium clip, which is left in the subcutaneous tissue and can be readily accessed in the future should it become necessary to close the AVF. Because the AVF is only 3 to 4 mm in diameter, it causes no hemodynamic problems, and routine closure is therefore not required.

Heparin is continued throughout the operative and postoperative period, and warfarin therapy is begun in the first postoperative day. External pneumatic compression devices are applied in the recovery room to further accelerate venous return and prevent recurrent thrombosis.

RESULTS

The results of treatment were categorized according to clinical outcome and the SVS/ISCVS clinical classification of chronic venous disease.[22] Outcome correlated directly with patency of the iliofemoral venous segment or the venous bypass. Fourteen patients with occlusive iliofemoral venous thrombosis were treated. Each had thrombus extending from the infrapopliteal veins through the iliac systems, and four had vena caval involvement. The conditions of 13 patients did not improve with anticoagulation. In one patient anticoagulant therapy was withheld because of an intracranial malignancy. Previous systemic fibrinolysis failed in six patients; two separate courses of intravenous thrombolysis failed in one patient. Iliofemoral thrombus (three involving the vena cava) was successfully treated in 11 of 14 patients, with patency restored or a patent bypass providing unobstructed venous outflow from the affected limb. These patients had either a good or excellent clinical outcome. Two of the treatment failures were persistent occlusion of the iliofemoral veins and vena cava, and one vena caval thrombosis, which developed 2 months after the operation.

In nine patients catheter-directed lytic therapy was attempted. In six of the nine patients, the catheters were properly positioned and successful lysis occurred, resulting in a good or excellent clinical outcome.

Nine patients underwent venous thrombectomy, five as a primary procedure and four after catheter-directed lysis. Four patients had an AVF and four underwent venous bypass to provide unobstructed venous drainage from the affected limb. Catheter-directed lysis failed in three of the nine patients who were surgically treated, and two patients underwent an adjunctive iliofemoral thrombectomy and bypass after successful lysis of infrainguinal thrombus. Two patients had residual obstruction after iliofemoral thrombectomy, one in the proximal common iliac vein and one with residual iliocaval thrombus. The patient with the intracranial malignancy initially had a good outcome following thrombectomy with AVF, but within 3 weeks required a cross-pubic bypass because of iliofemoral stenosis believed to be caused by intimal fibroplasia. Three months later, accelerated leg swelling developed as a result of vena caval thrombosis (anticoagulation was contraindicated). The bypass and AVF were dismantled. These three patients were placed in the poor clinical outcome category. In all five patients in whom unobstructed venous outflow was restored, a good or excellent result was achieved (mean follow-up, 38 months). None of the patients had symptomatic pulmonary embolism during therapy or hospitalization.

The cross-pubic venous bypass in one patient was dismantled because of vena caval thrombosis; two patients with cross-pubic venous bypass were monitored with venous duplex scanning for

40 and 63 months, respectively. Both had patent bypasses and remained symptom free.

Venous function studies (air plethysmography) were performed during follow-up in all patients capable of withstanding the study. Two patients died of metastatic cancer, and three were unable to undergo the test. Of the remaining nine patients, three were hemodynamically normal at 23, 40, and 63 months; five had mild-to-moderate venous insufficiency; and two had severe insufficiency.

DISCUSSION

The basic principles of treating iliofemoral venous thrombosis are (1) eliminate the thrombus from the common femoral vein (profunda branches) to the vena cava and as much of the thrombus from the superficial femoropopliteal veins as possible; (2) restore ipsilateral unobstructed venous drainage to the vena cava (correcting any intraluminal pathology or constructing an appropriate venous bypass); and (3) prevent rethrombosis (by means of aggressive anticoagulation, external pneumatic compression, and increasing flow velocity through the involved system with an AVF). Achieving and maintaining a patent and unobstructed iliofemoral venous system substantially reduced early and long-term morbidity.

Venous thrombectomy has not been a popular technique in the United States because of the poor results. Present-day venous thrombectomy, however, is a vastly improved procedure compared with techniques used in the late 1960s and early 1970s. Completion phlebography, correction of persisting intraluminal obstruction, and construction of a venous bypass and an AVF combined fistula with aggressive operation and postoperative anticoagulation therapy set the stage for a successful outcome.

Results of thrombolysis for iliofemoral venous thrombosis have also been disappointing. In view of the advanced degree of obstruction of the iliofemoral venous system, the large quantity of thrombus, and the minimal exposure of the lytic agent to the thrombus, it is easy to understand why the results of systemic thrombolysis for iliofemoral DVT have been poor. However, if the principles of intrathrombus delivery of fibrinolytic agents are applied, a successful outcome can be anticipated. This has been the case in the small series described herein. When the catheter is appropriately positioned, thrombolysis is successful. Occasionally, a lesion persists in the left common iliac vein at the point where it crosses beneath the right common iliac artery. I believe that this should be corrected either with transluminal techniques or by venous bypass. Transluminal techniques such as balloon angioplasty with or without stent grafting have been successful. However, these reports are preliminary and no long-term follow-up data are available. I am concerned that the repetitive arterial pulsation against the underlying venous stent will cause erosion over time, and therefore I have not used venous stents in this location.

None of my patients to date has had a clinically evident pulmonary embolism during therapy or the remainder of their hospitalization. Although a vena caval filter was in place in six of the patients at the time of treatment, three were placed previously and were occluded by caval thrombosis on presentation. Although previously inserted caval filters pose a technical challenge during venous thrombectomy, catheter-directed lysis through caval filters has not been difficult. Although the potential for bleeding during lysis through sites of filter attachment to the vena cava is a concern, transmural bleeding was not suspected or observed in any of the patients.

The patients reported on in this chapter represent the most extensive collection of acute venous thrombosis cases presenting during a 6-year period. This is a biased series because anticoagulation therapy was considered to have failed in most of these patients and they were referred from other services. Each patient had multilevel venous occlusion with thrombus extending from the lower leg through the common iliac vein, with vena caval involvement in 33%. The combined approach of catheter-directed thrombolysis and/or venous thrombectomy is conceptually unified and designed to eliminate thrombus, restore patency, provide unobstructed venous return, and prevent rethrombosis. An aggressive regional, multidisciplinary approach offers patients with the most severe form of DVT the possibility of substantially improved early and long-term prognosis compared with anticoagulation therapy alone.

REFERENCES

1. O'Donnell TF, Browse NL, Burnand KG, et al. The socioeconomic effects of an iliofemoral thrombosis. J Surg Res 22:483-488, 1977.
2. Cockett FB, Thomas L. The iliac compression syndrome. Br J Surg 52:816-821, 1965.

3. Haller JA, Abrams BL. Use of thrombectomy in the treatment of acute iliofemoral venous thrombosis in forty-five patients. Ann Surg 158:561-566, 1963.
4. DeWeese JA. Thrombectomy for acute iliofemoral venous thrombosis. J Cardiovasc Surg 5:703-712, 1964.
5. Lansing AM, Davis WM. Five-year follow-up study of iliofemoral venous thrombectomy. Ann Surg 168:620-628, 1968.
6. Plate G, Einarsson E, Ohlin P, et al. Thrombectomy with temporary arteriovenous fistula: The treatment of choice in acute iliofemoral venous thrombosis. J Vasc Surg 1:867-876, 1984.
7. Swedenborg J, Hagglog R, Jacobsson H, et al. Results of surgical treatment for iliofemoral venous thrombosis. Br J Surg 73:871-874, 1986.
8. Comerota AJ, Aldridge SC. Thrombolytic therapy for acute deep vein thrombosis. Semin Vasc Surg 5:76-81, 1992.
9. Hill SL, Martin D, Evans P. Massive deep vein thrombosis of the extremities. Am J Surg 158:131-136, 1989.
10. Lindner DJ, Edwards JM, Phinney ES, et al. Long-term hemodynamic and clinical sequelae of lower extremity deep vein thrombosis. J Vasc Surg 4:436-442, 1986.
11. Shull KC, Nicolaides AN, Fernandes e Fernandes J, et al. Significance of popliteal reflux in relation to ambulatory venous pressure and ulceration. Arch Surg 114:1304-1306, 1979.
12. Killewich LA, Bedford GR, Beach KW, Strandness DE. Spontaneous lysis of deep venous thrombi: Rate and outcome. J Vasc Surg 9:89-97, 1989.
13. Meissner MH, Manzo RA, Bergelin RO, Strandness DE. Deep venous insufficiency: The relationship between lysis and subsequent reflux. J Vasc Surg 18:596-605, 1993.
14. Elliot MS, Immelman EJ, Jeffrey P, et al. A comparative randomized trial of heparin versus streptokinase in the treatment of acute proximal venous thrombosis: An interim report of a prospective trial. Br J Surg 66:838-842, 1979.
15. Arnesen H, Hoiseth A, Ly B. Streptokinase or heparin in the treatment of deep vein thrombosis: Follow-up results of a prospective study. Acta Med Scand 211:65-71, 1982.
16. Jeffrey P, Immelman E, Amoore J. Treatment of deep vein thrombosis with heparin or streptokinase: Longterm venous function assessment [abst 520.3]. In Proceedings of the Second International Vascular Symposium, London, 1986.
17. Comerota AJ, Aldridge SC, Cohen G, et al. A strategy of aggressive regional therapy for acute iliofemoral venous thrombosis with contemporary venous thrombectomy or catheter directed thrombolysis. J Vasc Surg 20:244-254, 1994.
18. Eklof B, Juhan C. Revival of thrombectomy in the management of acute iliofemoral venous thrombosis. Contemp Surg 40:21-30, 1992.
19. Kistner RL, Sparkuhl MD. Surgery in acute and chronic venous disease. Surgery 85:31-43, 1979.
20. Loeprecht H. Angiosopie veineuse. Phlebologie 41:165-170, 1988.
21. Gruss J. Venous bypass for chronic venous insufficiency. In Bergan JJ, Yao JST, eds. Venous Disorders. Philadelphia: WB Saunders, 1991, pp 316-330.
22. Porter JM, Rutherford RB, Clagett GP, et al. Reporting standards in venous disease. J Vasc Surg 8:172-181, 1988.

84

Stents and Lytic Agents for Large Vein Occlusive Disease

MICHAEL D. DAKE, M.D.

The feasibility and efficacy of regional thrombolysis for the treatment of occluded native arteries and surgical bypass grafts are well documented in the literature. As a result of the success of thrombolysis, catheter-directed lytic infusions have become an integral part of the armamentarium for the nonoperative management of arterial disease. However, acceptance of similar techniques for use in the treatment of venous obstruction is not well established. Initial experience with the use of thrombolysis in the venous system suggests that regional thrombolysis may prove valuable.

The potential benefits of transcatheter infusions of lytic agents have been demonstrated in three broad categories of venous disease:
- Iliofemoral venous thrombosis
- Central venous obstruction
  Superior vena cava syndrome
  Inferior vena cava thrombosis
- Axillosubclavian venous thrombosis
  Spontaneous or effort-related thrombosis
  Secondary thrombosis resulting from devices such as catheters or pacemakers

REGIONAL THROMBOLYSIS FOR TREATMENT OF SYMPTOMATIC ILIOFEMORAL VENOUS THROMBOSIS

Lower extremity deep venous thrombosis (DVT) is a perplexing clinical problem that is associated with significant acute and chronic complications. Acutely there may be significant lower extremity symptoms including painful edema. In addition to the local discomfort associated with the presence of DVT, there is significant morbidity and mortality associated with pulmonary embolism that may complicate venous thrombosis. Also of considerable importance is the postphlebitic syndrome, a late complication of DVT affecting the involved extremity. The postphlebitic syndrome may only become apparent months to years after the episode of DVT. Long-term follow-up studies in patients with proved DVT have shown that more than 60% of patients develop some type of chronic problem such as edema, ulceration, or induration.[1]

One of the objectives of thrombolytic therapy for DVT is early treatment with complete lysis of thrombi to preserve vein valve function. To date, thrombolytic therapy for DVT usually consists of systemic infusions of a variety of plasminogen activators at various dosages for a period of time usually greater than 24 hours. In studies using systemic infusions, significant lysis has been reported in 48% to 83% of patients treated with thrombolytic agents.[1-10]

In a controlled multicenter study, 33 patients who had venographically proved iliofemoral thrombosis and symptoms for 2 to 3 days were treated for 3 days with one of three different thrombolytic regimens, two involving urokinase and one involving streptokinase.[9] The patients were studied with repeat venography after 3 days. Significant lysis with an improvement in venographic appearance was noted in 50% to 64% of patients; however, adverse effects consisting of hematuria, bleeding, and fever were noted in 18% to 45% of the patients in the urokinase group. However, it should be noted that other studies employing urokinase in venographically proved DVT recorded a lower incidence of complications. At the Cleveland Clinic approximately 80% of patients (n = 30) treated with urokinase had complete clot lysis proved by venography.[4] An additional 13% had partial lysis. Infusion time for urokinase averaged 26 hours. Nine of the 30 patients had a decrease in fibrinogen to levels below 100 mg/dl, but only one experienced a minor bleeding complication.

We have been impressed with the efficacy of regional transcatheter thrombolytic infusions for the treatment of axillosubclavian venous thrombosis. In a similar manner we have experienced success with central venous regional thrombolysis in the management of superior vena cava syndrome.[11] With this background we wanted to study the feasibility, safety, and efficacy of regional thrombolytic techniques applied to lower extremity DVT.

Any one of the following routes could be chosen to deliver thrombolytic agents to clots in the leg:

1. Arterial infusion into the affected lower extremity
2. Infusion into a foot vein with Ace wraps or cuffs employed to direct the drug into the deep veins
3. Popliteal vein puncture for transcatheter treatment of iliofemoral thrombus
4. Contralateral femoral vein puncture with passage of an infusion catheter over the caval bifurcation for treatment of iliofemoral thrombus
5. Transjugular placement of an infusion catheter for thrombolysis of iliofemoral clot

After experience with techniques 2 through 5, we selected the transjugular route for treatment of a consecutive series of patients with symptomatic iliofemoral venous occlusions. The transjugular route was chosen because of its potential technical advantages and patient comfort benefits during long infusions. The technique was used in 22 patients, all of whom had significant symptoms including painful edema. In 13 patients regional thrombolysis was initiated after systemic anticoagulation with heparin (mean, 7.9 days) failed to improve symptoms. Eight of the patients had chronic occlusion (mean, 1.4 years), which lasted up to 3 years. Complete lysis of the treated iliofemoral segments occurred in 16 patients after a mean infusion time of 27 hours. The mean total dose of urokinase was 3,600,000 IU. Fifteen patients had underlying lesions requiring balloon angioplasty and/or stent placement.

Following regional thrombolysis, symptomatic improvement with a decrease in unilateral leg swelling was evident in all but two patients. One patient developed heme-positive stools associated with a reduced hematocrit. The thrombolytic infusion was discontinued and there were no significant clinical sequelae. No other complications occurred. The fibrinogen level did not drop below 100 mg/dl in any patient. This initial experience suggests that regional thrombolysis in patients with symptomatic iliofemoral venous occlusions can be effective. Randomized controlled studies are necessary, however, to prove whether catheter-directed venous lysis will be more efficacious and associated with lower complication rates than are standard systemic intravenous infusions.

THROMBOLYSIS COMBINED WITH VASCULAR STENTS FOR THE TREATMENT OF SUPERIOR VENA CAVA SYNDROME

Results of percutaneous balloon angioplasty for the treatment of fibrous or elastic venous stenoses are often disappointing.[12-15] These lesions are notoriously difficult to dilate and have a high incidence of recurrence. Similarly, stenoses of hemodialysis fistulas and arterialized grafts tend to recur after balloon angioplasty because of their fibrotic nature.

The recent development of intravascular stents as adjuncts to balloon angioplasty offers a new possibility for improving the long-term results of nonoperative treatments for vascular disease. Intravascular stents are designed to provide a scaffolding that buttresses the vessel wall and maintains its patency after balloon angioplasty. This function can be critically important in preventing abrupt arterial closure following dilatation, which may be caused by angioplasty-induced dissections. Stents may also prevent vascular restenosis; however, because the longest reported clinical follow-up of arterial stenting is less than 5 years, there is no conclusive evidence that this is a definite benefit of stenting.

Designed primarily for clinical application in arteries, the experience with stents in the venous system is even more limited.[16-21] Venous stenting is usually restricted to a highly select group of patients who are poor surgical candidates or who have recurrent stenosis after previous surgery or angioplasty. Despite the relative inexperience with venous stenting, it is becoming increasingly clear that these percutaneous procedures are useful in reopening vessels compressed by extrinsic tumor. Although this has not yet been established, they may also prove to be beneficial as an adjunct to balloon angioplasty in the nonoperative treatment of failing hemodialysis conduits and other fibrotic or elastic venous stenoses.[17-19]

A detailed analysis of the various factors that must be considered when manufacturing a stent (e.g., materials, designs, and means of deployment) is beyond the scope of this discussion; however, certain current basic concepts allow for a few generalizations. The vast majority of stents under development and clinical evaluation are metallic; however, a number of projects using stents made of complex polysaccharide matrices and other bioresorbable substances are under investigation. Metals currently used in the manufacturing of stents include stainless steel, tantalum, and nitinol (nickel-titanium alloy). These metals have been fashioned into a spectrum of stent configurations including rigid tubes, flexible wire cylinders, and woven mesh designed to enhance various desired characteristics.

Regardless of the composition or design of the latticelike framework, all stents share one important characteristic—that is, they all provide sufficient radial force to resist the intrinsic elastic recoil of the vessel wall at the dilatation site. In arteries, stents can obliterate vessel recoil, which is known to limit the success of angioplasty and is associated with restenosis. Vascular stents may provide sufficient radial tension to tack down intimal flaps and effectively seal extensive dissections. This property allows stents to oppose extrinsic compression by tumor, elastic, or scarring processes.

In terms of current deployment methods, vascular stents are commonly characterized as either balloon-expandable or self-expanding. Balloon-expandable prostheses may be either rigid or flexible. An example of a rigid balloon-expandable stent is the Palmaz stent (Johnson & Johnson Interventional Systems Co., Warren, N.J.). This was the first vascular stent grafted FDA approval for clinical use. The stent is a 3 cm long stainless steel cylinder with a diameter of 3 mm. Longitudinal rows of rectangular slits are circumferentially etched through the wall of the cylinder. Minor modifications in this basic iliac stent design have been made for renal and coronary applications. The iliac stent is coaxially placed over an 8 mm outside diameter angioplasty balloon catheter. The stent is then crimped snugly over the balloon. The stent and balloon catheter assembly are then introduced through an angiographic sheath that has been placed through a previously dilated lesion. The angiographic sheath acts as a raceway to protect the stent and prevent migration as it is advanced to the site of deployment. When the stent is in a position bridging the lesion, the sheath is withdrawn past the balloon, the balloon is inflated, and the stent expands. On balloon inflation, each of the rectangular slits assumes a diamond shape as the stent progressively expands. Once full expansion of the device is confirmed fluoroscopically, the balloon is deflated and removed, leaving the stent in place. Subsequently the Palmaz stent may be balloon expanded up to 18 mm. At this diameter, however, there is significant foreshortening of the stent and a reduction in hoop strength. The range of preferred diameters for this stent is 8 to 12 mm.

The technical steps outlined for the Palmaz stent are essentially the same as for other balloon-expandable rigid or flexible stents. The flexible balloon-expandable stents include the Gianturco-Roubin (Cook, Inc., Bloomington, Ind.), Corvita (Cordis Corp., Miami, Fla.), Wiktor (Medtronic, Minneapolis, Minn.), and Strecker (Medi-Tech, Watertown, Mass.). The first three are composed of 0.009 to 0.011 inch tantalum or stainless steel wire. The stainless steel is type 316L, as is the Palmaz stent. Tantalum is used because it is more radiopaque than stainless steel. In most cases the wire is given a preliminary sinusoidal or other preformed shape before being wound over a cylindrical mold. The stents are mounted on balloon angioplasty catheters and deployed in a manner similar to the Palmaz stent. The Strecker stent has a somewhat different design. It is made of 0.009 inch tantalum wire woven into an open mesh of interlacing wire threads. The stent is balloon expandable; however, there is a unique method used to secure the device over the balloon prior to deployment. Two silicone sleeves are placed over the ends of the collapsed mesh to constrain the stent. As the balloon is inflated, the sleeves stretch as the stent is deployed. At full expansion, the stretched restraints release the stent. On deflation, the balloon and stent restraints collapse around the catheter shaft leaving the stent in place.

There are a few self-expanding metallic stents, the most notable being the Wallstent (Schneider Stent, Minneapolis, Minn.) and the Gianturco Z stent (Cook). Both of these stents are made of stainless steel; however, their designs and means of deployment are quite different. The Wallstent is a woven, springlike prosthesis that is available in various lengths and diameters. The stent is coaxially placed over a catheter, stretched to its minimum diameter, and then constrained by a rolling membrane. The catheter is advanced over a guidewire to a position bridging the lesion. A contrast medium is then introduced through a lumen that leads to the space subjacent to the constraining membrane. Once this space is expanded, it is possible to withdraw the membrane and unveil the stent. As the membrane is progressively rolled away from the tip of the catheter, there is significant foreshortening of the stent as it expands. Once fully deployed, the catheter is removed and balloon angioplasty may be performed if desired.

The Gianturco Z stent is composed of a series of stainless steel, diagonal, Z-shaped struts connected by suture material. The compressibility of the metallic struts allows the stent to be loaded into a delivery sheath, which has been placed across the site of deployment. Once inside the sheath, the stent is advanced to the lesion by a pusher device. After the optimal site for deployment is confirmed fluoroscopically, the pusher maintains its position as the sheath is withdrawn and the stent springs to expansion.

All of the aforementioned stents with the exception of the Gianturco-Roubin stent, which is designed primarily for coronary artery applications, have sufficiently high expansion ratios to make their use in veins feasible.

CLINICAL APPLICATIONS

To study the safety and efficacy of vascular stents for the treatment of venous obstruction unresponsive to balloon angioplasty (PTA), 98 patients with a variety of central and peripheral venous lesions involving the superior vena cava (SVC) (malignant, n = 25; nonmalignant, n = 11), inferior vena cava (n = 5), innominate-subclavian (n = 39), dural sinuses (n = 2), and extremity (n = 16) vessels were stented. All patients had significant symptoms including painful edema associated with a high-grade stenosis (>95% stenosis by diameter) (n = 47) or complete venous occlusion (n = 51).

In all cases stenting was combined with other percutaneous techniques including antecedent regional thrombolysis in 46 and PTA in 98. In all patients a significant pressure gradient and/or residual stenosis was observed after PTA alone. A total of 275 stents were implanted (mean, 2.8/patient) with complete (n = 90) or partial (n = 5) resolution of venous obstructive symptoms in 95 (97%). The stents have remained in place for up to 27 months (mean follow-up, 8.8 months). Stented segments have occluded in 10 patients; however, the secondary patency rate remains high (95%). One patient died 14 hours after the procedure and one had transient gross hematuria on a regimen of oral warfarin 2 months after stent placement.

Currently, most of the experience with venous stenting is in the setting of SVC syndrome.[16-21]

SVC syndrome is caused by a variety of diseases that obstruct the SVC. This obstruction typically causes progressive upper extremity, neck, and facial edema with dilatation of the superficial veins of the chest, neck, and arms. In this century the most common cause of SVC syndrome is malignant tumor, usually carcinoma of the lung extending into the mediastinum. Lymphoma and metastatic cancer are also responsible for a large number of SVC obstructions. Recently the increasing use of transvenous pacemaker leads and central venous catheters for cancer therapy, hemodialysis, parental nutrition, and long-term antibiotic therapy has caused an increase in the number of patients developing SVC syndrome.

If SVC obstruction occurs rapidly, the extent and adequacy of venous collateralization may be limited. The face, neck, and arms can swell to massive proportions. The increase in venous pressure may result in central nervous system disturbances, ocular and nasal conjunctival edema, facial cyanosis, dysphagia, upper airway obstruction, and bleeding from downhill esophageal varices. Traditionally SVC syndrome has been treated as a medical emergency. Nonspecific measures including elevation of a swollen extremity and administration of steroids may be helpful; however, in patients with an underlying malignancy, radiation therapy is usually instituted promptly. Radiation therapy is the mainstay for treating SVC syndrome caused by cancer. The effect of radiation may be noted soon after therapy is begun; however, the resolution of symptoms is gradual and is related to the cumulative dose and tumor radiosensitivity.

Thrombolytic therapy for SVC syndrome has been described in numerous case reports and in one series of 16 patients, 11 of whom had indwelling central venous catheters.[1] This form of treatment appears to be especially successful in relieving symptoms caused by SVC thrombosis associated with central venous catheters or pacemaker wires. It is much less effective in malignant disease where there is an extrinsic compression of the SVC and other central venous structures.

Multiple case studies in the literature report some benefits of balloon angioplasty used for the treatment of SVC obstruction; however, the results are variable, depending on the cause of SVC syndrome.[12-14] In isolated cases of SVC syndrome caused by malignant mediastinal disease, PTA of discreet SVC stenoses and occlusions has been noted to provide prompt symptomatic relief. In general, however, the results of balloon angioplasty alone are fair. The initial success is usually short-lived and restricted to focal lesions. This is often because the malignancy directly invades or extrinsically compresses the thin-walled vein, and any dilatation achieved by the inflated balloon is lost after the balloon is removed because of the recoil of abnormal tissue within or around the vein. Diffuse extrinsic constriction of central veins by mediastinal malignancy is particularly difficult to treat by PTA alone.

Surgical placement of a graft bypassing discreet SVC disease has been performed in selected patients with underlying malignancy; however, it requires an extensive operation to place a graft, which is susceptible to obstruction by local extension of tumor. A number of patients with malignant SVC syndrome have been treated with vascular stents.[16,20,21] The majority of these cases had discreet high-grade stenoses or focal total occlusions of the SVC. Most symptomatic and potentially life-threatening cases of SVC syndrome, however, often involve diffuse occlusion of numerous central veins including the SVC and the brachiocephalic, subclavian, jugular, and azygous veins. This diffuse disease is usually secondary to malignancy. Logistically, the percutaneous approach to this degree of massive thrombosis requires a combination of modalities including regional thrombolysis, balloon angioplasty, and stents for effective management. Although angioplasty and thrombolysis are important contributors to any success achieved, the emergence of vascular stents has provided the essential element necessary to potentially provide a more effective treatment for this difficult problem.

We have used intravascular stents to treat 25 patients with SVC syndrome caused by an underlying malignancy. All patients had significant symptoms including painful edema associated with a high-grade stenosis (>95% stenosis by diameter) (n = 10) or complete occlusion (n = 15) of the SVC. In all cases stenting was combined with other percutaneous techniques including antecedent regional thrombolysis in 14 and balloon angioplasty in 25. Complete resolution of the SVC syndrome occurred in 23 patients and partial resolution in two. In the latter, residual unilateral extremity edema was referable to nonstented, occluded caval tributaries.

In all patients significant pressure gradients and/or residual stenoses were observed after balloon angioplasty alone. Stents employed included the Palmaz stent in 65, the Wallstent in 15, and the modified Gianturco self-expanding Z stent in 1. The stents have remained in place for up to 24 months with a mean follow-up of 10.9 months. Stented segments occluded in five patients at 2 weeks, and at 2, 3, 7, and 12 months, respectively, after placement. In four patency was restored following regional thrombolysis and restenting of the lesion within the previously stented SVC. The stent occlusion that occurred at 12 months was diagnosed at another hospital and no attempts were made to determine the cause or reopen the SVC. In one patient, tumor overgrew the end of a stented segment 3 months after the stent was placed. This extension partially occluded subclavian and jugular tributaries to the stented innominate segment. After placement of an additional overlapping stent bridging the lesion, patency was restored without residual stenosis. Within 12 hours there was complete resolution of left upper extremity swelling and symptoms of cerebral edema. One patient in critical condition with far-advanced mesothelioma died 18 hours after a stent was placed in the SVC.

In a manner similar to their application in the SVC, vascular stents can be used to treat obstructions of the inferior vena cava resulting from tumor, retroperitoneal fibrosis, lymphadenopathy, or fibrotic postinflammatory reactions. Clinical experience with this application, however, is limited.[17]

The problem of failing hemodialysis access conduits is also being addressed by the use of vascular stents. This includes experience managing stenotic anastomoses, grafts, and venous outflow channels.[17-19] Initial results suggest that the use of stents in these lesions is usually only palliative treatment; however, the procedure appears safe and placement of these stents may extend the life of a failing dialysis access over what is currently possible by other means.[20-24] Larger trials in hemodialysis patients are clearly necessary before any definitive statements can be made regarding the benefit of vascular stents and their relative long-term patency and cost-effectiveness compared to surgical repair or other nonoperative approaches such as balloon angioplasty and atherectomy.

Along with the unique advantages that vascular stents afford interventionalists treating venous disease, there are a number of distinct problems and untoward effects associated with their use. Some of these are related to the generic use of stents and others are specific for applications in the venous system. In general, vascular prostheses require deployment mechanisms that allow the stents to be introduced into the vascular system and expanded to a desired diameter at a given site. Aside from local groin complications such as hematoma and bleeding related to obtaining sufficient vascular access to allow introduction of stents, general problems that may be encountered with the use of stents include migration of stents prior to or after deployment, placement of stents at the wrong location, thrombotic occlusion, stent infection with sepsis, inadequate expansion of stents because of resistant vascular lesions or extrinsic restraints, partial expansion of stents as a result of malfunction of the deployment device (e.g., balloon rupture or release mechanism dysfunction), vessel perforation, enhancement of a restenosis process, and mechanical stent compression after full deployment by extrinsic forces.

In addition, vascular stents are subject to some problems peculiar to their application in the venous system. In the treatment of malignant venous obstruction, tumor may grow through the interstices of stents or around the ends of stented segments to reocclude veins. Compared to arteries, veins are highly compliant and thin walled. This provides relatively little protection against adjacent extrinsic disease processes and normal kinesiologic forces, which apply pressures that may overcome the stent's intrinsic resistance to compression. Such clinical situations might include radiation fibrosis, inflammatory scarring, stents placed in constricted anatomic spaces subjected to repetitive or powerful mechanical forces, stents placed adjacent to bony prominences (May-Thurner syndrome), and stents in superficial locations commonly exposed to blunt trauma. The exact incidence of these stent-related problems is unclear and awaits further documentation.

REGIONAL THROMBOLYSIS FOR THE MANAGEMENT OF AXILLOSUBCLAVIAN OCCLUSION

Although the pathophysiologic processes responsible for spontaneous and secondary axillosubclavian thrombosis are distinctly different, clinical management strategies for both rely on the use of regional thrombolysis in combination with other techniques.[20-24,27] Recently this approach has received more attention because the incidence and morbidity of pulmonary embolism resulting from upper extremity venous thrombosis have become better defined and recognized. This increased awareness is due in part to the frequent use of central venous catheters in the management of a variety of conditions and the realization that pulmonary embolism secondary to catheter-induced upper extremity venous thrombosis is more common than was previously thought. A recent review of the literature identified a 12% incidence of pulmonary embolism in all patients with axillosubclavian venous thrombosis.[25] In addition, other studies suggest that pulmonary embolism may occur commonly in patients with central venous catheters but may be undiagnosed because the patients are generally asymptomatic.[26,27]

REFERENCES

1. Arnsen H, Hoiseth A, Ly B. Streptokinase or heparin in the treatment of deep vein thrombosis: Follow-up results of a prospective study. Acta Med Scand 211:65-68, 1982.
2. Duckert F, Muller G, Hyman D, et al. Treatment of deep vein thrombosis with streptokinase. Br Med J 1:479-481, 1975.
3. Elliot MS, Immelman EJ, Jeffrey P, et al. A comparative randomized trial of heparin versus streptokinase in the treatment of acute proximal venous thrombosis: An interim report of a prospective trial. Br J Surg 66:838-843, 1979.
4. Graor RA, Young JR, Risius B, et al. Comparison of cost effectiveness of streptokinase and urokinase in the treatment of deep vein thrombosis. Ann Vasc Surg 1:524-528, 1987.
5. Kakkar VV, Lawrence D. Hemodynamic and clinical assessment after therapy for acute deep vein thrombosis. Am J Surg 150:54-63, 1985.
6. Marder VJ, Soulen RL, Atichartakarn V. Quantitative venographic assessment of deep vein thrombosis in the evaluation of streptokinase and heparin therapy. J Lab Clin Med 89:1018-1029, 1977.
7. Rosch JJ, Dotter CT, Seaman AJ, et al. Healing of deep vein thrombosis: Venographic findings in a randomized study comparing streptokinase and heparin. Am J Roentgenol 1127:533-558, 1976.
8. Tsapogas MJ, Peabody RA, Wu KT, et al. Controlled study of thrombolytic therapy in deep vein thrombosis, Surgery 74:973-979, 1973.
9. Van de Loo JCW, Kriessmann A, Trubestein G, et al. Controlled multicenter pilot study of urokinase-heparin and in deep venous thrombosis. Thromb Haemost 50:660-663, 1983.
10. Zimmerman R, Epping J, Rasche H, et al. Urokinase and streptokinase treatment of deep vein thrombosis. Results of a randomized study. Haemostasis 16:9-10, 1986.
11. Gray BH, Olin JW, Groar RA, Young JR, Bartholomew JR, Ruschhaupt WF. Safety and efficacy of thrombolytic therapy for superior vena cava syndrome. Chest 99:54-59, 1991.

12. Rocchini AP, Cho KJ, Byrum C, et al. Transluminal angioplasty of superior vena cava obstruction in a 15-month-old child. Chest 82:506-508, 1982.
13. Sherry CS, Diamond NG, Meyers TP, et al. Successful treatment of superior vena cava syndrome by venous angioplasty. AJR 147:834-835, 1986.
14. Ali MK, Ewer MS, Balakrishnan PV, et al. Balloon angioplasty for superior vena cava obstruction. Ann Intern Med 107:856-857, 1987.
15. Capek P, Cope C. Percutaneous treatment of superior vena cava treatment. AJR 152:183-184, 1989.
16. Rosch J, Bedell JE, Putnam J, Antonovic R, Uchida B. Gianturco expandable wire stents in the treatment of superior vena cava syndrome recurring after maximum-tolerance radiation. Cancer 60:1243-1246, 1987.
17. Elson JD, Becker GJ, Wholey MH, Ehrman KO. Vena caval and central venous stenoses: Management with Palmaz balloon-expandable intraluminal stents. J Vasc Interv Radiol 2:215-223, 1991.
18. Zollikofer CL, Largiader I, Bruhlman WF, Uhlschmid GK, Marty AH. Endovascular stenting of veins and grafts: Preliminary clinical experience. Radiology 167:707-712, 1988.
19. Gunther RW, Vorwerk D, Klose KC, Bohndorf K, Kistler D, Mann H, Sieberth HG. Self-expanding stents for the treatment of a long venous stenosis in a dialysis shunt: Case report. Cardiovasc Intervent Radiol 12:29-31, 1989.
20. Charnsangavej C, Carrasco CH, Wallace S, et al. Stenosis of the vena cava: Preliminary assessment of treatment with expandable metallic stents. Radiology 161:295-298, 1986.
21. Putnam J, Uchida BS, Antonovic R, Rosch J. Superior vena cava syndrome associated with massive thrombosis: Treatment with expandable wire stents. Radiology 167:727-728, 1988.
22. Becker GJ, Holden RW, Rabe FE, et al. Local thrombolytic therapy for subclavian and axillary vein thrombosis. Radiology 149:419-423, 1983.
23. Fraschini G, Jadeja J, Lawson M, Holmes FA, Carrasco HC, Wallace S. Local infusion of urokinase for the lysis of thrombosis associated with permanent central venous catheters in cancer patients. J Clin Oncol 5:672-678, 1987.
24. Glanz S, Gordon DH, Lipkowitz G, et al. Axillary and subclavian vein stenosis: Percutaneous angioplasty. Radiology 168:371-373, 1988.
25. Horattas MC, Wright DJ, Fenton AH, et al. Changing concepts of deep venous thrombosis of the upper extremity: Report of a series and review of the literature. Surgery 104:561-567, 1988.
26. Machleder HI. Upper extremity venous thrombosis. Semin Vasc Surg 3:219-226 1990.
27. Zimmerman R, Morl H, Harenberg J, et al. Urokinase therapy of subclavian axillary vein thrombosis. Klin Wochenschr 59:851-856, 1981.

85

Update on Pulmonary Embolism

LAZAR J. GREENFIELD, M.D., and MARY C. PROCTOR, M.S.

Pulmonary embolism (PE) occurs in more than 500,000 patients annually and significantly contributes to the mortality rate of 142,000 to 200,000 deaths per year.[1] Although it can be the final event in a patient at the end stage of other diseases, it often develops in patients who would otherwise have survived. The clinical presentation of PE is frequently nonspecific, resulting in a missed or delayed diagnosis. As many as 60% of PEs found at autopsy had not been suspected prior to the patient's death. The physician should maintain a high level of suspicion for patients who present with signs or symptoms of PE as reviewed in the Urokinase Pulmonary Embolism Trial (UPET) including dyspnea, pleural pain, apprehension, tachypnea, tachycardia, and altered heart sounds.[2] Most patients respond well to standard therapy with intravenous heparin followed by 3 to 6 months of oral anticoagulation with Coumadin. However, approximately 10% to 12% of patients will die within the first hour or two without a prompt diagnosis and aggressive intervention. The challenge is to accurately identify the latter group.

We have developed and refined a classification system based on the physiologic changes that occur after PE to describe the level of severity (Table 1). Patients are classified as having minor, major, massive, or chronic recurrent PE. These levels are based on physical signs and symptoms, arterial blood gas values, the extent of pulmonary artery occlusion, and hemodynamic values. Patients with massive PE typically present in shock, require vasopressors and inotropes to maintain hemodynamic stability, and require emergency intervention. Acute myocardial infarction and overwhelming sepsis can mimic these findings, so the diagnosis must be confirmed, preferably by selective pulmonary angiography, which allows measurement of pulmonary arterial pressures.

INTERVENTIONS

The following four methods of treatment are currently in use: standard intravenous heparin and oral Coumadin, systemic or local thrombolytic infusion, operative embolectomy on cardiopulmonary bypass, and transvenous catheter embolectomy. Standard anticoagulation has proved effective in reducing morbidity and mortality from PE, and the majority of patients who are hemodynamically stable can be adequately treated this way. However, it may require several hours to become effective and does not reduce the embolic mass. It is indicated for patients in the minor category and for all patients in whom PE is suspected while awaiting confirmation of the diagnosis.

Several studies have demonstrated the efficacy of systemic[3,4] and local[5] infusions of thrombolytic drugs in reducing embolic mass and significantly improving the clinical status of

Table 1 Physiologic classification of patients with pulmonary embolism

Category	Signs and symptoms	Gases	Pulmonary artery occlusion (%)	Hemodynamics
Minor	Anxiety Hyperventilation	Pa_{O_2} <80 mm Hg Pa_{CO_2} <35 mm Hg	20-30	Tachycardia
Major	Dyspnea Collapse	Pa_{O_2} <65 mm Hg Pa_{CO_2} <30 mm Hg	30-50	CVP elevated, PAP >20 mm Hg Responds to resuscitation
Massive	Dyspnea Shock	Pa_{O_2} <50 mm Hg Pa_{CO_2} <30 mm Hg	>50	CVP elevated, PAP >25 mm Hg Requires pressors, inotropes
Chronic	Dyspnea Syncope	Pa_{O_2} <70 mm Hg Pa_{CO_2} 30-40 mm Hg	>50	CVP elevated, PAP >40 mm Hg Fixed low cardiac output

CVP = central venous pressure; PAP = pulmonary artery pressure.

those with major and massive PE. There are limitations, however, including the length of time required to lyse the thrombus and contraindications to the use of such agents in several clinical situations including the immediate postoperative period and in patients with gastrointestinal bleeding or stroke.[6] The risks of thrombolysis are serious, with hemorrhage being the major complication in addition to intracerebral bleeding and death.[7] The original multicenter trial also failed to show any improvement in the mortality rate.

Surgical embolectomy by thoracotomy as described by Trendelenburg was first successfully performed in the United States by Steenberg in 1958. The addition of cardiopulmonary bypass increased the survivial of patients undergoing this procedure,[8] although it remained a major insult under general anesthesia in patients already comprised. It also requires a specially trained staff and equipment that may not be available at many community hospitals on a 24-hour basis. If the patient must be transferred to a regional medical center, valuable time is lost. Reported success rates are highly variable because of patient selection criteria and differences in surgical technique. Mortality estimates range from 24% to 93%.[9,10]

Transvenous catheter embolectomy, first described by Greenfield et al.[11] in 1971, offers an effective, safe alternative for treatment of patients with massive PE. During the procedure, which is usually performed in the radiology suite under local anesthesia, emboli are removed from the pulmonary circulation until a critical threshold is passed, resulting in an increase in systemic blood pressure and cardiac output and frequently allowing the discontinuation of inotropes and vasopressors.

TECHNIQUE

Following successful animal studies, transvenous catheter embolectomy was initially attempted in 10 patients. Under local anesthesia, a cardiac catheter with a rigid cup attachment was inserted through the right femoral vein under fluoroscopic guidance, manipulated through the right side of the heart into the pulmonary artery, and juxtaposed with the embolus. Initial retrieval efforts were successful in 90% of these patients.[12] The catheter system was subsequently improved by providing steerability of the catheter tip to allow access to more lobar branches of the pulmonary artery. The procedure was further modified to include placement of a Greenfield vena caval filter to prevent recurrent PE, which occurred in two of the first 10 patients. In addition, the cup was changed to plastic.

The catheter is attached to a pistol-shaped handpiece with a "joystick" to control the steerable cup (Fig. 1). Access is obtained through the right femoral or jugular vein, although the jugular vein is now preferred because it avoids possible embolism from the femoral veins and the dissection is easier in the obese patient. The system is inserted through a longitudinal venot-

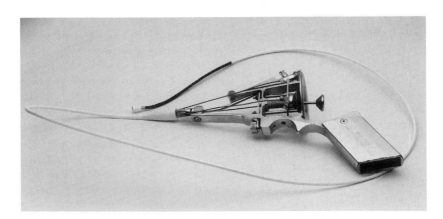

Fig. 1 The Greenfield embolectomy catheter is attached to a handle, which allows directional control.

omy and the radiopaque cup is advanced under fluoroscopic guidance through the right side of the heart. The handle is manipulated using the right hand while the left is used to advance the catheter and control direction. Medial angulation and anterior deflection are useful in passing the catheter from the right ventricle into the pulmonary artery. During the passage, some patients develop premature ventricular contractions or other rhythm disturbances, therefore ECG monitoring should be used throughout the procedure. Repositioning or withdrawal of the catheter usually corrects the arrhythmias. Entry into the left pulmonary artery is easiest while entry into the right main pulmonary artery is achieved by medial deflection of the cup as it reaches the superior edge of the heart shadow. Advancement can be improved by rotating the tip of the catheter. Alignment of the catheter cup with the embolus can be viewed by injection of a small bolus of contrast medium.

A large (30 ml) syringe is attached to the control handle using intravenous extension tubing. Once alignment is confirmed, an assistant withdraws the plunger of the syringe to create suction. If a vacuum is created, the embolus has been attached and the catheter should be withdrawn gently by the operator while the assistant maintains syringe suction. If there is a return of blood into the syringe, the blood should be returned and the cup repositioned until the embolus is attached. Repeated removals may be necessary to relieve obstruction. Frequent monitoring of pulmonary artery pressures and cardiac output is necessary to confirm effective clearing.[12] Systemic pressure will increase, the patient may regain consciousness, and vasopressors can be discontinued once a critical mass has been removed. Failure to increase cardiac output or the need for closed-chest massage are indications for placement of a vena caval filter and a switch to open embolectomy.

RESULTS

A total of 49 patients have been treated using catheter embolectomy: 10 with the early rigid cup and 39 with the improved device. There were 24 women and 25 men who had a mean age of 53 years. Twenty-eight procedures used the femoral approach and 1 the jugular. The procedure was successful in extracting thrombi in 76% of patients (39 of 49). Sixty-seven percent survived the initial hospitalization, whereas 53% (26 of 49) survived long term. Twenty-three patients have returned for follow-up, which ranged from 1 to 237 months (mean, 65.6 months). Four patients were classified with major PE, 35 with massive, and 10 with chronic recurrent embolism. There was an average reduction in mean pulmonary artery pressure of 8 mm Hg and a significant increase in mean cardiac output from 2.59 to 4.47 L/min. The complications are listed in Table 2, with wound hematoma in 15% being the most frequent. Cardiac arrest during angiography occurred in three early cases before the need to limit the volume of contrast medium injected was recognized. One agonal patient had a ventricular perforation with the use of the rigid steel cup, which has not occurred since the change to plastic. The success of the procedure was closely associated with the patient's clinical classification. It was 100% (4 of 4) in those with major PE, 83% (29 of 35) for massive PE, and 50% (5 of 10) for chronic PE. Inclusion of a small number of patients with major PE represents an extension of the indications for embolectomy. The procedure was performed at the request of pulmonary specialists to reduce the extent of pulmonary arterial occlusion to facilitate weaning of the patient from the ventilator. In each case the patient was able to be weaned within 6 hours of the procedure.

Patients with chronic recurrent PE have the poorest outcome from this procedure. Chronic emboli are firmly fixed to the arterial wall and are highly resistant to extraction. However, in approximately half of the cases, sufficient quan-

Table 2 Complications after catheter embolectomy (1970-1992)

Complications	No.	Percent
Wound hematoma	7	15
Pulmonary infarct	5	11
Recurrent deep venous thrombosis	3	7
Pleural effusion	2	4
Recurrent pulmonary embolism	2	4
Myocardial infarction	2	4
Pneumonia	1	2
Duodenal stump leak	1	2
Ruptured pulmonary artery (monitoring catheter)	1	2
Wound infection	1	2
Ventricular perforation	1	2

tities of fresh emboli were recovered to achieve hemodynamic improvement.

DISCUSSION

Treatment of massive PE requires prompt diagnosis and aggressive intervention. Both open embolectomy and thrombolytic therapy have high complication rates, are expensive, and require sophisticated equipment and medical monitoring. Transvenous catheter embolectomy can be safely conducted in the majority of medical facilities by radiologists and surgeons working jointly. The procedure is as effective as the other two but with a significantly better risk-benefit ratio. Some have attempted to modify the technique by eliminating the operative venotomy and substituting a percutaneous sheath to gain access to the jugular vein. Although this may be an appealing idea initially, it has potential for serious complications. Most of the emboli are captured in a folded position and may be sheared off by the edge of the sheath during withdrawal and reembolize, or the entire embolus may be knocked free. This does not occur with the open technique, as the vein is more compliant. In addition, use of the sheath may place the patient at risk for air embolism.

Use of the described technique is supported by reports of two other groups who have achieved success in individual cases and a larger series from Laennec Hospital. They have achieved technical success in 11 of 18 patients and a low morbidity rate of 28%. Their optimal results were associated with performance of the procedure within 48 hours of the onset of symptoms.[13]

Massive PE is a relatively rare event with two to three cases occurring at major medical centers on an annual basis. This makes outcome studies virtually impossible, but as further experience with this technique is reported, its proper role can be evaluated.

REFERENCES

1. Coon W. Venous thromboembolism. Prevalence, risk factors, and prevention. Clin Chest Med 5:391-401, 1984.
2. Urokinase Pulmonary Embolism Trial: A national cooperative study. Circulation 47(Suppl 2):1-108, 1973.
3. Goldhaber SZ, Kessler C, Heit JA, et al. Randomised controlled trial of recombinant tissue plasminogen activator versus urokinase in the treatment of acute pulmonary embolism. Lancet 2:293-298, 1988.
4. De Takats G. The urokinase pulmonary embolism trial. Am J Surg 126:311-313, 1973.
5. Rosenthal D, Evans RD, Borrero E, Lamis PA, Clark MD, Daniel W. Massive pulmonary embolism: Triple-armed therapy. J Vasc Surg 9:261-270, 1989.
6. Terrin ML, Goldhaber SZ, Thompson B. Selection of patients with acute pulmonary embolism for thrombolytic therapy. Thrombolysis in pulmonary embolism (TIPE) patient survey. Chest 95:279-281, 1989.
7. Jankel CA, McMillan JA, Martin BC. Effect of drug interactions on outcomes of patients receiving warfarin or theophylline. Am J Hosp Pharm 51:661-666, 1994.
8. Beall A, Cooley D. Surgical treatment of pulmonary embolism. Heart Bull 13:41-43, 1962.
9. Berger R. Pulmonary embolectomy with preoperative circulatory support. Ann Thorac Surg 16:217-227, 1973.
10. Paneth M. Pulmonary embolectomy: An analysis of 12 cases. J Thorac Cardiovasc Surg 53:77-83, 1967.
11. Greenfield LJ, Bruce T, Nichols N. Transvenous pulmonary embolectomy by catheter device. Ann Surg 174:881-886, 1971.
12. Stewart J, Greenfield LJ. Transvenous vena caval filtration and pulmonary embolectomy. Surg Clin North Am 62:411-429, 1982.
13. Timsit J, Reynaud P, Meyer G, Sors H. Pulmonary embolectomy by catheter device in massive pulmonary embolism. Chest 100:655-658, 1991.

SECTION X

Pioneers in Vascular Surgery

This section details the lives of Norman Freeman and Valentine Mott and discusses the influence of these two pioneers in vascular surgery.

86

Norman Freeman

JOHN E. CONNOLLY, M.D.

Norman Freeman was born in Philadelphia in 1903, the son of a prominent otolaryngologist and grandson of the renowned William W. Keen, Professor of Surgery at Jefferson Medical College from 1889 to 1921. His father died when Freeman was 17, and thereafter his grandfather exerted a major influence. Keen was the editor of the famous eight-volume *Keen's Surgery,* and although he was a pioneer of many general surgical procedures, he is often referred to as the "father of neurosurgery."

Freeman had an excellent education—secondary school at St. Paul's and college and medical school at Yale, where he received honors. He served a 2-year internship at the University of Pennsylvania under Isidor Ravdin, who recognized the brilliance of his student and arranged for him to spend 2 years as a National Research Council Fellow doing research with the famous Harvard Professor of Physiology, Walter B. Cannon. It was during those years that he became interested in the physiology of the vascular and sympathetic nervous systems and coauthored a number of papers with Dr. Cannon. He subsequently served a 3-year surgical residency under Edward D. Churchill at Massachusetts General Hospital, followed by a fourth year as a Dalton Fellow in Surgery.

In 1936 Ravdin brought Freeman back to his department at the University of Pennsylvania as the J. William White Assistant Professor of Surgical Research. Soon thereafter he was named Chief of Vascular Surgery at Pennsylvania Hospital, and beginning in 1937 he confined himself entirely to vascular surgery. It would appear that he was the first surgeon in the United States to do so.

During those prewar days Freeman was extraordinarily productive in his research, both in the laboratory and in the hospital. His studies, which were started in Boston and continued in Philadelphia, were on the physiology of peripheral blood flow, shock, gangrene, and the effects of the interaction of temperature, epinephrine, the sympathetic nervous system, and blood loss on them. Clinically his efforts were directed at the mysteries of Buerger's disease. He continued to pursue various clinical research interests during his 4 years of service in the Army Medical Corps, culminating in 1945 with his assignment as Chief of Surgery at DeWitt General Hospital in California, one of the three designated army vascular centers. There he pioneered reconstructive vascular surgical techniques. As an example, at that time arteriovenous fistulas were treated by quadruple ligation. His contribution was to divide the communications and reconstruct the vessels with restoration of blood flow. In 1946 he reported his success in 18 such cases to the American Surgical Association.[1]

After the war, he was persuaded to join the Department of Surgery at the University of California San Francisco rather than return to Philadelphia. The surgeon that the UCSF staff met in 1946 was a true physiologist, an innova-

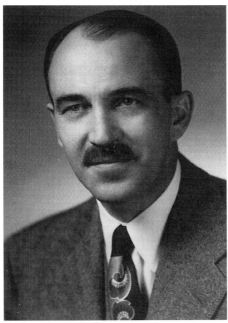

Norman Freeman

tive clinician, a teacher, and an investigator. At the same time, however, he was controversial because his temperamental qualities frequently brought him into conflict with authority. He was appointed Chief of the Vascular Clinic and given a room in the animal laboratory designated exclusively for vascular research. He also obtained grant funding to develop a vascular physiology research laboratory at the affiliated Franklin Hospital. His assistants during those days were Rutherford Gilfillan, Frank Leeds, and Jack Wylie, all of whom were surgical trainees who became interested in vascular surgery because of Freeman. Gilfillan went on to concentrate more on laboratory work, whereas Wylie and Leeds became outstanding clinicians. In 1951 Wylie, his pupil, performed the first aortoiliac endarterectomy in the United States,[2] followed within a few weeks by Freeman and Gilfillan.[3]

Freeman performed the first replacement of an abdominal aortic aneurysm with autogenous iliac vein on February 26, 1951.[4] This was 1 month before Dubost in Paris replaced an aortic aneurysm with a homograft, which has generally been considered the first aneurysmectomy. In 1952 he performed the first direct revascularization of a stenotic renal artery to effect a cure for renal hypertension by endarterectomy of the renal orifice through the open aorta.[5] In 1953 he reported the successful ligature of an aortic aneurysm in situ with distal flow reconstituted by the translocated splenic artery.[6] At about the same time he reported the first extra-anatomic bypass, a femorofemoral conduit that employed an eversion endarterectomized superficial femoral artery[1] (Fig. 1). Freeman, also in the 1950s, stimulated his associate Frank Leeds to pioneer endarterectomy of the profunda femoris artery for revascularization of the ischemic limb.[8] Another disciple of Freeman was Samuel Etheredge, of Oakland, California, who was inspired by Freeman's innovative spirit and encouragement to perform the first successful resection of a suprarenal aortic aneurysm on September 20, 1954.[9]

Freeman was forced to retire from active surgical practice for health reasons at the relatively young age of 59 and died of heart disease at age 72. It is of particular interest that he wrote an editorial in *California Medicine* in 1948[10] in which he addressed the question, "Is there room or actual need for vascular surgery as a specialty?" His answer was "yes, as long as the specialist takes advantage of his opportunities to contribute to the knowledge of the disorder he specifically treats." Thus he was more than 30 years ahead of the development of the specialty as we now know it.

To those of us who knew him well, Norman Freeman was a multifaceted person—at his best he was a genius who enhanced our knowledge and treatment of vascular surgery immensely.

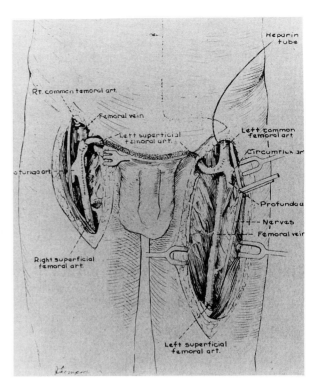

Fig. 1 First extra-anatomic bypass. Use of an eversion endarterectomized left superficial femoral artery for femorofemoral bypass.

REFERENCES
1. Freeman NE. Arterial repair in the treatment of aneurysms and arteriovenous fistulae, a report of eighteen successful restorations. Ann Surg 124:888-919, 1946.
2. Wylie EJ, Davies O. Experimental and clinical experiences with the use of fascia lata applied as a graft about major arteries after thromboendarterectomy and aneurysmorrhaphy. Surg Gynecol Obstet 93:257-272, 1951.
3. Freeman NE, Gilfillan RS. Regional heparinization after thromboendarterectomy in the treatment of obliterative arterial disease. Surgery 31:115-131, 1952.
4. Freeman NE, Leeds FH. Vein inlay graft in the treatment of aneurysms and thrombosis of the abdominal aorta. Angiology 2:579-587, 1951.

5. Freeman NE, Leeds FH, Elliott WC, Roland SI. Thromboendarterectomy for hypertension due to renal artery occlusion. JAMA 156:1077-1079, 1954.
6. Freeman NE, Leeds FH. Resection of aneurysms of the abdominal aorta with anastomosis of the splenic to the left iliac artery. Surgery 34:1021-1031, 1953.
7. Freeman NE, Leeds FH. Operations on large arteries. Calif Med 77:229-233, 1952.
8. Leeds FH, Gilfillan RS. Revascularization of the ischemic limb. Arch Surg 82:25-31, 1961.
9. Etheredge SN, Yee J, Smith JV, Schonberger S, Goldman MJ. Successful resection of a large aneurysm of the upper abdominal aorta. Surgery 38:1071-1081, 1955.
10. Freeman NE. Vascular surgery [editorial]. Calif Med 68:43-44, 1948.-

87
Valentine Mott

JESSE E. THOMPSON, M.D.

Valentine Mott, of New York City, was one of the most outstanding American surgeons during the first half of the nineteenth century. Although he worked in all areas of surgery, he was best known for his contributions to vascular surgery, which at that time consisted largely of arterial ligations and amputations.

Valentine Mott was born on August 20, 1785 in Glen Cove, Long Island, New York, the son of a physician, Dr. Henry Mott.[1] He received his secondary education at a private seminary and then enrolled for medical lectures in Columbia College, receiving his M.D. in 1806 at the age of 21. He spent the next year in the office of his cousin, Valentine Seaman, a prominent New York surgeon, and was persuaded to pursue a career in surgery.[2]

As was customary at that time, he decided to seek additional training in Europe. He proceeded to London where he registered as a pupil at Guy's Hospital on August 31, 1807. During the next 6 months he worked under Sir Astley Cooper, probably the most popular surgeon in London at that time.[3] Cooper's work, especially in arterial surgery, had a great influence on Mott. On June 22, 1808, at Guy's Hospital, Astley Cooper performed a carotid artery ligation for treatment of a cervical aneurysm in a 55-year-old man; the patient made a complete recovery and lived until 1821. This was the first successful use of ligation of the carotid artery to treat an aneurysm.[4]

Another of Cooper's famous operations was performed on June 25, 1817, when he treated a left external iliac aneurysm using ligation of the abdominal aorta. Although the patient died 40 hours after the operation, this was the first time the aorta had been ligated.[3] It remained for Rudolph Matas to perform the first successful ligation of the abdominal aorta in 1923, more than 100 years later.[5]

After further study in Edinburgh, Valentine Mott returned to New York and in 1810 was appointed Lecturer on Surgery and Demonstrator in Anatomy at Columbia College under the direction of Dr. Wright Post, another prominent New York surgeon who, in 1796, was the first American surgeon to tie the femoral artery in the femoral canal for popliteal aneurysm—this is known as the Hunterian ligation. Wright Post was also the first surgeon to successfully tie the subclavian artery, in 1817.[6]

In 1811 Mott was appointed Professor of Surgery at Columbia College. In 1813 Columbia College united with the College of Physicians and Surgeons of the University of New York to found a nearby medical college. The following year, at the age of 29, Valentine Mott was appointed to the chair of surgery at the new medical college, a position he held for 20 years, until 1834 when he resigned because of poor health.

He traveled in Europe over the next 7 years and on his return in 1841 was appointed to the new chair of surgery at the University Medical College of the University of New York, a new medical school. He held this position until 1853, when he retired at age 68 to become Emeritus Professor. He still carried on a respectable operating schedule, lectured, and taught medical students.[2,6]

In the ligation of arteries, Valentine Mott was without peer. No surgeon living or dead ever tied so many vessels so successfully.[3] These ligations were for a variety of reasons: as treatment for aneurysms, for relief of injuries such as gunshot or stab wounds, or to arrest tumor growth. At the time these operations were being performed, there was no anesthesia, no antisepsis, no asepsis, and no blood transfusion. Surgeons had to be quick, highly skilled, and well versed in surgical anatomy. Patients had to endure unbelievable amounts of pain. Inhalation anesthesia did not come into general use until after the first public demonstration of ether at the Massachusetts General Hospital on October 16, 1846. As preoperative medication, patients were usually given opium or some type of alcoholic beverage. Operations were carried out only when absolutely necessary, when all currently available conservative methods of treatment had failed.

It was not until 1867, when Lord Lister first published his paper on the antiseptic principle in the practice of surgery, that the era of infection control in surgery was inaugurated. Thus during most of Valentine Mott's career, not only were operations performed without anesthesia, but antisepsis was unheard of and infections were so common they were almost routine.

The operation that thrust Valentine Mott into prominence in the United States and internationally was the first ligation of the innominate artery, which he performed on May 11, 1818, for a traumatic subclavian aneurysm. The patient was Michael Bateman, a 57-year-old sailor, who was admitted to the New York Hospital on March 1, 1818, complaining of swelling of his right arm and shoulder. The diagnosis of right subclavian aneurysm was made. Mott's plan was to pass a ligature around the subclavian artery or around the innominate artery if the size of the mass should preclude the first procedure. One hour before the operation, the patient was given 70 drops of tincture of opium. The subclavian artery was found to be extensively inflamed, so Mott had no choice but to operate on the innominate artery. Mott stated, "A round silken ligature was now readily passed around it and the artery was tied about one-half inch below the bifurcation. The recurrent and phrenic nerves were not disturbed in this part of the operation. . . . I now made a knot in the ligature and with my forefingers, carried it down to the artery and drew it a little, so as partly to close its diameter and arrest the column of blood gradually. This was continued for a few seconds to observe the effect produced upon the heart and lungs; when no change taking place, it was drawn so as to stop the circulation entirely." The operation lasted approximately 1 hour. The patient did well immediately after the operation, but ulceration and sloughing later developed. Secondary hemorrhage occurred and the patient died on day 26 following the operation. An autopsy showed "the tripod of great vessels consisting of the innominate, subclavian and carotid arteries to the extent of nearly one inch was dissolved and carried away by the ulceration."[7,8]

The closing paragraph of Mott's published report is of interest. "The practicability and propriety of the operation appear to me to be satisfactorily established by this case: and although I feel a regret that none know who have not performed surgical operations in the fatal determination of it, and especially after the high and just expectations of recovery which it exhibited; yet I am happy in the reflection, as it is the only time it has ever been performed, that it is the bearer of a message to surgery, containing new and important results."[8] Mott was only 33 years of age when he wrote this.

Astley Cooper, commenting on Mott's operation on the innominate artery, states, "I would rather be the author of that one operation than of all I have ever originated."[2]

Although Mott's patient died, the first successful ligation of the innominate artery for subclavian aneurysm was performed by Andrew Woods Smyth at the Charity Hospital in New Orleans on May 15, 1864, 46 years later. The innominate, carotid, and vertebral arteries were all ligated. The patient lived for 11 years but returned to the hospital in 1875 with a large recurrent aneurysm. He underwent reoperation, at which time the sac was opened and plugged en masse. However, the patient died of hemorrhage within 48 hours. By 1908 Burns had collected 51 cases of innominate ligations with 11 recoveries.[9]

Another spectacular operation performed by Valentine Mott was the first successful ligation of the common iliac artery for an aneurysm of the external iliac artery. The patient was a 33-year-old male farmer who some 3 months earlier had fallen and sustained an injury. He developed a large right external iliac artery aneurysm, which was very painful. His operation was performed on March 15, 1827, at his home. "He cheerfully submitted to being placed upon a table of suitable height in a room which was well lighted." It was performed through a retroperitoneal approach and Mott commented that he took great pains to avoid entering the peritoneal cavity. The artery was ligated without incident and the wound healed perfectly. The leg remained warm and strong and when Mott saw the patient 2½ months after the operation, there was no evidence of aneurysm and there was a weak pulse in the right femoral artery distal to the ligature.[10]

In all, Mott performed 138 ligations of the great vessels for aneurysm repair. In addition to the one innominate artery ligation, this included 57 femoral, 51 common carotid, 10 popliteal, 8 subclavian, 6 external iliac, 2 external carotid, 1 common iliac, and 2 internal iliac ligations.[2] Astley Cooper said of him, "He has performed more of the great operations than any man living, or that ever did live."[6] Mott also reported that he had "closed with a fine ligature wounds of large veins of a longitudinal or transverse kind and even when an olive-sliced piece had been cut out."[2] Most of the early arterial ligations were simple ligations without division of the artery, and many patients died of hemorrhage when the ligature cut through. In Astley Cooper's successful case of carotid ligation, the artery was ligated and divided. Wangensteen and Wangensteen[11] give Emile Holman credit for pointing out the superiority of ligation with division over ligation alone.

In addition to his vascular operations, Mott performed 165 lithotomies for bladder stone retrieval and more than 1000 amputations.[12] He described a mandibular resection in 1822. He reported the first amputation at the hip joint in the United States in 1827. He performed the earliest resection of the clavicle for osteosarcoma in 1828. Mott's patients usually recovered. His operations were performed mainly at the New York Hospital, which had been founded in 1773.

Dr. Mott did not publish a great deal, other than a number of case reports. He was too busy operating to write a textbook or compile a surgical methodology. He was a polished gentleman of the old school, a good teacher, and popular with the students.

His solicitous attitude toward his patients in the days prior to the use of general anesthesia is exemplified by the following quotation: "How often when operating in some deep, dark, wound along the course of some great vein with thin walls, alternately distended and flaccid with a vital current—how often have I dreaded that some unfortunate struggle of a patient would deviate the knife a little from its proper course and that I, who fain would be the deliverer, should involuntarily become the executioner, seeing my patient perish in my hands by the most appalling form of death."[13,14]

Although Mott lived for some years after the advent of anesthesia, practically all of his notable work was done before the method came into vogue. But after the public demonstration of ether in 1846 at the Massachusetts General Hospital, he was quick to realize the significance of this event. Ether had not been very well accepted in Philadelphia, and in New York as well there was controversy over its use. Apparently the true acceptance of etherization in New York City came on December 8, 1846, when Dr. Mott removed a cluster of glands from the right axilla of a patient whose sufferings were "in part, averted entirely while the rest was greatly mitigated" by etherization.[15]

In the final 6 years of his life, Valentine Mott suffered from angina pectoris. He died on April 26, 1865, at the age of 80, with acute gangrene of the left lower leg; his death came 11 days after the assassination of Abraham Lincoln, who was a friend and correspondent.[2]

In honor of his enormous contributions to the field of surgery and his long association with the College of Physicians and Surgeons, an endowed professorship, the Valentine Mott Professorship, was established at the College of Physicians and Surgeons of Columbia University in 1930 through the generosity of Edward Harkness. The Valentine Mott Professor is the chairman of the department of surgery at the College of Physicians and Surgeons.

The first Valentine Mott Professor was Allen O. Whipple, who had no particular interest in vascular surgery but did perform splenorenal shunts after this procedure was developed by Arthur Blakemore. The second Valentine Mott Professor was George H. Humphreys II, a very distinguished cardiovascular and thoracic surgeon. The third Valentine Mott Professor was Keith Reemtsma, a vascular and cardiac transplant surgeon. The fourth and current Valentine Mott Professor is Dr. Eric A. Rose, a cardiovascular surgeon (Humphreys GH II. Personal communication, 1995).

These distinguished surgeons have continued the tradition of excellence established by Valentine Mott, a true pioneer in American vascular surgery.

I am deeply grateful to George H. Humphreys II, M.D., for providing material relating to New York hospitals, particularly the information concerning the Valentine Mott Professorships.

REFERENCES
1. Annan GL. Valentine Mott, 1785-1865, the Academy's third president. Bull N Y Acad Med 35:469-471, 1959.
2. Rutkow IM. Valentine Mott (1785-1865) the father of American vascular surgery: A historical perspective. Surgery 851:441-450, 1979.
3. Brock RC. The life and work of Astley Cooper. Edinburgh: E&S Livingstone, 1952.
4. Cooper A. Account of the first successful operation performed on the common carotid artery for aneurysm in the year 1808 with postmortem examination in the year 1821. Guys Hosp Rep 1:53-59, 1836.
5. Matas R. Ligation of the abdominal aorta. Ann Surg 81:457-464, 1925.

6. Garrison FH. Valentine Mott. Bull N Y Acad Med 1:209-214, 1925.
7. Mott V. Reflections on securing in a ligature the arteria innominata. Med Surg Register 1:9-54, 1818.
8. Cutter IS. Valentine Mott and ligation of the arteria innominata. Int Abst Surg 47:291-293, 1928.
9. Matas R. Surgery of the vascular system. In Keen WW, ed. Surgery: Its Principles and Practices. Philadelphia: WB Saunders, 1916, pp 17-350.
10. Mott V. Successful ligation of the common iliac artery. Am J Med Sci 1:156-161, 1828.
11. Wangensteen OH, Wangensteen SD. The Rise of Surgery. Minneapolis: University of Minnesota Press, 1978, p 258.
12. Garrison FH. History of Medicine. Philadelphia: WB Saunders, 1929.
13. Editorial. Valentine Mott (1785-1865) Manhattan surgeon. JAMA 199:40-41, 1967.
14. Mott V. Pain and anesthetics. In Military, Medical and Surgical Essays. Prepared for the United States Sanitary Commission 1862-1864. Washington, D.C.: 1865.
15. Trent JC. Surgical anesthesia, 1846-1946. J Hist Med 1:505-514, 1946.

Index

A

Abdominal aortic aneurysm (AAA)
  aortoenteric fistula and, 177
  common iliac artery aneurysms and, 178-179
  endovascular bifurcated graft for repair of, 127-132
  endovascular stent-graft repair of, 137-141
  EVT devices for, 124-126
  factors associated with growth of, 145-149
  femoral artery aneurysms and, 179
  genetic and biochemical factors in management of, 385-390
  graft aneurysms and, 178
  graft complications and, 178
  graft infection and, 177-178
  graft thrombosis and, 178
  intact, operative mortality for, 152-157
  laparoscopically assisted repair of, 133-134
  ligation treatment for; see Ligation treatment for abdominal aortic aneurysms
  Michigan Inpatient Data Base and, 150-152
  para-anastomotic aneurysm and, 176-177
  popliteal artery aneurysms and, 179
  remote aneurysms and, 178-179
  ruptured, operative mortality for, 157
  smoking and, 145-149
  standard resection of, late complications of, 176-180
  surgery for, 150-159
    Michigan Study Data Base for, 150-152
    prevalence and operative mortality of, 150-159
  thoracic aneurysms and, 179

ACAS; see Asymptomatic Carotid Atherosclerosis Study
Acetylsalicylic acid (ASA), 295-300
Acute iliofemoral venous thrombosis, surgical thrombectomy and regional catheter-directed urokinase for, 517-523
Adaptive intimal hyperplasia in experimental vein grafts, 402-403, 404
Adjusted-dose concept of low-dose heparin regimens, 290-291
Admitting privileges, vascular surgery and, 29-30
AEF; see Aortoenteric fistula
AFB; see Aortobifemoral bypass
Age, aortobifemoral bypass and, 197-200
Anastomotic hyperplasia, distal, superficial femoral vein as bypass graft and, 233
Anastomotic lesions, percutaneous transluminal angioplasty and, 223-227
Anesthesia
  carotid endarterectomy and, 322-323
  epidural, versus general anesthesia for infrainguinal bypass surgery, 217-222
  general, versus epidural anesthesia for infrainguinal bypass surgery, 217-222
Aneurysms
  abdominal aortic; see Abdominal aortic aneurysm
  aortic; see Aortic aneurysms
  arterial, endovascular treatment of, 115-123
  common iliac artery, 178-179
  endovascular treatment of, 107-141
  femoral artery, 179
  genetic and biochemical factors in management of, 385-390

Aneurysms—cont'd
  graft, 178
  iliac artery; see Iliac artery aneurysms
  inflammation and, 388
  para-anastomotic, 176-177
  popliteal artery, 179
  remote, 178-179
  surgery of, 143-213
  thoracic, 179
    stent-graft repair of, 135-136
  thoracoabdominal aortic; see Thoracoabdominal aortic aneurysms
Angioaccess surgery, upper extremity ischemia following, 463-467
Angiography, vascular surgery and, 24
Angioplasty
  angioscopy and, 94
  intraoperative iliac balloon, and stenting, infrainguinal bypass and, 32-36
  percutaneous transluminal; see Percutaneous transluminal angioplasty
Angioscopic thrombectomy, 92-93
Angioscopy, 91-101
  angioplasty procedures and, 94
  applications of, 91-94
  infrainguinal bypass surgery and, 250-259
    clinical experience in, 252-257
    endoluminal vein conduit preparation in, 255-256
    indications for, 250-251
    reoperative, 256-257
    technical aspects of, 251
  intraoperative, 91
  percutaneous, 91, 92
  vein graft, infrainguinal bypass surgery and, 245-249
Angioscopy-assisted in situ vein bypasses, 93-94
Anticoagulants, oral; see Oral anticoagulants

545

Antithrombotic therapy, oral anticoagulants and, 295-296
Aorta
  surgery of, 143-213
  visceral branches of, surgery of, 143-213
Aortic aneurysms, 116-121
  abdominal; *see* Abdominal aortic aneurysm
  aortic bifurcation angle and, 110-113
  endovascular aortic grafts and, 109-114
  iliac artery dimensions and, 110-113
  imaging of, 109-114
  infrarenal aortic tortuosity and length and, 110, 111, 112
  neck and cuff length and diameter and, 110, 111
  thoracic, stent-graft repair of, 135-136
  thoracoabdominal; *see* Thoracoabdominal aortic aneurysms
Aortic bifurcation angle, aortic aneurysms and, 110-113
Aortic disease, ischemic nephropathy and, 181-186
Aortic graft, endovascular, aortic aneurysms and, 109-114
Aortic graft infection, 437-442
  graft excision and extra-anatomic revascularization and, 437
  management of, 437
  treatment of, 437-441
Aortic prostheses, infected, deep and superficial lower extremity vein grafts and, 443-452
Aortic reconstruction
  elective, mortality after, 160-164
  multisystem organ failure after, 161, 162-163
  risk and cause of death after, 160-162
Aortic size, aortobifemoral bypass and, 197-200
Aortobifemoral bypass (AFB), age, sex, and aortic size in outcome of, 197-200
Aortoenteric fistula (AEF)
  abdominal aortic aneurysms and, 177
  diagnostic studies of, 193-194
  management of, 193-196
  surgical treatment of, 194-195
Aortoiliac aneurysms, 380-381
Aortoiliac occlusive disease, axillobifemoral bypass and, 204

Arterial aneurysms, endovascular treatment of, 115-123
Arterial emboli, paradoxical, 260-265
Arterial grafts
  infected prosthetic, gram-positive and gram-negative bacteria and, 397-401
  superficial femoral vein as bypass graft and, 235
Arterial injuries, endovascular stent-grafts and, 56-62
Arterial lesions, integrated self-expandable stent graft for, 37-45
Arterial ligation-bypass procedure in upper extremity ischemia, 464, 465
Arterial occlusive disease, limb-threatening, endoluminal stented grafts and, 46-55
Arterial prosthetic grafts, infected extracavitary, 453-458
Arterialization in infrainguinal bypasses, vein grafts and, 402-408
Arteriography, vascular surgery for impotence and, 470
Arteriomegaly, iliac, 383-384
ASA; *see* Acetylsalicylic acid
Association of Vascular Program Directors, 29
Asymptomatic Carotid Atherosclerosis Study (ACAS), 312-317, 359
Atherectomy
  intermittent claudication and, 268
  peripheral; *see* Peripheral atherectomy
Atherectomy device, Simpson; *see* Simpson atherectomy device
Atherosclerotic lesions, reversal of, 373-378
Auth Rotablator, 78-82
  complications and limitations of, 81-82
  indications for, 81
  results of, 81
  technique of, 78-81
A-V Impulse System foot pump, 509-511
A-V Impulse System technology
  plantar venous plexus and, 507-516
  postrevascularization edema and, 511-515
Axillobifemoral bypass (AxBF), 201-205
  aortoiliac occlusive disease and, 204

Axillobifemoral bypass (AxBF)—cont'd
  historical perspective of, 201-202
  results of, 202-203
  technical considerations of, 203-204
Axillosubclavian occlusion, regional thrombolysis for, 529

B
Bacteria, gram-positive and gram-negative, infected prosthetic arterial grafts and, 397-401
Bacteriology, infected prosthetic arterial grafts and, 398
Balloon angioplasty, intraoperative iliac, and stenting, infrainguinal bypass and, 32-36
Banding procedure in upper extremity ischemia, 464
Bifurcated graft insertion, endovascular, for abdominal aortic aneurysm repair, 127-132
Bifurcation graft repair, abdominal aortic anreurysms and, 124-126
Biochemical factors in management of aneurysms, 385-390
Bleeding time, early PTFE graft failure and, 409-415
Bypass
  angioscopy-assisted in situ, 93-94
  aortobifemoral, 197-200
  axillobifemoral, 201-205
  carotid-subclavian prosthetic, subclavian occlusive disease, 343-347
  distal, free flaps and, limb salvage and, 237-240
  femoropopliteal
    after failed balloon angioplasty, 85-90
    vein graft occlusion and, 416-418
  femorotibial, after failed balloon angioplasty, 85-90
  infrainguinal; *see* Infrainguinal bypass
  mesenteric, chronic mesenteric ischemia and, 434-435
  tibiotibial, for limb salvage, 241-244
Bypass graft, superficial femoral vein as, 228-236

C

Carotid artery disease, carotid endarterectomy and, 324
Carotid artery stenosis
 moderate, 359-364, 365-368
  results of, 366-367
  stroke and, 366-367
Carotid artery trauma
 diagnosis of, 428-429
 initial treatment of, 429
 management of, 427-432
 mechanisms of injury in, 427-428
 operative management of, 430-431
 patient selection in, 429-430
 postoperative care in, 432
Carotid endarterectomy (CEA)
 age and, 312-317
 anesthesia and monitoring in, 322-323
 associated medical conditions and, 325-326
 carotid artery disease and, 324
 carotid shortening during, 331-336
 clinical experience with, 314-315
 difficult, adjunctive techniques for management of, 322-326
 Johns Hopkins experience with, 315-316
 operative risks of, 313
 pathologic considerations of, 313-314
 previous surgery or radiation and, 324-325
 problems encountered during shunting in, 325
 unusual anatomy of, 323-324
Carotid endarterectomy flaps, Nd:YAG laser and, 327-330
Carotid shortening during carotid endarterectomy, 331-336
Carotid stump pressure, shunts and, 319
Carotid surgery, 305-355
 perioperative neurologic deficits after, 337-342
Carotid-subclavian prosthetic bypass, subclavian occlusive disease, 343-347
Catheter
 Trac-Wright; *see* Trac-Wright catheter
 transluminal extraction; *see* Transluminal extraction catheter

Catheter-directed urokinase, regional, acute iliofemoral venous thrombosis and, 517-523
Catheterization laboratory, vascular surgery and, 24-25
Cavernosography, dynamic infusion, vascular surgery for impotence and, 470
Cavernosometry, dynamic infusion, vascular surgery for impotence and, 470
CEA; *see* Carotid endarterectomy
Celiac arteries, reconstruction of, 206-213
Cerebrospinal fluid drainage, paraplegia and, 371
CEVG; *see* Corvita Endovascular Graft
Chronic mesenteric ischemia
 cause and diagnosis of, 433-434
 endarterectomy and, 434
 mesenteric bypass and, 434-435
 percutaneous transluminal angioplasty and, 435
 surgical treatment of, 433-436
Chronic venous insufficiency
 valve repair techniques for; *see* Valve repair techniques for chronic venous insufficiency
 venous ulceration and, 475-476
Cigarette smoking
 abdominal aortic aneurysms and, 145-149
 intermittent claudication and, 266-267
 vein graft failure and, 416-419
Claudication, intermittent; *see* Intermittent claudication
Combined obstruction/reflux, venous valve repair and, 505-506
Common iliac artery aneurysms, abdominal aortic aneurysms and, 178-179
Contracting potential of vascular laboratories, 287-288
Corvita Endovascular Graft (CEVG), 37-45
Credentialing, vascular surgery and, 29

D

Deep lower extremity vein grafts, infected aortic prostheses and, 443-452
Deep venous thrombosis (DVT)
 iliofemoral, 517-523

Deep venous thrombosis (DVT)—cont'd
 in pregnancy, 487-492
  anticoagulation in, 487-492
  clinical experience in, 491
  diagnosis of, 487-488
  Doppler ultrasound in, 488
  duplex ultrasonography in, 488
  incidence and pathophysiology of, 487
  noninvasive testing in, 488
  plethysmography in, 488
  results of, 491-492
  thromboembolic prophylaxis in, 490-491
  treatment of, 488-491
  vena caval filtration devices in, 487-492
Diagnostic modalities, noninvasive and less invasive, 283-303
Distal anastomotic hyperplasia, superficial femoral vein as bypass graft and, 233
Distal bypasses, free flaps and, limb salvage and, 237-240
Doppler ultrasound in deep venous thrombosis in pregnancy, 488
Duplex scanning, vascular surgery for impotence and, 470
Duplex ultrasonography in deep venous thrombosis in pregnancy, 488
DVT; *see* Deep venous thrombosis
Dynamic infusion cavernosography, vascular surgery for impotence and, 470
Dynamic infusion cavernosometry, vascular surgery for impotence and, 470

E

ECST; *see* European Carotid Surgery Trial
Edema, postrevascularization, A-V Impulse System and, 511-515
EDRF; *see* Endothelium-derived relaxing factor
Elective aortic reconstruction, mortality after, 160-164
Electroencephalogram (EEG), intraoperative, shunts and, 318-319
Embolism
 paradoxical arterial, 260-265
 pulmonary; *see* Pulmonary embolism

Endarterectomy
    carotid; see Carotid endarterectomy
    chronic mesenteric ischemia and, 434
    transaortic renal; see Transaortic renal endarterectomy
Endoluminal interventionist, vascular surgeon as, 16-26
Endoluminal stented grafts
    access and pathfinding in, 49-51
    assessment of, 51, 53
    clinical applications of, 46-48
    deployment of, 51, 52
    limb-threatening arterial occlusive disease and, 46-55
    Montefiore experience and, 51-54
    path dilatation in, 51
    placement and positioning of, 51, 52
    techniques for placement of, 48-54
Endoluminal vein conduit preparation in infrainguinal bypass surgery, 255-256
Endothelium-derived relaxing factor (EDRF), 373
Endovascular aortic grafts, aortic aneurysms and, 109-114
Endovascular bifurcated graft insertion
    for abdominal aortic aneurysm repair, 127-132
    follow-up of, 129
    patient selection for, 127
    procedure of, 127-129, 130
    results of, 130, 131
Endovascular procedures, 9-105
    for arterial aneurysms, 115-123
    impact of, on vascular surgery, 11-15
    intravascular ultrasound as adjunct to, 98-99
    vascular surgeons and, 63-66
Endovascular stent-grafts
    arterial injuries and, 56-62
    history of, 56-57
    in repair of abdominal aortic aneurysms, Sydney experience with, 137-141
    results of, 58-61
    techniques and devices in, 57-58, 59
Endovascular surgeon, 16-26

Endovascular Technologies (EVT) devices, 37
    abdominal aortic aneurysms and, 124-126
    bifurcation graft repair and, 125
    clinical experience with, 125
    FDA three-phase protocol for, 125
    problems with, 125-126
    technique of, 124-125
    tube graft repair and, 124-125
Endovascular treatment of aneurysms, 107-141
End-stage renal disease (ESRD), limb salvage and, 271
Epidural anesthesia versus general anesthesia for infrainguinal bypass surgery, 217-222
ESRD; see End-stage renal disease
European Carotid Surgery Trial (ECST), 307-311, 359, 365-368
European Journal of Vascular and Endovascular Surgery, 27
European Journal of Vascular Surgery, 27
EVT devices; see Endovascular Technologies (EVT) devices
Exercise, intermittent claudication and, 266
Extra-anatomic revascularization, aortic graft infection and, 437-442
Extracavitary arterial prosthetic grafts, infected, 453-458
Extrapleural T2 ganglion thoracic sympathectomy, transaxillary first rib resection with, 459-462

F
Failing vein grafts, percutaneous transluminal angioplasty and, 223-227
Familial Atherosclerosis Treatment Study (FATS), 374
Femoral artery aneurysms, abdominal aortic aneurysms and, 179
Femoral vein, superficial, as bypass graft, 228-236
Femoropopliteal bypass after failed balloon angioplasty, 85-90
Femoropopliteal bypass trial, MRC, vein graft occlusion and, 416-418
Femorotibial bypass after failed balloon angioplasty, 85-90

Fibrinogen
    interaction of, with vessel wall, 419
    vein graft failure and, 416-419
First rib resection, transaxillary, with extrapleural T2 ganglion thoracic sympathectomy, 459-462
Fistula, aortoenteric; see Aortoenteric fistula
Flap
    carotid endarterectomy, Nd:YAG laser and, 327-330
    free, distal bypasses and, limb salvage and, 237-240
    types of, free flaps, distal bypasses, and limb salvage and, 238
Fluoroscopy, vascular surgery and, 24
Free flaps, distal bypasses and, limb salvage and, 237-240
    flap types and, 238
    patient selection for, 237
    results of, 238
    vascular procedures and, 237
    wound types and, 238, 239
Freeman, Norman, 537-539
Free-standing multipurpose testing centers, 285
Free-standing vascular laboratories, 285
Funding, vascular laboratory, 285-288

G
General anesthesia versus epidural anesthesia for infrainguinal bypass surgery, 217-222
Genetic factors in management of aneurysms, 385-390
Graft
    aortic, infection of; see Aortic graft infection
    arterial, superficial femoral vein as bypass graft and, 235
    bifurcated, endovascular, for abdominal aortic aneurysm repair, 127-132
    bypass, superficial femoral vein as, 228-236
    complications of, abdominal aortic aneurysms and, 178
    endoluminal stented, limb-threatening arterial occlusive disease and, 46-55
    endovascular aortic, aortic aneurysms and, 109-114

Graft—cont'd
  endovascular bifurcated, for abdominal aortic aneurysm repair, 127-132
  failing vein, percutaneous transluminal angioplasty and, 223-227
  failures of, superficial femoral vein as bypass graft and, 230-231
  infected extracavitary arterial prosthetic, 453-458
  infected prosthetic arterial, gram-positive and gram-negative bacteria and, 397-401
  integrated self-expandable stent, 37-45
  intravascular, real-time intravascular ultrasound and, 99-100
  polytetrafluoroethylene; see Polytetrafluoroethylene graft
  subcutaneously tunneled, infrainguinal bypass wound complications and, 271-274
  subfascially tunneled, infrainguinal bypass wound complications and, 271-274
  transluminally placed endovascular, 12-14, 64
  vein; see Vein grafts
  venous, superficial femoral vein as bypass graft and, 235
Graft aneurysms, abdominal aortic aneurysms and, 178
Graft excision, aortic graft infection and, 437-442
Graft infection, abdominal aortic aneurysms and, 177-178
Graft thrombosis, abdominal aortic aneurysms and, 178
Gram-negative bacteria, infected prosthetic arterial grafts and, 397-401
Gram-positive bacteria, infected prosthetic arterial grafts and, 397-401

H
Hematologic evaluation, polytetrafluoroethylene graft and, 409-410
Heparin, low-dose; see Low-dose heparin regimens
Hyperplasia
  distal anastomotic, superficial femoral vein as bypass graft and, 233

Hyperplasia—cont'd
  intimal, in experimental vein grafts, 402-403, 404
Hypotension, paraplegia and, 370
Hypothermia, paraplegia and, 371

I
Iliac arteriomegaly, 383-384
Iliac artery aneurysms, 379-384
  aortoiliac aneurysms, 380-381
  common, abdominal aortic aneurysms and, 178-179
  iliac arteriomegaly, 383-384
  isolated, 381-383
  size criteria for, 380
Iliac artery dimensions, aortic aneurysms and, 110-113
Iliac artery occlusion, lytic agents for, 280-281
Iliac balloon angioplasty, intraoperative, and stenting, infrainguinal bypass and, 32-36
Iliac occlusions, percutaneous transluminal angioplasty and, 276
Iliac stenoses, percutaneous transluminal angioplasty and, 276
Iliofemoral venous thrombosis acute, 517-523
  regional thrombolysis for, 524-525
Impotence
  vascular surgery for, 468-474
    arteriography in, 470
    clinical presentation of, 469
    duplex scanning in, 470
    dynamic infusion cavernosometry and cavernosography in, 470
    invasive testing in, 470
    nocturnal penile tumescence in, 470
    patient selection for, 469-470
    technical approaches and results of, 472
    vascular involvement in, 471
    venous interruption and, 472
    vasculogenic, 471-472
Infected aortic prostheses, deep and superficial lower extremity vein grafts and, 443-452
Infected extracavitary arterial prosthetic grafts, 453-458

Infected prosthetic arterial grafts
  bacteriology and, 398-399
  gram-positive and gram-negative bacteria and, 397-401
  limb loss and, 398
  patient survival and, 398
  patients and methods of, 397-398
  results of, 398-399
  wound healing and, 398
Infection
  aortic graft; see Aortic graft infection
  graft, abdominal aortic aneurysms and, 177-178
Inflammation, aneurysms and, 388
Inflow sites for lower extremity tibiotibial bypass, 242
Infrainguinal bypass
  angioscopy and, 250-259
  arterialization in, vein grafts and, 402-408
  complications of, 271-274
  epidural versus general anesthesia for, 217-222
  intraoperative iliac balloon angioplasty and stenting and, 32-36
  vein graft angioscopy and, 245-249
Infrainguinal bypass wound complications, 271-274
Infrarenal aortic tortuosity and length, aortic aneurysms and, 110, 111, 112
Institution-based vascular laboratories, 285
Integrated self-expandable stent graft, 37-45
  delivery system of, 40
  materials and methods for, 38-41
  method of placement of, 41
  results of, 41-44
Intermittent claudication
  atherectomy and, 268
  exercise and, 266
  intervention for, 268-269
  natural history of, 391-396
  percutaneous transluminal angioplasty and, 268
  pharmacologic management of, 267-268
  smoking cessation and, 266-267
  surgical revascularization and, 268-269
  treatment of, 266-270
Internal carotid artery stenosis disease progression in, 360-362

Internal carotid artery stenosis—cont'd
  incidence of neurologic events in, 360, 361
  moderate, 359-364
  risk factors of, 362
Interventional radiology, vascular surgery and, 27-31
Intimal hyperplasia, adaptive, in experimental vein grafts, 402-403, 404
Intractable ulcers, radical excision for, 475-483
Intraoperative angioscopy, 91
Intraoperative iliac balloon angioplasty and stenting, infrainguinal bypass and, 32-36
Intravascular graft deployment, real-time intravascular ultrasound and, 99-100
Intravascular ultrasound (IVUS), 94-100
  as adjunct to endovascular interventions, 98-99
  applications for, 100
  clinical utility of, 95-100
  disease distribution and characterization of, 95-98
  intravascular graft deployment, 99-100
  real-time, intravascular graft deployment and, 99-100
  techniques of, 94-95
  value and limitations of, 91-101
Ischemia
  chronic mesenteric; see Chronic mesenteric ischemia
  lower extremity; see Lower extremity ischemia
  operative, paraplegia and, 370-371
  upper extremity; see Upper extremity ischemia
Ischemic nephropathy, 181-186
  and concomitant aortic disease, 181-186
  early outcome after combined repair of, 182-183
  late outcome after combined repair of, 183-185
  monitors of renal function in, 182
  pathophysiology of, 181-182
  patient population with, 182
IVUS; see Intravascular ultrasound

J
Journal of Endovascular Surgery, 27

K
Ketanserin, 477

L
Laboratories, vascular; see Vascular laboratories
Laparoscopically assisted abdominal aortic aneurysm repair, 133-134
Laser, Nd:YAG, carotid endarterectomy flaps and, 327-330
Legislation, self-referral, vascular laboratories and, 288
Lesion crossing, vascular surgery and, 21, 22
Ligation treatment
  for abdominal aortic aneurysms, 172-175
    clinical experience with, 172
    results of, 174
    technique of, 172-174
  Lymphazurin-assisted, lymphatic complications and, 484-486
  in upper extremity ischemia, 464
Ligation-bypass procedure, arterial, in upper extremity ischemia, 464, 465
Limb loss, infected prosthetic arterial grafts and, 398
Limb salvage
  free flaps and distal bypasses and, 237-240
  tibiotibial bypass for, 241-244
Limb-threatening arterial occlusive disease, endoluminal stented grafts and, 46-55
Low-dose heparin regimens, 289-294
  adjusted-dose concept of, 290-291
  low-molecular-weight, 291-292
Lower extremity ischemia
  advances in management of, 215-282
  vascular surgery versus thrombolysis for, 102-105
Lower extremity tibiotibial bypass, inflow sites for, 242
Lower extremity vein grafts, infected aortic prostheses and, 443-452
Low-molecular-weight heparin, 291-292
Loyola experience, perioperative neurologic deficits after carotid surgery and, 340-341

Lymphatic complications, treatment of, 484-486
Lymphazurin-assisted early ligation techniques, lymphatic complications and, 484-486
Lytic agents
  for iliac artery occlusion, 280-281
  indications for, 281
  for large vein occlusive disease, 524-530
  methods of, 280-281
  results of, 281

M
MARS; see Monitored Atherosclerosis Regression Study
Mesenteric arteries, superior, reconstruction of, 206-213
Mesenteric bypass, chronic mesenteric ischemia and, 434-435
Mesenteric ischemia, chronic; see Chronic mesenteric ischemia
Michigan Study Data Base, abdominal aortic aneurysm and, 150-152
Mobile vascular laboratories, 285-286
Monitored Atherosclerosis Regression Study (MARS), 374
Montefiore Medical Center
  endoluminal stented grafts and, 51-54
  infected prosthetic arterial grafts and, 397
Mortality
  after elective aortic reconstruction, 160-164
  effects of oral anticoagulants on, 298
  operative, for abdominal aortic aneurysm surgery, 150-159
Mott, Valentine, 540-543
MRC femoropopliteal bypass trial, vein graft occlusion and, 416-418
Multisystem organ failure (MSOF) after aortic reconstruction, 161, 162-163

N
NASCET; see North American Symptomatic Carotid Endarterectomy Trial
Nd:YAG laser ablation of carotid endarterectomy flaps, 327-330

Neck, revascularization across, using retropharyngeal route, 348-355
Nephropathy, ischemic; see Ischemic nephropathy
Neurologic deficits, perioperative, after carotid surgery, 337-342
Neurologic events in internal carotid artery stenosis, 360, 361
Nitinol stent, 38
Nocturnal penile tumescence, vascular surgery for impotence and, 470
Noninvasive diagnostic and therapeutic modalities, 283-303
Norfolk experience, intraoperative iliac balloon angioplasty and stenting and, 33-35
North American Symptomatic Carotid Endarterectomy Trial (NASCET), 307-311, 312-317, 359, 365
   degree of stenosis in, 308
   "moderate" patient in, 307-308

O

OAC; see Oral anticoagulants
Occlusive disease
   arterial, limb-threatening, endoluminal stented grafts and, 46-55
   large vein, stents and lytic agents for, 524-530
Office-based vascular laboratories, 285
Omnicath, 82-83
   complications of, 83
   indications for, 82-83
   results of, 83
   technique of, 82
Oral anticoagulants (OAC)
   acetylsalicylic acid and, 295-300
   antithrombotic therapy and, 295-296
   effects of, on death rates, 298
   effects of, on patency, 296-297
   effects of, on progression of disease, 297-298
   vascular surgical patients and, 295-300
Overexcitation injury, paraplegia and, 370

P

Para-anastomotic aneurysms, abdominal aortic aneurysms and, 176-177
Paradoxical arterial emboli, 260-265
   clinical experience with, 263-264
   diagnosis of, 262
   etiology and pathophysiology of, 260-262
   treatment of, 262-263
Paraplegia
   anatomy of spinal cord circulation and, 369-370
   cerebrospinal fluid drainage and, 371
   hypotension and, 370
   hypothermia and, 371
   operative ischemia and, 370-371
   overexcitation injury and, 370
   thoracoabdominal aneurysm repair and, 369-372
Parodi device, 118
Partial thromboplastin time (PTT), 413
Patches, carotid artery reconstruction and, 318-321
Patency, effects of oral anticoagulants on, 296-297
Penile tumescence, nocturnal, vascular surgery for impotence and, 470
Percutaneous angioscopy, 91, 92
Percutaneous transluminal angioplasty (PTA), 11-12, 63-66
   for aortoiliac disease, 275-278
   chronic mesenteric ischemia and, 435
   complications of, 276-277
   consequences of technical failure in, 277
   failed balloon angioplasty and, 85-90
   failing vein grafts and, 223-227
   iliac occlusions and, 276
   iliac stenoses and, 276
   indications for, 277-278
   intermittent claudication and, 268
   methods of, 275
   operative reconstruction after, 87, 88
   results of, 275-276
   versus surgery and conservative treatment, 277
Perioperative neurologic deficits after carotid surgery, 337-342
   Loyola experience with, 340-341
   operative procedure for, 339-340
   prevention of, 337-338
   recognition of stroke and, 338
Perioperative neurologic deficits after carotid surgery—cont'd
   stroke in operating room and, 339
   stroke in recovery room and, 339
   transient ischemic attack and, 339
   treatment of, 338-339
Peripheral atherectomy, 72-84
   Auth Rotablator and, 78-82
   Omnicath and, 82-83
   Simpson atherectomy device and, 72-75
   Trac-Wright catheter and, 77-78, 79
   transluminal extraction catheter and, 75-77
Plantar venous plexus, A-V impulse system technology and, 507-516
Plethysmography in deep venous thrombosis in pregnancy, 488
Pneumatic tourniquet occlusion techniques
   advantages of, 301
   applications of, 301
   research on, 302-303
   technique of, 301-302
   vascular applications of, 301-303
Polytetrafluoroethylene (PTFE) graft
   early failure of, bleeding time and, 409-415
   hematologic evaluation in, 409-410
   materials and methods of, 409
   results of, 410-412
Popliteal artery aneurysms, abdominal aortic aneurysms and, 179
Popliteal vein, superficial femoral vein as bypass graft versus, 232-233
Postphlebitic limbs, superficial femoral vein as bypass graft and, 233
Postrevascularization edema, A-V Impulse System and, 511-515
Postthrombotic reflux, venous valve repair and, 504-505
Postthrombotic valvular dysfunction in chronic venous insufficiency, 496-498
Postthrombotic valvular incompetence in chronic venous insufficiency, 499-501

Preexisting proximal occlusive disease, tibiotibial bypass for limb salvage and, 243
Pregnancy, deep venous thrombosis in; see Deep venous thrombosis in pregnancy
Primary valve reflux, venous valve repair and, 504
Primary valvular incompetence (PVI) in chronic venous insufficiency, 496, 497, 498-499
Prostaglandin E_1, 478
Prostaglandin I_2, 478
Prostheses, infected aortic, deep and superficial lower extremity vein grafts and, 443-452
Prosthetic grafts
  infected arterial, gram-positive and gram-negative bacteria and, 397-401
  infected extracavitary arterial, 453-458
Proximal occlusive disease, preexisting, tibiotibial bypass for limb salvage and, 243
PTA; see Percutaneous transluminal angioplasty
PTFE graft; see Polytetrafluoroethylene graft
PTT; see Partial thromboplastin time
Pulmonary embolism, 531-534
  interventions for, 531-532
  results of, 533-534
  technique of, 532-533
PVI; see Primary valvular incompetence

R

Radical excision for intractable ulcers, 475-483
Real-time intravascular ultrasound, intravascular graft deployment and, 99-100
Regional catheter-directed urokinase, acute iliofemoral venous thrombosis and, 517-523
Regional thrombolysis; see Thrombolysis, regional
Reimbursement, vascular laboratory, 285-288
Remote aneurysms, abdominal aortic aneurysms and, 178-179
Renal arteries, left and right, reconstruction of, 206-213

Renal endarterectomy, transaortic; see Transaortic renal endarterectomy
Renal failure, infrainguinal bypass wound complications in, 271-274
Renal function, monitors of, ischemic nephropathy and, 182
Reoperative infrainguinal bypass surgery, 256-257
Retroperitoneal approach, extended left, reconstruction of celiac, superior mesenteric, and left and right renal arteries using, 206-213
Retropharyngeal route, revascularization across neck using, 348-355
Revascularization
  across neck using retropharyngeal route, 348-355
  extra-anatomic, aortic graft infection and, 437-442
Rotablator, Auth; see Auth Rotablator

S

Saphenous hypertrophy, superficial femoral vein as bypass graft and, 233
Saphenous vein harvest, subcutaneous video-assisted, 67-71
Self-expandable stent graft, integrated, 37-45
Self-referral legislation, vascular laboratories and, 288
Sex, aortobifemoral bypass and, 197-200
Shunts, carotid endarterectomy and, 318-321, 325
Simpson atherectomy device, 72-75
  complications and limitations of, 74-75
  indications for, 73
  results of, 74
  techniques of, 72-73
Smoking
  abdominal aortic aneurysms and, 145-149
  intermittent claudication and, 266-267
  vein graft failure and, 416-419
Spinal cord circulation, paraplegia and, 369-370
St. Thomas' Atherosclerosis Regression Study (STARS), 374
Stanford experience with stent-graft repair of thoracic aortic aneurysms, 135-136

Stanozolol, 477
Staphylococcus aureus, graft infection and, 177
Staphylococcus epidermidis, graft infection and, 177, 178
STARS; see St. Thomas' Atherosclerosis Regression Study
Stasis changes, superficial femoral vein as bypass graft and, 232
Steal, diagnosis of, in upper extremity ischemia, 463
Stenosis
  moderate internal carotid artery, 359-364
  in North American Symptomatic Carotid Endarterectomy Trial, 308
  vein graft, 405-407, 418-419
Stent graft
  endoluminal, limb-threatening arterial occlusive disease and, 46-55
  integrated self-expandable, 37-45
  in repair
    of abdominal aortic aneurysms, 137-141
      endovascular, Sydney experience with, 137-141
      limitations of, 140-141
      results of, 137-138
      trombone technique of, 139-140
    of arterial injuries, 56-62
    of thoracic aortic aneurysms
      clinical data for, 136
      indications for, 135
      operative procedure of, 136
      results and complications of, 136
      Stanford experience with, 135-136
Stents
  for aortoiliac disease, 278-280
  indications for, 278-279, 280
  intraoperative iliac balloon angioplasty and, 32-36
  for large vein occlusive disease, 524-530
  nitinol, 38
  Palmaz series and, 279-280
  in prevention of failure of PTA, 278-279
  principles of, 278
  results of, 279-280
  thrombolysis and, for superior vena cava syndrome, 525-527
  Toronto series and, 279-280

STILE trial; see Surgery or Thrombolysis for the Ischemic Lower Extremity trial

Stroke
  moderate carotid artery stenosis and, 366-367
  in operating room, 339
  perioperative neurologic deficits after carotid surgery and, 338
  in recovery room, 339

Subclavian occlusive disease, carotid-subclavian prosthetic bypass and, 343-347

Subcutaneous video-assisted saphenous vein harvest, 67-71

Subcutaneously tunneled grafts, infrainguinal bypass wound complications and, 271-274

Subfascially tunneled grafts, infrainguinal bypass wound complications and, 271-274

Superficial femoral vein as bypass graft, 228-236
  analysis of graft failures in, 230-231
  anatomy and, 233, 234
  arterial grafts and, 235
  autogenous strategy for, 234-235
  case report of, 234
  contraindications to, 228
  distal anastomotic hyperplasia and, 233
  indications for, 228
  laboratory testing and, 232
  late structural changes in, 230
  morbidity and, 231-234
  versus popliteal vein, 232-233
  postphlebitic limbs and, 233
  results of, 229-231, 232
  saphenous hypertrophy and, 233
  stasis changes and, 232
  swelling and, 231-232
  techniques of, 228-229
  ulceration and, 232
  unusual grafts and, 233, 234
  venous grafts and, 235

Superficial lower extremity vein grafts, infected aortic prostheses and, 443-452

Superior mesenteric arteries, reconstruction of, 206-213

Superior vena cava syndrome, thrombolysis and vascular stents for, 525-527

Surgery or Thrombolysis for the Ischemic Lower Extremity (STILE) trial, lower extremity ischemia and, 102-105

Surgical revascularization, intermittent claudication and, 268-269

Swelling, superficial femoral vein as bypass graft and, 231-232

Sydney experience with endovascular stent-graft repair of abdominal aortic aneurysms, 137-141

Sympathectomy, extrapleural T2 ganglion thoracic, transaxillary first rib resection with, 459-462

T

T2 ganglion thoracic sympathectomy, extrapleural, transaxillary first rib resection with, 459-462

TAAAs; see Thoracoabdominal aortic aneurysms

Therapeutic modalities, noninvasive and less invasive, 283-303

Thoracic aneurysms, abdominal aortic aneurysms and, 179

Thoracic aortic aneurysms, stent-graft repair of, 135-136

Thoracic sympathectomy, extrapleural T2 ganglion, transaxillary first rib resection with, 459-462

Thoracoabdominal aortic aneurysms (TAAAs)
  incidence of, 165
  nonoperative management of, 165-171
  paraplegia and, 369-372
  rate of expansion of, 168, 169
  risk of rupture of, 166-168
  survival of patients with, 166, 167

Thrombectomy
  angioscopic, 92-93
  venous, acute iliofemoral venous thrombosis and, 517-523

Thromboembolic prophylaxis in deep venous thrombosis in pregnancy, 490-491

Thrombolysis
  regional
    for axillosubclavian occlusion, 529
    for iliofemoral venous thrombosis, 524-525

Thrombolysis—cont'd
  vascular stents and, for superior vena cava syndrome, 525-527
  vascular surgery versus, for lower extremity ischemia, 102-105

Thrombolysis Or Peripheral Arterial Surgery (TOPAS) trial, 102-105

Thrombosis
  deep venous; see Deep venous thrombosis
  graft, abdominal aortic aneurysms and, 178

Tibiotibial bypass for limb salvage, 241-244
  inflow sites for lower extremity bypass and, 242
  influence of bypass conduit on patency in, 242
  length of, 242
  noninvasive testing and, 243
  preexisting proximal occlusive disease and, 243
  progression of proximal disease and, 243
  techniques of, 243-244

TOPAS trial; see Thrombolysis Or Peripheral Arterial Surgery trial

Tourniquet, pneumatic, vascular applications of, 301-303

TPEG; see Transluminally placed endovascular graft

Trac-Wright catheter, 77-78
  complications and limitations of, 78, 79
  indications for, 77-78
  results of, 78
  technique of, 77

Transaortic renal endarterectomy, 187-192
  methods of, 187-188
  results of, 188-190

Transaxillary first rib resection with extrapleural T2 ganglion thoracic sympathectomy, 459-462

Transient ischemic attack, perioperative neurologic deficits after carotid surgery and, 339

Transluminal angioplasty, percutaneous; see Percutaneous transluminal angioplasty

Transluminal extraction catheter, 75-77
  complications and limitations of, 76-77
  indications for, 76
  results of, 76
  technique of, 75-76

Transluminal navigation, vascular surgery and, 21
Transluminally placed endovascular graft (TPEG), 12-14, 64
Trauma
　carotid artery; see Carotid artery trauma
　to large-sized and medium-sized veins, 423-426
　in vascular surgery, 421-491
　vertebral artery; see Vertebral artery trauma
Trombone technique of stent-graft repair of abdominal aortic aneurysms, 139-140
Tube graft repair, abdominal aortic anreurysms and, 124-126
Tumescence, nocturnal penile, vascular surgery for impotence and, 470

U

Ulceration
　superficial femoral vein as bypass graft and, 232
　venous; see Venous ulceration
Ulcers, intractable, radical excision for, 475
Ultrasonography, duplex, in deep venous thrombosis in pregnancy, 488
Ultrasound
　Doppler, in deep venous thrombosis in pregnancy, 488
　intravascular; see Intravascular ultrasound
University of Texas Southwestern Medical Center, neoaortoiliac system and, 448-451
Upper extremity ischemia
　arterial ligation-bypass procedure in, 464, 465
　banding procedure in, 464
　diagnosis of steal in, 463
　following angioaccess surgery, 463-467
　ligation procedure in, 464
Urokinase, regional catheter-directed, acute iliofemoral venous thrombosis and, 517-523

V

Valve reflux, primary, venous valve repair and, 504
Valve repair techniques for chronic venous insufficiency, 495-501
　diagnostic evaluation of, 495
　indications for, 495

Valve repair techniques for chronic venous insufficiency—cont'd
　postthrombotic valvular dysfunction in, 496-498
　postthrombotic valvular incompetence in, 499-501
　primary valvular incompetence in, 496, 497, 498-499
　results of, 498
　surgical technique of, 496
Valvular dysfunction, postthrombotic, in chronic venous insufficiency, 496-498
Valvular incompetence
　postthrombotic, in chronic venous insufficiency, 499-501
　primary, in chronic venous insufficiency, 496, 497, 498-499
Vascular applications of pneumatic tourniquet occlusion techniques, 301-303
Vascular laboratories
　changes in allowed indications for testing in, 286-287
　contracting potential of, 287-288
　decreasing workload and, 287
　funding and reimbursement of, 285-288
　policies and issues affecting, 286-288
　reduction in reimbursement rates for, 286
　self-referral legislation and, 288
　types of, 285-286
Vascular stents, thrombolysis and, for superior vena cava syndrome, 525
Vascular surgeon
　as endoluminal interventionist, 16-26
　endovascular procedures and, 63-66
Vascular surgery
　access to vascular lumen in, 18-20
　admitting privileges in, 29-30
　of aneurysms and aorta, 143-213
　angiography and, 24
　basic catheter/interventional skills of, 18-24
　catheterization laboratory and, 24-25
　credentialing in, 29
　endovascular procedures in, 28-29
　fluoroscopy and, 24

Vascular surgery—cont'd
　future of, 30-31
　history of, 27-28
　impact of endovascular technology on, 11-15
　for impotence; see Impotence, vascular surgery for
　interventional radiology and, 27-31
　lesion crossing in, 21, 22
　pioneers in, 535-543
　versus thrombolysis for lower extremity ischemia, 102-105
　transluminal navigation in, 21
　trauma in, 421-491
　treatment of target lesion in, 21-24
　wire introduction in, 21
Vasculogenic impotence, treatment of, 471-472
Vein
　large-sized and medium-sized, trauma to, 423-426
　saphenous, subcutaneous video-assisted harvest of, 67-71
　superficial femoral, as bypass graft, 228-236
Vein graft angioscopy, infrainguinal bypass surgery and, 245-249
Vein grafts
　adaptive remodeling in, 404-405
　arterialization in infrainguinal bypasses and, 402-408
　experimental, adaptive intimal hyperplasia in, 402-403, 404
　failing
　　effect of smoking and fibrinogen on, 416-419
　　percutaneous transluminal angioplasty and, 223-227
　lower extremity, infected aortic prostheses and, 443-452
　maladaptive intimal hyperplasia in, 404-405
　occlusion of, MRC femoropopliteal bypass trial and, 416-418
　stenosis of, 405-407, 418-419
　superficial femoral vein as bypass graft and, 235
Venous disease update, 493-534
Venous flow, basic mechanisms of, 507-508
Venous insufficiency, chronic; see Chronic venous insufficiency

Venous interruption, vascular surgery for impotence and, 472
Venous thrombectomy, acute iliofemoral venous thrombosis and, 517-523
Venous thrombosis, iliofemoral, regional thrombolysis for, 524-525
Venous ulceration
  chronic venous insufficiency and, 475-476
  compression and pharmacotherapy of, 476-478

Venous ulceration—cont'd
  direct treatment of, 479-482
  management of, 475-483
  surgical therapy for, 478-479
Venous valve repair, 502-506
  combined obstruction/reflux and, 505-506
  postthrombotic reflux and, 504-505
  primary valve reflux and, 504
Vertebral artery trauma
  injuries in, 431-432
  management of, 427-432
Vertebral surgery, 305-355

Video-assisted saphenous vein harvest, subcutaneous, 67-71

W

Wallstent, 38
Wire introduction, vascular surgery and, 21
Workload, decreasing, vascular laboratories and, 287
Wounds
  healing of, infected prosthetic arterial grafts and, 398
  types of, free flaps, distal bypasses, and limb salvage and, 238-240